AUTISM UNCENSORED

The Etiology of
Autism Spectrum Disorders

Alan Schwartz, M.D.

ISBN: 978-0-9983289-0-4

Library of Congress: 2016920050

Printed in the United States of America

First Edition

2 4 6 8 10 12

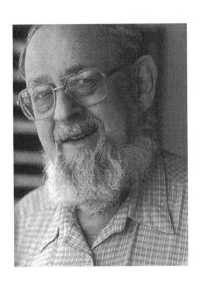

Dr. Bernie Rimland

This book is dedicated to the memory of Dr. Bernie Rimland, originator of the bio-medical approach to reversing autism and related disorders. He got us started in the right direction.

A heartfelt "Thank You" to my wonderful wife, Teresa, whose love bolstered me through trying times.

Contents

Prologue

"Nullius in verba"
("Take nobody's word for it")

— *The motto of London's Royal Society*

WE GET LIED *to a lot.* We were told that Saddam Hussein had "weapons of mass destruction." He didn't.

We were told by the Director of National Intelligence, William Clapper, that the National Security Agency did not wittingly collect information on millions of Americans. They did.

We have been told that that there is no epidemic of autism and that the apparent increase in the prevalence of this condition is simply due to better diagnostic awareness and additionally to changes in the diagnostic criteria. That's a falsehood.

We have been assured that vaccines are quite safe and effective and rarely cause serious side effects. That isn't true.

And we have also been repeatedly told by the Centers for Disease Control and Prevention (the CDC) that we don't know what causes autism, but, they assure us, whatever it is it isn't vaccines or mercury, and that isn't true either.

It is the purpose of this book to expose the nefarious campaign of lies and misinformation regarding immunization safety and the known etiologies of autism and related disorders, and by so doing allow appropriate research into the causes and treatments for these often devastating maladies to proceed.

In order to accomplish this task it was necessary to analyze the myriad studies that reveal the many factors that promote these related disorders and likewise expose the errors, misinformation and yes, even fraud in the so-called "negative" studies that purport to exonerate vaccinations and mercury as causative agents in these conditions.

We additionally needed to show that there is a lot more to the etiology of autism spectrum disorders than just immunizations and mercury. That is one reason this book is so long.

The bottom line is that autism spectrum disorders appear to be conditions arising in genetically vulnerable children who get inappropriately exposed to a variety of toxic substances, with dietary inadequacies and other factors playing key roles as well.

It was initially intended that the final chapters of the book would deal with the various beneficial treatments, supplements, therapies and techniques that have been shown to be successful in reversing autism spectrum disorders, but at about 500 pages without those final chapters it was decided to simply end the book at the completion of the chapters on etiology and then write a second volume regarding methods for improving and reversing autism, ADHD and other disorders on the autism spectrum. It is anticipated that that book will be published shortly.

Alan Schwartz

Part I
An Introduction to Autism and its Related Disorders

"We…give voice to those who believe that autism is an environmentally induced illness, that it is treatable, and that children can recover.… We believe that autism is the defining disorder of our age."

— *Mark Blaxill and Dan Olmstead, www.ageofautism.com*

Chapter 1
What is Autism?

"Education consists mainly of what we have unlearned."
— *Mark Twain*

AUTISM IS A *complex developmental disability that typically appears during the first three years of life. It was first described and named by Dr. Leo Kanner in his 1943 paper "Autistic Disturbances of Affective Contact."*[1]

Kanner borrowed the term "autism" (actually "autismus") from Eugene Bleuler, a renowned Swiss psychiatrist, who also coined the term "schizophrenia," and who had used the word "autismus" to describe certain self-directed behaviors seen in some adult schizophrenics. However, Dr. Kanner, who authored a textbook on child psychiatry and who founded the first child psychiatry clinic in the U.S., did not consider childhood autism to be a prodrome for or a variety of schizophrenia.[2]

The vast majority of autistic children are normal in appearance. They often exhibit bizarre (stereotypical) behaviors and interests and typically have problems communicating and socializing. One of the eleven children that Dr. Kanner listed in his seminal paper was Donald T., a five-year-old boy whose father described as "happiest when he was alone...drawing into a shell and living within himself... oblivious to everything around him.

"Donald had a mania for spinning toys, liked to shake his head from side to side and spin himself around in circles, and he had temper tantrums when his routine was disrupted."[3]

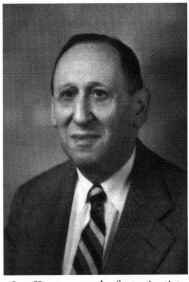

Leo Kanner was the first scientist to name and clearly define autism.

Leo Kanner was the first scientist to define autism clearly. Autism manifests as a disorder that affects not only the functioning of the brain, but also the intestinal tract, the immune system, and other bodily processes, and unless appropriate interventions are instituted early in the course of this condition, its manifestations are likely to remain throughout life.

The first epidemiological study done to determine the prevalence of autism was carried out in 1966 by Victor Lotter twenty-three years after Kanner first described this disorder. Mr. Lotter surveyed the autistic population in Middle-

---

1   *Nervous Child.* 1943; 2, 217-250.
2   Leo Kanner's 1943 paper on autism: Commentary by Gerald Fischbach; Fri, 07 Dec 2007; www.simonsfoundation.org
3   Ibid.

sex, England and found a prevalence rate of 4.5 per 10,000 children. This works out to one out of every 2,222 births.[4]

In 1970, Treffert published the first study that evaluated the prevalence of autism in the U.S. and found it to be 1 in 10,000.[5]

In California in the 1970s, 100-200 *new* cases of autism were reported annually. However, in 1998, 1,425 *new* cases were reported to the public school system (a 700 percent increase). And the following year, that number had jumped to 1,944. These increases were disproportionate to the population growth.

In New Jersey, the number of autism cases reported increased from 241 in 1991 to 1,634 in 1997 (an 800 percent increase).[6]

In Great Britain, the autism numbers climbed 700 percent from 1988 to 1999.[7] In studies prior to 1988, the estimated prevalence of classical autism was about 4-5 cases (+/-1) per 10,000 births. This number rose to 17 cases per 10,000 births by 2001, and if autism spectrum disorders (like Asperger's syndrome and PDD-NOS) were included in the statistics, the incidence jumped to 63 per every 10,000 children. [8] In Japan the rate of autism in the 1980s was 5-16 per 10,000 births and rose to 21.1 per 10,000 by 1996.[9]

In 2003 autism and its associated behaviors and manifestations were estimated to have occurred in 2-6 children for every 1,000 births.[10] This averages out to about one child in every 160-500 births. Between 2003 and 2007, a period of just four years, the incidence of parent-reported cases of autism spectrum disorders doubled according to a 2007 survey of 82,000 respondents by the National Survey of Children's Health.

Autism is four to five times more prevalent in boys than girls and knows no racial, ethnic, or social boundaries. Data from the Centers for Disease Control in 2009 indicated that the chances of an infant born in 1998 developing some form of autism spectrum disorder *by the age of 8 years* (data for 2006) were a frightening 1 in 110, and since boys are more at risk for developing autism and ADHD, the risk for boys at that time was even higher: one in 58-70. This translated into 2.6 percent of all male children born in the U.S. in 1998. And this is not just a U.S. problem, for as we have noted, countries around the world (like the United Kingdom and Japan) are also reporting dramatic increases in autism.

And the news gets even worse. On March 29, 2012 the CDC announced that the autism prevalence in fourteen sites across the U.S. had risen 23 percent from the 2006 figure and now affected 1 in 88 children and 1 in 64 eight-year-old boys born in the year 2000, with the greatest rise occurring in the black (42 percent) and Hispanic (29 percent) population. The rise among white children was 16 percent.

The prevalence for girls overall was 1 in 252 (approximately five times less than for boys). The prevalence rate varies from state to state with Alabama having the lowest figure (1 in 210) and Utah having the highest (1 in 47 children and 1 in every 32 boys!).[11]

In South Korea, the 2011 estimated autism prevalence in children aged 7-12 years was found to be even higher than in Utah, affecting 1 in 33 children or 2.64 percent of the population of school-age children.[12]

While family income and educational levels do not affect the likelihood of autism's occurrence, certain environmental influences most certainly do. And poverty does influence the course of autism, as many autistic children born to low income families are unable to access the resources necessary to address this malady.

---

4   Lotter 1966.

5   Treffert, D.A. "Epidemiology of infantile autism." *Arch Gen Psychiatry*. May 1970; 22(5):431-8

6   *JAMA*. 2001; 285:1183-85

7   *British Medical Journal*. 2001; 322:460-63

8   *News Telegraph* July 8, 2001

9   *Japanese Journal of Infectious Diseases*. 2001; 54: 78-79

10   Centers for Disease Control and Prevention, 2003

11   CDC Morbidity and Mortality Weekly Report. March 29, 2012 & http://www.medscape.com/viewarticle/761162

12   *American Journal of Psychiatry*. May 8, 2011; published online and http://esciencenews.com/articles/2011/05/09/prevalence.autism.south.korea. estimated.1.38.children

Autism is currently classified as a mental illness, and is listed as such in the DSM-IV manual. (See Appendix I for the DSM-IV criteria that describe the symptoms of autism and specify how it is diagnosed). However, there is a great deal of evidence that autism should not be classified solely as a mental illness, because it is also a systemic inflammatory condition that affects the digestive tract, the central nervous system, and often the immune system as well.

Autism is not a "disease," as such, with every afflicted individual manifesting the same symptoms that arise as a consequence of the same causal factors. Rather, it is a "syndrome," a collection of commonly observed manifestations, with each individual's unique biochemistry, lifestyle stresses, environmental exposures, and genetic make-up influencing the course and prognosis of this potentially devastating condition.

In other words, *each person with an autism spectrum disorder has his or her own unique version of this malady*, which means that what may benefit one individual may not benefit the next. This also implies that each autistic individual must be "worked up" medically to determine what specific factors are influencing his or her particular condition. It is only in this way that autism can be reversed. And it can often be reversed!

Are Autistic Children Retarded?

Usually no, but many may fit the criteria for retardation if they are not treated appropriately or early enough in life. Many autistic children, once "normalized," are as smart as non-autistic children, and many seem to be more intelligent than average.

It is also not really possible to measure accurately the IQs of autistic children who appear to be disconnected from the world around them, who may not communicate well, and who are distracted by various sensory inputs that the majority of us would have no difficulty in suppressing.

Consider Tito, a low functioning teenage autistic boy described in the March 2005 edition of *National Geographic* magazine.[13] He was initially diagnosed as being mentally retarded. He remains unable to speak and avoids eye contact, and he still makes unintelligible grunts and moans and rocks and flaps his hands.

He was taken to many doctors in his native India by his "determined mother" who, through "relentless, sometimes unorthodox training" was able to "break through the barrier of silence, teaching Tito to add and subtract, to enjoy literature, and eventually to communicate by writing." He is now extremely articulate when he writes out his answers to questions. For example, when asked why he moves around so much, he wrote, "I know it looks different, but I got into this habit to find and feel my own scattered self."

Tito catalogued his thoughts in a book he wrote between the ages of eight and eleven (*Beyond the Silence,* published in England in 2000 and in the U.S. in 2003 under the title *The Mind Tree*). In this work, he describes "the cacophony of disconnected information arriving through his senses and his profound struggle to control his own body and behavior."[14] He described two "selves," one a thinking self "filled with learnings and feelings," and the other an "acting self" that was "weird and full of actions" over which he had no control.

Tito is still autistic, but despite his disabilities and bizarre behaviors, he is clearly not mentally retarded.

Nevertheless, there are certain children born with particular genetic disorders, like Rett Syndrome, Fragile-X Syndrome, and others, who may manifest autistic-like symptoms, and who do indeed appear to be truly mentally retarded. These named genetic syndromes will be discussed later in this narrative, but they make up only a minority of those diagnosed with autism or related disorders.

Even the IQ scores of high-functioning autistic children appear to be poor predictors of their academic abilities, according to a recent study.[15] In this study 27 of the 30 children had discrepancies between their predicted and actual performance scores, and 60 percent *tested higher* than predicted on at least one of the academic tests.

---

13   Shreeve, James. p. 22-23
14   Ibid.
15   Estes, Annette et al. *J of Autism and Develop. Disorders.* Nov 2, 2010

"As many as 70 percent of individuals with ASD are now thought to have intellectual ability in the average to above average range," write the study authors.[16]

> *"Autism is a very big spectrum, ranging from people with severe handicaps to high functioning individuals ...The best course of action for mild autism, Aspreger's or ADHD is the same: help the child to understand their strengths.*
> *Focus on things they are good at."*
>
> — *Temple Grandin, Ph.D.; recovered autistic; 3-5-13, at a lecture in Bozeman, Montana*

What Is a Savant?

A savant is a person with remarkable cognitive abilities or talents, but usually in only one area of functioning. Often this "talent" is disproportionate to the individual's overall functioning or disability. Occasionally, the talent or ability is so remarkable that it would be highly unusual to find it even in a non-impaired individual.

Examples of such remarkable gifts include prodigious memory, like the ability to recall exact dates and events, or a photographic memory of things read, or the ability to play a piece of music perfectly after only hearing it played once, or having an unusual artistic talent, or the facility to calculate large number multiples, square roots, or additions almost instantly. Perhaps the strangest and most controversial savant ability ascribed to only a few autistic individuals is that of extra-sensory perception. Bernard Rimland described several children who allegedly had this ability.

One does not need to have any impairment to have savant-like abilities. Eidetic memory, the ability to remember literally everything that one has read or experienced, has been demonstrated in individuals without any obvious mental impairment; however, most examples of savant syndrome are noted in the autistic population (about 50 percent of all savants are autistic) and in the neurologically disabled population (the other 50 percent of all savants). Since there are more disabled than there are autistics, the incidence works out to about 10 percent of all autistics and less than 1 percent of the disabled population.

A Multiple-Talented Young Savant

Jacob Barnett, who at age fourteen months attempted to calculate the volume of a cereal box, lost all speech by age two and no longer responded to others socially for a period of time. He was diagnosed as being autistic. He recovered his lost skills, however, to blossom as a child prodigy with a photographic memory and a high IQ (172) who taught himself Braille in one day, is advanced in higher mathematics, skipped seven grade levels and was enrolled at Indiana University at age twelve. Years earlier, he was able to play a Beethoven piece he had heard only once, having had no music training. He hopes to become an astrophysicist.

Savants tend to be male (6:1 male predominance), and a lot of the savant skills tend to emanate from the right hemisphere. It is not clear what factors are responsible for creating this mysterious condition, or why it is so common in male autistic individuals.[17]

Are There Different Kinds of Classical Autism?

Yes. When autism was first described by Dr. Leo Kanner of Johns Hopkins Hospital in 1943 (he categorized the symptoms after observing only eleven children with this condition), the incidence was estimated to be 1-2 in every 10,000 births.

---

16   Ibid.

17   Treffert, D.A. "The savant syndrome: an extraordinary condition. A synopsis: past, present, future." *Philos Trans R Soc Lond B Biol Sci.* 2009; 364 (1522): 1351–7. doi: 10.1098/rstb.2008.0326 and McMullen, T. "The savant syndrome and extrasensory perception." Dec 1991; *Psychol Rep* 69 (3 Pt 1): 1004–6. doi:10.2466/PR0.69.7.1004-1006. PMID 1784646. "D.A. Treffert, following B. Rimland, cited examples which he states show ESP to be occurring in certain autistic savant children. The evidence is questioned on the ground that it is hearsay, uncorroborated by independent scrutiny."

At that time, the disorder seemed to be evident shortly after birth in most children so diagnosed. This type of *birth-onset autism* is but one variety of *classical autism*. The incidence of birth-onset autism does not appear to have increased any prior to 1973, and since that time, it has risen much less rapidly than has delayed-onset autism. (See graph below).[18]

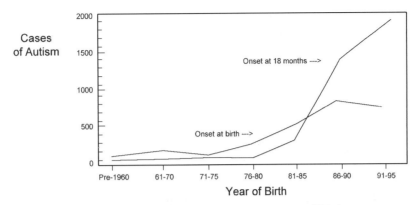

Figure 1.1. U.S. Cases of Autism vs. Year of Birth:
Autistic children who behaved normally before 18 months vs. those with no normal period
(birth onset) California Dept. of Health Services Data

The kind of autism that predominates today, as can be appreciated from the above graph, differs from Dr. Kanner's classical birth-onset autism (AKA "infantile-onset" or "Kanner autism") in that the symptoms of most autistic children born in recent years do not appear right after birth, but rather much later in the child's development—generally between one and two years of age (sometimes sooner, sometimes later, the average age being eighteen months).

This variety of classical autism is called *delayed-onset* or *regressive autism* and appears to be epidemic. The incidence of regressive autism, as we have noted, is frighteningly high and increasing.

As Dr. Bernard Rimland put it in his *Autism Research Review International* paper, "data collected by the Autism Research Institute since the 1960s reveal that the onset of autism at 18 months is a recent development."[19]

Parent reports show that from the 1960s through the early 1980s, children autistic from birth outnumbered by 2 to 1 those with delayed onset at eighteen months. Starting in the early 1980s, when the MMR triple vaccine was introduced[20], the picture has *reversed*; now the onset at eighteen months children outnumber the onset at birth by 2 to 1.

The U.S. Centers for Disease Control and Prevention (CDC) reported that the prevalence of autism spectrum disorders in the United States in eight-year-old children in 2006 was approximately 1 percent of the population, or 1 out of every 110 children eight years of age. These statistics weren't published until December 2009. The autistic children who were eight years of age in 2006 were born in 1998 when many immunizations given to babies were still preserved with mercury-containing thimerosal. The relevance of this will be discussed in a later chapter.

As we have previously pointed out, the prevalence of autism continues to rise and is 1 in 88 children born in 2000, also a time when the children were getting frequent toxic doses of thimerosal (49.6 percent mercury by weight) preserved vaccines.

Children with regressive autism often appear to develop normally for the first year of life, and sometime after that age, they appear to regress or else fail to progress developmentally. Speech may start normally and then regress or cease or may not start at all. Normal behaviors, like finger pointing, may never be noted. See Chapter 3 for a more

---

18   *Autism Research Review International*, 2000, Vol. 14, No. 1, page 3; based on the responses to ARI's E-2 checklist, which has been completed by thousands of autism families.
19   Ibid.
20   In the United States, the MMR vaccine was licensed in 1971 and the second booster dose was introduced in 1989. (Wikipedia)

detailed accounting of the symptoms and characteristics of autism.

Autism-like manifestations can be seen in many conditions, including those who have suffered injury to the brain. Certain other named conditions associated with autism will be discussed in later chapters.

There are also syndromes classified as being on the *autism spectrum*, because they share many, but not all, of the observed symptoms of autism. These Autism Spectrum Disorders (ASDs) include attention deficit disorder with (ADHD) or without (ADD) hyperactivity, Tourette's syndrome, Asperger's Syndrome and others. These disorders will also be discussed in more detail in the next chapter.

"By 1985 the incidence of regressive autism had equaled that from birth. By 1997 both types had increased although the regressive form was now >75 percent of the total occurrence. This suggests that an acquired condition was overtaking birth defects or purely genetic conditions."[21]

Is Autism Genetic?

Yes, in part, but environmental influences appear to be the primary influence in this regard. In earlier studies of identical (mono-zygotic) twins, it was found that if one child has autism, there is up to an 88 percent chance that the second twin will also be autistic. The incidence of autism in fraternal (non-identical, dizygotic twins) was said to be about 30 percent. This demonstrates that there clearly are both genetic and environmental components to autism.[22]

However, "the largest and most rigorous twin study to date" (nearly 400 twins), that attempted to better define the genetic vs. the environmental influences in autism, led to some surprising results. The study found that environmental factors accounted for more than half of the susceptibility to autism (55-58 percent), while genetics factors could only account for about 38 percent of the risk of getting autism.

"A boy with a fraternal (not identical) twin with autism spectrum disorder had a 31 percent chance of also having the disorder, while a boy with an identical twin with the disorder had a 77 percent chance of sharing it. In girls, the concordance was 50 percent in identical twins and 36 percent for fraternal pairs."

Neil Risch, senior author of this paper and director of the Institute for Human Genetics at the University of California San Francisco, stated, "Autism had been thought to be the most heritable of all neurodevelopmental disorders, with a few small twin studies suggesting a 90 percent link. It turns out the genetic component still plays an important role, but in our study, it was overshadowed by the environmental factors shared by twins."

The study was conducted jointly by scientists at the UCSF Institute for Human Genetics and Stanford University among others.[23]

It is likely that most, if not all, autistic individuals harbor genetic defects (mutations—variations in how genes and proteins are constructed) that increase the likelihood of their acquiring autistic symptoms, and these inherited or acquired variances are often unique in each individual.

It appears that many genes are involved in fostering the autistic state. However, having such genetic propensities doesn't necessarily cause a child to become autistic because it is apparent that environmental factors also play a key (and likely a predominant role) in promoting this condition.

For example, if a child has a genetic defect in detoxifying a neurotoxic metal like mercury, there is evidence that he or she will be more prone to developing autistic symptoms after ingesting foods that are high in mercury, like tuna, or

21   Ewing, G. *N Am J Med Sci*; Jul 2009; 1(2).
22   Betancur, C. et. al. *Am J Hum Genet*. 2002 May; 70(5): 1381–1383 and Greenberg, D.A. et al. "Excess of twins among affected sibling pairs with autism: implications for the etiology of autism." *Am J Hum Genet*. 2001; 69:1062–1067 and Rosenberg, Rebecca E. et al. "Characteristics and Concordance of Autism Spectrum Disorders among 277 Twin Pairs." *Arch Pediatric Adolescent Medicine*. Oct 2009; 163: 907 - 914.
23   Hallmayer, J. et al. "Genetic Heritability and Shared Environmental Factors among Twin Pairs with Autism." *Arch Gen Psychiatry*. July 2011; doi: 10.1001/arch gen psychiatry. July, 2011.76.

by being injected with a mercury-containing substance like thimerosal. If such a susceptible child is not exposed to excessive amounts of mercury during infancy, then he or she may never develop the symptoms of autism or ADHD, despite having a genetic propensity for this condition.

Is Autism Reversible?

The short answer is yes, but unfortunately, not in all cases, and not always completely.

Conventional wisdom suggests the opposite, however. It is thought by many in the medical field that autism is an irreversible condition that will last a lifetime, but which may be helped to some extent by certain drugs that are used to control symptoms and by the use of certain therapies, like ABA and speech therapy. Many parents are told that they should love their child, but prepare to have him or her institutionalized because "nothing can be done."

The Autism Research Institute (among many others) disagrees. It alleges that by using its protocols, many autistic children can be "recovered," and by that, it means that these formerly autistic children will improve to such an extent that they will no longer fit the criteria for autism. These children can live normal lives. They can socialize, communicate, and do well scholastically. They can marry, have families, and hold jobs.

The Autism Research Institute (ARI) has data to support this contention. It has received reports on more than 1,000 children who've recovered from autism using intensive combined interventions. Its website (www.autism.com) provides before and after video clips of many of these children.

But reversing autism in some means that not every person with autism or who is on the autism spectrum can have his or her behavioral, biochemical, and other abnormalities completely reversed. Nevertheless, the good news is that virtually all true autistics can be improved in functioning to some degree, but due to the uniqueness of each individual's biochemistry, his or her environmental exposures and genetic weaknesses, and the age at which therapy is started, not all can be helped sufficiently to reverse their condition completely.

> *"(Our son) was diagnosed at two of the premier institutions on the West Coast: UC San Francisco and Oregon Health Sciences University. It was genetic. There's nothing we can do about it. It was lifelong.*
> *"Institutionalization was likely, and we'd be lucky if he ever talked. It was a prognosis of doom that no parent could bear."*
>
> *— J.B. Handley (parent of an autistic boy) Frontline interview; e-pub 4-29-10 http://www. wellsphere.com/autism*

There is evidence suggesting that the earlier the intervention, the greater the likelihood of success in this regard. The National Research Council analyzed intervention models for young children with autistic disorders and concluded that intensive early intervention "makes a clinically significant difference for many children. Children who had early intervention had better outcomes."

The study, published online in the journal *Pediatrics*, examined an intervention called the Early Start Denver Model, which combines applied behavioral analysis (ABA) teaching methods with developmental "relationship-based" approaches. The study found significant gains in IQ, communication, and social interaction using this approach.[24]

Unfortunately, poverty plays a detrimental role in the prognosis of autism. Being born poor or to a less educated, minority, or foreign-born mother makes it more likely that an autistic child will be low functioning from the start and will fail to improve. This is likely due in part to the fact that neither the parent nor the schools will have the resources necessary to help these children.[25]

---

24   "Early Intervention for Toddlers with Autism Highly Effective." November 2009.
25   Fountain, Christine et al. "Six Developmental Trajectories Characterize Children with Autism." *Pediatrics*; originally published online April 2, 2012.

What Is the Prevalence of Autism?

Part of the difficulty in determining autism prevalence rates has to do with how autism is defined. Does one just count those with symptoms of classical autism? Or should the enumeration also include other disorders on the autism spectrum like Asperger's Syndrome, ADHD, and other developmental disorders? Criteria for defining this disorder needed to be established.

The prevalence of autism, as has been mentioned, was first measured in the 1960s in Great Britain.[26] The criteria for diagnosing autism were first established in 1980, and have been revised several times since then.[27] According to the Centers for Disease Control and Prevention (the CDC), the best estimate of the prevalence of autism "for decades" was 4-5 children out of every 10,000 births.[28]

Since the early 1990s, special education programs in the U.S. have been required to report how many children diagnosed with an autism spectrum disorder (ASD) received such services, and these numbers may be falsely low as some ASD children would not have been counted, "because some children receive special education for a particular need, like speech therapy, and not for a classification of autism."[29]

In order to get a better handle on the true prevalence of autism, the CDC partnered with the American Academy of Pediatrics to establish an "Autism A.L.A.R.M to educate physicians about ASDs."[30]

According to the CDC, the autism rate in 2004—to include Asperger's and Pervasive developmental disorder (PDD)—varied from 2 to 6 per 1,000 individuals or as many as 1 in 166 children.[31]

The following graph shows the prevalence of autism in eight-year-old children from various states in the U.S. in 2002 and 2006.[32] It is important to note that the children who were eight years old in 2002 were born in 1994 and those eight years old in 2006 were born in 1998.

Thimerosal-preserved vaccines were in general and increasing use during those years. In 2006, on average, approximately 1 percent or one child in every 110 in the eleven Autism & Developmental Disabilities Monitoring (ADDM) sites was classified as having an ASD (approximate range: 1:80 to 1:240 children [males: 1:70; females: 1:315]).[33]

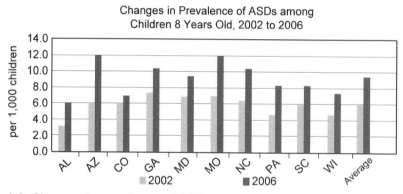

Figure 1.2. Changes in prevalence of ASDs among children 8 years old. 2002-2006

26   Lotter, V. "Epidemiology of autistic conditions in young children. Some characteristics of the parents and children." *Soc Psychiatry.* 1966; 1:124-37
27   American Psychiatric Association. *Diagnostic and Statistical Manual of Mental Disorders*, 3rd ed. Washington (DC): APA; 1980. American Psychiatric Association. *Diagnostic and Statistical Manual of Mental Disorders*, 4th ed, text revision. Washington (DC): APA; 2000.)
28   CDC .gov website: Autism Developmental Disabilities Monitoring Network report
29   Ibid.
30   American Academy of Pediatrics. The National Center of Medical Home Initiatives for Children with Special Needs. Autism A.L.A.R.M. [cited 2006 Nov]. http://www.medicalhomeinfo.org/health/Autism percent20downloads/Autism Alarm.pdf.)
31   Ibid.
32   www.cdc.gov/ncbddd/autism/index.html
33   CDC website: Ibid.

Alarming Statistics from the CDC

- *One out of every 54 boys has been diagnosed with an autism spectrum disorder & one out of every 252 girls!*

- *About 730,000 individuals between the ages 6 and 21 have an ASD!*

- *Approximately 13 percent of children have a developmental disability, ranging from mild disabilities such as speech and language impairments to serious developmental disabilities, such as intellectual disabilities, cerebral palsy, and autism.*

- *"In the more recent National Survey of Children's Health (NSCH), parents reported that 1 in 50 school-age children (2 percent) have an autism spectrum disorder. This strongly suggests that we are significantly underestimating prevalence and that autism is an urgent public health issue requiring a national public health response."[34]*

Are there reasons to question the CDC data?

Yes! For many years, the CDC appears to have been manipulating data to obfuscate the actual incidence of autism. The CDC, together with the Department of Health and Human Services, formed a tracking entity called the Autism & Developmental Disabilities Monitoring network (ADDM), which encompasses "a group of programs funded by (the) CDC to determine the number of people with autism spectrum disorders (ASDs) in the United States."[35]

The ADDM is also tasked with the goal of describing the population of children with autism spectrum disorders, comparing ASD prevalence in different groups of children and different areas of the country, and identifying changes in ASD prevalence over time.[36]

The CDC has data on children with autism going back at least to 1988, but strangely, the ADDM autism data analysis doesn't start until 1992. This is a serious omission as the detailed data the CDC compiled from Brick Township in New Jersey from 1988 to 1995 are vital in helping us appreciate the significant parallels between the introduction of the new thimerosal-containing immunizations (Haemophilus influenza B [HIB] and hepatitis B in 1990 and 1991 respectively) and the prevalence of autism. Although the CDC *did not publish this data*, Sallie Bernard of Safe Minds was able to acquire much of the unpublished data from CDC employees.[37]

The Brick township data was very accurate. The CDC paid clinicians to conduct personal diagnostic interviews of *all* suspected cases of autism in a specified population in Brick Township between the years 1988 and 1995.

And what they found was startling!

There were *no cases of full spectrum autism in children born prior to 1990*, but for children born in 1993, the full syndrome rate had climbed to 1 in 128! The overall rate for children with all autism spectrum disorders was 1 in 225 for children born before 1991, and this increased to over 1 in 80 for children born in 1992. Importantly, two new thimerosal preserved vaccines were introduced during that time period, the HIB vaccine (Hemophilus Influenza B) and the Hepatitis B vaccine.

One might ask why the CDC declined to publish these important reports that our taxpayers had paid for. Were they suspecting a vaccine-autism link?

Autism has always been listed as a "mental disorder," (although, as we have stated, it is clearly a lot more than that), and the criteria for diagnosing this disorder are listed in a publication known as the *Diagnostic and Statistical Manual of Mental Disorders* (the DSM). When the revised third edition of this manual (DSM III revised) was published in 1987, it updated the criteria for autism, and renamed the condition "autistic disorder."

34   http://www.autismspeaks.org/science/science-news/autism-major-piece-child-mental-health-picture
35   CDC.gov
36   Ibid.
37   safeminds.org

The DSM manual was revised again in 1994 (DSM IV) and it now categorized Asperger's Syndrome along with autism as pervasive developmental disorders (PDDs), and it also expanded the initial autism symptom threshold from thirty months (DSM III revised) to thirty-six.

For some reason, the ADDM researchers decided to group together all the pervasive developmental disorder diagnoses into one "lump" for analysis instead of separating the various diagnoses as autism, Asperger's Syndrome, PDD-NOS, etc. This unnecessary conglomeration of PDD conditions created confusion regarding the true prevalence of autism, and perhaps it was designed to.

The ADDM reviewers also constantly changed the states that they were analyzing. These ADDM reviews track how many eight-year-olds are diagnosed with autism and associated disorders in a given birth year. These reports generally aren't available for the public to review until 2-5 years after the report year listed.

The 2000 report for children born in 1992 listed just six states in the ADDM network, but the report that followed in 2002 (children born in 1994) listed fourteen states. These reports are supposed to come out every two years, but the 2004 report (for children born in 1996) was strangely buried in an appendix that appeared in the 2006 report (which was not available until December 2009). The 2006 report for children born in 1998 included just eleven states because the researchers had eliminated 2 of the 6 states in the 2000 group and 4 of the 14 in the 2002 group.

By comparing autism prevalence in different state cohorts over time, the CDC had succeeded in masking the true rise in autism. The CDC did this by removing states with high or rising rates of autism (NJ, UT, WV, AR), and it should be noted that two of these states (NJ and WV) had the largest rates of autism increase between 2000 and 2002.

The CDC also added in Alabama in 2002, which at the time had one of the lowest autism rates in the country, and later added Philadelphia County, Pennsylvania and Colorado, which also had very low autism rates.

As Mark Blaxill of Safe Minds states, "It doesn't take a degree in statistics to figure out that if you remove the states with the highest rates in the sample, the average rates will go down; similarly, if you add in states with low autism rates, the average will fall even further."[38]

The CDC did not release the 2000 and 2002 reports until February 2007. In comparing the trends in autism rates, the CDC concluded that the prevalence of autism for children born in 1992 (the 2000 report) was 6.7 autistic children per 1,000 and the prevalence for children born in 1994 (the 2002 report) was just 6.6. It would thus appear that the prevalence of autism was not rising and might have even fallen slightly. But that would be a false assumption because the CDC did not compare the same six states analyzed in the 2000 report.

The CDC inappropriately added in eight other states with *low* prevalence rates for autism in the 2002 report in order (one suspects) to make the prevalence rates appear to stabilize. What they should have done, of course, was compare the prevalence rates in just the six states analyzed for the children born in 1992 with the children born in those same states in 1994.

Mark Blaxill of Safe Minds actually did that analysis and found that, "A true 'apples to apples' comparison of the sites included in both studies would have shown a 10 percent increase in those 6 sites over the two year period."[39]

Was the CDC manipulating its data because it knew that autism rates were actually rising and it feared that others might suspect the vaccine program as the culprit?

And what about the 2004 report buried in the appendix of the 2006 report? According to Mark Blaxill, "Based on an honest comparison, between 2002 and 2004, the autism rate rose by 31 percent."[40] That dramatic increase in prevalence may be why the CDC did not want to publish the 2004 report, but when the 2006 statistics confirmed that the

---

38   Blaxill, Max. "Lies, Damned Lies and CDC Autism Statistics." Dec 23, 2009. Safe Minds.org
39   Ibid.
40   Ibid.

explosive rise in autism cases could not be hidden any longer, the CDC realized it had no choice but to publish the results.

Keep in mind that the CDC estimate of autism as 1 in every 110 children born in 1998 represents data from a group of states with varying rates of autism prevalence. Since the autism incidence is much higher in males, the CDC estimates would put the overall prevalence of autism in boys born in 1998 at 1 in 70.

However, as we have stated, some states have even higher rates than that. Mark Blaxill estimated that the autism rate for white males born in Missouri in 1998 is 1 in 45 and in Arizona is 1 in 42![41] That's quite an epidemic!

Why some children in certain states are at higher risk for autism will be discussed in later chapters.

Is the Prevalence of Autism Really Increasing?

Yes! Absolutely! As has been mentioned, the reported prevalence of autism has increased dramatically in the last thirty years, and not just in the U.S.[42] The incidence of autism by age six in California has increased from fewer than 9 in 10,000 for children born in 1990 to more than 44 in 10,000 for children born in 2000[43] to 91 per 10,000 in 2008.[44]

The following graph illustrates this rise up to the year 2000 for different age groups.

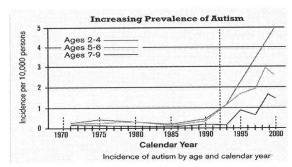

Figure 1.3. Life Extension Foundation article on vitamin D and autism

Please note the *delayed rise* in autism incidence in the older populations. This clearly demonstrates that variances in diagnostic criteria cannot account for the increased incidence of autism because, at any given moment in time, the criteria would be the same for all populations.

Here's another graph showing the same effect in children in Minnesota.

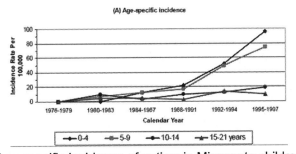

Figure 1.4. Age specific incidence of autism in Minnesota children at different ages & calendar years.

---

41   Ibid.
42   http://www.cdc.gov/cdcgrandrounds/archives/2014/april2014.htm
43   *Science Daily.* January 2009
44   CDC 2009 report.

These data *prove* that the rise in autism is real and is not caused by better diagnosing or changing diagnostic criteria.

Nevertheless, there is currently still some debate and a great deal of skepticism about whether the prevalence of autism is actually increasing or whether the apparent increase is simply due to better diagnosis, earlier diagnosis, population shifts and/or a change in the criteria for making the diagnosis of autism.[45]

While some of the rise in the prevalence of autism is certainly attributable to better screening and a revision of the diagnostic criteria (King and Bearman found that only 25 percent of the increase in autism diagnosis could be attributed to these factors), changes in the practice, inclusion criteria, and methodology involved in diagnosing autism cannot and do not account for the huge numbers of individuals now being classified as autistic.

A look at the graphs above clearly supports this contention. From 1990 through 1997, there was no change in the criteria for diagnosing autism, and improved screening for autism was in its infancy, yet the dramatic rise in autism cases starting in 1988 is clear. The year 1985 is, perhaps not coincidentally, also the year when the first of a new series of HIB vaccines were introduced, although they were routinely administered to babies only after 1990.

HIB stands for Haemophilus Influenza B (a bacterium that can produce serious infections in infants), and the immunization series (four shots-often preserved with thimerosal, a mercury-containing preservative, in the 1990s) was recommended to be given during the first two years of life (usually at two, four, six, and eighteen months of age).

Equally relevant is the fact that the delay in escalation of cases of autism in the older populations of children reflects what one would expect if the rise were due to an increase in *new* cases of autism starting in infancy.

If better screening of children with autism or a change in the criteria for diagnosing autism were the only reason for this dramatic rise in reported cases, then we would expect to see an equal (or even greater[46]) rise in the number of children reported with autism in the older populations, but we don't!

Autism prevalence then rocketed upward in the late 1980s and 1990s after the HIB and hepatitis B vaccines were introduced. Both contained mercury in toxic amounts (by both EPA and FDA standards) and the hepatitis B vaccine, given on the first day of life, also contained neurotoxic aluminum.

In the "Report to the Legislature on the Principle Findings from the Epidemiology of Autism in California: A Comprehensive Pilot Study," the author concluded: "There is no evidence that a loosening in the diagnostic criteria has contributed to increased number of autism clients...we conclude that some, if not all, of the observed increase represents a true increase in cases of autism in California...a purely genetic basis for autism does not fully explain the increasing autism prevalence. Other theories that attempt to better explain the observed increase in autism cases include environmental exposures to substances such as mercury; viral exposures; autoimmune disorders; and childhood vaccinations."[47]

Mark Blaxill, MBA, analyzed the autism data in California and published his study "The Changing Prevalence of Autism in California" in the April 2003 edition of the *Journal of Autism and Developmental Disorders*. He also refuted the suggestion of some researchers that the huge rise in diagnosed cases of autism was due to "diagnostic substitution," and countered that "This hypothesized substitution is not supported by proper and detailed analyses of the California data."

Mr. Blaxill went on to analyze further reported rates of autism throughout the United States as well as in the United Kingdom.[48] His analysis again showed that the *alleged epidemic of autism is real* and further refuted the notion that the dramatic increase in reported cases of autism was due merely to better diagnosis or expanded diagnostic criteria.

---

45   King, M.; Bearman, P. "Diagnostic change and the increased prevalence of autism." *International Journal of Epidemiology.* 2009. 38(5):1224-1234; doi:10.1093/ije/dyp261.

46   Since the diagnosis of autism is often not made until a child is 4-8 years of age or older, we would actually expect to see more autism in the older populations if the autism epidemic skeptics were correct, but we don't!

47   Byrd, Robert. M.I.N.D. Institute; UC Davis, October 2002.

48   "What's going on? The Question of Time Trends in Autism." Public Health Reports; Nov-Dec 2004

In a 2005 study, "National Autism Prevalence Trends From United States Special Education Data," published in the journal *Pediatrics* (March 2005), author Craig Newschaffer, Ph.D. of Johns Hopkins University concludes that his study "shows that the rise in the incidence of autism is real, and that the greatest increase took place between 1987 and 1992, which matches the timing of the near tripling of vaccines given to our children and the tripling of mercury within those vaccines."

And still further evidence to support the contention that this epidemic of newly diagnosed autism cases is real comes from a study published in the January 2009 issue of the journal *Epidemiology*, authored by researchers at the U.C. Davis M.I.N.D. Institute.[49]

By analyzing data collected by the State of California Department of Developmental Services (DDS) from 1990 to 2006, as well as the United States Census Bureau and State of California Department of Public Health Office of Vital Records, which compiles and maintains birth statistics, the two researchers were able to determine that less than 1/10th of the estimated 600-700 percent increase in the number of reported autism cases could be attributed to the inclusion of milder cases of autism. Only 1/20th of the increase could be attributed to earlier age at diagnosis.

Although the authors do caution that, "Other artifacts have yet to be quantified, and as a result, the extent to which the continued rise represents a true increase in the occurrence of autism remains unclear." However, Professor Hertz-Picciotto apparently does believe that the rise in autism prevalence is real, because she also declares that, "It's time to start looking for the environmental culprits responsible for the remarkable increase in the rate of autism in California."

Currently, a majority of the research money devoted to finding the cause of autism is directed at looking for *genetic* mutations, and that research is certainly important. However, these study results suggest that the research emphasis should shift from funding primarily genetic studies to also adequately underwriting studies evaluating *environmental factors* and their relationship to this epidemic of autism because genetic factors cannot account for and do not cause epidemics.

Suspected environmental influences that are likely culprits responsible for this epidemic include immunizations, toxic chemical exposures, changes in gut micro-organisms, chronic infections, auto-immune reactions, as well as other potentially noxious agents.

Conclusions:

- The major part of the dramatic increase in autism diagnoses that started in the mid to late 1980s is not factitious and represents a true epidemic.
- Delayed onset (regressive) autism has been increasing since the 1970s and now accounts for most of those diagnosed with autism.
- Since genetic factors, which clearly play a major role in promoting autism, cannot account for and do not cause epidemics, we must identify the environmental influences that are involved in triggering this epidemic.

The evidence is now clear that most cases of autism are caused by adverse environmental influences that "exploit" certain genetic "propensities."

"There is no more unscientific position in public health today than the fiction that rising autism rates come from better diagnosing."

— *Mark Blaxill, MBA*

---

49   Professor Irva Hertz-Picciotto and the U.C. Davis Department of Public Health Sciences (Lora Delwiche)

"There is no question that there has got to be an environmental component here."

— Tom Insel, head of autism research at the NIH

How is Autism Diagnosed and By Whom?

There are no medical tests that are specific for autism. Autism is currently diagnosed according to *arbitrarily defined criteria* as listed in either the DSM-V manual (edition V of the *Diagnostic and Statistical Manual of Mental Illnesses of the American Psychiatric Association*) or the ICD-10 code book (ICD-10 refers to the 10th edition of the *International Classification of Diseases*).

The diagnosis of autism based on the DSM-V criteria is determined after interviewing the parents or other caregivers and observing the child (although parental reports of the child's behavior have been found to be accurate and may substitute for direct observation).[50] Certain laboratory and non-medical tests may also be used to aid in helping to confirm the diagnosis.

Literally, anyone who can read and who understands the diagnostic criteria can diagnose autism; however, the diagnosis is usually made by pediatricians, especially those trained in developmental pediatrics, psychiatrists, psychologists, and pediatric neurologists.

Very often, other professionals, who are familiar with autism, such as speech therapists, teachers, occupational therapists, physical therapists, social workers, and others are quite capable of diagnosing autism. An experienced observer, from any discipline, is, therefore, generally able to make an accurate diagnosis. However, state authorities generally specify who may officially make the diagnosis.

Not uncommonly, it is parents who first suspect autism in their children and have to convince their pediatricians of the correctness of their suspicions.

At What Age Is Autism Usually Diagnosed?

A research team of scientists at the U.C. Davis Mind Institute closely observed a series of babies, half of whom had siblings previously diagnosed as being autistic. The children were followed for a three-year period and assessed at ages 6, 12, 18, 24, and 36 months of age. The children were evaluated using standard diagnostic tools like the Autism Diagnostic Observation Schedule (ADOS) and the Autism Diagnostic Interview-revised (ADI-R).

The scientists recorded each instance of eye contact, babbling, and smiling in each infant and were not told which babies had autistic siblings and which ones did not. They found that there were significant differences by the end of the first year of life (but not by six months of age) between those babies who would later be diagnosed as being autistic compared to those who developed normally. The children who would later be diagnosed as being autistic showed significant delays in sociability and communicative behaviors by the end of the first year of life.[51]

The study suggests that many, or even most, autistic children could be diagnosed prior to their first birthday; however, although some children are indeed suspected of having an autism spectrum disorder by twelve months of age, the average age of diagnosis for boys with autism is at 5-7 *years* of age, and girls with autism are often misdiagnosed, not diagnosed at all, or are diagnosed at a much later age than are boys.[52]

This is unfortunate because, as has been mentioned, there is evidence showing that early intervention results in bet-

---

50   The CDC's Fact Sheet: "MMWR—Parental Report of Diagnosed Autism in Children Aged 4–17 Years, United States, 2003–2004" found that their two large parental surveys provided data "within the range reported from other studies using other study methods."
51   Ozonoff, S. et al. *J. of the Amer. Acad. of Child & Adolescent Psychiatry*. March 2010.
52   David Rose, health correspondent and Rachel Carlyle; timesline@co.uk; is.qd/7MN3j

ter outcomes in autistic children. A March 2012 CDC report on autism prevalence also noted that only 12 percent of autistics were diagnosed before age three in 1994, but this figure increased to 18 percent by the year 2000.[53]

British researcher Richard Mills of Research Autism states that "Girls are less likely to have language delay than boys with autism, so that all the right boxes get ticked when they are toddlers and their autism can get missed."

"Autistic girls are also more likely to be outwardly social when they are younger, whereas boys are less so," he added.

In a study published later in 2010, Dr. Mills reviewed the diagnoses of 60 female patients at a psychiatric hospital who were routinely screened for autism and found that the diagnosis of autism was missed in 11 of the 60 "possibly because most tests were developed around male characteristics of autism," he concluded.[54]

Dr. Mills also believes that another reason why autism is missed or misdiagnosed in girls is because it is assumed that it is a rare condition in females, and so doctors are less likely to consider it.

What Causes Autism?

The etiology of autism is complex, to say the least, and will be discussed in detail in Parts II and III of this book. What needs to be emphasized here is *what does not cause autism*, and that is the autistic child's parents.

In his 1943 paper, Leo Kanner, first described the condition that he named "infantile autism," and in that paper, he also noted what he regarded as a lack of parental affection for autistic children.

In his 1949 paper on the same subject, he went further and attributed autism to a "genuine lack of maternal warmth" and the "refrigerator mother" theory of autism was born.

In formulating this now-rejected theory, Dr. Kanner appears to have ignored the fact that the non-autistic siblings of the autistic children that he described presumably would have been exposed to the same lack of warmth and affection as were their autistic kin. This would suggest that Kanner was "putting the cart before the horse." Autistic children often appear "detached" and poorly responsive to affection and nurturing. Many do not like to be held or cuddled. A child who does not seem to respond to or even rejects his parents' nurturing attempts is, therefore, less likely to be snuggled.

Bruno Bettelheim (August 28, 1903 – March 13, 1990), a famous Austrian-born, American child psychologist, promoted Kanner's "refrigerator mother" theory for many years, and summarized his thoughts in his 1967 book *The Empty Fortress: Infantile Autism and the Birth of the Self*, which reemphasized his position that "cold," unnurturing parents, especially moms, are to blame for autism.

These misanthropic parents were described as being aloof or absent and not wanting to hold or lovingly interact with their children. The "affection deprivation" theory of Kanner & Bettelheim was very popular from the 1950s through the 1970s, and became the accepted explanation for autism.[55] Some physicians to this day still quote the theory as if it were factual [personal experience of author]. But it is not. There was and is no evidence to support this theory, and it is currently rejected by mainstream medicine.

One of the reasons for this rejection was the publication of a book in 1964 by a disgruntled parent, a naval psychologist named Bernard Rimland, who knew that the affection deprivation theory of Kanner and Bettelheim had to be wrong, because he himself was the parent of an autistic boy (Mark), and both he and his wife were good parents who loved and nurtured that child.

Dr. Rimland's book, *Infantile Autism: the Syndrome and Its Implications for a Neural Theory of Behavior*, opened the eyes of many to a possible biomedical and behavioral approach for evaluating and treating this malady. In so doing,

---

53   http://www.medscape.com/view article/761162
54   Ibid.
55   Severson, Katherine DeMaria; Aune, James Arnt; Jodlowski, Denise (2007). "Bruno Bettelheim, Autism, and the Rhetoric of Scientific Authority" in Osteen, Mark. *Autism and Representation*. Routledge. pp. 65-77.

he was also challenging Bettelheim's "poor parenting" hypothesis, and although Bettelheim, as has been noted, reaffirmed his stand in his book, *The Empty Fortress*, published three years after Rimland's book appeared, his parent-disparaging theory was already losing favor in the scientific community. The "death knell" for the Freudian school of thought that blamed parents for virtually all of their children's dysfunctions was fast approaching.

Bernard Rimland made it his life's work to find the causes of autism and to establish therapies that would help both the afflicted children and their loved ones. Over the years, he amassed a huge database of autism research and case histories and founded both the Autism Society of America (ASA) and the Autism Research Institute (ARI), which now itself underwrites a good deal of autism research and education and also sponsors autism conferences that are generally held twice yearly in the U.S.

Dr. Rimland was a strong supporter of Applied Behavioral Analysis (ABA), a very successful educational therapy pioneered by Norwegian-born psychologist Ivar Lovaas at UCLA, who died in August 2010. ABA has helped many autistic children improve their communication and social skills.

Dr. Rimland also advocated the supplementation of required nutrients, special diets that eliminated reactive foods, the elimination of toxic metals and other toxic substances via avoidance and chelation, and the normalization of intestinal microbes by a variety of means. All of these approaches have benefited many autistic children.

Dr. Rimland, the "father" of the biomedical approach to evaluating and treating autism, also recruited many top researchers into the ranks of the Autism Research Institute, either as founding members or as lecturers at the ARI sponsored DAN! (Defeat Autism Now) conferences.

Bernard Rimland died at age seventy-eight on November 21, 2006. His son Mark, although not completely recovered, is a successful artist.

What Medical Services Do Autistic Children Require?

Children with autism are more likely than their non-autistic peers to exhibit behavioral and conduct problems, ADHD symptoms, speech delay, anxiety, allergies, and a variety of other medical concerns.

A 2006 study by James Gurney and colleagues published in the *Archives of Pediatric and Adolescent Medicine*[56] revealed the increased broad medical needs of children with autism as compared with non-autistic children. Autistic children were found to require significantly more medical care, medications, educational and mental health services, and more physical, occupational, and speech therapy than their non-autistic counterparts.

Notably, autistic children almost always require special education services, which may entail the hiring of a private aide to assist the children while in class. Some older children and many adults with autism require lifelong institutional care. All these needs are expensive. Very expensive!

What Are the Estimated Costs to Families and Society of Raising an Autistic Child?

Bob Wright, of *Autism Speaks*, estimates that some families can spend "$40,000-$50,000 *a year* for therapies for each autistic child, and a few spend a lot more."[57]

A more analytical answer to this question can be found in the April 2007 issue of the medical journal, the *Archives of Pediatrics and Adolescent Medicine*.

Michael Ganz, M.S., Ph.D. and the Harvard School of Public Health analyzed data from the medical literature and national surveys to summarize the average direct medical and non-medical costs of autism projected over a lifetime. These costs included behavioral therapies, prescription medications, adult care and special education, and excluded

---

56   Vol. 160; pp 825-30
57   Roberts, Deborah et al. ABC News.com; April 9, 2009.

medical and non-medical costs that would likely have been incurred by individuals without autism. Cost estimates for each five-year interval starting at age 3 and ending at age 66 were provided. Direct costs (both medical and non-medical) and indirect costs were considered separately.

Dr. Ganz stated that, "*Direct medical costs*, like physician evaluations and behavioral therapy, are quite high for the first five years of life (average of around $35,000 per year), start to decline substantially by age 8 years (around $6,000/year) and continue to decline through the end of life to around $1,000." He found that these "direct medical costs constitute almost 10 percent of total estimated costs over a lifetime and behavioral therapy itself account(ed) for 6.5 percent of these total costs."

"*Direct non-medical costs*," Dr. Ganz continues, "like child or adult care and home modifications, vary (from) around $10,000 to approximately $16,000/year during the first 20 years of life, peak in the 23- to 27-year age range (around $27,500/year) and then steadily decline to the end of life to around $8,000 in the last age group. These direct non-medical costs account for 31 percent of the total life-time costs of caring for an autistic individual."

"*Indirect costs* also display a similar pattern, decreasing from around $43,000 in early life, peaking at ages 23 to 27 years (around $52,000) and declining through the end of life to $0." Lost productivity and other indirect costs were found to account for about 59 percent of autism-related costs over a lifetime.

According to the Ganz study, the direct and indirect costs to society of caring for one autistic person from childhood through old age is an astounding 3.2 million dollars, with much of this cost attributable to lost productivity and adult care.

The estimated direct and indirect cost for the entire U.S. population of autistic individuals is thought to be about 35 billion dollars each year.[58]

These cost estimates *do not include* the loss of family income when one parent or caregiver has to stop working in order to care for an autistic child, nor do they include the physical, emotional, and financial stresses that raising an autistic child bring to bear on their families, which in turn can lead to bankruptcies, divorces, and even behavioral problems in the often less-focused-on siblings of the autistic child. By 2025, the projected cost to society of this autism epidemic is projected to reach one trillion dollars annually![59]

Who Pays for These Evaluations and Therapies?

The staggering financial burden of having to evaluate, treat, educate, and care for an autistic child is borne by the state and local governments, the local school district, by the parents, and to a lesser degree, by some health insurance companies.

Every state has its own rules and regulations regarding what services it covers. When states, local municipalities, and school districts are stressed financially, many of these services are subject to reductions or outright cuts. Private medical insurance may cover some of the costs of laboratory testing, therapies and drugs, but parents are often responsible for underwriting a large part of this financial burden out of their own pockets.

When these autistic children become adults, society may have to bear the burden of maintaining them (through Social Security disability benefits, for example), and those costs will be crippling!

Do Any Risk Factors Increase the Chances of Giving Birth to an Autistic Child?

Yes. These risk factors include extremely premature birth with neurological damage, having close relatives with autism or related disorders, giving birth at an older age, nutrient deficiencies, and exposures to certain toxic substances, infectious agents, and others.

---

58   Ganz, M.L. "The costs of autism." In Moldin, S.O.; Rubenstein, J.L.R., eds. *Understanding autism: From basic neuroscience to treatment.* 1st Edition. Boca Raton (FL): CRC Press; 2006 p. 475-502.

59   https://tacanowblog.com/2016/04/01/the-new-autism-prevalence-rate-is-not-a-cause-for-celebration/

Extremely Premature Birth

Researchers found that of the 219 British and Irish children studied who were born in 1995 before the 26th week of pregnancy, 8 percent (1 in 13) met the criteria for autism spectrum disorders at age 11, compared to none of the 153 classmates born full-term that same year and used as a comparison group.

However, of the 56 pre-term children who were found to have no cognitive impairment at age 6, none were found to have autism or related conditions when re-evaluated at age 11. In contrast, 18 percent of the 34 children with moderate to severe cognitive impairment at age 6 were diagnosed as autistic (or as having a pervasive developmental disorder, not otherwise specified) at age 11.[60]

Having an Older Father

As men age, the DNA in their sperm is more subject to mutation. Studies show that men over 50 have twice the risk of having a child with autism compared to men under 30. The risk quadruples for men over 55.[61]

Having a Close Relative with either Schizophrenia or Bipolar Disorder

Two studies, one in Denmark and the other of Swedish and Israeli populations, show a significantly increased risk for autism in a child (2.5-12 times) if a parent or sibling has either schizophrenia or bipolar disorder, indicating that these three disorders may share common etiological factors.[62]

Having a Mother with an Autoimmune Disorder Like Type I Diabetes, Rheumatoid Arthritis, or Celiac Disease

The maternal brain is protected from antibody-mediated damage by the blood-brain barrier, whereas the fetal brain is exposed to all maternal antibodies. Some mothers produce antibodies against brain tissue. There is evidence that brain-reactive antibodies from the mother can lead to autism spectrum disorders in the offspring. Perhaps 15 to 20 percent of autism cases could be explained by this mechanism. A 2009 Danish study concluded that the risk for autism more than doubles for children of women with one of these disorders.[63]

Birth Order and Interval Between Pregnancies

One study found that "in families with a single affected child, autism risk increases with each birth. In families that have more than one child with autism, middle children have the highest risk, according to the study."[64]

Two studies found that children born within a year of an older sibling have a more than threefold higher risk of developing autism than those born at least three years apart.[65]

Other risk factors, like exposures to toxic substances and immunizations, will be discussed in more detail later in this book.

Induced Labor

Obstetricians often induce labor in mothers-to-be who are past their due date and not in labor, if labor is slow in progressing, or if there are problems with the baby or mother's health. Almost a quarter of all births in 2008 were induced. However, this procedure is not without risk.

---

60   Marlow, Neil, M.D. *J of Pediatrics*; Online; January 8, 2010 & Larsson H.J. et al. "Risk factors for autism: perinatal factors, parental psychiatric history, and socioeconomic status." *Am J Epidemiol.* 2005 May 15; 161(10):916-25; discussion 926-8.
61   http://us.mg205.mail.yahoo.com/neo/launch?partner=sbc
62   Sullivan, P.F. et al. "Family History of Schizophrenia and Bipolar Disorder as Risk Factors for Autism." *Arch Gen Psychiatry.* 2012; 69(11):1099-1103. and Larsson, H.J. et al. "Risk factors for autism: perinatal factors, parental psychiatric history, and socioeconomic status." *Am J Epidemiol.* 2005 May 15; 161(10):916-25; discussion 926-8.
63   Atladóttir, H.O. et al. *Pediatrics.* 124, 687-694 (2009)
64   Martin, L.A; Horriat, N.L.. PLoS One. 2012; 7, e51049 and http://sfari.org/news-and-opinion/news/2013/autism-symptoms-more-severe-in-later-born-children
65   Cheslack-Postava, K. et al. Pediatrics. 2011; 127, 246-253. PubMed and American Society of Human Genetics conference in San Francisco in November 2012.

The results of a study published in *JAMA Pediatrics* in August 2013 revealed that inducing or augmenting a mother's labor with Pitocin slightly increased the chances of that child becomg autistic.

"Mothers who had induced or augmented labor were 13-16 percent more likely to have a child with autism. If a mother had both methods used on her, the child was 27 percent more likely to be diagnosed with autism during childhood."[66]

It is possible and even likely that this increased autism risk may be related to the reason the labor needed to be induced and not to the inducing agent itself. More research into this area needs to be done. Correlation does not prove causation.

"Mental disorders are known to affect 13 percent—20 percent of children and cost society an estimated $247 billion annually…. The prevalence of many child mental health conditions is increasing over time.

The current (CDC) report[67] (5-16-13) found the most common child mental health conditions among children aged 3-17 years to include:

- *Attention-deficit/hyperactivity disorder (6.8 percent)*
- *Behavioral or conduct problems (3.5 percent)*
- *Anxiety (3.0 percent)*
- *Depression (2.1 percent)*
- *Autism spectrum disorders (1.1 percent).*

Some Other Risk Factors for Autism[68]

- Fetal Distress during delivery
- Circumcision prior to age 5 doubles the risk of developing autism[69]
- Maternal Thyroid hormone deficiency[70]
- Maternal Diabetes
- Maternal hypertension (high blood pressure)
- Maternal obesity
- Maternal exposure to the Rubella (German Measles) virus
- Maternal exposure to air pollution during pregnancy
- Low folic acid (a B vitamin) levels in the pregnant mother
- Maternal antibodies against the fetal brain
- Preeclampsia during pregnancy[71]
- Placental insufficiency[72]
- Low levels of vitamin D during pregnancy and at birth (see Table 1.1)[73]

66   http://www.cbsnews.com/8301-204_162-57598203/induced-labor-may-increase-risk-of-autism-in-offspring/
67   "Mental Health Surveillance among Children in the U.S. from 2005-2011." http://www.autismspeaks.org/science/science-news/autism-major-piece-child-mental-health-picture
68   http://www.usatoday.com/story/news/nation/2013/08/12/autism-labor-induction/2641391/
69   Frisch, M. et al. *JRSM*; 1-8-15 pub. online
70   *Annals of Neurology*; August 2013; Roman G, et al.
71   Walker, Cheryl et al. "Childhood risks of autism from genetics and the environment." *JAMA Pediatrics*. Dec 2014. Vol. 168, No. 12.
72   Ibid.
73   http://www.vitamindwiki.com/Most+Autism+Risk+factors+are+associated+with+low+ vitamin+D+-+March+2014.

VitaminDWiki has highlighted those autism risk factors that are also associated with low levels of Vitamin D.

Table 1.1. Risk factors associated with low levels of vitamin D

Factors Studied that increase risk for autism Factors with an asterisk are associated with low levels of vitamin D.	**Actual Risks** **Based on more than 100 scientific papers published over the past 20 years, here is how selected factors are believed to affect the likelihood of autism.**	
Identical twin is autistic*	+8,300% added risk	About 36% to 95% of these children expected to develop autism
Injury to the cerebellum at birth	+3,800	About 37% developed autism
Fraternal twin is autistic*	+2,100	Up to 31% expected to develop autism
Premature by 9 or more weeks*	+630	Less than 3% of these children expected to develop autism
Conceived within 12 months of another older sibling's birth*	+240	
Pregnant mom caught in a hurricane zone*	+200	
Sibling is a science or engineering major in college	+200	
Emigration at time of pregnancy	+130	
Father older than 60*	+100	
Mother or father with mental illness*	+100	
Living within 0.19 miles of a freeway*	+90	
Maternal depression*	+50	
Air pollutants, including mercury*	+40	
Father older than 40	+40	
Mother older than 35	+30	
Birth month	No statistically significant risk	
Premature by 3-8 weeks	No statistically significant risk	
Antidepressant use during pregnancy	No statistically significant risk	

Chapter 2
Autism Spectrum Disorders (ASDs)

"I know in my heart that man is good, that what is right will eventually triumph,
and there is purpose and worth to each and every life."

— *Ronald Reagan*

WHAT ARE PERVASIVE *Developmental Disorders?*

Autism today is categorized as a mental/neurological disorder (although it clearly is a lot more than that), and represents one of the five conditions previously listed (DSM-4) under the general heading of Pervasive Developmental Disorders (PDDs). These also include:

1. Asperger Syndrome
2. Rett Syndrome
3. Childhood Disintegrative Disorder [CDD]
4. Pervasive Developmental Disorder, Not Otherwise Specified [PDD-NOS] (a catch-all category)

These, together with attention deficit disorders with or without hyperactivity (ADD/ADHD), tic disorders (including Tourette syndrome), certain other syndromes and obsessive and compulsive disorders (OCD), were (until 2013) classified as disorders on the autism spectrum, because they all overlap in both symptomatology and, in many cases, in commonly seen laboratory and physiological abnormalities.

What Is Asperger Syndrome?

A year after Dr. Kanner's paper, in which he elucidated the manifestations of the condition that he called "Early Infantile Autism," a German scientist named Hans Asperger was describing a milder variant of this condition, which has ever since born his name. Asperger Syndrome-afflicted individuals exhibit high functioning and intelligence, but their social abilities are limited, as is their spectrum of interests.

Individuals with Asperger Syndrome often focus on one keen area of interest to the exclusion of all others. Their conversations are often limited to this one area of interest, which itself may or may not change in time. They often have difficulty reading the "body language" of others. They may be awkward socially. They may be clumsy physically. This makes them targets for bullying at school. The criteria for making this diagnosis are listed in Appendix III. The incidence of Asperger syndrome in males is perhaps 15 times greater than it is for females.

The new and controversial DSM-5 criteria published in May 2013 has dropped Asperger syndrome as a distinct classification and has included it (along with PDD-NOS and childhood disintegrative disorder) under the umbrella of Autism Spectrum Disorder.[1]

The incidence of Asperger's is much higher in boys than in girls, and ranges from c 2:1 to 4:1 with some claims as high as 16:1. Eliminating Asperger syndrome as a distinct diagnosis and renaming it as simply an "autism spectrum disorder" will now make it impossible to do research or track prevalence changes in this condition.[2]

What Is Rett Syndrome?

Rett syndrome is a true progressive *retardation* disorder, first described by the Austrian physician Andreas Rett in 1966, that occurs almost exclusively in females and, like classical autism, is relatively rare (occurring in one out of every 10,000 to 15,000 births). It is caused by an identified genetic defect (usually a mutation of the MECP2 gene), which results in autistic symptoms appearing after 6-18 months of age.

Children with this disorder often wring or mouth their hands and exhibit severe mental and developmental deficiencies. They withdraw socially, appear not to recognize their parents or others, and exhibit severe coordination and communications impairments. They have no verbal skills. Many are unable to ambulate. Seizures are common. Many have small heads and small brains (in contrast to most autistic children who have normal to large brains). Many have curved spines (scoliosis), short stature, and intestinal disorders. Physical, occupational, and speech therapies are of limited help in improving their functioning.

There is currently no cure for this condition; however, there is hope. A recent study showed that giving mice that were bred with a Rett Syndrome-like genetic defect a bone marrow transplant (after their bone marrow was first sterilized with radiation) seemed totally to reverse the adverse manifestations of the syndrome.

Mice that received the bone marrow transplant of brain microglial cells but did not have their bone marrow irradiated were not helped by the procedure. The microglial cells increased lifespan, normalized breathing, increased body weight, and improved locomotor activity in the mice.

Of course, what works in a mouse model may not apply to humans, so further studies must be done in this regard.[3]

As of May 2013, Rett Syndrome is no longer classified as an autism spectrum disorder.[4]

What is Childhood Disintegrative Disorder (CDD)?

Diagnostic Criteria for Childhood Disintegrative Disorder:[5]

A. Starting from ages 2-10, acquired skills are lost almost completely in 2 of 6 of these functional areas: 1-expressive language; 2-receptive language; 3-self care and social skills; 4-control over bowel and bladder; 5-play skills; 6-motor abilities.

B. Lack of normal function or impairment also occurs in at least 2 of the following 3 areas: 1.social interaction, 2. communication, and 3. Repetitive behavior and interest patterns.

In 1908, a Viennese remedial educator named Theodore Heller described an autism-like syndrome that he called "Dementia Infantilis" in the *Journal of Research and Treatment of Juvenile Feeblemindedness*.[6] This later was renamed childhood disintegrative disorder (CDD).

1   American Psychiatric Association (2000). "Diagnostic criteria for 299.80 Asperger's Disorder (AD)." *Diagnostic and Statistical Manual of Mental Disorders.* (4th, text revision) ISBN 0-89042-025-4. http://www.behavenet.com/capsules/disorders/asperger.htm, *and* Klin, A "Autism and Asperger syndrome: an overview." *Rev Bras Psiquiatr.* 2006; 28 (suppl 1): S3–S11.] http://en.wikipedia.org/wiki/DSM-5
2   Mattila, M.L. et al. "An epidemiological and diagnostic study of Asperger syndrome according to four sets of diagnostic criteria." *J Am Acad Child Adolesc Psychiatry.* 2007; 46 (5): 636–46 and David Rose, Times Online; 2-6-10.
3   "Wild-type microglia arrest pathology in a mouse model of Rett syndrome." Noël C. Derecki et al. *Nature* (2012) doi: 10.1038/nature10907; Published online; 18 March 2012
4   http://www.graceforrett.com/rett-syndrome/r168x/the-dsm-5-in-plain-english-is-rett-syndrome-autism/
5   Note: the CDD diagnostic criteria are the same as the criteria for diagnosing regressive autism
6   Heller, T. "Dementia Infantilis, Zeit Schrift fur die Erforschungund Behandlung des Jugen Lichen Schwansinns." 1908; 2:144-165.

Very few children who have an autism spectrum disorder (ASD) diagnosis meet the criteria for childhood disintegrative disorder (CDD). An estimate based on four surveys of ASD found that fewer than 2 children in 100,000 with ASD could be classified as having CDD. This suggests that CDD is a very rare form of ASD. It, like autism and ADHD, has a strong male preponderance. It is not clear what causes this condition, but an etiology similar to that of delayed onset (regressive) autism is suspected.

Symptoms may appear by age 2, but the average age of onset is between 3 and 4 years. Until this time, the child has age-appropriate skills in communication and social relationships. The somewhat longer period of normal development before regression helps differentiate this condition from delayed onset (AKA regressive-) autism. This appears to be a variant of classical delayed onset autism, however, and it is indeed now categorized as just "autism spectrum disorder" in the new DSM-V criteria (as of May 2013). The term "childhood disintegrative disorder" will no longer be used.

What Is Tourette Syndrome?

French physician Georges Gilles de la Tourette first described this condition, which appropriately bears his name, in an article he wrote over 100 years ago. In the article, "he described nine individuals who, since childhood, had suffered from involuntary movements and vocalizations as well as compulsive rituals or behaviors."[7]

Tourette syndrome is considered by many to be one of the autism spectrum disorders because many overlaps in symptomatology are noted in both conditions. For example, tics are more common in the autistic population as compared to non-autistics, and obsessions, compulsions, inattention, impulsivity, hyperactivity, anxiety, and mood variability are commonly observed in all these maladies.[8]

To be diagnosed as having Tourette syndrome, one must have vocal tics as well as motor tics; however, this distinction appears to be somewhat artificial, as a greater percentage of close relatives of those with Tourette syndrome compared to non-Tourette syndrome individuals exhibit an increase in motor tics, indicating that tic disorders have a genetic as well as an environmental component and range from mild: those with just a few motor tics, to severe: those with frequent motor and vocal tics.

A rare cause of Tourette syndrome has been found recently. A mutation in the histidine decarboxylase (HDC) gene was discovered in a family with Tourette syndrome. The gene in question makes a somewhat defective version of the HDC enzyme, which converts histidine in the brain into the neurotransmitter histamine. How and why this mutation promotes Tourette syndrome is not clear as yet, but these findings may lead researchers into a better understanding of this syndrome, and these findings may ultimately lead to a more successful therapy for this condition than currently exists.[9]

Be that as it may, those with Tourette syndrome, as is true of all syndromes on the autism spectrum, can often benefit by many of the same therapies that benefit autistic children.

What Are ADD & ADHD?

The acronym ADD stands for attention deficit disorder (no hyperactivity). ADHD is attention deficit disorder with hyperactivity. Children with these disorders have trouble paying attention, focusing, making good eye contact, and remembering what has been said to them. They are easily distracted and often impulsive. If also hyperactive/impulsive, they may be fidgety, in constant motion, moody, quick to anger or to cry, and some may be aggressive at times. They are frequently poor at reading body language. Many have learning disabilities.

In 1845, Dr. Heinrich Hoffman wrote a children's book entitled *The Story of Fidgety Phillip*. In the book, Phillip's behaviors mirrored those of children with hyperactivity disorder. Sir George Still, in 1902, published a series of lectures to England's Royal College of Physicians in which he described children with impulsivity and behavior concerns whose symptoms would have been consistent with a diagnosis of ADHD today.

---

7   www.tourettesyndrome.net
8   Ibid.
9   Catelan, B.L. et al. "Histidine decarboxylase activity causes Tourette syndrome…" *Neuron.* 2014; Jan 8; 81(1) 77-90.

But the criteria (as defined by DSM-IV) for making the diagnosis of ADD/ADHD are actually rather arbitrary and they change over time. [See Appendix III]. However, they have been superseded by the current (since 2013) DSM-V criteria. One positive change is the ability now to be allowed to diagnose ADHD in a child who has autism or other pervasive developmental disorders like Asperger syndrome.

Prior to 2013, although some 29-70 percent of people on the autism spectrum fulfill all the criteria for ADHD (which is often the major concern for the parents), clinicians were forbidden to make that diagnosis in these individuals according to DSM-IV criteria. This profoundly limiting stricture presupposes that an individual may not have these two conditions at the same time.

However, a recent prospective study by researchers at the Kennedy Krieger Institute found that nearly one third of the autistic children, 4-8 years of age and followed since they were toddlers, had both autism and ADHD, and those with both diagnoses had more severe cognitive defects.[10]

Another change in DSM-V is in the subcategories of ADD/ADHD. Currently, ADHD individuals are catalogued as being primarily hyperactive and compulsive, primarily inattentive, or exhibiting both concerns.

However, the current committee of three work-group members (all academics and *none* with clinical experience) evaluating these possible changes isn't even sure that the subtypes are valid. Why? Because nine studies show that the response to medications is the same in children diagnosed with either the inattentive or combined sub-types, and more importantly, because these subtypes "are not stable over time."

"A child's ADHD subtype might change many times over the years, and less than 40 percent of children maintain the same diagnosis at two time points."[11] The work-group definers have not yet considered that individuals can also *vary in the severity* of their condition from time to time in formulating their diagnostic criteria for these most subjectively defined maladies.

In pointing out the problems with the somewhat arbitrary diagnostic criteria currently in existence, which require that in order to be diagnosed as ADHD, a child must demonstrate or satisfy a minimum of 12 symptoms or criteria, Dr. Gabrielle Carlson, Director of Child and Adolescent Psychiatry at the State University of New York at Stony Brook, stated to the three non-clinician work-group members, "We don't really give a crap about ten symptoms vs. 12 symptoms, because people…want help for problems, and if you're a decent clinician, you're used to…hearing what the symptom constellation sounds like, and what's important is how impairing those particular symptoms are."[12]

In other words, what is really critical in all these conditions isn't the somewhat arbitrary diagnostic name we assign to them; the dysfunctions are the concern that must be addressed. However, because the specific diagnosis is invariably a critical necessity in allowing access to insurance-covered medications and services for the affected individual, it is best to allow clinicians some leeway in making the diagnosis of autism or ADHD in children with sub-threshold symptoms so that their dysfunctions can be appropriately managed.

In the words of Dr. Carlson, "I also think you have to understand that you're making clothes for people who have to wear them, and if you don't have a place for us to put the kids that we see, there are unintended consequences of where those kids get put."[13]

As with autism, ADD/ADHD disorders are syndromes, not diseases. Each child has his or her own mix of genetic predispositions and environmental triggers, which is why *what works for one will not necessarily benefit others*. And as is true in autism (and most other conditions for that matter), there is a spectrum of severity from mild to extreme.

---

10   Lao, P.; Landa, R. "Association between severity of behavioral phenotype and comorbid attention deficit hyperactivity disorder symptoms in children with autism spectrum disorders." *Autism: The Interntnl J and Practice*. Jun 5, 2013.
11   *Pediatric News*; Vol. 43, No. Dec 12 2099:1.
12   Ibid.
13   Ibid.

A number of studies have shown associations (co-morbidities) between ADHD and Oppositional Defiant Disorder (one third to one half of all hyperactives—mainly boys), Conduct Disorder (20-40 percent), speech problems, and learning disabilities.[14]

One study "found up to 80 percent of 11 year-old boys with ADHD were at least two years delayed with learning disabilities."[15]

The diagnosis of ADD or ADHD is generally made by qualified medical personnel, like physicians, and psychologists, often by using a questionnaire, like the Connor's Scale (see Appendix II). There is a Connor's scale for teachers and also for parents (both have short and long versions).

And as is true in autism, ADD and ADHD occur more often in males, and the incidence appears to be increasing. "The American Psychiatric Association states in the Diagnostic and Statistical Manual of Mental Disorders (DSM-IV-TR) that 3 percent-7 percent of school-aged children have ADHD. However, studies have estimated higher rates in community samples."[16]

According to the CDC, recent data from surveys of parents indicate that:

- Approximately 9.5 percent of children 4-17 years of age (5.4 million) have been diagnosed with ADHD as of 2007. That's almost one in ten, and the percentage of children with a parent-reported ADHD diagnosis increased by 22 percent between 2003 and 2007. "Disorders of neurobehavioral development affect 10-15 percent of all births," confirm researchers at the Harvard School of Public Health and New York's Mount Sinai.

- Rates of ADHD diagnosis increased an average of 3 percent per year from 1997 to 2006 and an average of 5.5 percent per year from 2003 to 2007.

- Boys (13.2 percent) were more likely than girls (5.6 percent) to have ever been diagnosed with ADHD, and rates of ADHD diagnosis increased at a greater rate among older teens as compared to younger children.

- Prevalence of parent-reported ADHD diagnosis varied substantially by state, from a low of 5.6 percent in Nevada to a high of 15.6 percent in North Carolina.

- As of 2007, parents of 2.7 million youth ages 4-17 years (66.3 percent of those with a current diagnosis) report that their child was receiving medication treatment for the disorder.

- Rates of medication treatment for ADHD varied by age and sex; children aged 11-17 years of age were more likely than those 4-10 years of age to take medication, and boys are 2.8 times more likely to take medication than girls.

- In 2007, geographic variability in the percent of children taking medication for ADHD ranged from a low of 1.2 percent in Nevada to a high of 9.4 percent in North Carolina.

- In 2003, geographic variability in prevalence of medication treatment ranged from a low of 2.1 percent in California to a high of 6.5 percent in Arkansas.

- About 5 percent of children had ADHD without Learning Disability (LD), 5 percent had LD without ADHD, and 4 percent had both conditions.

- Parents of children with a history of ADHD report almost 3 times as many peer problems as those without a history of ADHD and are almost 10 times as likely to have difficulties that interfere with friendships (20.6 percent vs. 2.0 percent).

- Children with ADHD, compared to children without ADHD, were more likely to have major injuries (59 percent vs. 49 percent), hospital inpatient (26 percent vs. 18 percent), hospital outpatient (41 per-

---

14   Hinshaw 1992; Biederman et al. 1991 & 1987; Sprich 1991; Munir et al. 1987; Barkley 1990a; Lahey et al. 1987, etc.
15   McGee, Williams, et al. (1989).
16   http://www.cdc.gov/ncbddd/adhd/data.html

cent vs. 33 percent), or emergency department admission (81 percent vs. 74 percent)

- Using a prevalence rate of 5 percent, the annual societal "cost of illness" for ADHD is estimated to be between $36 and $52 billion, in 2005 dollars. It is estimated to be between $12,005 and $17,458 annually per individual. The total excess cost of ADHD in the U.S. in 2000 was $31.6 billion.

- Workers with ADHD are absent from work more days per month than are those without ADHD.[17]

Many physicians and scientists believe that the dramatic rise in ADHD diagnosed children, which parallels that of autistic children, is a reflection of many of the same biochemical dysfunctions that are commonly seen in autistic children as well. ADHD, in most cases, appears to be due to a similar combination of genetic predispositions and adverse environmental influences.

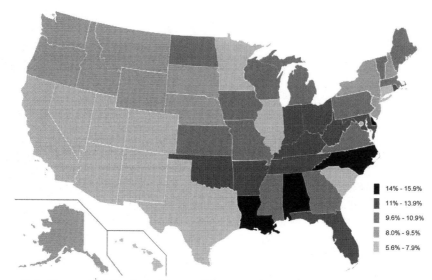

Figure 2.1. Percent of Youth 4-17 ever Diagnosed with Attention-Deficit/Hyperactivity Disorder by state: National Survey of Children's Health, 2007.[18] The apparent increased ADD/ADHD risk in the north and southeast USA may represent diminished vitamin D production secondary to decreased sunshine exposure.

What Causes ADD/ADHD?

The causes of this condition appear to be similar to those that promote autism, and both conditions share many traits. A combination of genetic factors and environmental insults are likely to underlie the entire autism spectrum of conditions, including ADHD and ADD. These will be discussed in later chapters in more detail. We will now review just a few of the many likely factors that have been associated with promoting or exacerbating hyperactivity and attention deficits.

Vitamin D Deficiency

Children with ADHD have been shown in one study to be deficient in vitamin D (c. 21 ng/ml on average) as compared to their non-ADHD peers (c. 35 ng/ml on average). Vitamin D is a hormone-like vitamin that plays a major role in normalizing brain function. See Figure 2.1.[19]

---

17   Ibid.
18   Ibid.
19   Goksugur, S.B. et al. "Vitamin D Status in Children with Attention Deficit Hyperactivity Disorder." *Pediatric Int.* 2014 Jan 13. doi: 10.1111/ped.12286.

Frequent Ear Infections?

One such influence is having frequent ear infections as a child. These are common in children with both autism and ADHD. Professor Jean Hébert of the Albert Einstein School of Medicine did a mouse study that "provides the first evidence that a sensory impairment, such as inner-ear dysfunction, can induce specific molecular changes in the brain that cause maladaptive behaviors traditionally considered to originate exclusively in the brain."[20]

A Cell Phone Connection?

The offspring of pregnant mice exposed to continuous cell phone radiation during their seventeen days of gestation had impaired memory, were hyperactive, and showed reduced transmissions in the prefrontal cortex of the brain. The researchers worried that, "the exposure of cellular telephones in pregnancy may have a comparable effect on the fetus and similar implications for society."[21]

In another study, this time involving fetal rats exposed to cell phone radiation three times a day for up to sixty minutes at a time for just three weeks, the scientists found that *all* the irradiated rats, as compared to the non-exposed control group, had brain abnormalities including increased levels of oxidative stress and neurotransmitter abnormalities.[22]

These cell phone radiation risks appear to apply also to humans. An analysis of data from almost 13,000 children revealed that exposure of the fetus to cell phone radiation as well as to the child after delivery appeared to increase dramatically the risk of that child experiencing behavioral difficulties in early childhood.

If a pregnant woman used a cell phone just 2-3 times a day, she significantly increased the likelihood that the exposed child would experience symptoms of hyperactivity, conduct disorder, emotional lability, and difficulty forming relationships by the time the child reached school age. This risk increased if the child in question was also a cell phone user prior to age seven.[23]

The results of this study were confirmed in a larger second study that evaluated data from nearly 29,000 children. As in the previous study, "children whose mothers used cell phones while pregnant were 40 percent more likely to have behavioral problems," and this risk "rose to 50 percent if the children were cell phone users themselves."[24]

The developing brain of the fetus and young child appear to be especially sensitive to the adverse effects of microwave radiation from cell phones, and likely from cell phone towers, Wi-Fi transmissions, smart meters, and related electromagnetic "smog" as well. The alarming implications of the aforementioned studies suggest that children and pregnant women in particular should not use cell phones.

> *Every 900 milliseconds, whether you are using the phone or not, your cell phone has a spike in radiation because it is looking for a signal from the tower.*
>
> — *Dr. Devra Davis, Ph D.*[25]

The Diet Connection

It is clear from dozens of studies and thousands of parent reports that certain foods and food additives, like artificial colors and preservatives, can adversely affect behavior, academic performance, and cognitive function. This subject will be discussed in greater detail in Chapters 29, 30, and 31.

---

20   Antoine, M.W. et al. "A Causative Link Between Inner Ear Defects and Long-Term Striatal Dysfunction." *Science*. Sept 2013.

21   Taylor, H. et al. *Scientific Reports*. March 15, 2012: 2; 312.

22   *Electromagnetic Biology and Medicine*. January 23, 2012.

23   *Epidemiology*. 2008 July. 19(4): 523-9.

24   www.mercola.com & *J of Epidem. and Community Health*. December 7, 2010.

25   www.electromagnetichealth.org

Acetaminophen During Pregnancy

A recent well-done study published online in *JAMA Pediatrics* (February 24, 2014, Zeyan Liew, et al.) found that women who used acetaminophen (AKA paracetamol—Tylenol™ and other brands) during pregnancy were significantly more likely to have children with ADHD and hyperactivity (hyperkinesis). The highest risk (68 percent increased risk) in this regard was for women who took acetaminophen during both the second and third trimesters of pregnancy.[26] These findings were confirmed in a recent New Zealand study. Thompson JM, et al. Associations between acetaminophen use during pregnancy and ADHD symptoms measured at ages 7 and 11 years.[27] We will have more to say about acetaminophen later in this narrative.

Toxins in the Environment Can Contribute to ADHD and Cognitive Dysfunction

Prenatal Mercury

Many industrial chemicals have been linked to developmental and neurological disorders in children. Philippe Grandjean, MD and Philip Landrigan identified 12 of these and "postulate that even more neurotoxicants remain undiscovered."[28]

Researchers evaluated 279 children living in the Canadian arctic for levels of methyl mercury, certain endocrine disrupting chemicals called PCBs (polychlorinated biphenyls) and lead at birth and at school age (average age 11 years). They found that the concentration of mercury in the child's cord blood correlated with later problems with attention and disruptive behavior as did lead.

The investigators concluded that to their knowledge, "this study is the first to identify an association between prenatal methyl mercury and ADHD symptomatology in childhood and the first to replicate previous reported associations between low-level childhood lead exposure and ADHD in a population exposed to lead primarily from dietary sources."

A second study in 2012 confirmed the prenatal mercury exposure-ADHD linkage.[29]

Childhood Lead Exposure

There is clear and consistent research linking childhood lead exposure in a dose dependent manner to not only low IQ but also attention problems, aggressive behavior, sleep difficulties, irritability, decreased appetite, developmental delays, and low energy, as was confirmed by the aforementioned study. A child's *current blood level of lead* has also been shown to correlate with his or her ADHD symptom scores.[30]

Polychlorinated Biphenyls (PCBs)

PCBs are a class of chemicals once widely used for a variety of industrial uses. They are endocrine disruptors and can cause cancer in humans as well as neurotoxicity and immune suppression. They were forbidden to be manufactured after 1978; however, products containing PCBs are still around, including electrical insulation and equipment, paints, plastics, carbonless copy paper, and others. PCBs are very stable and don't break down in the environment appreciably. They can still be released from hazardous waste sites, and they may currently be found at low levels in some drinking water, fish, and breast milk.

"Newborn monkeys exposed to PCBs showed persistent and significant deficits in neurological development, including visual recognition, short-term memory, and learning," according to the Environmental Protection Agency, and "Studies in humans have suggested effects similar to those observed in monkeys…including learning deficits and changes in activity," the agency states.[31]

---

26   http://archpedi.jamanetwork.com/article.aspx?articleid=1833486
27   HYPERLINK "http://www.ncbi.nlm.nih.gov/pubmed/25251831" \o "PloS one." PLoS One. 2014 Sep 24;9(9)
28   Neurobehavioural effects of developmental toxicity; The Lancet Neurology; Vol 13, No.3, 330-338, March 2014
29   Boucher, O. et al. *Environmental Health Perspectives*. 2012; 10: 1456-61 *and* Sagiv, S.K. et al. *JAMA Pediatrics*. Dec 2012, Vol 166, No. 12.
30   Boucher, Ibid.
31   http://www.epa.gov/wastes/hazard/tsd/pcbs/pubs/effects.htm

Phthalate Exposure

Phthalates (THAL-ates) are also endocrine-mimicking chemicals found commonly in plastic containers, car interiors, pacifiers, and children's toys. They have been shown to somewhat feminize male fetuses (increased risk of penile abnormalities like hypospadias, as well as testicular dysgenesis and low and abnormal sperm counts later in life). A recent Korean study also showed "a strong positive association between phthalate metabolites in urine and symptoms of ADHD among school-age children."[32]

Arsenic

Arsenic, linked to reduced cognitive function in schoolchildren, is found in chicken meat (chicken feed is often supplemented with arsenic), rice, and, occasionally, water. It is still being released through different agricultural applications. Two Monsanto plants were placed on the EPAs superfund list as priorities to be cleaned up for their release of arsenic laden waste.[33]

Toluene

Maternal exposure has been linked to brain development problems and attention deficits in the child, according to the EPA and OSHA. Toluene is found in paints, fragrances, glues, nail polish, automobile emissions, and cigarette smoke.[34]

Pesticides

Organophosphate pesticides like chlorpyrifos, diazinon, Malathion, and dimethoate have been linked to developmental disorders, learning difficulties, and ADHD. They are all neurotoxins that interfere with the enzyme (acetylcholinesterase) that breaks down the neurotransmitter acetylcholine. This results in continuous overstimulation of the brain leading to neurological dysfunction. These pesticides also cause cancer, reproductive harm, and Parkinson's disease, and they kill wildlife like salmon and frogs.[35]

Manganese

Manganese is a nutrient needed in only small amounts. Excess manganese, as found in some soy formulas for babies, can be neurotoxic and lead to ADHD and diminished intellectual function.[36]

Fluoride

Fluoride found in toothpaste and fluoridated water has been shown in at least thirty-two studies to be neurotoxic to children, as manifested by lower IQ scores and attention deficits.[37]

Tetrachloroethylene

This substance is a solvent used to dry clean clothes and for other purposes. Nurses, hairdressers, and beauticians are often at risk for exposure. It is a known carcinogen that is linked to ADHD and aggressive behavior.[38]

Flame Retardants

The now banned flame retardants known as PBDEs (polybrominateddiphenyl ethers) are still present in a good deal of old furniture and have been linked to neurodevelopmental disorders in children.[39]

---

32   Bung-Nyun, Kim et al. "Phthalates Exposure and Attention-Deficit/Hyperactivity Disorder in School-Age Children." *Biological Psychiatry.* Vol. 66, Issue 10, p. 958–963, Nov 15, 2009.

33   http://oawhealth.com/2015/06/22/silent-neurotoxin-pandemic-11-chemicals-affecting-childrens-brain-development-2/

34   Ibid.

35   Ibid.

36   Ibid.

37   Ibid.

38   Ibid.

39   Ibid.

Are There Different Subtypes of ADD?

Yes. Dr. Daniel Amen (a psychologist with offices in Newport Beach, California) has identified seven subtypes of ADD over the twenty-plus years of his practice and has performed tens of thousands of brain scans (SPECT) on individuals with this disorder in order to help identify each type of ADD. This is important as each type requires its own therapy in order to improve functioning in an individual. An individual may manifest more than one type of ADD.

All of the subtypes exhibit at least three of the five following symptoms: short attention span, distractibility, disorganization, procrastination, and impulse control issues.

The seven subtypes of ADD, according to Dr. Amen, are:

Type 1. Classical ADD (ADHD): Children with this subtype tend to be hyperactive and restless. They are disorganized, inattentive, and are easily distracted. They have short attention spans and often act impulsively. SPECT scans show low activity in the brain. Children may respond well to stimulant medications like amphetamine and Ritalin.

Type 2. Inattentive ADD: These individuals are not hyperactive or impulsive, but (as with Classical ADD) they have short attention spans, are easily distracted, and somewhat disorganized. They tend to be slow moving and are often lost in their own thoughts. SPECT scans show low activity in the brain. Stimulant meds may be helpful.

Type 3. Overfocused ADD: These individuals tend to dwell on negative thoughts and behaviors and have difficulty shifting their attention. "They tend to worry, hold grudges, and when things don't go their way, they get upset," says Dr. Amen. They are often oppositional and argumentative and don't respond well to stimulant medications that may worsen their symptoms.

Type 4. Temporal Lobe ADD: This subtype is characterized by anger outbursts, irritability, inflexibility, aggressive behaviors, and memory and learning problems. Children may or may not be hyperactive but often exhibit many of the behaviors of Classical ADD like distractibility and short attention spans. Stimulant medications tend to worsen their symptoms.

Type 5. Limbic ADD: Individuals with this subtype of ADD tend to be moody and mildly depressed. They have low energy and often feel hopeless and worthless. They have difficulty paying attention and exhibit many of the other ADD characteristics. They may or may not be hyperactive.

Type 6. "Ring of Fire" ADD: Dr. Amen finds that individuals with this disorder have too much going on everywhere in the brain. They are often cyclically moody, oppositional, angry, distractible, and inattentive. They often exhibit certain autistic traits like hypersensitivity to noise, bright lights, and touch.

Type 7: Anxious ADD: This subtype manifests in people who have the symptoms of anxiety, nervousness, tension, a tendency to predict the worst, and have trouble with timed-tests or don't like speaking in public, along with all the other ADD symptoms.[40]

Dr. Amen has created a free questionnaire on his website that allows individuals to determine which subtype of ADD they have. He has devised specific therapies for each of these subtypes.[41]

What Is PDD-NOS?

Pervasive Developmental Disorder—Not Otherwise Specified

This is a catch-all category of developmental disorder that is defined as being a disorder that shares some of the characteristics of autism and the other pervasive development disorders, but not enough to fit the criteria of autism, Tourette syndrome, Rett syndrome, or Asperger syndrome.

---

40   From Dr. Amen's website at: http://www.elevated existence .com/blog/2014/01/04/dr-daniel-amen-healing-the-7-types-of-add/
41   http://www.elevatedexistence.com/blog/2014/01/04/dr-daniel-amen-healing-the-7-types-of-add/#sthash. nVb0Zafz.dpuf

It is sometimes referred to as atypical autism, atypical PDD, or atypical personality development. The children so diagnosed vary in the clinical manifestations of their own particular developmental disorder, which makes doing research on this poorly defined syndrome difficult. Some children given this diagnosis early in life are later categorized as being autistic, and some children are given this diagnosis because of reticence on the part of the clinician (or parent) to label the child as being autistic.[42]

PDD-NOS has been omitted as a diagnosis in DSM-5 as of May 2013, so children who formerly fit the DSM-4 diagnostic criteria will now be categorized as just "autism spectrum disorder."

---

42   Author's experience.

Chapter 3
Common Characteristics of the Autistic Child

"All differences in the world are of degree and not of kind,
because oneness is the secret of everything."

— *Swami Vivakananda*

What Are the Common Behavioral Characteristics Noted in Autism?

AUTISTIC CHILDREN VARY *in what dysfunctions they exhibit, and these may also vary in intensity and frequency over time. Not all autistic individuals exhibit all the listed manifestations of this disorder, but the following characteristics and behaviors are commonly observed:*

Problems in Socialization

Autistic individuals often don't interact well or appropriately with others. They may be interested in other people, but not know how to relate, play, or talk to them. Severely autistic children may almost totally ignore others. Many prefer to be by themselves. They often avoid eye contact. They generally have difficulty understanding other people's feelings and are usually not able to discuss their own feelings.

Problems in Communication

Autistic children may never develop language, or may develop it only to lose it for a period of time, or may develop language skills very slowly or later than usual. Some exhibit *echolalia*: the tendency to repeat words or phrases that they have just heard. Some can memorize whole passages from movies they have seen or songs that they have heard, but not understand what they are parroting.

This disorder appears to be due in some autistics to a relative deficiency in the production of *creatine* (KREE-uh-teen), an energy molecule found throughout the body and essential for speech and communication.[1]

Metallothionein (met-TALLO-thigh-oh-neen) dysfunction is also implicated in this regard and will be discussed in a later chapter.

Restricted Patterns of Behavior and Interests

Autistic children are often limited in their interests and activities, and generally exhibit little or no imaginative activity. They tend not to be able to play "pretend" games. They often prefer to play with just one toy or a part of a toy. For example, many autistic children enjoy watching objects spin or move and become fascinated with the wheels on toy cars and trucks. They may not point to objects to show interest.

---

1   Gene Reviews© Cerebral Creatine Deficiency Syndromes; Saadet Mercimek-Mahmutoglu, MD; http://www.ncbi.nlm.nih.gov/books/NBK3794/

Difficulty Adapting to New Situations

Autistic children often get upset when they have to change their routine. They may scream, yell, cry, or throw tantrums.

Repetitive Behaviors (also called "stimming" or self-stimulating behaviors)

These include jumping up and down, making noises, flapping the hands and arms, turning the head side to side or banging it, moving the fingers in unusual and repetitive ways, flipping a switch off and on repetitively, rocking, and many others.

Bizarre Behaviors

Some autistic children will regard an object or person out of the corner of their eye rather than looking straight at that person or object. Some autistic individuals will hold their fingers close to their eyes while moving their fingers. Some will purposefully injure themselves by biting their own body parts or by banging their heads. Toe walking is not uncommon. Some like to be swaddled tightly. Some make strange sounds or laugh inappropriately.

Signs of Intestinal Disturbances

Many autistic children will press their abdomens against furniture or other objects in order to relieve their intestinal discomfort. Many have bloated abdomens, diarrhea, and/or infrequent bowel movements (constipation), which are often foul-smelling. About 40-60 percent of autistic children experience these signs of intestinal dysfunction.

Many have intestinal yeasts and bacteria that produce neurotoxic substances. This will be discussed in greater detail later in this narrative. About 20 percent show hypertrophic (overgrown) lymph nodes in the intestinal tract (nodular hyperplasia—see picture) and about 40-60 percent show evidence of inflammation and even ulcerations throughout the GI tract.[2]

Many autistic children have problems with digestion and the assimilation of nutrients. Some show signs of malnourishment, and some have retardation in their growth as a result.

A research study presented at the 2010 Pediatric Academic Societies Annual Meeting in Vancouver, Canada clearly demonstrated the association between autism and serious gastrointestinal disease in children. This study analyzed data on over 1100 autistic children aged 2-18 years from 15 treatment and research centers in the United States and Canada.

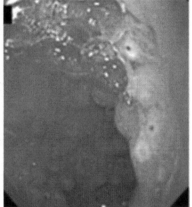

Lymphoid Nodular Hyperplasia

Forty-five percent of these children had chronic intestinal symptoms including abdominal pain (59 percent), diarrhea (43 percent), nausea (31 percent), and bloating (26 percent). Seventy percent of the children with intestinal complaints also had sleep problems as opposed to just 30 percent of the autistic children with no abdominal complaints.[3]

In 2012, Dr. Daniel Coury and colleagues published a review article in the journal *Pediatrics* in which they acknowledge that, "Gastrointestinal complaints are a commonly reported concern for parents and may be related to problem behaviors and other medical issues such as dysregulated sleep…. Despite the magnitude of these issues, potential GI problems are not routinely considered in ASD evaluations," they maintain.

---

2   Wakefield, A.J. et al. *Am J Gastroenterol* 95:2285–2295, 2000. Sabra, A. et al. "Ileal-lymphoid-nodular hyperplasia, non-specific colitis, and pervasive developmental disorder in children." *Lancet* 352:234–235, 1998. Horvath, K. et al. "Gastrointestinal abnormalities in children with autistic disorder." *J Pediat* 135:559–563, 1999. Black, C. et al. "Relation of childhood gastrointestinal disorders to autism: nested case-control study using data from the UK General Practice Research Database." *Br Med J* 325:419–421, 2002.
3   "GI Symptoms in Autism Spectrum Disorders (ASD): An Autism Treatment Network Study."

They also point out that, "Endoscopic analyses of children with ASD and GI symptoms have revealed the presence of a subtle, diffuse inflammation of the intestinal tract."

They caution that children with autism often show evidence of increased intestinal permeability ("leaky gut") and that disruption of the optimal gut organism milieu needs to be evaluated and corrected, because "dysbiosis" can present as adverse intestinal and behavioral symptoms. They acknowledge the gut-brain connection, and suggest appropriate ways to work up and treat an autistic child who manifests intestinal symptoms.[4]

In a 2013 study, scientists at the UC Davis Mind Institute found that autistic children were six to eight times more likely to have food sensitivities, bloating, constipation, and diarrhea than typically developing children.[5]

Obsessive and Compulsive Behaviors

Autistic children may line up toys and other objects, or be upset if routines or the order of things are disrupted.

Anxiety

Anxiety appears to be a very common concern in autistic children. They are often anxious in crowds, or where there are loud noises or too many distractions or when routines are changed.

Decreased Pain Sensitivity

Children with autism are often described as being less sensitive to painful stimuli. One genetic cause of this is a partial deletion of the 22nd chromosome, which can cause a condition known as Phelan-McDermid Syndrome. Other genetic disorders that can result in pain tolerance include Rett Syndrome, duplication of of chromosome region 15q 11-13, Smith Magenis Syndrome, and Fragile X Syndrome. If a child with autism manifests pain tolerance, a genetic workup would be appropriate.[6]

Another theorized cause of pain tolerance in autistic individuals is the presence of food-derived opioid peptides that are common in this condition. These will be discussed at greater length in Chapter 29. A 2009 study of 187 autistic children showed that pain sensitivity could be improved with a combination of free fatty acids and vitamin E. (This will be discussed in more detail shortly.)

Attention Deficits and Hyperactivity

Autistic children are often easily distracted and unable to focus or concentrate. They often don't make good eye contact. Many are very active. Officially, the diagnosis of autism precludes also being labeled as having ADHD (or ADD); however, this artificial restriction, as has been previously pointed out, makes no sense as autistic individuals often fit the criteria for the diagnosis of attention deficit with hyperactivity and probably share many of the same biochemical and genetic predispositions as do children with ADHD.

This problem, as in children with just ADHD or ADD disorders, may be due in part to commonly seen dysfunctions in the methionine synthase gene. Methionine synthase is an enzyme found in the cell membrane that functions in the transfer of methyl groups (a carbon with three hydrogen atoms attached) to cell membrane-bound phospholipids. When this methyl group transfer does not occur at the appropriate rate, then certain calcium channels (regulated by glutamate receptors) don't open sufficiently, and when calcium doesn't enter the neuron in sufficient amounts, then the cell is insufficiently stimulated. The end result is lack of attention and focus. This will be discussed in more detail in a later chapter.

---

4   Coury, Daniel et al. "Gastrointestinal Conditions in Children with Autism Spectrum Disorder: Developing a Research Agenda." *Pediatrics.* Vol.130. Supplement 2. Nov 1, 2012; p. S160-S168; (doi: 10.1542/peds.2012-0900N)

5   Pedersen, T. et al. "Autism linked to digestive problems." Psych Central. http://psychcentral.com/news/2013/11/09/autism-linked-to-digestive-problems/61822.html

6   http://sfari.org/news-and-opinion/conference-news/2012/society-for-neuroscience-2012/mice-mimic-pain-tolerance-seen-in-phelan-mcdermid-syndrome

Sleep Disturbances

Many autistic children don't sleep well, or long enough; many wake way too early in the morning. This is often a major problem and concern for their tired parents.

Hypersensitivity to Sensory Stimuli

Many autistic children are sensitive to loud sounds, crowd noise, bright lights, certain textures, and touch. Some like to be swaddled tightly. Others have problems with the tastes and textures of certain foods. Most are extremely picky eaters who crave carbohydrate-rich foods and refuse to eat other, more nutritious foods. Children with autism are often overwhelmed by too much sensory input. Crowd noises and loud noises in general are common sources of anxiety for autistic individuals. Sensory issues are often related to dysfunctions in a class of proteins known as the *metallothioneins* (me-TAL-oh-THIGH-oh-neens). Their function will also be discussed in more detail later in this narrative.

> *"Our brains are wired differently.*
> *We take in many sounds and conversations at once.*
> *I take over a thousand pictures of a person's face when I look at them.*
> *That's why we have a hard time looking at people."*
>
> — *Carly Fleishmann, autistic teen*

Tics

Tics are *involuntary* purposeless movements or inappropriate vocalizations and are much more common in autistic individuals. It is estimated that 20-30 percent of autistic children experience tics, which may manifest as rapid eye blinking, facial grimacing, throat clearing, and sniffing.

Tics may also present as more complex behaviors such as jumping, touching people or things, twirling about, and tapping. They may additionally materialize as vocalizations like yelping, shouting, and grunting, the uttering of words or phrases (including obscene words), and repeating sounds or words just heard, including one's own (echolalia).

They can be exhausting, embarrassing, and adversely affect social interactions, as tics are often a source of annoyance to others. Tics can wax and wane, and their intensity and frequency are affected by mood, stress, sufficiency of sleep, physical activity, focus, and a variety of environmental influences. Tic disorders tend to run in families, may be evident throughout life, and sometimes respond to medications.[7]

Restricted Dietary Desires

Autistic children are often carbohydrate addicts and are frequently extremely picky in their food choices. This makes it difficult to provide them with appropriate meals and adequate nutrition. Many crave gluten and casein-containing foods, which have addictive potentials in those children who do not metabolize well the morphine-like peptides (gliadorphin, casomorphin, and others) that derive from these foods. This will be discussed at length in Chapter 29.

Seizures

Seizures are not a characteristic symptom in most autistic individuals, but they do occur more frequently in autistics than in the non-autistic population.

The prevalence of epilepsy (two or more non-febrile seizures) in those diagnosed with an autism spectrum disorder is widely estimated to be between 5-38 percent, whereas only 1-2 percent in the general population will develop epileptic seizures. Seizures may start at any age from infancy through adulthood, and are the leading cause of death

---

7   Canianto, R. Vivanti, G. "Tics and Tourette Syndrome in autism spectrum disorders." *Autism*. 2007; 11 (91): 19-28.

in adults with autism spectrum disorders. Individuals with genetic abnormalities, intellectual disabilities, and brain malformations are more likely to have seizures.[8]

Increased inflammation is commonly observed in autistic individuals. Brain inflammation has been proposed as a possible cause of seizures in autism. Tufts University researchers Theoharis C. Theoharides and Bodi Zhang hypothesize that brain mast cell (a type of immune cell) activation "due to allergic, environmental and/or stress triggers could lead to focal disruption of the blood-brain barrier and neuro-inflammation, thus contributing to the development of seizures."[9]

Researchers Richard Frye and Daniel Rossignol have a different theory. They implicate mitochondrial disorders, frequently found in autistic individuals, as possible promoters of seizures and other manifestations commonly seen in autism.[10] Mitochondrial disorders in autism will be discussed further shortly.

So it appears that factors associated with autism, like neuro-inflammation and mitochondrial defects, may trigger epileptic seizures, and the reverse may also be true.

Researcher SallyAnn Wakeford of the University of Bath's Department of Psychology discovered that "adults with epilepsy are more likely to have a greater number of characteristics of autism and Asperger syndrome." These characteristic include such autistic traits as impaired communication and social interaction and restricted and repetitive interests. These findings need to be confirmed.[11]

Coordination difficulties and muscle weakness

These symptoms are not seen in all autistic children, but do occur in autistics more frequently than in non-autistic children.

Loss of Skills They Once Had

Many parents report that their autistic child will seem to have developed normally up to a certain age, generally between 1 and 2 years, and then either fail to progress or actually lose some of the abilities, like speech, focus, sociability, and eye contact, that the child previously possessed. This deterioration in function often occurs shortly after an immunization has been administered.

Wandering

Deaths associated with wandering remain a leading cause of fatalities among children and adults with autism. Severely affected individuals may wander away from home, school, day care, camps, or other settings if not properly supervised, and they don't recognize the dangers they face in so doing. Tragically, deaths by drowning or by vehicular collision are not uncommon.

Preliminary information from the 2011 Interactive Autism Network Study "found that roughly half of the children with autism attempt to wander/elope from safe environments, such as home, school, and public settings."[12]

What Laboratory and Metabolic Abnormalities Are Commonly Observed in Autistic Children?

There are certain characteristic metabolic abnormalities that are frequently found in children with autism and related disorders. Many of these are not unique to autism spectrum disordered individuals, and none of these is diagnostic for autism or related conditions. Please note that not all autistic children will be found to have every one of these abnormalities, and not all are readily measurable in non-research laboratories.

---

8   http://www.tacanow.org/family-resources/seizures/ and Frye, Richard E. *J Am Acad Child Adolesc Psychiatry.* 1990 Jan; 29(1):127-9.

9   *Journal of Neuroinflammation.* 2011, 8:168.

10   *Pediatr Res.* 2011 May; 69(5 Pt 2): 41R–47R.

11   http://www.medicalnewstoday.com/articles /260649.php

12   http://us.mg201.mail.yahoo.com/neo/launch?. partner=sbc

There is a lot of evidence that autistic children are under high oxidative stress. This stress derives from both increased free radical production and diminished antioxidant protection. Free radicals are electron-stealing substances, also known as "oxidizing agents," that damage tissues and organs. Antioxidants act as sacrificial lambs that donate their electrons to free radicals, and by so doing, neutralize them.

Chronic inflammation is also a characteristic condition found in most autistic individuals. It will be discussed at greater length subsequently.

Many autistic children are affected adversely by mutations in a variety of enzymes that serve to transport methyl groups and sulfur along essential metabolic pathways. A "methyl group," it may be recalled, is a molecule that contains three hydrogen atoms attached to one carbon atom. These "transmethylation" and "transsulfuration pathways" will be discussed in more detail in a later chapter of this book. A depiction of these pathways is illustrated in Appendix II.

Characteristic Metabolic Abnormalities Commonly found in Autism

Persistence of Measles Virus after the MMR Vaccine?

The unfairly maligned Dr. Andrew Wakefield and others have presented some compelling data in regard to measles persistence following the MMR vaccine, although there is, to say the least, a great deal of controversy in the scientific community concerning the accuracy of this data. This controversy will be discussed in more depth in later chapters.

Elevated Serum Copper to Zinc Ratio

This elevation is seen in 85 percent or more of autistic children (the average ratio in autistics is 1.63), according to data accumulated at the Pfeiffer Clinic. The optimal ratio (as seen in non-autistic individuals) is about 1.15. One of the functions of the metallothioneins is to regulate the levels and ratio of copper and zinc.

The Pfeiffer Clinic, in Naperville, Illinois, under the direction of Dr. James Walsh, Ph.D., has collected extensive laboratory data on over 6,000 patients with autism. Some of this data was presented at the American Psychiatric Association meeting in New Orleans in 2001. One study compared the copper to zinc ratios of 503 autistic children to that of 25 controls. The differences were significant to $p<.0001$ (less than a 1 in 10,000 chance that results were due to chance).[13]

Elevated Free Copper

Dr. Walsh has also found elevated free (unbound) copper to be significantly higher in autistic children than in controls. Free copper is an oxidizing agent and can damage organs and tissues. It also inactivates the metallothionein enzymes and depletes glutathione. In comparing autistic children to matched controls, Dr. Walsh found that the autistic group had significantly higher levels of unbound (free) serum copper ($p<.01$). This contributes to high oxidative stress.[14]

Low Levels of Ceruloplasmin

Ceruloplasmin (SER-you-low-PLAZ-min) is a copper-binding enzyme that protects the body from copper's free-radical attack. Autistic individuals tend to have lower levels of this protective protein. Copper is an essential mineral, but too much of a good thing isn't. Excess copper can act as a free radical and thereby damage organ systems throughout the body. Individuals born with the non-autistic genetic disease known as Wilson's Syndrome, exhibit elevated levels of free copper, early-onset organ dysfunction, and premature demise.

Deficient Metallothionein (met-TAL-owe-THIGH-oh-neen) Levels

In another study done at the Pfeiffer clinic, autistic children were found to have *significantly lower metallothionein levels* compared to controls ($p<.0092$[15]).[16]

---

13   Also Faber, S. et al. "The plasma zinc/serum copper ratio as a biomarker in children with autism spectrum disorders." *Biomarkers*. Mar 2009; 11:1-10.
14   Ibid.
15    $p<.0092$ means the probability of this difference occurring by chance is less than 92 occurrences out of every 10,000 tests. Anything less than 500 chances out of 10,000 (5 chances out of 100) is considered to be significant.
16   Walsh; Ibid.

The Great Plains Lab can measure metallothionein levels; however, only types I and II are measurable in serum. Type III (brain metallothionein) and Type IV (gut metallothionein) cannot be readily measured because they are not easily, or safely, accessible.

Metallothioneins are detoxifying enzymes and also antioxidants. Diminished levels will increase oxidative stress. Most toxic metals are excreted bound to metallothionein proteins after large exposures, so low levels of metallothioneins (or dysfunctional metallothioneins) would be expected to diminish a person's detoxification ability.[17] (The metallothionein connection to autism will also be discussed in greater detail in Chapter 6.)

Metallothionein Dysfunction

There are a number of ways that metallothionein proteins can become dysfunctional, even if they are found in sufficient number. This will be discussed in more detail in Chapter 6.

Methionine and SAM (S-Adenosyl Methionine) Deficiency

These substances were found to be low in many autistic children in a 2008 study by J. Suh and colleagues. Methionine is an important amino acid. It is obtained from protein sources in the diet and can also be manufactured in the body from homocysteine. It is transformed by an enzyme into SAM (S-adenosyl methionine), an important "methyl donor" that is of primary importance in many chemical reactions in the body, including the manufacture of certain neurotransmitters.[18]

Inactive folic acid (a B vitamin) becomes activated by changing its methylene group to a methyl group. The enzyme that catalyzes this transformation (abbreviated MTHFR) is often not optimal in children with ADHD and autism.

With the assistance of another enzyme (methionine synthase), the methyl group on the folic acid is then passed to cobalamin (B12) to form *methyl*cobalamin and from *methyl*cobalamin to homocysteine, which is transformed into methionine, an important amino acid. Many autistic children have an impaired ability to transfer the methyl group from the methyl folic acid to cobalamin. Not surprisingly, these children do well when supplemented with methylcobalamin.

This pathway ends in the manufacture of the amino acid *cysteine*, which can then be transformed by other mechanisms into proteins like the *metallothioneins* or into *glutathione* or *taurine*.

Elevated Adenosine and SAH (S-Adenosyl Homocysteine)

S-adenosyl homocysteine (SAH) can be *reversibly* transformed enzymatically into homocysteine, a potentially harmful amino acid, which in turn, via a variety of chemical steps, is either converted back to methionine or further transformed into cysteine, an amino acid essential in the production of metallothioneins and glutathione. When folate methylation is impaired or vitamin B12 is deficient, as is common in autistic children, then homocysteine is insufficiently converted to methionine and tends to form SAH at an increased rate.[19]

Low Levels of Cysteine

Cysteine is an important amino acid used in making taurine, proteins, and enzymes like the metallothioneins. Autistic children tend to have lower levels of cysteine than do non-affected children according to researcher Jill St. James. See Figure A. 1. in Appendex II.

---

17   Ibid.
18   Ibid. and Suh, J. et al. "Altered Sulfur Amino Acid metabolism in Immune Cells of Children Diagnosed with Autism." *Amer. J. of Biochemistry and Biotechnology.* 2008; 4(2): 105-113.
19   Walsh; op cit 2001 and Suh, J. et al. "Altered Sulfur Amino Acid metabolism in Immune Cells of Children Diagnosed with Autism." *Amer. J. of Biochemistry and Biotechnology.* 4(2): 105-113; 2008

Low Levels of Glutathione

Glutathione is the body's most potent antioxidant and is the most abundant antioxidant in the brain. It also helps in the detoxification of mercury and other toxic metals. Low levels impair the body's ability to protect against heavy metals and free radicals (potentially damaging oxidizing agents). Autistic spectrum individuals tend to have low levels of glutathione.[20]

Glutathione has a limited capacity to detoxify heavy metals like lead and mercury, according to William Walsh. If more than 10 percent of the glutathione is bound to these toxic metals, any additional toxic metals are transferred to the metallothionein proteins. The speed of these detoxification reactions is increased by up to 50 percent when sufficient selenium is present.[21]

Glutathione exists in two forms: the active (reduced) form and the inactive (oxidized) form. Autistic children and their parents tend to have more of the inactive form and less of the active. Both groups also tend to have higher levels of homocysteine and S-adenosyl homocysteine. These deviations from the norm are signs of inflammation and oxidative stress.[22]

Low Levels of Selenium

Selenium is a trace mineral that is also important in normalizing thyroid function, and it is a cofactor for an important antioxidant. It also seems to offer protection against viral infections and cancer, and sufficiency is required, as we have just stated, for optimal detoxification speed to occur.[23]

High Urinary Isoprostanes

Isoprostanes are markers for *increased oxidative stress*, in this case lipid peroxidation (*oxidation of fats in the body*). Elevated levels imply either increased oxidative stress from free radicals and/or diminished antioxidant protection or both.[24]

Oxidative Stress: Elevated Levels of Free Radicals Causing Oxidative Damage

It is widely believed that oxidative stress plays a key role in causing autism. Many of the aforementioned biochemical abnormalities are associated with increases in oxidative damage to fats and vascular tissues (as compared to controls).[25] The first evidence of oxidative damage to the autistic brain and resulting neurodegeneration was published in 2008.[26] There are now at least 115 studies that found an association between oxidative stress and ASDs.[27]

Dr. Shaw, biochemist and head of the Great Plains Lab, believes that "untreated autism may be neurodegenerative with oxidative damage causing loss of brain cells and IQ (and that) antioxidant therapy may be necessary throughout the life of a person diagnosed with an autism spectrum disorder."[28]

In an attempt to clarify and quantify the relationship between oxidative stress-related blood biomarkers and autism spectrum disorders, a systematic literature review was carried out by a team of Italian researchers.

They found evidence supporting the view that oxidative stress is associated with autism spectrum disorders. "The ASD patients showed decreased blood levels of reduced glutathione (27 percent), glutathione peroxidase (18 per-

---

20   Suh, J.; Walsh, W. et al. *American Journal of Biotechnology and Biochemistry*. 2008; 4(2): 105-113.
21   Walsh; op cit 2001 *and* Suh, J et al. "Altered Sulfur Amino Acid metabolism in Immune Cells of Children Diagnosed with Autism." *Amer. J. of Biochemistry and Biotechnology*. 4(2): 105-113; 2008.
22   *J Autism Dev Disord*. 2008 Nov; 38(10): 1966-75.
23   Ibid.
24   Ming, X. et al. "Increased excretion of a lipid peroxidation biomarker in autism." *Prostaglandins, Leukotrienes and Essential Fatty Acids*. Vol. 73, Issue 5, Nov 2005, p. 379-384.
25   Practico, Walsh et al. *Archives of Neurology*. Vol. 63: October 2006; 1161-4.
26   Evans, et al. *American J of Biotechnology and Biochemistry*. 4(2):61-72, 2008.
27   Rossignol, D.A. *and* Frye, R.E. *Molecular Psychiatry*. 2012 17: 389f.
28   Shaw op cit 2001.

cent), methionine (13 percent), and cysteine (14 percent) and increased concentrations of oxidized glutathione (45 percent) and adenosine relative to controls...."[29]

Other studies found that autistic children had lower antioxidant nutrients like vitamins C and E and Coenzyme Q10, higher organic toxins and heavy metals, and a higher production of nitric oxide, a free-radical oxidizing gas.[30]

Evidence of Abnormally-Increased Inflammation

A review of 437 publications that examined immune dysregulation or inflammation in ASD found an association in 415 (95 percent). Inflammation refers to the condition whereby the immune system is activated with a consequent release of various inflammatory mediators, like interleukin 6 and TNF-alpha, that attract certain immune cells to the site of inflammation. Inflammation may manifest as swelling (edema), dilated blood vessels (redness and heat), and even pain. One of the many markers of inflammation in the body is a substance known as C-Reactive Protein (CRP).[31]

Inflammation is not always apparent or sensed by the individual, however. It is the body's normal response to infection or injury and serves a beneficial purpose thereby, but inflammation can be inappropriate and misfocused and can cause a great deal of harm if it is chronic or occurs at the wrong time. And it appears that one of the inappropriate times for inflammation to occur is during pregnancy. A study by researchers at Columbia University College of Physicians and Surgeons found that inflammation in the mother during pregnancy, as evidenced by elevations of C-Reactive Protein, increased the risk for autism in the child by up to 43 percent, and *the higher the C-Reactive Protein, the greater the autism risk.*[32]

It is recommended now that pregnant women be injected with the influenza vaccine *any time* during the pregnancy, but a study published in 2011 suggests that this may not be a wise idea. Investigators at Ohio State University analyzed the immune reaction of women who received the trivalent influenza vaccine during their pregnancy and found that they experienced a significant and rapid inflammatory response as evidenced by significant elevations of C-Reactive Protein.

They noted that, "a tendency toward greater inflammatory responding to immune triggers may predict risk of adverse outcomes... (and that)... further research is needed to confirm that the mild inflammatory response elicited by vaccination is benign in pregnancy."[33]

In other words, there is insufficient research now to determine whether giving a woman an influenza immunization during her pregnancy is safe for the baby, especially when that injection contains neurotoxic mercury!

What about inflammation in the baby itself? Does that also promote autism? Are autistic children more likely to be inflamed?

A number of researchers have attempted to answer these questions. Scientists at Tufts University found that, "Autism spectrum disorder children respond disproportionally to stress and are also affected by food and skin allergies. Corticotropin-releasing hormone is secreted under stress and together with neurotensin (a neurotransmitter) stimulates mast cells (a type of immune cell) and microglia (a type of mast cell found in the brain) resulting in focal brain inflammation and neurotoxicity."

Neurotensin has been shown to be increased in the serum of children with autism. It contributes to inflammation via several mechanisms, including stimulating mast cells to release some of their mitochondrial DNA, which induces inflammation.

29   Frustaci, A. et al. "Oxidative stress-related biomarkers in autism: systematic review and meta-analyses." *Free Radic Biol Med.* 2012 May 15; 52(10): 2128-41. & James, S.J. et al. "Metab. Biomarkers of increased oxidative stress...in children with autism." *Am J Clin Nutr.* Dec 2004. 80(6): 1611f.

30   McGinnis, W.R. "Oxidative stress in autism." *Alt Ther in Hlth & Med.* Nov-Dec 2004. 10(6): 22f.

31   Rossignol, D.A. *and* Frye, R.E. *Molecular Psychiatry.* 2012 17: 389f.

32   Brown, A.S. et al. "Elevated maternal C-reactive protein and autism in a national birth cohort." *Mol Psychiatry.* 2013 Jan 22. doi: 10.1038/mp.2012.197.

33   Christian, L.M. et al. "Inflammatory Responses to Trivalent Influenza Virus Vaccine among Pregnant Women." *Vaccine.* Nov 8, 2011; 29(48): 8982–8987.

There are certain enzymes called "TOR" (targets of rapamycin) that play a role in many functions, including promoting inflammation. A particular gene mutation (PTEN), shown to be associated with a higher risk of autism, stimulates the TOR enzymes as does neurotensin. This can result in enhanced mast cell secretion and activation of the brain mast cells (microglia), which in turn results in brain inflammation.[34]

A research team at Johns Hopkins "recently demonstrated the presence of neuroglial and innate neuroimmune system activation in brain tissue and cerebrospinal fluid of patients with autism, findings that support the view that neuroimmune abnormalities occur in the brain of autistic patients and may contribute to the diversity of the autistic phenotypes. The role of neuroglial activation and neuroinflammation are still uncertain but could be critical in maintaining, as well as in initiating, some of the CNS abnormalities present in autism."[35]

A possible remedy to help quench this "fire in the brain" is a natural substance called *luteolin*, which inhibits the TOR enzymes, mast cells and microglial cells, and which might therefore prove to be beneficial to those with autism spectrum disorders.[36]

The long-term effects of luteolin are not known, however. It appears to have endocrinological effects, and so should be used with caution in pre-pubescent children.[37]

Dysfunctional DPP IV

DPP IV (Dipetidyl Peptidase IV) is an intestinal enzyme that helps break down peptides, which are small protein fractions that come from foods. An inability to break down certain peptides from gluten, casein, and soy results in the elevation of certain potentially neurotoxic, m*orphine*-like peptides that form in the gut (like casom*orphin*, gliad*orphin*, derm*orphin*, etc).

These have narcotic-like (similar to morphine) properties. When they are absorbed, they may adversely affect neurological and immunological function, and they promote constipation. Children are often "addicted" to the foods that promote these morphine-like peptides, and so they often crave and consume them to the exclusion of other foods.

The same enzyme (DPP IV) also appears on the surface of certain immune cells and serves to signal the cell into activity. When this enzyme is dysfunctional, the immune system is compromised.[38]

Evidence of Immune Dysfunction and Autoimmune Disease

There appears to be a genetic predisposition in autistic children to having an autoimmune condition. Families with an autistic child were shown to be twice as likely to have a close relative with an autoimmune condition as other families, even those with a non-autistic child with an autoimmune condition.[39]

According to researchers at the University of California, "Published findings have identified widespread changes in the immune systems of children with autism, at both systemic and cellular levels. *Brain specimens from autism subjects exhibit signs of active, ongoing inflammation,* as well as alterations in gene pathways associated with immune signaling and immune function.

Moreover, many genetic studies have indicated a link between autism and genes that are relevant to both the nervous system and the immune system. Alterations in these pathways can affect function in both systems. Together, these reports suggest that autism may in fact be a systemic disorder with connections to abnormal immune responses.[40]

---

34   Theoharides, T.C. et al. "Focal brain inflammation and autism." *Journal of Neuroinflammation.* 2013; 10:46.

35   Pardo, C. et al. "Immunity, neuroglia and neuroinflammation in autism." *International Review of Psychiatry.* Dec 2005; 17(6): 485–495.

36   Theoharides, T.C. et al. "Focal brain inflammation and autism." *Journal of Neuroinflammation.* 2013; 10:46.

37   http://www.sciencedaily.com/releases/2013/07/130715151158.htm?utm_source=feedburner&utm_medi um=email&utm_campaign=Feed percent3A+sciencedaily+ percent28Science Daily percent3A+Latest+Science+News percent29

38   Aytac, U. et al. "CD26/dipeptidyl peptidase IV: a regulator of immune function and a potential molecular target for therapy." *Curr Drug Targets Immune Endocr Metabol Disord.* 2004 Mar; 4(1):11-8.

39   Sweeten, T.L. et al. "Increased prevalence of familial autoimmunity...in PDD." *Pediatrics.* 2003.

40   Careaga, M. et al. "Immune dysfunction in autism: a pathway to treatment." *Neurotherapeutics.* 2010 Jul; 7(3):283-92.

Carla Lintas and colleagues found that, "A dysregulated immune response, accompanied by enhanced oxidative stress and abnormal mitochondrial metabolism seemingly represents the common molecular underpinning of not only autism but also Rett syndrome and Down syndrome as well."[41]

The neurotoxin mercury appears to play a role in promoting immune dysfunction and autoimmune reactions. This has been well established in various mouse studies, with some varieties being more prone to developing autoimmune dysfunctions than others.

In mice, "Ethylmercury, the active compound in thimerosal and other medical substances, induces in a dose-dependent pattern all the features of systemic autoimmunity that have been described after exposure to mercuric chloride," (an inorganic form of mercury) according to a study published in the journal *Toxicology and Applied Pharmacology.*[42]

The evidence that thimerosal, a preservative in many multi-dose vaccine vials, plays a key role in the development of autism will be presented in subsequent chapters.

Mouse studies are all well and good, but does mercury also induce autoimmunity in humans? The answer appears to be yes.

In a Brazilian study published in 2004, the researchers examined three groups of natives living in three distinct areas in Brazil and exposed to various amounts of mercury (methyl- and inorganic), and as was found in the aforementioned mouse study, their risk of having autoantibodies to cellular structures (the nucleus and the nucleolus) was mercury-dose dependent. That is to say, the greater the mercury exposure, the greater was the incidence of autoimmune disease.[43]

Antibodies to Myelin Basic Protein

Myelin is the insulation that shields nerve cells. Antibodies to myelin basic protein would be expected to promote neurological dysfunction. These auto-antibodies are seen in over 80 percent of autistic individuals. Antibodies to other brain proteins have also been found.[44]

Other Harmful Antibodies

Many children with autism have antibodies against VIP (vasoactive intestinal peptide), a small signaling molecule produced by intestinal cells. VIP has many functions, including preventing autoimmunity. *Autoimmune dysfunctions, manifesting as, for example, the production of auto-antibodies that "attack" certain brain proteins, are common in autistic children.*[45]

Table 3.1 lists a number of studies that found a variety of auto-antibodies against several central nervous system proteins in children with autism spectrum disorders. In the Connolly study referenced in Table 3.1, IgG anti-brain autoantibodies were present in 27 percent of children with ASD and in only 2 percent of controls, and IgM anti-brain autoantibodies were found in 36 percent of children with ASD and in none of the controls. In the Mostafa studies referenced below, the level of anti-brain autoantibodies were directly correlated with the severity of the autism.

41   Lintas et al. *Neurobiol Dis.* 2010.

42   Havarinasab, S. et al. "Dose-response study of thimerosal-induced murine systemic autoimmunity." 2004; 194:169–179.

43   Silva, Ines A. et al. "Mercury exposure, malaria, and serum antinuclear/antinucleolar antibodies in Amazon populations in Brazil: a cross-sectional study." *Environ Health.* 2004; 3: 11.

44   Singh, V.K. et al. "Antibodies to myelin basic protein in children with autistic behavior." *Brain Behav Immun.* 1993 Mar; 7(1):97-103.

45   Delneste, Y. et al. "Vasoactive intestinal peptide synergizes with TNF-alpha in inducing human dendritic cell maturation." *J Immunol.* 1999 (Sep. 15); 163(6):3071 ff.

Table 3.1. Autoantibodies against CNS proteins reported in ASD patients

Antibody (Ab) specificity	Reference
Antibodies to neuron-axon filament proteins (NAFP)	Singh et al. *Pediatr Neurol* 1997;17(1):88 – 90.
Abs to cerebellar neurofilaments	Plioplys et al. *Neuropediatrics* 1989 (May); 20(2):93ff.
Abs to myelin basic protein	Singh et al. *Brain Behav Immun* 1993;7(1):97 – 103.
Antibodies to caudate nucleus	Singh et al. *Neurosci Let* 2004 (Jan. 23); 355 (1-2): 53ff
Antibodies to serotonin receptor	Singh et al. *Biol Psychiatry* 1997 (Mar.15);41(6): 753ff.
Abs to brain endothelial cells	Connolly et al. *J Pediatr* 1999;34(5):607ff.
Antibodies to brain tissue	Todd et al. *Biol Psychiatry* 1988 (Mar. 15); 23(6):644ff.
Abs to anti-ribosomal P proteins*	Mostafa et al. *J NeuroInflamm.* 12-21-11; 8(1); 180
Antineuronal antibodies*	Mostafa et al. *Eur J Paediatr Neur.*1-5-12; (e Pub)
*Correlated with severity of autism Adapted from Table 1, P. Ashwood, J. Van de Water / Autoimmunity Reviews 3 (2004)	

IgG Food Allergies

"IgG" stands for immunoglobulin G, one of several classes of antibodies that immune cells produce. Unlike immunoglobulin E (IgE) antibodies, which cause rapidly manifesting allergic reactions like asthma and anaphylaxis, IgG allergies promote *delayed* sensitivity reactions and are common in the general population. Autistic children in particular are more often adversely affected by these allergies than are their non-autistic peers. IgG reactions may manifest as behavioral abnormalities like ADD or ADHD, as intestinal dysfunctions like irritable bowel, or in many other ways.[46]

IgG food allergies may be tested for by drawing some blood from an arm vein and sending the serum to an appropriate lab for ELISA testing. Traditional allergy skin tests (scratch, prick, and RAST) will not detect these allergies. This will be discussed at greater length in Chapter 31.

Metal Allergies

These have been demonstrated in children with autism. The Melissa Foundation describes two children with elevated antibodies to thimerosal (50 percent ethyl mercury), one of whom also reacted to aluminum and thiosalicylate (the other half of the thimerosal molecule). Most vaccines, even today, contain trace amounts of thimerosal. It is conceivable that allergies to thimerosal or aluminum may play a role in promoting autism in addition to their neurotoxic effects. Further research is needed in this regard.[47]

Toxic Metal Overload

This is a controversial topic in conventional medicine, but it really shouldn't be. The evidence is clear that autistic children harbor much higher levels of toxic metals, like mercury, than do non-autistic children. This was clearly demonstrated by brain autopsy on autistic children who had died in accidents. *Dr. Bradstreet found*

46   Jyonouchi, H. et al. "Impact of innate immunity in a subset of children with autism spectrum disorders: a case control study." *J Neuroinflamm* 2008; 5: 52.

47   http://www.melisa.org/metals-disease/case-reports/autism

mercury levels to be 8 times higher in autistic children than in non-autistic youth. Upwards of 92 percent of autistic children show abnormally elevated levels of toxic metals. This concern will be discussed at greater length later in this narrative.[48]

Gut Dysbiosis

Dysbiosis refers to an imbalance in the type and/or amount of gut organisms sufficient to cause harm. Intestinal bacteria, protozoans, and yeasts may promote intestinal irritation and leaky gut; they may produce toxic substances and interfere with the proper digestion and assimilation of nutrients from foods. Dysbiosis is usually diagnosed on a comprehensive digestive stool analysis test (CDSA), and further clues to its presence may be discerned on a microbial organic acid test (usually evaluated on a sample of urine or blood). The role that microorganisms in the gut play in promoting autism will also be addressed in more detail in Chapter 32.

G-Protein Abnormalities

The role these "molecular switches" might play in promoting autism will be revealed in Chapter 8.

Peroxisomal Disorders

Peroxisomes are tiny organelles found in virtually all cells in the body. They have many functions including the shortening (by *β-oxidation*) of very long chain fatty acids so that they may be metabolized in the mitochondria (the tiny "energy factories" in cells) for the production of energy. There is evidence that peroxisomes in autistic patients don't degrade these very long chain fatty acids well. This results in decreased energy production and the accumulation of very long fatty acids in the membranes of cells.

Peroxisomes also play a role in the formation of the myelin nerve sheath, essential for proper nerve conduction.

Dr. Patricia Kane and her husband Edward measured the fatty acid profile in the lipid membrane of red blood cells in fifty autistic children and found a characteristic excess accumulation of several kinds of very long chain fatty acids indicative of a peroxisomal disorder.

According to Patricia Kane, "The accumulation of renegade or very long chain fatty acids reflects blocked detoxification and methylation pathways, and may be characteristic in autism, PDD, seizure disorders, stroke, neurological disease and states of neurotoxicity."[49]

She showed, via a case history, that the peroxisomal disorder was apparently reversible in a two-year-old boy with autism whose symptoms improved rapidly as a result of targeted nutritional interventions.[50]

Under-Methylation

This is seen in approximately 95 percent or more of autistic children and, according to Dr. William Walsh of the Pfeiffer Treatment Center, is characterized by *low levels* of the neurotransmitters dopamine, epinephrine, and norepinephrine, elevated levels of histamine, and a tendency to have depression, oppositional defiant disorder, and OCD (obsessive and compulsive traits).[51]

Methylation refers to the acquisition of a molecule called the "methyl group," which consists of a carbon atom attached to three hydrogen atoms (abbreviated-CH3).

Methylation reactions are vital to our biological processes. They are necessary for the formation (and destruction) of certain neurotransmitters; they determine whether or not a particular gene is active (able to produce a protein) or not. They have necessary functions in supporting the immune system, and they play a key role in the pathways that are often disrupted in autistic individuals.

---

48   Bradstreet, J. et al. *Journal of American Physicians and Surgeons.* Vol. 8. No. 3. Fall 2003.
49   http://www.ageofautism.com/2009/07/solving-the-autism-puzzle-the-fatty-acid-question-and-big-fat-neurons.html
50   Kane, P.; Kane, E. "Peroxisomal Disturbances in Autism Spectrum Disorder." *The Journal of Orthomolecular Medicine.* Vol. 12, 4th Quarter 1997.
51   http://www.walshinstitute.org/uploads/1/7/9/9/17997321/the_collision_of_undermethylation_epigenetics_and_oxidative_stress_in_autism_spectrum.pdf

Under-methylation is often due to mutations in certain enzymes. One of these aberrant enzymes is abbreviated MTHFR (Methylene TetraHydroFolate Reductase). This enzyme functions by changing the "methylene" group in the methyl*ene* THF (a type of folic acid-one of the B vitamins) molecule to a "methyl" group.

Methylene THF then becomes 5-*methyl* tetrahydrofolate. The 5-methyl THF then passes the methyl group to vitamin B12 (under the influence of another enzyme known as methionine synthase), and by so doing, changes the B12 into an active form called *methyl*cobalamin.

*Methyl*cobalamin then immediately donates its newly acquired methyl group to homocysteine, thereby converting homocysteine into methionine. Hence, the methyl group is passed around, like a football, from folic acid to vitamin B12 to homocysteine. This process is called "trans-methylation" by chemists.

The end result and purpose of all this methyl transferring is the synthesis of methionine and the elimination of homocysteine, a potentially harmful amino acid.

The synthesis of methylcobalamin, the active form of vitamin B12, also requires adequate amounts of glutathione (GLUE-tuh-thigh-OWN) and SAMe (S-adenosyl methionine-also made from methionine).

Some children with autism lack that part of the methionine synthase molecule that binds to SAMe. This causes problems in the synthesis of methyl cobalamin. Children with autism often have high levels of mercury and other substances that inhibit the production of glutathione and SAMe. The result is an additional diminishment in the production of methyl cobalamin. It's no wonder, therefore, that supplementing the missing methyl cobalamin to autistic children is so often productive.

Over-Methylation

It isn't clear what causes this problem, which occurs in less than 5 percent of autistic children and is characterized, according to Dr. Walsh, by an overabundance of dopamine, epinephrine, and nor-epinephrine as well as low blood histamine. He is "absolutely certain…that methionine and/or SAMe usually harm low-histamine (over-methylated) persons…but are wonderful for high-histamine (undermethylated) persons." The reverse is true for those with elevated histamine levels (undermethylated persons), who thrive on methionine, SAMe, Ca, and Mg…but get much worse if they take folates & B-12, which can increase methyl trapping.

Conditions that Dr. Walsh feels are associated with over-methylation include: anxiety/panic disorders, anxious-depression, hyperactivity, learning disabilities, low motivation, "space cadet" syndrome, paranoid schizophrenia, and hallucinations.

A 2010 study established a link between methylation and autism and suggested that blocking the methylation of certain genes might reverse autistic symptoms, and that drugs that "influence the methylation state of genes could reverse autism's effects."[52]

Pyrrole (PIE-roll) Disorder

This genetic defect is found in about 25-35 percent of autistic children and may be diagnosed when elevated levels of *kryptopyrroles* (also called HPL [haemopyrrollactam] complex or "mauve factor") appear in the urine. Kryptopyrroles are actually a complex made up of pyrrole rings that should have been incorporated into the hemoglobin molecule but weren't. Hemoglobin is the red-colored substance that carries oxygen inside of red blood cells (erythrocytes).

Pyrrole disorder is associated with increased loss of vitamin B6 (pyridoxine [peer-i-DOX-een]) in *active* form, called pyridoxine-5-phosphate (P5P) and zinc in the urine, and to a lesser degree, chromium, manganese, and magnesium.

---

52   Nguyen, A. et al. FASEB (published online) August 2010; 101(8):3036-51.

The loss of these nutrients disables many enzyme systems including the metallothioneins. This condition is also known as *kryptopyrroluria* (CRIP-toe-PIE-roll-YOUR-ee-uh). It is common for those who have inherited this disorder also to excrete substances known as coproporphyrins (COP-row-POUR-for-ins) into the urine.

Pyrrole Disorder is diagnosed by finding elevated kryptopyrroles in urine. Positive kryptopyrrole levels for children under ten are those above 0.65 micromoles per liter. For children over 10, any excretion above 0.75 micromoles/liter is positive, and for adults, values over 1 micromole/liter are significant.

Pyrrole Disorder is also commonly found in individuals with depression, anxiety, oppositional defiant disorder, schizophrenia, bipolar disorder, and ADD/ADHD.

Symptoms of pyrrole disorder vary but may include: abdominal pain, poor stress control, nervousness, anxiety, depression, mood swings, severe inner tension, episodic anger, agitation, poor short-term memory, frequent infections, inability to tan, poor dream recall, abnormal fat distribution, and sensitivity to light and sound. Many of these symptoms are commonly seen in autistic individuals.

The good news is that by supplementing with zinc (c 30-60 mg per day for adults) and B6 *as P5P* (c 50 mg per day) this problem can be overcome.[53]

Nutritional Deficiencies

Malabsorption of nutrients is a common concomitant of metallothionein (MT) dysfunction, as are *dysbiosis* (an overgrowth of undesirable intestinal microorganisms) and impaired digestive function. Malabsorption is seen in approximately 85 percent of autistic children. This plus an inadequate diet can lead to a variety of nutritional deficiencies that can be measured directly or indirectly, utilizing blood and urine tests.

A common clinical (picture) of male predominance, autism, sensory issues, low muscle tone, coordination difficulties, food allergy, and GI symptoms emerged in a study of 187 children with a neurological inability to speak (verbal apraxia) that is common in children with autistic regression. "Low carnitine (20/26), high antigliadin antibodies (15/21), gluten-sensitivity HLA alleles (10/10), and zinc (2/2) and vitamin D deficiencies (4/7) were common abnormalities. Fat malabsorption was identified in 8 of 11 boys screened.[54]

"All the children received vitamin E + polyunsaturated (omega-3) fatty acid supplementation," and the results were remarkable. "181 families (97 percent) reported dramatic improvements in a number of areas including speech, imitation, coordination, eye contact, behavior, sensory issues, and development of pain sensation."

The theory behind this therapy is that the fatty acid membranes of cells in autistic children get damaged by free radicals (oxidation) secondary to inflammation and that vitamin E protects these sensitive and vital fatty acids form this "lipid peroxidation."

The best form of vitamin E to use in this regard is *mixed natural tocopherols*. Omega 3 fatty acids are found in fish and krill oils.

Other Genetic Enzyme Errors

Many genetic mutations have been found in autistics, including dysfunctions in the enzyme catechol [CAT-uh-coal] O-methyl transferase (COMT).

This enzyme transfers a methyl group to the catecholamine hormones (which are also neurotransmitters) dopamine, epinephrine, and norepinephrine, and by so doing, inactivates them. If this function is impaired, then imbalances in these neurotransmitter hormones result.

53   McGinnis, W. et al. *Alt. Therapies in Health and Medicine.* Vol. 14, No.2, Mar 2008.
54   Morris, C.R.; Agin, M.C. *Altern Ther Health Med.* 2009 Jul-Aug;15(4):34-43.

Genetic testing of many of the enzymes along the trans-methylation, trans-sulfuration, and other pathways can lead to a better understanding of the underlying chemistry that promotes autistic behaviors.

These pathways are pictured in Appendix II. In many cases, genetic mutations in these pathways can be bypassed. This will be discussed briefly in the section on "Genetic Bypass," an approach promoted by Dr. Amy Yasko in Chapter 33.

Table 3.2 summarizes a study by Dr. Jill St. James of 20 autistic and 33 non-autistic ("neurotypical") children performed at Arkansas Children's Hospital in which she compared the levels of key molecules that are formed along the trans-methylation and trans-sulfuration pathways in these two groups. As can be seen, the profiles of the autistic children were quite abnormal.[55]

Table 3.2. Study by Dr. Jill St. James of 20 autistic and 33 non-autistic ("neurotypical") children performed at Arkansas Children's Hospital

Molecule	Neurotypical Children	Autistic Children
Methionine (µmol/L)	30.6 ± 6.5	19.3 ± 9.7
SAM (nmol/L)	90.0 ± 16.2	75.8 ± 16.2
SAH (nmol/L)	20.1 ± 4.3	26.1 ± 5.4
Homocysteine (µmol/L)	6.3 ± 1.2	5.4 ± 0.9
Adenosine (µmol/L)	0.28 ± 0.16	0.39 ± 0.19
Cysteine (µmol/L)	210 ± 18.5	163 ± 14.6
Total Glutathione (µmol/L)	7.9 ± 1.8	4.1 ± 0.5
Oxidized Glutathione (nmol/L)	0.3 ± 0.1	0.55 ± 0.2
GSH/GSSG Ratio	25.5± 8.9	8.6 ± 3.5

SAM is S-adenosyl methionine, an important donor of methyl groups; GSH is the abbreviation for reduced (active) glutathione, a vitally important antioxidant and detoxifying agent; GSSG is oxidized (inactive) glutathione.

Elevated Testosterone

Increased pre- and post-natal levels of testosterone and other androgen (male hormone) metabolites have been noted more frequently in autistics than in the non-autistic population.[56]

Testosterone appears to increase the toxicity of thimerosal, the mercury-containing preservative found in many immunizations.[57]

One of the manifestations of this prenatal elevation of testosterone is a change in the finger length ratio of the second (index) finger compared to the fourth (ring) finger.

Compared to controls, children with autism, attention deficit hyperactivity disorder (ADHD), oppositional defiant disorder (ODD), and non-specific developmental disorder (PDD-NOS) have a shorter index finger relative to their ring finger, according to research published in the journal *Developmental Medicine and Child Neurology.*

These results indicate "that higher fetal testosterone levels may play a role, not only in the origin of autism, but also in the aetiology of PDD–NOS and of ADHD/ADD."[58]

---

55   St. James J, et al. Metabolic biomarkers of increased oxidative stress and impaired methylation capacity in children with autism. Am J Clin Nutr, 2004 Dec;80(6):1611-7.

56   Geier, David; Kerns, Janet. "Understanding the Medical Basis and Treatment of Patients Diagnosed with an Autism Spectrum Disorder…" U.S. Autism and Asperger Assoc. Conf. April 30-May 3, 2009.

57   Boyd, Haley http://www.flcv.com/hgsynerg.html

58   De Bruin, E. et al. "Differences in finger length ratio between males with autism, pervasive developmental disorder–not otherwise specified, ADHD,

Elevated Growth Hormones and Growth Factors

Autistic boys and those on the spectrum have been found to have higher levels of growth hormones and other growth factors like *insulin-like growth factors 1* and 2 (IGF1 & IGF2), as well as *insulin-like growth factor binding protein and growth hormone binding protein.*

It is difficult to measure human growth hormone directly as it is not produced consistently throughout the day. IGF1 is considered by many to be a reliable surrogate marker for the sufficiency of human growth hormone.

It isn't clear whether this overproduction of growth factors is a reason why autistic children often have larger brains and heads than do their non-autistic peers or why they tend to have larger weight to height ratios.

Interestingly, the bone age of autistic children is not advanced compared to their non-autistic peers, nor is their sexual maturation, and both these findings would be expected in children with elevated growth hormones. This seeming inhibition of growth factor effects may be due to the compensating increase in binding proteins that inactivate the hormones attached to them.[59]

Increased Concentrations of Specific Urinary Porphyrins (PORE-fur-ins)

Heme is a substance that is manufactured in the liver, kidneys, and immature red blood cells that makes up part of the red hemoglobin molecule that functions to transport oxygen from the lungs to all the cells of the body.

Its manufacture from chemical precursors is illustrated in Figure 3.1. Certain toxic metals, like mercury and lead, can inhibit several steps in this process and cause the production of chemical products (*metabolites*) known as *porphyrins.*

The presence of certain specific porphyrins—coproporphyrin (COP-row-PORE-fur-in), precoproporphyrin, and pentacarboxyporphyrin (PENT-uh car-BOX-ee PORE fur-in)—in abnormally elevated concentrations in the urine and in specific ratios has been shown in at least nine studies to correlate with the presence of these toxic metals, and in particular, mercury.[60]

The Nine Porphyrin Studies

1. Bowers, M. A., Aicher, L. D., Davis, H. A., and Woods, J. S. 1992. "Quantitative determination of porphyrins in rat and human urine and evaluation or urinary porphyrin profiles during mercury and lead exposures." *J. Lab. Clin. Med.* 120:272–281.

2. Pingree, S. D., Simmonds, P. L., Rummel, K. T., and Woods, J. S. 2001. "Quantitative evaluation of urinary porphryins as a measure of kidney mercury content and mercury body burden during prolonged methlmercury exposure in rats." *Toxicol. Sci.* 61:234–240.

3. Rosen, J. F., and Markowitz, M. E. 1993. "Trends in the management of childhood lead poisonings." *Neurotoxicology.* 14:211–217.

4. Woods, J. S. 1995. "Porphyrin metabolism as indicator of metal exposure and toxicity." In: Goyer, R. A., Cherian, M. G., eds. *Handbook of experimental pharmacology: Toxicology of metals—Biochemical aspects.* Vol. 115, pp.15–92. Berlin: Springer-Verlag.

5. Woods, J. S. 1996. "Altered porphyrin metabolism as a biomarker of mercury exposure and toxicity." *Can. J. Physiol. Pharmacol.* 74:210–215.

6. Woods, J. S., Echeverria, D., Heyer, N. J., Simmonds, P. L., Wilkerson, J., and Farin, F. M. 2005. "The association between genetic polymorphisms of coproporphyrinogen oxidase and an atypical porphyrinogenic response to mercury exposure in humans." *Toxicol. Appl. Pharmacol.* 206:113–120.

and anxiety disorders." *Developmental Medicine & Child Neurology.* Vol. 48. Issue 12. Dec 2006, pp 962–965.

59   Mills, J.L. et al. "Elevated levels of growth-related hormones in autism and autism spectrum disorder." *Clin Endocrinol* (Oxf). 2007 Aug; 67(2):230-7.

60   Woods 1966; Woods and Kardish 1983; Bowers et al. 1992; Pingree, et al 2001; Woods et al. 1993; Woods et al. 2005; Rosen and Markowitz, 1993.

7. Woods, J. S., and Kardish, R. M. 1983. "Developmental aspects of hepatic heme biosynthetic capability and hematotoxicity—II. Studies on uroporphyrinogen decarboxylase." *Biochem. Pharmacol.* 32:73–78.

8. Woods, J. S., Martin, M. D., Naleway, C. A., and Echeverria, D. 1993. "Urinary porphyrin profiles as a biomarker of mercury exposure: Studies on dentists with occupational exposure to mercury vapor." *J. Toxicol. Environ. Health.* 40:235–246.

9. Woods, J. S., and Miller, H. S. 1993. "Quantitative measurement of porphyrins in biological tissues and evaluation of tissue porphyrins during toxicant exposures." *Fundam. Appl. Toxicol.* 21:291–297.

In addition, two studies have also demonstrated that removing toxic metals like lead and mercury by a process known as chelation results in a diminishment of these biomarker porphyrins.[61]

Also, three recent studies have shown that autistic children showed *significantly* increased biomarker porphyrins indicative of mercury toxicity relative to controls.[62]

1. Nataf, R., Lam. A., Lathe, R., Skorupka, C. 2006. "Porphyrinurea in Childhood Autistic Disorders: Implications for Environmental Toxicity." *Toxicol. Appl. Pharmacol.* 214(2):99-108.

2. Geier, M., Geier. D. 2006. "A prospective assessment of porphyrins in autistic disorders: a potential marker for heavy metal exposure." *Neurotox Res.* Aug. 10(1):57-64]

3. Geier, M., Geier. D. "A Prospective Study of Mercury Toxicity Biomarkers in Autistic Spectrum Disorders." *Journal of Toxicology and Environmental Health, Part A*, 70: 1723–1730, 2007.

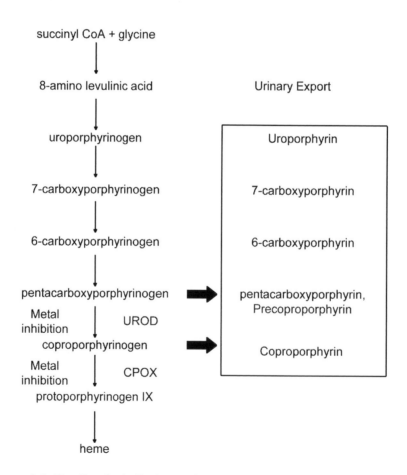

Figure 3.1. The Porphyrin Pathway: from Succinyl CoA & Glycine to Heme

61   Geier & Geier 2006 (see below) *and* Gonzalez-Ramirez, et al. "Sodium 2,3-dimercaptopropane-1-sulfonate challenge test for mercury in humans: II. Urinary mercury, porphyrins and neurobehavioral changes of dental workers in Monterrey, Mexico. *J.Pharmacol Exp. Ther.* 1995: 272: 264-74.

62   Geier & Geier 2006; Geier & Geier 2007; *and* Nataf et al. 2006.

Deficient Cholesterol

This may surprise some people. Most lay persons (and not a few physicians) regard cholesterol as a "harmful" substance, and believe that the less of it we have the better. Actually, nothing could be further from the truth. We cannot live without cholesterol. It is the precursor to all the steroid hormones and to vitamin D. It is necessary for our brains to function optimally. It plays a vital role in digestion, and it provides other important physiological benefits. *Mercury inhibits the production of Coenzyme A, necessary for the formation of cholesterol.*

The Smith-Lemli-Opitz Syndrome (SLOS) is a rare genetic disorder that involves impaired cholesterol biosynthesis, and in which autism symptoms are almost universally seen. Supplementing these children with cholesterol actually improves their functioning.[63]

A study published in 2006 was undertaken to determine whether low cholesterol levels would also be found in non-SLOS autistic children. The researchers measured the cholesterol levels in 100 autistic children and discovered that low levels (less than 100 mg/dL: below the 5th percentile) were found in 19 percent of the children.[64]

William Shaw, Ph.D., and director of the Great Plains Laboratory in Lenexa, Kansas, repeated this study in 40 children with autism and found similar results.[65]

Low Vitamin D Levels

Low levels of vitamin D2 (25- hydroxyl vitamin D) have been found in many autistic children. According to John Cannell, co-author of a study linking vitamin D deficiency and autism, "Five studies (from groups around the world) have shown that vitamin D deficiency is high among autistic children. One study showed that the higher the vitamin D level, the less severe the autism (and vice-versa)."[66]

"One Spanish study," Cannell stated, "looked at psychological development in 4-year-olds and then looked at mom's vitamin D levels when pregnant. It found a direct relationship between D deficiency and abnormalities in psychological development. Another Australian study found that the lower the mom's D levels during pregnancy, the more likely the child was to have speech difficulties."

In his own study, Cannell measured the amount of vitamin-D forming ultraviolet B radiation in each state and found that the greater the amount of UVB radiation, the less the incidence of autism. "Arizona has three times less autism than Maine," Cannell said. "This is the first time there has been such a clear association shown between autism and surface UVB radiation."

Support for this theory comes from observations of Somali children who have migrated to Sweden and Minnesota, relatively colder climates where they had less sun exposure than they did in Somalia. Less sun exposure and dark skin means less vitamin D is manufactured and, therefore, D deficiency is likely to be more prevalent. Children in Somalia have little or no autism, but this condition became common when they moved to Minnesota and Sweden.[67]

Researchers measured the vitamin D levels in 117 adult psychiatric outpatients. The patients with the lowest levels suffered from autism, schizophrenia, and depression. The ten who had autism had the lowest levels of vitamin D. This finding was confirmed in a Faroe Islands study of young adults with autism. Males with autism and their siblings had lower levels of vitamin D and 88 percent of the ASD population was deficient in D.[68]

Low levels of vitamin D, which is essential for optimal immune system function, have also been linked to an increased incidence of auto-immune disorders, including diabetes, multiple sclerosis, and thyroid disease.

63   Richard Kelley of Johns Hopkins. "Inborn Errors of Cholesterol Biosynthesis." *Adv. Pediatr.* 2000; 47:1-53.
64   Tierney, E. et al. 2006. "Abnormalities of Cholesterol Metabolism in Autism Spectrum Disorders." *Am J Med Genet Part B* 141B:666-668.
65   http://www.greatplainslaboratory.com/home/eng/cholesterol.asp
66   Cannell, J.J. "Autism and vitamin D." *Med Hypotheses.* 2008; 70(4):750-9.
67   Bejerot, S.; Humble, M. "Increased occurrence of autism among Somali children—does vitamin D deficiency play a role?" *Tidsskr Nor Laegeforen.* 2008 Sep 11; 128(17):1986-7 *and* Fernell E, et al. "Serum levels of 25-hydroxyvitamin D in mothers of Swedish and of Somali origin who have children with and without autism." *Acta Paediatr.* 2010; 99:743–7.
68   Kočovska, E. et al. "Vitamin D in the General Population of Young Adults with Autism in the Faroe Islands." *J Autism Dev Disord.* Jun 14, 2014.

But how does vitamin D reduce the risk of autism?

A likely answer is that it protects the body from excess mercury and other toxic substances as well as from oxidative stress by dramatically increasing the production of glutathione, the body's premier antioxidant detoxifier.[69]

Dr. Cannell recommends that mothers "should take adequate amounts of D before (they) even plan to conceive a child—5,000 IU per day—and continue during pregnancy and while breastfeeding. If (a mother) is not taking that amount, the breastfeeding infant should take 1,000 IUs daily. Formula-fed infants need an extra 600 IUs daily. Once weaned, the infant needs to take vitamin D—1,000 IUs per day for under 25 pounds; 2,000 IUs for up to 50; and 3,000 for 50 to 75 pounds."[70]

Elevated Serotonin Levels

Serotonin is a well-known neurotransmitter that is also manufactured in the gut and in platelets. Elevated blood and platelet levels of serotonin are seen in about 25-30 percent of all autistic children.[71]

In 2005, scientists at Vanderbilt University discovered that certain *rare* genetic variations (mutations) in *some* autistic children can disrupt the function of a serotonin transporter molecule.[72]

In March 2012, the Vanderbilt researchers, using a mouse model that expressed most of these same variations, discovered that they promoted both a diminishment in the amount of serotonin available to the brain synapses as well as an increase in the levels of serotonin found in the blood (in the platelets). And more to the point, the mice exhibited socialization and communication impairments as well as repetitive behaviors that parallel those commonly observed in autistic children.[73]

Inability in Many Autistic Children to Transform Certain B Vitamins into Their Active Form

Folic Acid (Vitamin B9)

This B vitamin, it may be remembered, must be transformed from its inactive form (methyl*ene*-tetrahydrofolate) to its active functional form (5-*methyl*-tetrahydrofolate) by way of an enzyme abbreviated MTHFR, which may manifest as a number of less effective mutations. One such variant (A1298C) has been shown in two studies to correlate with symptoms of inattention and ADHD. This enzyme variant is less able to "activate" folic acid.[74]

The kind of folic acid found in vitamin pills is usually a synthetic variety that differs chemically from the natural forms found in foods, like 5-formyl tetrahydrofolate (AKA folicin), for example.

---

69   Garcion, E. et al. "New clues about vitamin D functions in the nervous system." *Trends in Endocrinology and Metabolism.* April 2002, Vol. 13, Issue 3, 1, p. 100-105

70   http://newhope360.com/retail-science/does-vitamin-d-deficiency-raise-autism-risk

71   Schain, R.J.; Freedman, D.X. (1961). "Studies on 5-hydroxyindole metabolism in autistic and other mentally retarded children." *J Pediatr.* 58:315-20. *and* Anderson, G.M. et. al. (1990). "The hyperserotonemia of autism." *Ann N Y Acad Sci* 600:331–340 *and* Cook, E.H. Jr. (2001). "Genetics of autism." *Child Adolesc Psychiatr Clin N Am*10:333–350 *and* Cook, E.H., Leventhal, B.L. (1996). "The serotonin system in autism." *Curr Opin Pediatr.* 8:348–354.

72   Blakely, R.D., et al (2005). "Biogenic amine neurotransmitter transporters: just when you thought you knew them." *Physiology* (Bethesda) 20:225–231 *and* Blakely, R.D., et al (1998) "Regulated phosphorylation and trafficking of antidepressant sensitive serotonin transporter proteins." *Biol Psychiatry* 44:169 –178.

73   Veenstra-VanderWeele, J. et al; "Autism gene variant causes hyperserotonemia, serotonin receptor hypersensitivity, social impairment and repetitive behavior." Proceedings of the National Academy of Sciences. 2012; DOI:10.1073/pnas.1112345109. Cook, E.H.; Leventhal, B.L. "The serotonin system in autism." *Curr Opin Pediatr* 1996 (Aug); 8(4):348 – 54. *and* Cook E.H. "Autism: review of neurochemical investigation." *Synapse.* 1990; 6(3):292 – 308. *and* Betancur, C. et al. "Serotonin transporter gene polymorphisms and hyperserotonemia in autistic disorder." *Mol Psychiatry* 2002; 7(1):67 – 71.

74   Gokcen, C. et al. "Methylenetetrahydrofolate Reductase Gene Polymorphisms in Children with Attention Deficit Hyperactivity Disorder." *Int J Med Sci* 2011; 8(7):523-528 *and* Krull, K.R. et al. "Folate Pathway Genetic Polymorphisms are related to Attention Disorders in Childhood Leukemia Survivors." *J Pediatr.* 2008Jan; 152(1):101-5.

Vitamin B6 (Pyridoxine and Pyridoxal)

Vitamin B6 is needed for over 100 metabolic reactions. It is inactive unless converted to its active state, P5P (pyridoxal 5- phosphate). The enzyme that performs this task may be dysfunctional in some autistic children. For example, P5P is a necessary cofactor in the conversion of inactive folic acid (methylene tetrahydrofolate) to its active form (methyl tetra hydrofolate) and in the conversion of homocysteine to cystathionine. If B6 isn't converted to P5P, abnormally high levels of B6 may be found in the blood.[75]

The enzyme that assists in this transformation of pyridoxine to P5P is called pyridoxal kinase, and aberrant forms of this enzyme in many autistic children hamper this activation process. If pyridoxine (B6) is not converted efficiently to P5P, then pyridoxine levels remain high in the bloodstream while levels of P5P are consequently low, and that is exactly what was confirmed by James Adams and fellow researchers at Arizona State University.

They found that unsupplemented "children with autism had a 75 percent higher level of total vitamin B6 than did the controls" (p=0.00002). "These results," they continue, "are consistent with previous studies that found that:

(1) *Pyridoxal kinase* had a very low activity in children with autism, and as a result...

(2) *Pyridoxal 5 phosphate* (P5P) levels were unusually low in children with autism.

"Thus," they add, "it appears that the low conversion of pyridoxal and pyridoxine to P5P results in low levels of P5P, which is the *active* cofactor for 113 known enzymatic reactions, including the formation of many key neurotransmitters...."

This, they conclude, "may explain the many published studies of benefits of high-dose vitamin B6 supplementation in some children and adults with autism."[76]

Vitamin B12 (Cobalamin)

This B vitamin exists in four chemical forms: *cyano*cobalamin (the *synthetic* form commonly found in vitamin pills), *methyl*cobalamin, *hydroxo*cobalamin, and *adenosyl cobalamin*.

Many children with autism and ADHD have difficulty making *methyl*cobalamin because their enzymes are structurally less effective in their ability to catalyze the reactions necessary for the methylation of cobalamin or because they are dietarily deficient in required nutrient cofactors or are less able to activate pyridoxine (Vitamin B6) by converting it to P5P.

Jill St. James and colleagues at the Arkansas Children's Hospital Research Institute published a study that found that autistic children differ markedly from their non-autistic peers in regard to their plasma levels of several breakdown products (called "metabolites") of the various substances involved in the chemical pathway illustrated in Figure A.1 (the Trans-methylation and Trans-Sufuration Cycles) which depicts the transfer of a methyl group from folic acid to cobalamin to homocysteine, etc. This transmethylation/trans-sulfuration pathway ultimately results in the production of the antioxidant detoxifier glutathione.

Supplementing autistic children with both folinic acid (a more bioavailable form of folic acid) and injectable *methyl*cobalamin resulted in improvements in the children's biochemical status, and many improved clinically as well.

The researchers concluded that "significant improvements observed in transmethylation metabolites and glutathione redox status (refers to having more of the beneficial reduced form of glutathione) after treatment suggest that targeted nutritional intervention with methylcobalamin and folinic acid may be of clinical benefit in some children who have autism." [77]

---

75   Adams et al. "Abnormally high plasma levels of vitamin B6 in children with autism not taking supplements compared to controls not taking supplements." *J Altern Complement Med.* 2006 Jan-Feb;12(1):59-63.

76   Adams, J. et al. "Abnormally high plasma levels of vitamin B6 in children with autism not taking supplements compared to controls not taking supplements." *J Altern Complement Med.* 2006 Jan-Feb; 12(1):59-63.

77   "Efficacy of methylcobalamin and folinic acid treatment on glutathione redox status in children with autism." *Am J Clin Nutr.* 2009 January; 89(1):

Lower Concentrations of Proteins in Autistic Children's Hair and Nails

This finding, which likely reflects dietary inadequacies, was confirmed by a study in Chenai, India. The researchers also found that levels of nitric oxide, an oxidizing gas produced by the lining of blood vessels, was higher in autistic children than in controls, consistent with the notion that autistic children are subject to higher levels of oxidative stress.

Nitric oxide can react with a particular amino acid found in most proteins called tyrosine. The attachment of nitrogen to proteins is called "nitration." The researchers also found evidence of oxidized fats and increased nitration of hair and nail proteins in the autistic children. They found that, "Lower protein content and higher percentage of nitration in the hair and nails of autistic children correlated with their degrees of severity." [78]

Abnormal Placentas

"More than 95 percent of placentas from infants who were among the greatest risk of developing autism contained abnormal cells known as 'trophoblast inclusions,'" according to a recent study. "Trophoblasts are specialized cells present in fetal tissue and form the conduit for interaction between mother and fetus. Trophoblast inclusions are not normal and are marked by cell clusters that will look like the tissue is folded within the placenta.

"Researchers believe that trophoblast inclusions are a symptom of altered physiology or genetic predisposition, particularly because they are already associated with other genetic chromosomal abnormalities that are likely triggered by environmental exposures." [79]

Low Levels of Lithium and Iodine on Hair Analysis

These low levels were found in a study by James Adams and colleagues. It is not clear, however, that hair analysis provides accurate information regarding the adequacy or lack thereof of these nutrients. [80]

Mitochondrial Disorders and Dysfunctions

The mitochondria are tiny energy-making organelles found in almost all cells. There are a number of studies pointing to mitochondrial dysfunction as a causative mechanism in promoting autism. One study found that 32 percent of children with autism had abnormal mitochondrial function. These dysfunctions can be identified by looking for certain novel phospholipid biomarkers of autism. [81]

Of 153 publications that examined mitochondrial dysfunction in ASD, 89 percent reported an association. "The prevalence of mitochondrial disorders in the general population of ASD was 5.0 percent (95 percent confidence interval 3.2–6.9 percent), much higher than found in the general population (≈ 0.01 percent)." [82]

Mitochondrial dysfunctions may be inherited or may be acquired secondary to adverse environmental exposures. Mercury, for example, has been shown to induce mitochondrial dysfunction, which results in depletion of the energy molecule known as ATP (adenosine triphosphate). In addition, mercury causes depletion of the antioxidant detoxifier known as glutathione and reduces oxidative defenses, resulting in oxidative stress and increases in the oxidation of lipids (fats). All these dysfunctions and sequelae are commonly seen in autistic children. [83]

425–430.

78   Lakshmi, Priya; Geetha, A. "A biochemical study on the level of proteins and their percentage of nitration in the hair and nail of autistic children." *Clin Chim Acta.* 2011 May 12; 412(11-12):1036-42.

79   http://www.naturalhealth365.com/autism_news/autism_risk.html?goback= percent2Egde_1799831_member_247149321. Anderson, G.M. et al. "Placental Trophoblast Inclusions in Autism Spectrum Disorder." *Biol Psychiatry.* 2007; 61:487– 491.

80   Adams, J.B. et al. "Analyses of toxic metals and essential minerals in the hair of Arizona children with autism and associated conditions, and their mothers." *Biological Trace Element Research.* Vol. 110, 2006, 193-209.

81   Pastural, E. et al. "Novel plasma phospholipid biomarkers of autism: Mitochondrial dysfunction as a putative causative mechanism." *Prostaglandins Leukot Essent Fatty Acids.* 2009 Oct; 81(4):253-64.

82   Rossignol, D.A.; Frye, R.E. *Molecular Psychiatry.* 2012 17: 389f.

83   Houston, M.C. "Role of mercury toxicity in hypertension, cardiovascular disease, and stroke." *J Clin Hypertens* (Greenwich). 2011 Aug; 13(8):621-7.

Thimerosal is a mercury-containing preservative found in some vaccines. A recent study compared the effect of exposing cell lines from autistic and non-autistic children to thimerosal at levels two orders of magnitude *lower* than those used in vaccines. The authors found that the abnormally functioning cells in the autistic children were unable to maintain their reserve capacity to make energy when exposed to thimerosal. Reserve capacity loss can lead to cell death. The normally functioning cells, when exposed to thimerosal, did not lose their reserve capacity.[84]

The researchers then pretreated the subgroup of cells with abnormally-functioning mitochondria to N-acetyl cysteine (NAC), a precursor of glutathione. When these cells were exposed to the ethyl mercury found in thimerosal, they did not lose their reserve capacity to make energy. These findings provide support for the use of NAC to help mediate the oxidative stress seen in autistic individuals and suggest a mechanism whereby immunizations with thimerosal might potentiate the likelihood of developing an autistic disorder.[85]

The authors conclude that, "the epidemiological link between environmental mercury exposure and an increased risk of developing autism may be mediated through mitochondrial dysfunction and support the notion that a subset of individuals with autism may be vulnerable to environmental influences with detrimental effects on development through mitochondrial dysfunction."[86]

Abnormal Levels of Epidermal Growth Factor

Epidermal growth factor is a substance secreted by cells that stimulates their growth and multiplication. *Low levels* have been found in the serum of adults with high functioning autism and *increased levels* were found in autistic children.[87]

Deficient phenolsulfotransferase enzyme (PST)

This enzyme, *important in the detoxification cycle*, was found to be low in virtually all autistic children tested by Rosemary Waring.[88]

Oxalate Excess

Oxalates, including oxalic acid, are substances found in foods like nuts, berries, spinach, and chocolate. They may also be made by our own bodies and by certain fungi (like aspergillus and penicillium) and possibly by yeasts like Candida as well. Dr. William Walsh, director/owner of the Great Plains Lab, measured the urine oxalate values of 100 autistic children and compared these to the levels in 16 control children.

He found that autistic children had on average much higher levels than did the control group (as depicted in this graph). Eighty-four percent of the autistic children had oxalate values outside the normal range. None of the control children did. These findings were confirmed in a 2012 European study.[89]

The elevated oxalate found in autistic children appears to be doing harm. Susan Owens, the head researcher at the Autism Research Institute's Autism Oxalate Project, discovered that *a low oxalate diet benefited many children with autism*. Improvements were noted in gross and fine motor skills, expressive speech, counting ability, sociability, cognition, handwriting, and sleep, among others.[90]

In addition to a low oxalate diet, high oxalate levels may be lowered by supplementing each meal with calcium citrate. The calcium part of the molecule binds oxalate in the intestine so that it cannot be absorbed and citrate inhibits the absorption of oxalate.

84   Rose, S. et al. "Increased susceptibility to ethylmercury-induced mitochondrial dysfunction in a subset of autism lymphoblastoid cell lines." *J of Toxicology*; 2015 online; http://dx.doi.org/10.1155/2015/573701

85   Ibid.

86   Ibid.

87   Suzuki, K. et al. *Biol. Psychiatry* 2007, 62: 267 f. *and* Ii, E. et al. *J Autism Dev. Disord* 2010.

88   Waring, R.H.; Klovrza, L.V. "Sulphur Metabolism in Autism." *Journal of Nutritional and Environmental Medicine* 10, 25–32 (2000).

89   Konstantynowicz, Jerzy et al. "A potential pathogenic role of oxalate in autism." *Europ J of Paed Neurology*; September 2012; 16(5): 45f.

90   http://www.greatplainslaboratory.com/home/eng/oxalates.asp and https://www.linkedin.com/pub/susan-owens/4/11b/a36

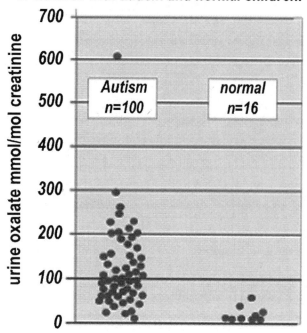

Figure 3.2. Oxalate Excess[91]

A beneficial gut microbe, Oxalobacter formigenes, "eats" oxalates in the GI tract and degrades them into safer substances. Individuals who consume a lot of oxalate with no apparent harm may be the lucky hosts to a healthy supply of intestinal Oxalobacter bacteria. A company (Oxthera Products) is seeking approval to sell this beneficial organism as a drug to treat elevated oxalate levels in individuals with autism and other conditions. Excess levels of oxalates in the body may also be caused by deficiencies in certain B vitamins (B1, B5, and B6) and by too much glycine or vitamin C.[92]

The following websites list foods and their oxalate levels, plus a great deal more information on this important subject.

- http://www.greatplainslaboratory.com/home/eng/oxalates.asp
- http://www.nutrition-healing.com/lowoxalate.html
- http://www.lowoxalate.info/food_lists/alph_oxstat_chart.pdf

An informative oxalate brochure from the Great Plains Lab may be downloaded at: http://www.Greatplainslaboratory.com/home/eng/brochures/OAT Oxalates.pdf

---

"About 1 in 6 children in the U.S. had a developmental disability in 2006-2008, ranging from mild disabilities such as speech and language impairments to serious developmental disabilities, such as intellectual disabilities, cerebral palsy, and autism."[93]

---

91   http://www.greatplainslaboratory.com/home/eng/oxalates.asp.
92   http://www.nutrition-healing.com/lowoxalate.html
93   CDC website (Sept 2013) http://www.cdc.gov/ncbddd/autism/data.html

What other findings are commonly seen in autistic children?

Large Heads

Since 1983, Dr. Margaret Bauman, a neurologist at Harvard Medical School, and her colleagues have been studying brain tissue obtained from autopsies of eleven autistic children and adults.

They found that, in general, the brains of autistics are larger and heavier than those of non-autistic individuals. Large heads are particularly characteristic of male children with delayed-onset but not early-onset autism. It is not clear why this is so.[94]

One of the four metallothioneins (MT-3) directs the "pruning" of excess brain cells, allowing the growth of new cells (see Chapter 6). Dr. Bauman's team noted a *greater number* of smaller, immature cells in the limbic system of the brain, which processes emotions. The cerebellums of these autistic individuals had 30-50 percent *less* cells, particularly Purkinje (per-KIN-gee) cells, than expected. The cerebellum functions to help coordinate motor activity and helps make predictions about future movements.

The researchers also found that parts of the frontal lobes were *larger* than normal. The dopamine-sensitive frontal lobes are involved with higher mental functions like the ability to choose from among a variety of options, the ability to suppress socially unacceptable actions, and the ability to "determine similarities and differences between things and events."[95]

Amygdala Dysfunction

It is commonly observed that autistic children don't read facial expressions well. Scientists, like Dr. Ruth Amaral at U.C. Davis, suggest that this disability can be traced to a dysfunction in the amygdala (uh-MIG-duh-luh), a part of the brain that responds to faces and the angle of gaze. Her husband, David Amaral, also of UC Davis, and his colleague Cynthia Mills Schumann found that "the autistic *amygdala* appears to undergo an abnormal pattern of postnatal development that includes early enlargement and ultimately a reduced number of neurons."[96]

Frontal Lobe Impairment

The ability to shift attention *unconsciously*, a cerebellar ability, is normal in autistic children, but if they are asked *consciously* to shift their attention from one task to another, they are unable to do this because the conscious shifting of attention involves the frontal lobes that appear to be somewhat impaired in this regard.

The structural differences found in autistic individuals on autopsy include short, dense, under-developed brain cells and other abnormalities that coincidentally are observed where levels of metallothioneins are highest, like the amygdala, hippocampus, and pineal gland.[97]

Reduced Thickness of Hand Bones

Autistic boys have unexplained reductions in the thickness of their metacarpal (hand) bones, which is consistent with childhood or even intrauterine vitamin D deficiency.[98]

Subtle Facial Differences

In a study published in the October 14, 2012 issue of *Molecular Autism*, researchers compared 17 points on the faces of 64 boys with autism with those of 41 typically developing boys, aged 8-12 years old, using a 3-D camera system.

---

94   Wu, Nordahl; Wu, Christine et al. "Brain enlargement is associated with regression in preschool-age boys with autism spectrum disorders." *PNAS* Oct 2011; http://www.pnas.org/content/early/2011/11/14/1107560108.abstract?sid=c037d64e-727a-4686-aee2-5dececd67b5b

95   Wikipedia & Sources: Dr. Margaret Bauman, Harvard Medical School, Ruth Carper, The Laboratory for Research on the Neuroscience of Autism

96   *The Journal of Neuroscience*, July 19, 2006, 26(29):7674-7.

97   Ibid.

98   Hediger, M.L. et al. "Reduced bone cortical thickness in boys with autism or autism spectrum disorder." *J Autism Dev Disord.* 2008; 38:848–56.

What was found was that (as compared to non-autistic peers) children with autism had:

- Wider eyes

- A "broader upper face"

- A shorter middle region of the face—including the nose and cheeks

- A wider mouth and philtrum (the dimple between the upper lip and nose)

- Other distinct differences in severely affected autistic children when compared with mildly autistic children.[99]

Increased Intestinal Permeability ("Leaky Gut")

Twenty-one autistic children with *no evidence of intestinal disorders* were given an intestinal permeability test (IPT), and an increased intestinal permeability was found in 9 of the 21 (43 percent), but in none of the 40 control children.[100]

A later study confirmed these findings. Abnormal intestinal permeability was found in 38 percent of autistics and 21 percent of their relatives, but in only 5 percent of "normal" subjects. "The IPT alterations found in first-degree relatives suggest the presence of an intestinal (tight-junction linked) hereditary factor in the families of subjects with autism," the authors concluded.[101]

Positive Response to Oxytocin in Some Autistic Children

Oxytocin is a hormone that improves social functioning in individuals. Although autistic children have not been shown to have lower levels of oxytocin than their non-autistic peers, there is some evidence that supplemental oxytocin can improve social functioning in autistic individuals (and non-autistic individuals as well).[102]

---

99   Aldridge, Kristine et al. *Molecular Autism*; Oct 14, 2012.
100   D'Eufemia, P. et al. Acta Paediatrica. 1996; 85: 1076f.
101   *J Pediatric Gastroenterol Nutr*. Jul 28, 2010.
102   http://www.pnas.org/ content/111/33/12258; & Sikich, et al.; Hollander 2007 & Gaustella, et al. 2010.

Chapter 4
Other Medical Conditions that Can Mimic Autism

"There's a reason I am the way I am, and there's a reason I was born to you."
— *Dean Koontz,* Relentless

WHAT IS TUBEROUS *Sclerosis (Tuberous Sclerosis Complex)?*

This rare, currently untreatable genetic disorder is seen in all sexes, races, and ethnic groups and may manifest at any age. It causes those afflicted to develop non-cancerous tumors in many organs, including the brain. It is not surprising, therefore, that seizures, mental retardation, delayed development, and behavior problems are seen frequently in those with this condition, and perhaps as many as 45 percent with TS exhibit the characteristics of autism. Conversely, about 14 percent of autistics *who also have seizures* may be diagnosable with tuberous sclerosis. It isn't clear why this association occurs. About 50 percent of those with TS have normal intelligence.

The skin, liver, kidneys, and other organs are commonly affected. Symptoms may start in the first years of life, or may be delayed. The potato-like tuberous tumors that appear in the brain often harden (sclerose), hence the name.

A wide variety of skin abnormalities may occur in individuals with TS. Most cause no problems but are helpful in diagnosis. Some cases may cause disfigurement, necessitating treatment. The most common skin abnormalities include:

- Hypomelanic macules ("ash leaf spots"), which are white or lighter patches of skin that may appear anywhere on the body and are caused by a lack of the skin pigment, melanin, the substance that gives skin its color. These "ash-leaf spots" are seen best with an ultraviolet light.

- Reddish spots or bumps, called facial angiofibromas (also called adenoma sebaceum), which appear on the face (sometimes resembling acne) and consist of blood vessels and fibrous tissue.

- Raised, discolored areas on the forehead called forehead plaques, which are common and unique to TSC and may help doctors diagnose the disorder.

- Areas of thick leathery, pebbly skin called shagreen patches, usually found on the lower back or nape of the neck.

- Small fleshy tumors called ungual or subungual fibromas that grow around and under the toenails or fingernails and may need to be surgically removed if they enlarge or cause bleeding. These usually appear later in life (ages 20 – 50).

- Other skin features that are *not unique* to individuals with TSC include molluscum fibrosum or skin tags, which typically occur across the back of the neck and shoulders, café au lait (ka-FAY-aw-LAY) spots, which are flat tan marks, and poliosis, which is a tuft or patch of white hair that may appear on the scalp or eyelids.

Tuberous Sclerosis is caused by mutations in either or both of two genes named TSC-1 and TSC-2. Although children can inherit the defective gene or genes from either parent with this disorder (*if one parent has TS, then there is a 50 percent chance that a child born to that parent will have the disorder*), most cases of TS arise as spontaneous mutations in the aforementioned genes which, if normal, would direct the cell to manufacture two proteins known as hamartin and tuberin. These proteins in turn are essential in inhibiting the action of an enzyme known as mTOR (mammalian Target Of Rapamycin) which regulates cell growth.

In those afflicted with TS, the mutations in the aforementioned genes don't allow for normal mTOR regulation, and "this leads to abnormal differentiation and development, and to the generation of enlarged cells, as are seen in TSC brain lesions."[1]

Tuberous sclerosis is often suspected in children with seizures, delayed development, and Shagreen's spots or other skin lesions (ash leaf spots and angio-fibromas). The diagnosis is generally made by an MRI or CT scan of the brain or an ultrasound examination of other organs.[2]

What Is Prader-Willi Syndrome (PWS)?

This condition, which sometimes presents with autism-like symptoms, is due to a genetic abnormality on chromosome 15. It occurs equally in males and females and all races at a rate of about one in 15,000 births and is the most common known genetic cause of potentially life-threatening *obesity* in children.

The commonly observed symptoms include low IQ (average is c 70), low muscle tone, small and incomplete genitalia, a compulsive tendency to overeat, behavior abnormalities, and short stature (unless treated with growth hormone). Some individuals have normal IQs but also usually have learning disorders. Affected individuals tend to have gentle and loving personalities.

Infants born with this condition are generally small and underweight for their gestational age and exhibit poor muscle tone and don't suck well. At about 2-5 years of age, they begin to eat excessively and tend to gain lots of weight unless their diet is strictly supervised and limited.

The behavioral concerns in these children that are also observed in some autistic children include anxiety, compulsive behaviors, a tendency not to want normal routines changed, and a tendency to have repetitive thoughts or verbalizations. They may collect and hoard possessions, and may become disproportionately upset or angry when frustrated.

The genetics of PWS are interesting in that the region affected on the 15th chromosome (called "q12") is only active on the father's chromosome 15. Children normally inherit one chromosome 15 from the father and another from the mother.

In 75 percent of the cases of PWS, the abnormality in the father's chromosome 15 is a deletion (absence) of the q12 portion, which is essential for normal development. The mother's chromosome 15, even if entirely normal, does not correct this condition.

In the other 25 percent of cases, the child inherits both chromosome 15s from the mother, and since the maternal q12 portion is inactive, the child will develop PWS. In rare cases, the father's chromosome 15 is present, but due to an imprinting defect, is unable to foster the creation of the necessary proteins to prevent PWS from occurring.[3]

Prader-Willi Syndrome is currently not curable and is diagnosed based on the symptoms and genetic tests.

---

1   NIH.org
2   "Tuberous Sclerosis Fact Sheet." NINDS. NIH Publication No. 07-1846; Hunt, A. Shepherd, C, "A prevalence study of autism in tuberous sclerosis." *J Autism Dev Disord*, 1993, Jun; 23 (2):323-39; Smalley, S.L. "Autism and Tuberous Sclerosis." *J Autism Dev Disord*, 1998 October; 28 (5): 407-14.
3   www.pwsausa.org

What Is Angelman's Syndrome?

An English physician named Harry Angelman first described three children with this disorder in 1965. Symptoms include severe developmental delays, seizures, absence of speech, puppet-like jerky movements, walking and balancing disabilities, and a tendency to laugh inappropriately.

As in autism, hand and arm flapping are common, but in contradistinction with autistic children, who tend to have normal sized or larger than normal heads and brains, children with Angelman's syndrome often have small heads and brains (microcephaly). Early on, children with this disorder may be misdiagnosed as being autistic or as having cerebral palsy. Most children with this disorder are normal in appearance.

As in the Prader-Willi syndrome, the defect in this malady, which may occur in either sex, also has to do with an abnormal chromosome 15. The incidence, about one in 15,000 births, is also similar to that in the Prader-Willi syndrome; however, in Angelman's Syndrome, the defect occurs on the *maternally* donated 15th chromosome and the responsible genetic defect in most instances has been identified as a deletion of the *UBE3A gene.*

This gene codes for an enzyme that transfers a small protein called *ubiquitin* to certain target proteins that need to be degraded (destroyed). In Angelman's Syndrome, these target proteins are insufficiently degraded and their accumulation, through an as yet unknown mechanism, is suspected to promote the dysfunctions noted in Angelman's Syndrome.

The Angelman Syndrome Foundation (www.angelman.org) is a good source of up-to-date information and research on this currently incurable genetic defect. Individuals with this syndrome will require lifelong care. Genetic testing is necessary to confirm the diagnosis.

What Is the Smith-Lemli-Opitz Syndrome (SLOS)?

The Cholesterol Connection

Cholesterol, as we have mentioned, is a much maligned molecule. The current medical view is that it is best to have as little cholesterol as possible because elevated levels of cholesterol are associated with an increased risk of cardiovascular disease. However, low levels of cholesterol have also been found to cause problems like an increased cancer risk and an increase in depression and suicidality.

In 1993, the genetic inability to manufacture cholesterol in the liver was found to be the defect responsible for the abnormalities found in the Smith-Lemli-Opitz syndrome, which was named after the three geneticists who first described it in three boys in 1964.

Cholesterol is in reality an essential nutrient. We get it from eating cholesterol-containing foods like red meat, cream, and eggs, but most of the cholesterol in our body is manufactured in the liver. Cholesterol is essential for digestion. It appears in the bile and helps emulsify fats. It is found in cell membranes where it performs essential functions. It is particularly important for normal brain development, and it is the precursor to all the steroid hormones, including testosterone, estrogen, progesterone, DHEA, and hydrocortisone. We cannot live without cholesterol.

The immediate precursor to cholesterol in the body is a compound called 7-dehydrocholesterol (7-DHC). The enzyme that is missing or abnormal in children with SLOS is called 7-DHC reductase. It converts 7-DHC into cholesterol. Children with SLOS, therefore, tend to accumulate excessive amounts of 7-DHC (which is also a precursor to vitamin D) and to have very low levels of cholesterol (generally less than 50 mg/dL = milligrams per deciliter.[4] The "optimal" level of cholesterol is 100 mg/dL or more.)

Children born with this syndrome tend to have many abnormalities, like delayed growth and development, feeding problems, mental retardation, constipation, and a variety of malformations, including small heads and brains (mi-

---

4   A gram is about a fifth of a tsp. A milligram is one thousandth of a gram. A liter is a volume slightly larger than a quart. A deciliter is one tenth of a liter.

crocephaly), extra fingers and toes, low set ears, webbed toes, genital abnormalities in boys, like undescended testes and hypospadias (a condition in which the urethra opens at the bottom of the penis instead of at the end), drooping eyelids, cataracts, narrow stomach outlet (pyloric stenosis), scoliosis, osteoporosis, small thumbs and chin, and a cleft palate, among others. They may also have heart, lung, kidney, and liver defects.

Many SLOS children have symptoms that parallel those seen in many autistic children, like communication difficulties, delayed speech, behavioral issues like outbursts and self-abuse, inability to sleep, impaired immunity, and sensitivity to textures and the environment. Children with SLOS often benefit from cholesterol supplementation. Recently, low levels of cholesterol were found in some autistic children whose symptoms also improved after cholesterol supplementation.[5]

Some SLOS children have only one or two minor defects while others exhibit most of the abnormalities mentioned. Generally, the lower the cholesterol level, the more severe are the presentation and symptoms of this disorder. Some children have actually been found to have no detectable level of cholesterol at all! Children born with severe forms of this disorder may live only a short time. Others can live normal lifespans, especially if treated with cholesterol-containing supplements and foods.

The syndrome is diagnosed clinically and by finding abnormally low levels of cholesterol and elevated amounts of 7-DHC on lab testing. It is transmitted as an autosomal recessive disorder. This means that it is necessary to have abnormalities or deletions in both the 7-DHC reductase genes (one from each parent) in order to have the syndrome. Each of the parents carries the abnormal gene, but the normal gene is protective and prevents the expression of this disorder in the mother and father.

The incidence of SLOS is about one in 20,000 births. The testing for 7-DHC levels can be performed only at certain labs (see www.smithlemliopitz.org). Supplementation with cholesterol (either synthetic or via pasteurized egg) appears to help alleviate some of the symptoms of this disorder and may extend life. It does not cure the condition, however.[6]

The Smith-Lemli-Opitz Foundation is an excellent source of information about this disorder, and its website (www.smithlemliopitz.org) lists labs that are able to test for this disorder, sources of synthetic cholesterol for supplementation, support for SLOS families, and information on current research.

What Is Neurofibromatosis?

There are three related incurable conditions that fall under the heading of neurofibromatosis (NF, AKA Von Recklinghausen's Disease), and all involve genetic abnormalities that induce tumors to grow on nerve cells. NF occurs in one of every 4,000 births.

NF Type I usually presents at birth and manifests as skin changes (tumors or "café-au-lait spots"[7]), nerve tumors, and bony deformities. A small minority of children with Type I neurofibromatosis exhibit signs of ADHD and autism. It is not clear whether this association occurs any more often than it would in the general population. There are conflicting reports in this regard (see ref. below). Learning difficulties are not uncommon in NF Type I. The genetic abnormality in this disorder involves a defective gene (found on chromosome 17) that codes for a protein known as neurofibromin.

This condition may be mild with only skin manifestations apparent, or severe with nerve tumors that cause pain and affect function. Some people can have hundreds of small tumors. Life expectancy is generally normal in most of the afflicted.[8]

5   Tierney, E. et al. "Abnormalities of cholesterol metabolism in Autism." *Am J Med Gen*; Sep 5, 2006; 141B:666f.

6   www.smithlemliopitz.org

7   These tan flat areas may appear anywhere on the skin. It is not unusual for unaffected individuals to have one or two. Finding five or more of these "coffee with cream" spots greater than 1.5 cm in greater diameter is usually a sign that NF Type I is present.

8   Williams, P. Gail and Joseph Hirsch, "Brief Report: The Association of Neurofibromatosis Type 1 and Autism." *J of Autism and Devel. Disorders*; (28) No.6; December 1998; Mouridsen, S.E. et al. "Neurofibromatosis in infantile autism and other types of childhood psychoses." *Acta Paedo Psychiatr*, 1992; 55 (1): 15-18; Ferner, R.E. "Neurofibromatosis 1 and neurofibromatosis 2: a twenty first century perspective." *Lancet Neurol.* 2007; 6:340-351.

NF Type II, which is less common than Type I NF, generally manifests during the adolescent years with acoustic (ear) nerve-related symptoms like ringing in the ears (tinnitus), hearing loss, and poor balance. Tumors elsewhere in the brain and spinal cord may also occur, for which surgery is often necessary. Café-au-lait spots occur as in Type I NF, and other manifestations include cataracts, balance and vision problems, and headaches. This type is not associated with autism. The genetic defect in this condition occurs on chromosome 22.[9]

Both Type I and Type II NF are autosomal dominant conditions, meaning if one parent has NF, there will be a 50 percent chance that any child of theirs will have the condition.

The rarest type, called *Schwannomatosis*, effects Schwann cells which encase nerves and act as insulators. Tumors, called Schwannomas, develop in these Schwann cells, which can cause intense pain. This type is also not associated with autism.

These three conditions arise due to specific genetic mutations and may occur spontaneously (50 percent) or be passed down from affected parent to child. The only treatments available are surgery to remove tumors, radiation therapy to shrink tumors, and certain medications to relieve pain. These therapies only provide symptomatic relief, as they do not cure these conditions.

What Is Williams Syndrome (WS) AKA Williams-Beuren or Elfin Faces Syndrome?

This rare (up to 1 in 20,000) neuro-developmental disorder was first identified in 1961 by Dr. J. Willams of New Zealand and is caused by a deletion of approximately 26 genes from the long arm of chromosome 7. Children who are born with Williams Syndrome appear to have diminished intelligence (average IQ is 70) and have distinctive features like a thin, pixie-like face with a low nasal bridge.

WS children generally appear cheerful and are typically not frightened of strangers. They have fair to good language skills, often have perfect pitch, are often left-handed, and tend to hyper-focus on the eyes of someone they are interested in. WS children are often overly sensitive to certain frequencies and intensities of sound, a symptom that they share with many autistic children. Many exhibit increased anxiety.[10]

The characteristic "Williams personality" is described in the literature as "a love of company and conversation combined, often awkwardly, with a poor understanding of social dynamics and a lack of social inhibition."[11]

WS individuals may have a narrowing of the large artery (the aorta) that leaves the heart (supravalvular aortic stenosis), other abnormally small caliber major arteries, high blood pressure (due to the narrowed arteries), and heart murmurs. Episodic elevations of blood calcium levels may occur.

Individuals with WS share a number of similarities with autistic children. In addition to sound sensitivity (hyperacusis) and anxiety, both disorders tend to have more individuals who exhibit inflexibility, ritualism, obsessiveness, developmental delays, attention deficits, cognitive disabilities, and savant abilities.

The syndromes differ, however, in many respects. WS individuals tend to be very social. They make good eye contact, have rich vocabularies, and like to converse, although their conversation often jumps from one topic to another. Autistics often appear to prefer living in their own world, they often don't make good eye contact, and they have difficulties in communicating orally. Autistics generally have normal to above average IQ scores, whereas WS people have lower intelligence quotients.

There is no cure for Williams Syndrome. Some WS adults may be able to work in a structured environment. Most will need adult support throughout their lives. A geneticist should be consulted if Williams Syndrome is suspected so

9   Ferner Ibid.

10   Martens, M.A., Wilson, S.J., Reutens, D.C. (2008). "Research Review: Williams syndrome: a critical review of the cognitive, behavioral, and neuroanatomical phenotype." *J Child Psychol Psychiatry* 49 (6): 576–608.

11   Dobbs, David (July 8, 2007). "The Gregarious Brain." *New York Times.* http://www .nytimes.com/2007/07/08/magazine/08sociability-t.html. Retrieved 2007-09-25.

that appropriate genetic testing can be done to confirm the diagnosis. Contact the Williams Syndrome Association for more details.[12]

What Is the Fragile-X Syndrome (FXS)?

The Fragile X syndrome is the most commonly seen (1 out of 4600 births) cause of inherited mental retardation. As is true of most disorders, its presentation ranges from mild (some learning difficulties) to severe (significant cognitive impairment, seizures, and developmental delays).

This X-linked recessive syndrome, which has three subtypes, is transmitted via an abnormal X chromosome donated by the mother. The abnormal fragile-X chromosome contains a mutated gene called FMR1 which, if *not* mutated, would code for a protein (FMRP/Fragile-X Mental Retardation Protein) that normalizes cell signaling in the brain.

Mutations in this gene (which typically consist of an excess number of repeats [>200] of the CGG sequence, which codes for a particular amino acid in the FMRP protein) induce the silencing of the gene by a process called "methylation." This silencing prevents the production of the Fragile-X Mental Retardation protein, the absence of which manifests as "overactive transmitters that send out too much information."[13]

The "X" and "Y" chromosomes are the sex chromosomes. Females have two X chromosomes and males have one X and one Y chromosome, so if a male child inherits the abnormal X chromosome from his mother, he will manifest the symptoms of Syndrome X because the Y chromosome does not code for the FMR1 gene and is, therefore, unable to protect the child from the consequences of the mutated gene. Female children who inherit the abnormal X chromosome from their mother will also receive a normal "protective" X chromosome from their father and will either be not affected at all or minimally affected (learning disabilities, slight decrease in cognitive function).

A minority (15-33 percent) of individuals with the Fragile-X diagnosis will qualify as being autistic using the Childhood Autism Rating Scale (CARS). Conversely, about 2-6 percent of autistic individuals will be found upon testing to carry the Fragile X gene.[14]

Many of the commonly observed symptoms of the Fragile X Syndrome like hand flapping, hand biting, poor eye contact, social anxiety, and shyness are also commonly noted in autistics. However, most boys with FXS are quite social, as opposed to those with autism, who generally prefer social isolation. Boys with FXS are almost always mentally retarded and, at puberty, commonly develop unusually large testes. Other physical characteristics seen in many (but not all) fragile-X afflicted individuals include large ears, an elongated face, and high arched palate.

Don Bailey and coworkers found that 25 percent of the boys with FXS also were autistic and that when a boy had both diagnoses, his IQ appeared to be lower than that found in boys with just one of the two diagnoses. This study was confirmed by others.[15]

Interestingly, levels of the Fragile X protein (FMRP) *did not correlate* with the presence or absence of autism, indicating that *the autism component's additive effect was likely due to other genetic and/or environmental factors.*[16]

Although there is currently no treatment available for Fragile X Syndrome individuals, there is hope that a proposed new treatment may someday be able, at least partially, to correct this condition.

MIT neuroscientist Mark Bear hypothesized that a class of drugs known as mGluR5 inhibitors might one day be able to reverse some of the pathology underlying not only Fragile X Syndrome disease but perhaps even autism itself.

12   Finn, Robert (1991). "Different Minds." *Discover Magazine* (June 1991). http://www.nasw.org/finn/ws.ht ml; Pinel, J. P. J. (2008). *Biopsychology* (7th ed.). Boston: Allyn & Bacon; Gillberg, C. and Rasmussen, P. "Brief Report: Four Case Histories and a literature review of Williams Disorder and Autistic Behavior." *J of Autism and Devel. Disorders*. 24:381-392, 1994.

13   Myrick, L.K. et al. "Independent role for presynaptic FMRP revealed by an FMR1 missense mutation associated with intellectual disability and seizures." *PNAS*. Published online January 5 2015 doi:10.1073/pnas.1423094112.

14   www.fragilex.org

15   Bailey, D. et al. 2001 *Journal of Autism and Dev Disorders* 31(2): 165-174; Rogers, S. et al. 2001 *Journal of Developmental & Behavioral Pediatrics* 22(6): 409-417.

16   Bailey, D. et al. 2000. *J of Autism and Dev Disorders*. 30(1): 49-59.

Bear has experimented with a type of mouse that harbors a fragile-x protein-like gene that causes the mouse cells to manufacture the abnormal FMRP protein, which, by some unknown mechanism, interferes with learning. The production of certain specific proteins is essential for normalizing basic cellular processes involved with memory, and inhibitors of the mGluR5 gene are theorized to be of possible help in this regard.

Dr. Bear realized that drugs that inhibit the mGluR5 gene already existed, and by adjusting protein levels with these drugs, it might just be possible to reverse this condition.

Dr. Bear has founded Seaside Therapeutics to research this possibility further. Testing of an mGluR5 inhibitor drug (from Merck) on Fragile X patients was scheduled to start in 2011.[17]

Unfortunately, a trial of Seaside Therapeutics' fragile-x test drug, *arbaclofen*, had to be suspended prematurely in 2013 for lack of funding. The drug appeared to be helping many children with the condition, but did not appear to help with the symptom of social withdrawal, which was the one specific endpoint of the trial.

One mother, whose son was one of the trial participants, found arbaclofen to be extremely beneficial. "The drug trial proved to be life changing," she wrote. "It was a double blind trial, nothing changed during the placebo time…everything changed when he went on the real thing. For the first time ever, my son said, unprompted…"I love you mom."[18]

Sudden discontinuation of *baclofen*, a related drug, can initiate withdrawal symptoms similar to those seen in benzodiazepine or alcohol dependence withdrawals.[19]

What Is the Landau-Kleffner Syndrome (LKS)?

The Landau-Kleffner Syndrome is a rare and very mysterious condition. It is seen in normally-developing children with normal hearing between the ages of 3 and 7 years, and it presents inexplicably as the sudden or gradual onset of an inability to understand the spoken word (auditory agnosia). This progresses and eventually affects the child's spoken (expressive) language, which may regress to a complete loss of the ability to speak. The child becomes mute. Abnormal brain electrical activity and seizures (seen in 70-80 percent) are common in most LKS children, and these symptoms start at about the time the auditory agnosia is noted. Many have prolonged nighttime seizure-like electrical discharges (status epilepticus), and the longer these persist, the longer the time between onset and recovery.[20]

LKS children appear to have normal intelligence, and most are able to communicate by writing or by using sign language. By the age of 15, most of those afflicted do not show any further signs of abnormal brain activity or seizures. The ability to speak and understand language may return in whole or in part in a few, but difficulties comprehending and speaking often persist into adulthood. LKS is not believed to be an inheritable disorder.

Children with LKS are not autistic, but the sudden regression in spoken language abilities seen in these children parallels in some ways the regressions seen in delayed onset autism. In both conditions, abnormal EEGs and seizures are common (much less so in autism). Pain insensitivity, aggression, poor eye contact, dislike of change, and sleep problems are other symptoms that are shared in the two conditions.[21]

The similarities have led to speculation that there may be a physiological relationship between them.[22] Teresa Binstock has suggested a possible viral connection and encourages further research in this regard.[23] Researcher A. Connolly and colleagues, in a study published in *The Journal of Pediatrics*,[24] demonstrated that children with autism and an LKS variant syndrome had increased amounts of both serum IgG and IgM auto-antibodies to certain brain proteins as compared to control patients.

17   Langreth, Robert. "Mark Bear's Fight to Decode Autism." *Forbes Magazine*. Dec 06, 2010.
18   http://www.socialjusticesolutions.org/2013/05/16/what-happens-when-a-drug-trial-ends-and-a-childs-health-fails/
19   http://en.wikipedia.org/wiki/Baclofen
20   Robinson, R.O. et al. *Developmental Medicine and Child Neurology*. 2001; 43:243–247.
21   www.autism.com
22   Mantovani, John. *Developmental Medicine & Child Neurology*. (2000) 42:5:349-353.
23   www.autismworld.com
24   1999, Vol. 134, Issue 5. p. 607-613.

The authors conclude that, "The presence of these antibodies raises the possibility that autoimmunity plays a role in the pathogenesis of language and social developmental abnormalities in a subset of children with these disorders."

Conclusions: We have shown that autism is not just a "psychiatric condition." It is a highly complex systemic illness that affects the immune system, the brain, and the gut. This implies that to have any hope of reversing this condition, it will be necessary to address all of the biochemical and physiological abnormalities associated with this disorder.

In addition, it will be essential that exposures to possible environmental autism "triggers" be reduced or eliminated.

In Part II of this book, we will discuss some of the genetic factors associated with autism, and there are many. The numerous likely environmental causes of autism and ADHD are revealed in Part III.

The reader will soon learn that the scientific investigations into the factors that have given rise to this devastating epidemic of damaged children and adults have been marred by deceitful and flawed studies, corrupt politicians, and conflicted scientists, individuals, corporations, and institutions.

We believe that the information presented in this book will show, beyond a reasonable doubt, that this is so. The reader must decide for him- or herself whether or not we have proven our case.

Part II
The Etiology of Autism and ASD
The Genetic Component

"All things appear and disappear because of the concurrence of causes and conditions. Nothing ever exists entirely alone; everything is in relation to everything else."

— *Buddha*

Chapter 5
The Basics

"The world isn't ready for some people when they show up,
but that shouldn't stop anyone."

— *Ashly Lorenzana*

WHY DO WE *Believe that Genetics Plays a Role in Autism?*
The evidence that suggests that autism (and related conditions) have a genetic component is very strong. It comes from the fact that identical twins, as compared to fraternal twins or non-twin siblings, are much more likely both to be autistic, if either one is, and from research into the mutations in genes that appear to be involved in promoting this condition.

There is clearly no one genetic defect that causes autism, but rather, it is the interplay of a variety of undesirable mutations coupled with adverse environmental influences that appear to be the causative factors that promote the autistic state.

The next three chapters will delve into the role some of the genetic mutations so far investigated play in this regard.

What Is DNA (DeoxyriboseNucleic Acid)?

The template that determines the position of each amino acid in every protein is encoded in our DNA (found in the chromosomes located in our cell nuclei). DNA is shaped like a twisted ladder, and the frame and rungs are constructed of chains of substances called nucleotides. When the body desires that a particular protein be made, part of the DNA untwists and the unsilenced genes in that segment are then able to transfer their chemically-coded information to ribosomes, cellular structures that assemble the desired protein.

What Is RNA?

The transfer of the genetic information from DNA to ribosomes is accomplished by utilizing the unique properties of RNA (RiboseNucleic Acid), a molecule with a structure similar to that of DNA, which is able to copy the desired genetic information from the DNA and then travel to the ribosome, where the genetic information for creating the desired protein is transferred.

What Are Nucleotides?

Nucleotides are substances making up the structure of DNA molecules. DNA contains two chains of nucleotide molecules, which themselves consist of three parts: the phosphate group that binds the nucleotides in each chain together, a sugar, and a base section that attaches one chain to its twin. These are depicted schematically in the diagrams below.

There are only four different nucleotides in DNA, and they are designated by the letters C, G, A, and T (for cytosine, guanine, adenine, and thymine). It takes three pairs of these to form the code for a particular amino acid. As it turns out, adenine only bonds with thymine, and cytosine only bonds with guanine. Relatively weak hydrogen bonds hold the two strands of DNA together, and this allows the DNA strands to separate when the cell divides or if a segment of the DNA needs to be unraveled so that its code may be copied and transferred to the ribosomes, the protein assembling components of the cell.

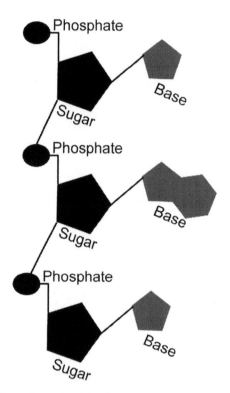

Figure 5.1. A section of a polynucleotide chain with each individual nucleotide bonded together.

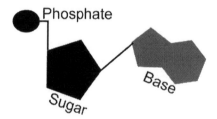

Figure 5.2. The basic unit of a polynucleotide chain is the nucleotide.

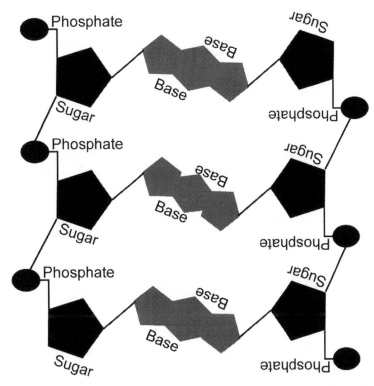

Figure 5.3. Typical DNA strand with one nucleotide chain bonded with another.

What Are Genes?

A gene is simply a segment of the DNA molecule that contains the complete code for one or more proteins. The coded instructions are copied by a messenger RNA molecule and taken to the ribosome, the "factory" of the cell, where the proteins are assembled from available amino acids.

How Does All of This Work?

Not all amino acids are used to make proteins, but there are about twenty that are so utilized. The order in which these amino acids appear in the proteins is vital to their functioning. If the wrong amino acid is substituted for the optimal one, or is simply missing, or if the correct amino acid is replicated too many times, a dysfunction is likely to result.

This can occur if there are mutations in the DNA genes. These may be thought of as being akin to errors in spelling. A word is misspelled if a wrong letter is substituted for the correct one or if a correct letter is missing (deleted) or repeated too many times. In the same way, a protein can be "misspelled" if the wrong amino acid in a sequence is substituted for the correct one, or if an amino acid is deleted or repeated too many times, and this can affect its function adversely.

Mutational mistakes in the placement of one or more of the four DNA nucleotides may be inherited or may arise due to exposure to toxic chemicals or radiation.

Geneticists refer to these genetic "misspellings" (mutations) as polymorphisms, a word that means "many shapes". Very often, there is only one misspelling (mutation) in the DNA due to the wrong nucleotide. This is called a single nucleotide polymorphism or SNP, (pronounced "snip") which will result in an abnormal protein or enzyme being formed.

SNPs are generally listed by the code letter for the optimal nucleotide followed by a number that represents where in the protein structure the substitution has taken place. That number is followed by the code letter for the undesired nucleotide, the one that causes the mutation. See Appendix II for more information and illustrations in this regard.

What Is Epigenetics?

A gene does not have to be mutated in order for one's genetic instructions to be adversely affected. Normally, genes are turned on and off in the body as they are needed or not. Negative environmental factors, like exposures to certain toxic substances, for example, can inappropriately prevent or increase the silencing of genes, which can have untold undesirable consequences not only for the individual so affected, but also for his or her progeny, as these acquired abnormalities that are able to switch genes off and on can persist and be passed on from one generation to the next. Epigenetics is the science that studies the factors that switch genes off and on.

A recent landmark study has shown that newly acquired genetic information in the form of RNA may be carried by cellular entities called "exosomes," which can then be passed directly from body cells to sperm cells, thereby adding a new non-DNA pathway to our understanding of the genetic inheritance of traits.[1]

What Genetic Abnormalities Are Common in Autism?

The following chapters go over some particularly relevant genetic abnormalities. A good review of the many other rare genetic abnormalities associated with autism may be seen at: http://www.ncbi.nlm.nih.gov/books/NBK1442/

---

1   Cossetti, Cristina et al. "Soma-to-Germline Transmission of RNA in Mice Xenografted with Human Tumour Cells: Possible Transport by Exosomes." *PloS One* 2014; 9(7):e101629. Epub 2014 Jul 3. PMID: 24992257.

Chapter 6
The Metallothionein Connection

"Don't let your baggage define your travels, each life unravels differently."
— *Shane Koyczan*

WHAT ARE METALLOTHIONEINS *(met TAL-low-THIGH-oh-neens)?*

The theory that may best explain and account for most of the features and characteristics noted in autistic individuals is that of metallothionein (MT) dysfunction or deficiency in association with oxidative damage.

It is suspected that MT dysfunction plays a role in many, but not necessarily all, autistic individuals, and it is clear that many other genetic influences as well as environmental stressors also play key roles in promoting this often devastating condition.

In February 2000, William Walsh, Ph.D. and director of the Pfeiffer Treatment Center came to the conclusion that "most autistic patients exhibit evidence of diminished metallothionein (MT) activity and (that)…many of the classic features of autism can be explained by a compromised metallothionein system."[1]

The metallothionein family of metal-binding proteins is found throughout the body. They are short, linear, S-shaped chains of amino acids and are rich in *cysteine*, an amino acid that is capable of binding to toxic metals like mercury and lead. Each metallothionein molecule (depicted below) can bind up to seven zinc ions and thirteen copper ions.

What Do Metallothioneins Do?

The metallothioneins function to:

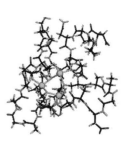

- Regulate zinc and copper levels in the blood. Autistic individuals tend to have abnormally high copper to zinc ratios in their serum.

- Detoxify mercury and other harmful metals. Autistic individuals tend to have higher levels of mercury (and probably many other toxic substances) than do non-autistics.

- Regulate the development and function of the immune system. Impaired immune function is common in autistics.

- Regulate the development and pruning of brain neurons. This can lead to larger brains, a characteristic of autism.

---

1   Walsh, W.J., Usman, A., and Tarpey, J. "Disordered Metal Metabolism In a Large Autism Population." Proceedings of the Amer. Psych. Assn.; New Research: Abstract NR109, New Orleans, May, 2001.

- Prevent yeast overgrowth in the GI tract. Intestinal yeast and bacterial overgrowth are commonly observed in autistic individuals.

- Produce enzymes that break down casein and gluten (DPP-IV). Impaired DPP-IV (dipeptidyl peptidase IV) enzymatic function in the intestine leads to an increase in abnormal morphine-like peptides that are commonly noted in autistics.

- Respond appropriately to intestinal inflammation. It is believed that autistic individuals exhibit intestinal inflammation and its associated side effects (like "leaky gut") at higher rates than do non-autistic individuals.

- Produce stomach acid. Maldigestion and impaired breakdown of foods will occur with reduced production of stomach acid (hydrochloric acid), which can lead to malnutrition and food allergies. These are common findings in autistic individuals.

- Regulate taste and texture discrimination on the tongue. Extreme fussiness about the taste and texture of foods is also a characteristic found in most autistic children.

- Normalize hippocampal function and behavior control. The hippocampus is a brain structure that plays a role in long-term memory, spatial awareness, and possibly behavior inhibition. Dysfunctions in this area are characteristic of the autism population.

- Normalize the development of emotional memory and socialization. Dysfunctions in these areas are also typically noted in autistic individuals.

Do Autistic Children Tend to Have Low Levels of Metallothioneins?

Yes. Dr. Walsh found that autistic children tend to have significantly less metallothionein proteins than do age-matched controls.

The chart on the following page illustrates this relative deficiency.

Metallothioneins may also be found in sufficient amounts in autistic indivduals, but may be inactivated or disabled by a variety of mechanisms or they may be dysfunctional as a result of improper structure (mutations).

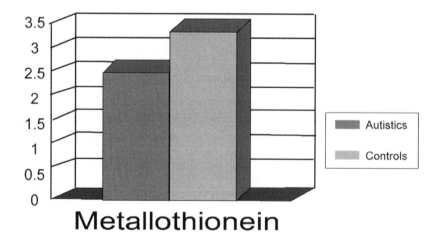

Figure 6.1. Low Metallothionein Levels in Autism $p < 0.0092$[2]

---

2   From: "An Epigenetic Model of Autism and a Warning Regarding Risperdal." Autism One Conference, Chicago, Illinois: May 2012

What Are the Factors that Disable (Inactivate) the Metallothioneins?

Dr. Walsh hypothesizes that autistic children probably have a genetic or acquired defect in the function, quantity, or activity of the metallothionein (MT) proteins. That is to say autistic children may have a deficiency or defect (a mutation) in the structure of the MT proteins that would make them less effective in their function and/or they might have normal MT proteins that have been rendered less functional, secondary to adverse environmental influences.

Examples of known biochemical factors that are capable of disabling metallothionein proteins include:

- Severe zinc depletion. Zinc, an essential component of the metallothionein molecule, is itself regulated by metallothioneins, and zinc depletion inactivates these essential proteins. Zinc is an important trace mineral that is also necessary for activating many fundamental biochemical reactions in the body that regulate immune function, hunger, taste sensation, digestion, metallothionein function, and other important processes.

- Abnormalities in the glutathione antioxidant system. Glutathione (GLUE-tuh-THIGH-own) is an important antioxidant peptide (a small protein) that also plays a key role in detoxification. It is composed of just three amino acids: glycine, cysteine, and glutamine. Anything that interferes with the transmethylation or transsulfuration cycles[3] may reduce the production of cysteine, glutathione, and the metallothioneins.

- A deficiency in cysteine. Cysteine ("SIS-tee-een") is an amino acid, and one of only four that contains a sulfur atom. It is a necessary part of many proteins (like the metallothioneins) and peptides (like glutathione). It also represents a necessary step in the manufacture of other important substances in the body. Cysteine is obtained both from the diet as well as being created as part of the trans-methylation pathway, which is often defective in children with autism and ADHD as we shall see.

- Malfunction of metal regulating elements.

- Genetic inherited modifications in the structure of the metallothionein proteins (mutations). It is likely that autism propensity is not determined by a single genetic defect, but rather by several genetic variances.

- Toxic metals like mercury, lead, and cadmium. According to Vanderbilt Univ. School of Medicine researcher M.C. Houston, "Mercury binds to metallothioneins and substitutes for zinc, copper, and other trace metals, reducing the effectiveness of metalloenzymes."[4]

- Even excess copper, an essential nutrient, has been shown to disable the metallothionein proteins temporarily.

- Pyrrole chemistry disorders. These can promote the loss of zinc and vitamin B6 into the urine.

- Impaired functioning of an antioxidant enzyme called super oxide dismutase (SOD). There are several varieties of this enzyme.

- Free radicals, emotional stress, infection, and inflammation may also deplete metallothioneins.

What Are the Four Varieties of Metallothioneins, and What Functions Do They Perform?

MT-I and MT-II are found throughout the body and function to regulate zinc and copper levels, promote the development of neurons and synaptic connections, normalize immune function, and detoxify heavy metals. MT-IV is found in the GI tract and functions in part as a barrier to the entry of toxic metals like mercury and lead.

MT-III functions to rid the brain of excess neurons during early infancy when the brain has an overabundance of small, densely-packed neurons. MT III eliminates the excess neurons, and by so doing, allows the remaining neurons to develop normally and make appropriate synaptic connections.

---

3   These terms refer to the transfer of methyl (a carbon with three attached hydrogen atoms) or sulfur molecules from one substance to another.

4   "Role of mercury toxicity in hypertension, cardiovascular disease, and stroke." *J Clin Hypertens* (Greenwich). 2011 Aug; 13(8):621-7.

As Dr. Walsh states in his book *Metallothioneins and Autism:* "An early MT-III dysfunction would be expected to result in (a) incomplete pruning (elimination of unwanted neurons), (b) areas of densely packed small neurons, and (c) increased brain volume and head diameter. All of these phenomena have been observed in autism."[5]

MT proteins are found in high levels in the hippocampal region in the brain, an area important in learning, memory, and behavior control. MT proteins are also found in the amygdala, a region important in the development of socialization skills and emotional memory.

Impaired MT function in early childhood would thus be expected to result in regressions in speech, behavior, socialization, and cognition if the damage were done when those particular areas of the brain were developing, generally before the age of three years.

According to Dr. Walsh, "After the age of 3, the brain may have matured sufficiently so that environmental insults can no longer provoke autism."[6]

MT proteins are also found to be abundant in the pineal gland, which manufactures melatonin, a master regulating hormone, and which is essential for normalizing sleep cycles. Many autistic children have sleep disturbances, and melatonin has been found in a number of studies to be helpful in this regard.

Mice with deficient MT proteins have an increased incidence of seizures and a severely impaired immune system; both concerns are seen at increased frequency in autism.

MT proteins ferry zinc, an essential element in immune functioning, to peripheral tissues, including the immune cells in the thymus and lymphoid system. If zinc is not transported in sufficient amount, the cellular immunity is weakened. This results in overproduction of a transcription factor associated with inflammation called NF kappa-B and the release of inflammatory mediators like Interleukin 6 (IL-6), which in turn overstimulate the humoral antibody response.

Metallothioneins are also excellent antioxidants. Macrophages and neutrophils are immune cells that kill germs like bacteria and viruses by releasing toxic substances, including hydrogen peroxide. After an infection with bacteria or viruses, there is an increased amount of this peroxide left behind that must be neutralized by enzymes like the metallothioneins. *Impaired metallothionein function would, therefore, be expected to leave a child vulnerable to the effects of vaccines and to be hypersensitive to a variety of infectious agents.*

Metallothioneins are "heavy metal magnets." They bind these toxic elements tightly and render them relatively harmless. Deficiencies in metallothionein functioning would, therefore, be expected to lead to an increased burden of these dangerous substances, and that, indeed, is what we find in autistic children.

Metallothionein proteins are found at very high concentrations in intestinal linings. There they "capture" any heavy metals that are present in the gut, which discards its mucosal cells every 3-10 days. If MT proteins are deficient in the GI tract, heavy metals are more readily able to enter the bloodstream and disable important enzyme systems. MT proteins are also found in high concentrations in the liver, kidney, and the blood-brain barrier.

Since it is impossible to avoid exposures to heavy metals, especially in today's toxic environment, an efficient MT system is essential for good health. The average adult ingests 20 mcg of mercury each day (much more if we eat certain fish) of which about 1 mcg is absorbed into the bloodstream.

The metallothioneins also bind to copper and regulate its absorption into the bloodstream. Once absorbed, copper is bound to ceruloplasmin, a copper-binding protein. Autistic children tend to have increased copper in the bloodstream and decreased ceruloplasmin. This results in an excess of free copper, an oxidizing agent that can damage organ systems and inactivate metallothionein from functioning.

---

5   p. 11
6   Ibid. p. 12.

Excess copper has been shown to be associated with hyperactivity, learning difficulties (short-term memory failure, trouble concentrating), anxiety, and impulsive behaviors, all of which are commonly seen in autistic children.

Metallothioneins also function in the synthesis of certain digestive enzymes (carboxypeptidase and aminopeptidase), which help break down food proteins, including gluten and casein. The MT proteins donate zinc, which activates DPP IV, a gut enzyme that breaks down gliadorphin, casomorphin, and other morphine-like toxic peptides that form when certain foods, like dairy (casein), gluten-containing grains, and soy are ingested. Elimination of gluten, casein, and soy from the diet of most autistic children often results in marked improvements in functioning.

Researcher Karl Reichelt has found increased amounts of gliadorphin, casomorphin, and other opioid-like peptides in the urine of autistic children as opposed to non-autistic controls. This will be discussed in more detail later in this book.

Metallothioneins are found on the tongue and normalize sensations of taste and texture. Autistic children are often incredibly sensitive to the taste and texture of foods that they sample, which makes them incredibly "picky" eaters.

In the stomach, metallothioneins protect against inflammation, enhance the production of stomach acids, and activate digestive enzymes. Low stomach acid output results in an inadequate production of secretin from the duodenum. Secretin is a hormone that stimulates the pancreas to "dump" its digestive enzymes into the digestive tract.

Sub-optimal hydrochloric acid production in the stomach will, therefore, result in a diminished output of secretin, which in turn results in insufficiently broken down food proteins, which may then leak through the gut mucosa and promote food allergies. Impaired hydrochloric acid and secretin production will also result in the insufficient digestion and assimilation of many nutrients necessary for optimal physiological functioning. Despite some allegedly negative studies, secretin remains an effective remedy for a significant number of autistic children.

Impaired MT function also offers us an explanation for the predominance of autism and ADHD in males. It has been found that the "female hormones," estrogen and progesterone, induce the manufacture of metallothioneins, so females would be expected to have higher levels of metallothioneins than males and, thus, be offered some protection in this regard. Testosterone, a "male hormone," has been shown to enhance the toxic effects of mercury, which again places males at a biochemical disadvantage.[7]

If the MT system isn't functioning properly, then impairment of the brain, liver, and kidneys may result, and a dysfunctional immune system, digestive tract, and problems with learning, behavior, speech, socialization, and impaired enzyme functioning are likely to occur.

The Pfeiffer Clinic approach has been to treat autistic children with high copper to zinc ratios with an initial supplement of zinc ("Pfeiffer Primer III") for 6-8 weeks followed by an amino acid supplement ("MT Promoter II"). During the zinc-loading phase, amino acids, glutathione, and selenium should be withheld. A too rapid reduction in copper sometimes causes increased stimming and irritability. Dosing the zinc in a pulsatile manner often reduces these potential side effects.[8]

The Pfeiffer Clinic practitioners also attempt to identify intestinal bacterial imbalances and correct these. They also remove the toxic metals using chelation or clathration protocols and supplement with appropriate nutrients and digestive enzymes. This methodology has resulted in improved functioning in up to 90 percent of autistic children; however, there are some who get no benefit or who have had side effects (increased stimming, graying of hair, etc).

---

7   Geier, M., Geier, D. "Testosterone: A Key to Understanding Mercury-Autism Link." *Autism Research Review.* Vol. 19, No. 1, 2005.
8   Walsh, W.J. et al. *Metallothioneins and Autism.* 2nd ed. Naperville, IL: Pfeiffer Treatment Center, 2002.

Chapter 7
Other Genetic Abnormalities Associated with Autism Spectrum Disorders

"There is very little difference in people, *but that little difference makes a big difference.*"

— *W. Clement Stone*

WHAT ARE METHYLATION *Dysfunctions?*

Methylation refers to the addition of a methyl group to another molecule. A methyl group, as has been stated, is simply a carbon atom with three hydrogen atoms attached. Very often, this methyl group is passed like a football from one molecule to another, a process that biochemists refer to as "trans-methylation." These important reactions are carried out with the assistance of enzymes, all of which are proteins, and proteins are simply collections of amino acids joined end-to-end.

Why Are Trans-Methylation Pathways Relevant to Autism?[1]

Folic acid (also known as "methyl*ene* tetrahydro folate") is one of the "B vitamins" and has several forms, but unfortunately, it is inactive (non-functional).

To make this B vitamin useful the "methyl*ene* portion of the molecule must be transformed ("reduced" chemically speaking) to a methyl group. This is done with the assistance of the enzyme methylene tetrahydrofolate reductase (MTHFR), which converts the inactive folic acid molecule (methyl*ene* tetrahydrofolate) into the active, functional molecule 5-<u>methyl</u> tetrahydrofolate.

methyl group

5-methyl tetrahydrofolate then is able to donate its methyl group to cobalamin, another name for vitamin B12, turning it into *methyl* B12 (also known as *methyl* cobalamin).

This is accomplished with the assistance of yet another methyl passing enzyme (methionine synthase (MS), which first transfers the methyl group from the methylated folic acid to the B12 molecule and thence from the methylated B12 molecule to homocysteine, thereby converting it into methionine, a vitally important amino acid. The end result of these rapid chemical reactions is an increase in methionine and a consequent decrease in homocysteine, a potentially harmful amino acid.

---

1   See Figure 3.1. The Trans-methylation and Trans-Sufuration Cycles in Chapter 3.

When methionine is not being synthesized in sufficient amounts due to dysfunctions in either the MTHFR enzyme or the methionine synthase enzyme (or an insufficiency in the diet), a great many biochemical abnormalities may, and often do, result.

For example, methionine is necessary in the manufacture of cysteine, one of the amino acids found in large amounts in the metallothionein proteins and in glutathione. With insufficient cysteine, it is possible that not enough metallothioneins and glutathione are made. Without enough metallothioneins and glutathione, antioxidant protections are impaired and detoxification of harmful substances declines.

Glutathione is an extremely vital substance that helps combat free radical damage in the body (i.e., it is an antioxidant). It also activates a variety of enzyme systems (including the metallothioneins) and is a premier detoxification agent in its own right (it helps remove mercury and other toxic metals).

SAM (S-adenosyl methionine) is also made from methionine and is another important methyl-donating molecule. It is particularly important in melatonin (the sleep hormone) and neurotransmitter production. When genes are methylated, they "turn off." That is, they are unable to code for proteins. SAM plays a role in this regard as well. If synthesis of methionine is reduced (or is insufficient in the diet), then SAM production also declines. SAM is often effective therapeutically for such conditions as depression and arthritis.

What Effects Do Common Mutations in the MTHFR (5, 10-Methylene Tetrahydrofolate Reductase) Enzyme Have in Autistic Children?

"Overall the data show an increased risk of autism spectrum disorders associated with common mutations affecting the folate/methylation cycle."

— *Marvin Boris,* J Amer Phys & Surg *(9); No.4 Winter 2004*

Research shows an increased risk of autism associated with certain MTHFR mutations. Two common ones are the C677T and the A1298C SNPs.

These mutations, which may be inherited or acquired, have been shown to promote the risk of having attention deficit disorder and hyperactivity (ADHD), and are seen in autism at a greater frequency than in non-autistic controls.

Marvin Boris and colleagues retrospectively examined the lab data of 168 consecutive referrals to their facility of children with confirmed diagnoses of either autism or PDD. All the children had a DNA evaluation to determine the frequency of the C677T and A1298C polymorphisms.

What they found was that the C677T mutation was significantly more common in autistic children than in controls, and, surprisingly, the A1298C was more common in controls, but that autistics had significantly more combined mutations (both the C677T and the A1298C) than did controls.

The authors conclude that "Overall the data show an increased risk of autism spectrum disorders (ASD) associated with common mutations affecting the folate/methylation cycle."[2]

Other Evidence that Mutations in MTHFR Promote Attention Disorders

"Preliminary data imply a strong relationship between MTHFR polymorphisms and the inattentive symptoms of ADHD in survivors of childhood (leukemia)."

— J Pediatr. *2008 Jan; 152(1):101-5*

---

2   Boris, M. et al. *J of American Physicians and Surgeons.* Vol. 9; No.4; Winter 2004:106-108.

The chemotherapy used to treat cancers, like childhood leukemia, can damage the DNA. This is one way that acquired mutations may occur. Children who survive acute lymphocytic leukemia (ALL) after chemotherapy appear to have a high risk of developing the inattentive sub-type of ADHD.

A study published in the journal *Pediatrics,* January 2008, sought to clarify whether particular mutations in MTHFR enzymes could account for the variations in ADHD that develop in a high percentage of children after chemotherapy.

What they found was that 11 of the 48 children (c 23 percent) had scores consistent with an attention disorder. "Patients with genotypes related to lower folate levels (11 out of 39; 39.2 percent) were more likely to have ADHD. The A1298C genotype appeared to be the predominant linkage to the inattentive symptoms, leading to a 7.4-fold increase in diagnosis, compared with a 1.3-fold increase for the C677T genotype. Age at diagnosis and sex were not associated with inattentiveness."

The authors conclude that their "Preliminary data imply a strong relationship between MTHFR polymorphisms and the inattentive symptoms of ADHD in survivors of childhood ALL."[3]

Defects in the MTHFR enzyme (that activates folic acid) cannot always be overcome by providing more folic acid; however, if the active form of folic acid is provided (5 methyl tetrahydrofolate), then the mutation may be successfully bypassed.

What Are Methionine Synthase (MS) Mutation Dysfunctions and How Do They Promote Autism?

This ubiquitous enzyme plays at least two major roles in the biochemistry of the body. In both reactions, it synthesizes methionine, an important amino acid, from homocysteine by attaching a methyl group to homocysteine.

Methionine synthase (meh-THIGH-oh-neen SIN-thase) is found in most cells of the body where it is responsible for transferring the methyl group from either SAM or 5-methyl THF (active folic acid) to cobalamin (inactive vitamin B12) and thence to homocysteine. The addition of a methyl group to homocysteine converts that substance into methionine.[4]

Homocysteine can also be *reversibly* converted to SAH (S-adenosyl homocysteine) with the help of the enzyme SAHH and an adenosine molecule.

If one follows the trans-methylation pathway,[5] it is apparent that methionine can be converted to SAM (S-Adenosyl Methionine), which can then be converted to SAH (S-adenosyl homocysteine), which can be *reversibly* converted back to homocysteine. Since SAH can be turned into homocysteine and homocysteine can be converted back into SAH (if there is enough adenosine handy), a failure of methionine synthase to convert homocysteine to methionine will result in a decrease in methionine production,and an increase in the conversion of homocysteine to SAH.

As has been pointed out in Chapter 3 (Table 3.2), elevated levels of SAH and low levels of methionine are precisely what we find in many autistic children.

Decreased methionine synthase activity will also result in a decreased production of S-adenosyl methionine, and low levels of this important methyl donor are indeed noted in autistic children at increased frequency (Table 3.2).

The problem with excess SAH is that it *inhibits methylation reactions* and *decreases methionine synthase activity*. This promotes a vicious cycle where decreased MS activity causes an increase in SAH which in turn inhibits MS activity. The end result is reduced DNA methylation, which may manifest as alterations in gene expression, decreased melatonin production, and impaired development.[6]

---

3   J Pediatr. 2008 Jan; 152(1):101-5.

4   Muratore, C.R., Deth, R. *PLoS One.* 2013; 8(2): e56927. Published online 2013 February 20. doi: 10.1371/journal .pone.0056927 PMCID: PMC3577685. Age-Dependent Decrease and Alternative Splicing of Methionine Synthase mRNA in Human Cerebral Cortex and an Accelerated Decrease in Autism.

5   See Figure A.1. The Trans-methylation and Trans-Sufuration Cycles.

6   Deth, Richard; Waly, Mostafa. "Effects of Mercury on Methionine Synthase: Implications for Disordered Methylation in Autism." Fall Defeat Autism

"Methionine synthesis activity is important for normal attention, (and) a decrease in its activity may contribute to ADHD."

— Richard Deth, PH.D.

The second known function of MS (methionine synthase) was revealed by Ph.D. biochemists Richard Deth (pro-nounced "deeth") and his coworker Mostafa Waly. They discovered that the MS enzyme is also located snaking through the membranes of neurons (brain cells) in the region of a receptor (the D4 receptor) for the neurotransmitter dopamine. This is illustrated in figure 7.1. Part of the MS enzyme is located outside the membrane. Part is within the membrane, and part is in the interior of the cell.

Dopamine has many functions in the brain and is necessary for the maintenance of focus and attention. In order to exert its affects on a brain cell, a dopamine molecule must first attach to the D4 receptor. The docking of dopamine to this receptor initiates a series of biochemical changes in the cell that ultimately result in the opening of a channel that allows calcium to enter the cell.

The role of methionine synthase (MS), remember, is to transfer the methyl group from methylated folic acid (5-meth-yl tetrahydrofolate) to B12 (cobalamin) and then to a homocysteine molecule, which in this instance is located in the D4 receptor. This reaction converts the homocysteine molecule into methionine, which can then donate the newly acquired methyl group to a membrane substance called a phospholipid.

Ethanolamine (ETH-uh-NOLE-uh-meen) is one such phospholipid. When ethanolamine is methylated (receives a methyl group) the membrane of the cell becomes more fluid.

Another methionine-containing molecule (labeled MET 313 in figure 7.1) located in the part of the MS molecule that appears inside the cell is also able to donate a methyl group to ethanolamine. This reaction happens quite rapidly-up to 50 times per second![7]

In this diagram (fig. 7.1) of the Dopamine D4 receptor the methionine synthase enzyme (an essential part of the recep-tor) is depicted as a protein with a lot of hairpin turns winding in and out of the cell. One end (upper left) terminates in an -NH2 group and the other in a –COOH group. The hypervariable portion will tend to promote attention deficits if it contains seven or more repeats of a particular sequence of amino acids. The phospholipids are depicted as circles (the "head-groups") attached to fatty acids (the wiggly lines). The cytoplasm comprises all the substances inside the cell.[8]

The addition of methyl groups to the nearby phospholipids causes an increase in the spacing between phospholipid head-groups and alters the fluid properties of the membrane in the region surrounding the receptor.

According to Dr. Deth, "The activity of membrane proteins located near the D4 receptor can be modulated by this phospholipid methylation, and this "solid-state signaling" mechanism has been implicated in the molecular mecha-nism of attention."[9]

"Proline-rich segments [proline (PRO-lean) is an amino acid] present in the cytoplasmic portion of the receptor (the part inside the cell membrane) in all species allow it to serve as a docking site for signaling proteins that become targets for phospholipid methylation-based modulation.

"In humans and other primates, the D4 receptor possesses anywhere from 2 to 11 additional proline-rich repeat seg-ments (see diagram above), and a higher number of repeats (i.e., seven or more), as has been mentioned, brings an increased risk of attention-deficit hyperactivity disorder (ADHD). Thus methionine synthase activity is important for normal attention (and focus), while a decrease in its activity may contribute to ADHD."[10]

Now! TM 2003 Conference. Portland, Oregon. October 3-5, 2003.
7   Deth; Ibid.
8   From Deth, R. and Waly, M. Ibid.
9   LaHoste, G.J., Swanson, J.M., Wigal, S.B., Glabe, C., Wigal, T., King, N., & Kennedy, J.L. (1996) *Mol. Psychiatry* 1, 121-4.
10   Deth, R.C. *Molecular Origins of Human Attention.* Boston, MA: Kluwer Academic Publishers, 2003.

Heavy metals and thimerosal, a mercury-containing preservative still used in immunizations, may interfere with the ability of growth factors like IGF-1 to promote development by impairing their control over methionine synthase.

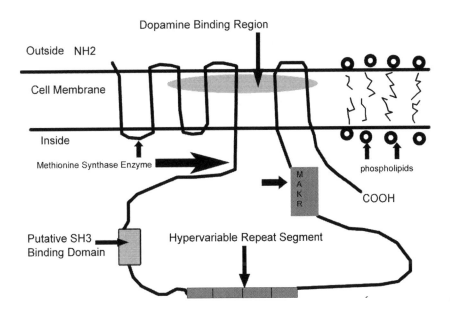

Figure 7.1. The MS enzyme snaking through membranes of neurons in the region of the D4 receptor for the neurotransmitter dopamine. [11]

What Are COMT (Catechol O-Methyl Transferase) Mutation Dysfunctions, and How Do They Promote Autism?

As was previously discussed, (COMT) aids in transferring a methyl group, donated by SAM (S-Adenosyl Methionine), to dopamine, epinephrine, and nor-epinephrine. Chemists call these substances catecholamines (CAT-uh-COAL-uh-means).

"Methylating" these neurotransmitters *inactivates* them. Epinephrine (also called adrenalin) and norepinephrine are also manufactured by the adrenal gland, and dopamine is also made by certain intestinal cells, so the catecholamines may be considered to be both neurotransmitters (when made in the brain) and hormones (when made in the body).

Many children with autism or attention disorders may possess aberrant forms of the COMT enzyme (it has several variations) and either under-methylate (minimally inactivate) or over-methylate (over-inactivate) the catecholamine neurotransmitters.

These variances in COMT functioning cause neurotransmitter imbalances that effect mood, attention, and activity. Individuals with low enzyme (COMT) activity will tend to have higher levels of dopamine, epinephrine, and norepinephrine. Those with overactive COMT enzymes will have low levels of these substances.

What Is Dopamine?

Arvid Carlsson won the 2000 Nobel Prize in physiology or medicine for his discovery of dopamine's role as a neurotransmitter. Dopamine has many effects both in and outside of the central nervous system. One of its main functions is to inhibit the release of the hormone prolactin. Dopamine also helps coordinate and control our movements.

---

11   Adapted from diagram in Deth & Waly study (Ibid).

The death of dopamine-generating neurons is commonly associated with Parkinson's disease. In addition, dopamine plays a vital role in memory, attention, and problem solving.

Dopamine is commonly associated with the brain's "pleasure system." It stimulates feelings of enjoyment and motivates us to do, or continue doing, certain activities, like eating and engaging in sexual activities. Even anticipating something pleasurable will cause the release of dopamine. It is the *neurotransmitter of desire.*

Low levels of dopamine (brought about by drugs or otherwise), are associated with a decline in *desire* for pleasurable activities; however, if pleasurable activities do occur, they are enjoyed just as much.

A normal variant of the gene for catechol-O-methyl transferase "has been shown to affect cognitive tasks broadly related to executive function, such as response inhibition, abstract thought and the acquisition of rules."[12]

Dopamine also helps us prioritize which objects or events are likely to be important in both pleasurable and potentially harmful ways. Major disruptions in the dopamine system have been associated with psychoses, including schizophrenia.

An interesting way to assess dopamine levels clinically is to count the number of blinks per minute. The average number of blinks is 15-30 per minute. The blink rate has been found to vary with the amount of dopamine present: the more dopamine, the more the blinking rate and vice versa.

What Is Epinephrine's Role?

Epinephrine (also called "adrenalin") is implicated in arousal, whether this takes the form of anxiety, excitement, or fear. Within the body, adrenaline acts in such a way as to maintain an activated state, allowing a higher state of energy to be produced.

What Is Norepinephrine's Role?

Norepinephrine functions to improve memory and attention and allows us to inhibit certain behaviors via its stimulation of certain specific neuronal receptors (alpha 2 adrenergic receptors). It is also produced (like epinephrine) in the adrenal glands in response to stress.

Many studies implicate nor-epinephrine neurotransmitter system dysfunctions in causing attention deficit disorders. It is likely that insufficient stimulus of the norepinephrine receptor in the brain promotes attention deficits. This disorder may be due to inadequate production of norepinephrine or to abnormalities in the receptor for this hormone.

---

12   Wikipedia

Chapter 8
G-Alpha Protein Abnormalities and the Vitamin A Connection

"There is in us all that line that prevents us from fully understanding those who are different."

— *Leon Uris*, QB VII

WHAT ARE G-ALPHA *Proteins?*

The G-alpha proteins (also called Guanine [GWA-neen] nucleotide-binding proteins or simply "G proteins") are a family of enzymes located just *under* the cell membrane, which are coupled to receptors located *on* the cell membrane.

They function as "molecular switches" that turn on and off a variety of other necessary chemical reactions in the cell. The G-proteins were discovered and their functions elucidated by scientists Alfred Gilman and Martin Rodbell, which won them the Nobel Prize in Physiology and Medicine in 1994.

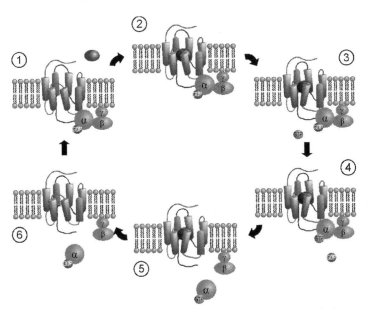

Figure 8.1. Activation cycle of G-proteins by G-protein-coupled receptors.[1]

---

1   Wikipedia

What Is the Connection Between G-Protein Abnormalities and Autism?

In 1999, Dr. Mary Megson of the University of Virginia presented her research findings in regard to how G-alpha protein abnormalities in *genetically susceptible children* promote the autistic state.[2]

Her article, "Is autism a G-alpha protein defect reversible with natural vitamin A?" was published in the journal *Medical Hypothesis* in 2000.[3]

Dr. Megson discovered that G-alpha protein receptors on the surface of cells were disrupted in autistic children with *genetic susceptibilities to this defect*. The abnormal G-alpha protein receptors found in autistic children were also associated with defective receptors for retinoids (vitamin A and its chemical relatives) in the brain and intestinal tract.

Vitamin A is necessary for vision, the prevention of night blindness, sensory perception, immune function, language processing, and attention. Autistic children typically have concerns regarding sensory issues, language processing, and attention. Many show signs of immune system dysfunctions as well.

Children of families with a history of night blindness, pseudo-hypo-parathyroidism, or an adenoma (a benign tumor) of the thyroid or pituitary gland were found to be more prone to this G-alpha protein abnormality.

What Is the Connection Between G-Protein Abnormalities, Pertussis, and Measles Immunizations and Autism?

Dr. Megson found a connection between the measles and pertussis (whooping cough) vaccinations and G-alpha protein defects.

She discovered that the *pertussis endotoxin* found in the DPT[4] vaccine (normally injected at 2, 4, 6, and 18 months of age) separates the G-alpha protein from retinoid (vitamin A) receptors. It also promotes a chronic auto-immune reaction (an infiltration of a kind of white blood cell called a monocyte) in the deep layer (lamina propria) of the gut lining (mucosa).

This in turn leads to a chemical disconnect of the G-alpha protein pathways and the regulating retinoid (Vitamin A) switch, which then results in the non-specific branch of the immune system being turned on. Unfortunately, *without the proper functioning of the retinoid switch, the immune system can't be turned off!* The end result is an inflamed intestinal tract.

The measles virus, a component of the MMR vaccination (typically injected at 12-15 months of age and again at 4-5 years of age), also plays a role in the G-alpha protein problem.

The measles vaccination is associated with lower vitamin A levels, and only vitamin A *in its natural form* as cis-retinoic acid, and not as beta-carotene or Vitamin A Palmitate, can activate the retinoid receptors.[5]

Dr. Megson found that there is an important difference between natural vitamin A ("cis-retinoic acid-found in fish oils) and the synthetic vitamin A palmitate found in infant formulas and commercial vitamins.

The artificial vitamin A palmitate binds the free G-alpha protein, and by so doing, deactivates the "off switch" for multiple metabolic pathways involved in vision, cell growth, hormonal regulation, and the metabolism of lipids (fats), proteins, and glycogen, a storage form of glucose.

The antibodies to the measles virus that form as a result of the measles or combined measles, mumps, and rubella (MMR) immunization may also disrupt the "molecular glue" that connects one cell to another, which is so essential

---

2   Defeat Autism Now Conference, 1999
3   (54)6: 979-983.
4   Since c. 2001-2004 the DTaP vaccine has been used instead of the DPT, and has much less endotoxin than does the DPT immunization.
5   Sporn, M., Roberts, A., Goodman, D. *The Retinoids: Biology, Chemistry and Medicine.* Raven Press, 1994: 231.

to cell-to-cell communication and gut mucosal integrity. The absorption of vitamin A from the intestinal tract requires an intact gut mucosal surface, the right acidity (pH) and the presence of bile.

Is There a Way to Bypass This Genetic Abnormality?

Fortunately, Dr. Megson was able to find a simple and inexpensive solution for this biochemical dilemma: cod liver oil and urocholine (Bethanecol).

This protocol has been used in over 500 patients without any side effects. In the first phase, loading with vitamin A in its natural form (preferably from toxin-free cod liver oil) is started and continued for 2-3 months. This is followed by the introduction of *Bethanecol*, a parasympathetic nervous system stimulator that promotes the utilization of vitamin A in cells. Bethanecol can only be obtained by prescription from a licensed medical practitioner.

This treatment is especially effective for those experiencing any of the following symptoms: malabsorption, divergent gaze, speech delay, dry skin, poor social skills, night blindness, soft stools, and dry eyes.

Table 8.1. The recommended dosage of mercury & *dioxin-free cod liver oil*

20-30 lbs	850-1250 IU
31-45 lbs	2500 IU
46-75 lbs	3750 IU
76-125 lbs	5000 IU
>125 lbs	7500 IU

Good brands of cod liver oil include Nordic Naturals, Eskimo 3, Pharmax, Carlson's, and Kirkman's. Quality fish oils should have little or no fishy smell and be certified dioxin and mercury free.

Bethanecol comes as thin, scored 10 mg tablets. They can be halved or quartered or crushed and dissolved in water. Bethanecol remains stable in a watery solution for at least thirty days. Don't start the Bethanecol until the child has been on the cod liver oil for at least two months. Continue the cod liver oil while on the Bethanecol.

Table 8.2. Suggested oral daily dosages of *bethanecol* are as follows:

Less than 5 years	start with 2.5 mg
5-8 years	start with 5-7.5 mg
Above 8 years	start with 10 mg
Maximum dosage is	12.5 mg

If the initial dosage of bethanecol doesn't result in signs of improved functioning, then the dose may be increased by increments of 2.5 mg per dose to maximum of 12.5 mg. *A sign of too much bethanecol is constricted pupils.*

Part III
The Environmental Connection to Autism and ASD

"All truth passes through three stages:
First it is ridiculed,
Second, it is violently opposed, and
Third, it is accepted as self-evident."

— *Arthur Schopenhauer (1788-1860)*

Chapter 9
The Immunization Link—General Principles

"Whenever you find yourself on the side of the majority,
it is time to pause and reflect."

— Mark Twain

WHAT THEORIES AND *Evidence Underlie the Supposition that Immunizations Might Be a Causative Factor in Autism?*

It has been suggested by various researchers that:

1. The mercury-containing preservative, thimerosal, (AKA Merthiolate and thiomersal) found as a preservative in many immunizations (especially prior to 2001) promotes the autistic state. Mercury is a known neurotoxin, and starting in the late 1980s, babies and young children in the U.S.A. were receiving more and more immunizations each year, which increased their cumulative mercury load. The supposition is that certain children have inherently defective mechanisms for removing toxic substances like mercury and lead, which places these children at especially increased risk. As we shall see, there is overwhelming evidence to support this contention.

2. The pertussis toxin found in the DPT (and to a lesser extent in the DTaP) immunizations, could promote autism by uncoupling G-alpha proteins from the retinoid (vitamin A) receptor (as per Dr. Megson).

3. The measles immunization, a component of the MMR vaccine, which contains live attenuated viruses, could promote autism by lowering vitamin A levels, by disrupting the tight junctions between the cells that line the intestinal tract (as per Dr. Megson) and by other means (to be discussed).

4. The measles virus vaccination could promote autism in some children by inducing autoimmune reactions that could negatively affect brain function. This will also be addressed subsequently.

5. In some children, the measles component of the MMR immunization appears to induce abnormal overgrowth of the lymphoid follicles (collections of immune cells) that line the intestinal tract and, through auto-immune and other mechanisms, promote the autistic state. This theory has been largely attributed to the inappropriately maligned Dr. Andrew Wakefield, and is supported by many knowledgeable practitioners and other research and will be discussed at greater length in subsequent chapters.

6. The MMR (measles, mumps, and rubella) immunization may disrupt the balance between two amino acids: glycine and glutamate (glutamic acid), and this imbalance may damage neurons and promotes autism. The Center for Promoting Optimal Outcomes™, LLC alleges to have evidence supporting this view.

7. The use of acetaminophen (Tylenol, etc., but not ibuprofen) in conjunction with the MMR has been shown to increase significantly the risk of becoming autistic.

8. Adjuvants (additional substances like aluminum and squalene), which are and have been added to certain vaccines, have neurotoxic potential and may act in a synergistic fashion with other known neurotoxins like mercury.

9. There is a significant association between the onset of the dramatic rise in autism and the parallel rise in the number of immunizations that children were being given, and in particular, with the immunizations preserved with thimerosal, a mercury-containing preservative and with those that contain aluminum.[1]

10. There is evidence that demonstrates a significant increase in autism and ADHD in those children who have been immunized vs. those who haven't been. Evidence to support this contention comes from a number of studies, including the unmanipulated Verstraeten study (to be discussed later), the Generation Rescue Study, the Hepatitis B study, and from the observation that unvaccinated populations have an extremely low risk of autistic spectrum disorders.

11. Many parents have noted the onset of autistic symptoms and developmental regression in their child in close temporal proximity to a recently given immunization. This information comes from many thousands of anecdotal reports to physicians and other healthcare providers and from data compiled by the Autism Research Institute.

12. Antibiotics may also cause harm and promote autism. Many babies and young children receive antibiotics for ear infections or for other reasons. Antibiotics invariably deplete beneficial gut bacteria and allow the overgrowth of harmful organisms, which in turn may promote inflammation and prime the body for a pro-inflammatory response. Subsequent immune challenges from infections or immunizations might then trigger brain inflammation that results in autism.

13. Conjugate vaccines, like the HIB (Hemophilus Influenza B) and pneumococcal and meningococcal vaccines, may promote autism by "tricking" the body into utilizing certain immune cells to react to the carbohydrate coating on these bacteria. Doing so bypasses the normal blunted immune response of babies and young children to carbohydrate antigens. This blunted response may be protective in that it diminishes the likelihood of auto-immune reactions, which antibodies to carbohydrate substances appear to promote. There is evidence for antibodies to carbohydrate structures in the brain, and the rise in autism prevalence parallels the introduction and increased use of the HIB and other conjugate vaccines.

Do Any Studies Compare Vaccinated and Unvaccinated Children With Regard to Autism Risk?

Yes and no. There are several studies and anecdotal reports that come close, but the CDC, which has the data to accomplish this task (Vaccine Safety Datalink), steadfastly refuses to do or publish such a study. What follows is the best that we have thus far.

The Generation Rescue Study

On June 26, 2007, the results of a phone survey commissioned by Generation Rescue and conducted by "SurveyUSA" were released. The survey, based on interviews of almost 12,000 households, involving 17,674 children, compared vaccinated and unvaccinated children in nine counties in Oregon and California and found that for the 9,000 or so boys aged 4-17 evaluated, vaccinated boys were two and a half times more likely to have neurological disorders compared to their unvaccinated peers.

Vaccinated younger boys were 224 percent more likely to have attention deficit disorder and 61 percent more likely to have autism. For the older population of boys, aged 11-17, the vaccinated boys were 158 percent more likely to have a neurological disorder compared to the unvaccinated males in this age group. They were also 112 percent more likely to have autism and 317 percent more likely to have ADHD.

---

1   McDonald, Michael E. and Paul, John F. "Timing of Increased Autistic Disorder Cumulative Incidence." *Environmental Sci Technol.* 2010. 44, 2112-2118.

The older boys, who were born during the 1990s, would have been exposed to a greater number of immunizations preserved with thimerosal than were boys born after 2003, and they were found to have a higher incidence of autism and neurological disorders. The methodology used by the researchers "closely mirrored that used by the Centers for Disease Control and Prevention (the CDC) to establish the national prevalence for neurological disorders like (ADHD), Asperger's Syndrome, (PDD-NOS) and autism."[2]

For female children evaluated in this study, no significant neurodevelopmental association was found between those who had been vaccinated and those who hadn't. This may have been due to the fact that autism is 4-5 times more common in males than in females and that autism spectrum disorder females, as we have pointed out, are often not diagnosed as having this disorder, or are misdiagnosed, or are diagnosed much later than are males with autism spectrum disorders.

The CDC has conducted similar phone surveys to ascertain the prevalence of autism and found them to be reliable.[3]

This phone survey study is not without its limitations and needs to be repeated on a larger scale to confirm or rebut the startling findings. Generation Rescue, the sponsor of this study, encourages this, and it suggested that the CDC or other governmental agency conduct a larger nationwide survey comparing vaccinated and unvaccinated children in regard to possible adverse neurological outcomes.

In 2006, three members of Congress from both parties—Carolyn Mahoney (D), Maurice Hinchey (D), and Ron Paul (R)—sponsored a bill titled "The Comprehensive Comparative Study of Vaccinated and Unvaccinated Population Act of 2006" (H.R.2832), which would have required the NIH to complete this research. The bill was introduced June 22, 2007, but was referred to the Sub-Committee on Health, where it died and so never became law.

Representative Carolyn Mahoney reintroduced the bill (H.R.3069) in June 2009 with three Republican and five Democratic cosponsors, and it was again referred to committee, this time the House Committee on Energy and Commerce, where it apparently died an untimely death. It was introduced again in 2013, and has suffered the same fate again.

One must ask what forces are rallied against doing this research. Are we afraid to find out the truth about vaccinations and neurodevelopmental harm? The answer appears to be "Yes," and the reasons for this are not that difficult to discern and will be discussed later in this narrative.

The Amish

The majority of the Pennsylvania Dutch population does not routinely immunize their children, according to Dr. Frank Noonan, a family practitioner in Lancaster County Pennsylvania, who has treated autistic families and their children for over twenty-five years. Indeed, "Among the Amish in Lancaster County, Pennsylvania, investigators found that only 16 percent of children aged 6 months to 5 years were fully immunized."[4]

"I have not seen autism with the Amish," Dr. Noonan states. "You'll find all the other stuff, but we don't find the autism. We're right in the heart of Amish country and seeing none, and that's just the way it is."[5]

Dan Olmsted also investigated the Amish population of Lancaster County in Pennsylvania for evidence of autism in their children. Based on the national incidence of autism, he calculated that there should be 130 autistic children in the Amish community he surveyed. He did find four. Three of these had been vaccinated and the fourth had been exposed to high levels of mercury from a power plant.[6]

---

2   http://www.generationrescue.org/resources/vaccination/cal-oregon-unvaccinated-survey/

3   http://web.archive.org/web/20061107223258/http://www.cdc.gov/od/oc/media /transcripts/ASD *MMWRfactSheet.pdf*

4   Wenger EK, et al. "Underimmunization in Ohio's Amish: Parental Fears Are a Greater Obstacle than Access to Care." *Pediatrics*; Pub. Online June 27, 2011 http://pediatrics.Aappublica-tions.org/content/early/2011/06/23/peds.2009-2599.full.pdf+ html

5   "The Age of Autism; Amish Bill Introduced; Expected to show that vaccination is associated with autism." Published: July 28, 2006 at 10:35 AM by Dan Olmsted, UPI Senior Editor.

6   Kennedy, Robert F. Jr. "Deadly Immunity." *Rolling Stone.* Jun 20, 2005.

In another study, researchers mailed 1000 questionnaires regarding immunization beliefs to randomly selected Amish residents of Holmes County, Ohio. However, only 37 percent chose to respond. Of the respondees, 68 percent stated that all of their children had received at least one vaccination; 17 percent had at least one child who had received at least one vaccination, and 14 percent had never immunized their children. Reasons for not vaccinating or incompletely vaccinating were mostly related to vaccine side-effect concerns. This study suffers from the unusually poor response rate to the survey questionnaire. Also of note, the survey did not address the autism rate among the Amish in the population surveyed.[7]

Homefirst Medical Services

The late Dr. Mayer Eisenstein, Medical Director of Homefirst Medical Services, a large Chicago-based medical practice, did not believe that the alleged benefits of immunizations outweighed their risks. He encouraged his clientele not to get immunized or have their children immunized. He contended that he had treated upwards of 30,000 children in his practice over the years and states that, "I don't think we have a single case of autism in children delivered by us who never received vaccines."[8]

The Israeli-Ethiopian Population Study

Jews have traditionally lived in Ethiopia for millennia. They have lived largely in the Gondar province and called themselves Beta Israel. In the early 1980s, Ethiopia made the practice of Judaism illegal and banned the teaching of Hebrew. Jews were actively discriminated against and lived largely in very poor and unsanitary conditions. Ethiopians, in general, including the impoverished Jewish community, were by and large unvaccinated.

A large exodus of Ethiopian Jews to Israel occurred between 1989 and 1991, and today over 36,000 Jews of Ethiopian descent live in Israel.

A study was published in 2003 by Kamer, Zohar, and others, which reviewed a national registry of Israeli Jewish children who had been diagnosed with pervasive developmental disorder (PDD-largely autism), 1004 in all.

The investigators analyzed the prevalence of PDD[9] in subgroups of Israeli children in the years from 1983 to 1997 and made a remarkable discovery. Of the 11,800 Ethiopian children who had been born abroad and had not received the usual childhood vaccinations, *not one had been diagnosed with a pervasive developmental disorder*. There was no autism!

Of the 15,600 children of Ethiopian descent who had been *born in Israel* and had been given the usual childhood vaccinations, the prevalence of PDD (8.3/10,000 population) was similar to that noted in the Israeli population overall (9 cases/10,000 population).[10]

Comment: As Dr. Yazbak points out, "This review is as close as anyone can get to an unvaccinated versus vaccinated study without undertaking such a study, and a Zero PDD count among Ethiopian-born children in Israel should be convincing enough that the issue is by no means settled, as some would like us to believe."[11]

The Verstraeten (et al.) Study

Additional powerful evidence that vaccines and mercury cause autism comes from a CDC-sponsored study by Thomas Verstraeten (et al.) which, prior to devious statistical manipulation by Verstraeten under the direction of the CDC, showed significant and dramatic increased risks for autism, ADD/ADHD, and other neuro-developmental disorders in babies who were exposed to maximum amounts of thimerosal by three months of age as compared to babies who had received no immunizations by that age. This study will be discussed in detail later in this narrative.

---

7   Wenger Op. Cit.
8   Olmsted, D. Ibid.
9   PDD is pervasive developmental disorder and includes autism.
10   Kamer, A., Zohar, A.H., Youngmann, R., Diamond, G.W., Inbar, D., Senecky, Y. "A prevalence estimate of pervasive developmental disorder among Immigrants to Israel and Israeli natives." *Soc Psychiatry Psychiatr Epidemiol.* 2004 Feb; 39(2):141-5.
11   http://www.vaccinationnews.com/20110121AutismVaccinationImmigrantsYazbakFE

The Gallagher (et al.) Hepatitis B Study

Researchers at New York's Stony Brook University Medical Center analyzed information obtained from the National Health Interview Survey 1997-2002 data-sets to estimate the effects of the Hepatitis B vaccination on autism spectrum disorder (ASD) risk among boys aged 3-17 with shot records, adjusted for race, maternal education, and two parent-household.

They found that boys who received the hepatitis B vaccine during the first month of life had an almost threefold risk of being diagnosed with an autism spectrum disorder compared to boys who received the vaccination later or who were never vaccinated to hepatitis B. The risk was greatest for non-white boys.[12]

It should be pointed out that *all the boys* who were evaluated in this study and were immunized with the hepatitis B vaccine at one month or less *would have received the vaccine preserved with thimerosal.* Thimerosal was not removed from this vaccine until after 2003. (Thimerosal was listed as an ingredient at 25 mcg/dose in this product in the 2003 PDR.) A three-year-old boy in 2002 would have been immunized in 1999 if he had the first hepatitis B vaccination at age one month or less.

It is common for babies to receive their first dose of hepatitis B vaccine on the day of their birth and a second dose at the one-month checkup. The hepatitis B vaccine did contain aluminum as an adjuvant and still does. Aluminum is neurotoxic and, when combined with mercury from thimerosal, is additionally much more toxic.

In the next several chapters, we will present convincing evidence linking mercury and thimerosal with autism.

"Don't let schooling interfere with your education."

— *Mark Twain*

---

12   Gallagher, C.M. et al. "Hepatitis B Vaccination of Male Neonates and Autism." *Annals of Epidemiology.* Vol. 19, No. 9 ABSTRACTS (ACE) September 2009: 651-680. p. 659.

Chapter 10
The Evidence Linking Thimerosal and Mercury to Autism

"Only the small secrets need to be protected.
The big ones are kept secret by public incredulity."

— *Marshall McLuhan*

WHAT IS THIMEROSAL *(also called Thiomersal)?*

Thimerosal (thigh-MER-oh-sal) is a mercury-containing preservative with antibacterial and anti-fungal properties. The mercury in thimerosal is readily metabolized in the body to an organic form known as "ethyl" mercury (generally written as one word: "ethylmercury").

Thimerosal was invented and patented in 1927 and marketed several years later by the pharmaceutical giant Eli Lilly and Company as Merthiolate. It is still (2015) found in multi-dose vaccines (like most multi-dose influenza vaccines and certain tetanus booster sera), skin test antigens, tattoo ink, and a variety of over-the-counter and prescription products like some nose sprays and eye drops.

Thimerosal is extremely toxic and can poison by inhalation and even by direct contact with the skin.[1]

It has been found to be very toxic to animals and was banned from the market as an over-the-counter topical antiseptic for humans in 1982 because of harmful side effects. It continues to this day (2015) to be found in vaccines for influenza and diphtheria/tetanus boosters, and was present in virtually all childhood vaccines (except the MMR and polio vaccines) prior to 2001.

It is an *unstable* molecule that readily breaks down in the presence of oxygen and copper (both found in the human body and in all mammals) into highly toxic ethyl mercury and thiosalicylate.[2]

Research has shown that thimerosal is slowly *bactericidal* (kills bacteria) and is mainly *bacteriostatic* (doesn't kill the organism but prevents its growth). According to Engley, a scientist in the biological department at Camp Detrick in Maryland, "This bacteriostasis is even nullified by the presence of many types of sulfur compounds...*body fluids* and other organic matter."[3]

Thimerosal is also not a particularly good preservative because, as has been stated, *it spontaneously breaks down and loses its potency over time.*

---

1   Clarkson, T.W. "The three modern faces of mercury." *Environ Health Perspect.* (2002) 110 (S1): 11–23.
2   Kharasch, 1932. "Stabilized Bactericide and Process of Stabilizing It." U.S. Patent 1,862,896.
3   Engley, F.B. 1950. "Evaluation of Mercury Compounds as Antiseptics." *Ann NY Acad of Sc* 53:1970206.

Its method of action involves the mercury portion of the molecule reacting with the sulfhydryl group (a sulfur attached to a hydrogen atom) of bacterial enzymes.

Unfortunately, these same sulfur hydrogen groups are plentiful in the human body, including in human serum, which consequently binds to the thimerosal and thereby lessens its ability to inhibit bacterial enzymes.

Thimerosal tends to settle to the bottom of vaccine vials, which if not shaken prior to use will cause the individual receiving the vaccine to receive less or more thimerosal than is recommended by the pharmaceutical manufacturer.

Thimerosal is also *more toxic to human and animal cells than it is to bacteria.*[4]

> *"You couldn't even construct a study that shows thimerosal is safe. It's just too darn toxic. If you inject thimerosal into an animal, its brain will sicken. If you apply it to living tissue, the cells die. If you put it in a petri dish, the culture dies. Knowing these things, it would be shocking if one could inject it into an infant without causing damage."*
>
> — *Professor Boyd Haley*

What Studies Demonstrated the Safety and Efficacy of Thimerosal?

A Relevant Timeline

1927: Thimerosal was first synthesized by Morris S. Kharasch and a patent was applied for and granted (in collaboration with Eli Lilly and Co.).[5]

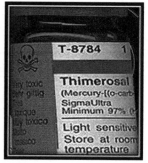

1930: The first evaluation of thimerosal (brand name: "Merthiolate") was conducted prior to its release in 1930 by Eli Lilly and Company, which still owns the patent rights to the product.

In this initial "safety study" by Smithburn and colleagues, thimerosal was given *intravenously* (up to 50 cc of a *1 percent solution*), not to healthy volunteers, but to twenty-two patients with meningococcal meningitis, an extremely serious and often fatal condition that can also cause neurological damage in any survivors. There was no control group!

Seven of the patients were followed for only one day, because *they were all dead by the second day!* The remaining fifteen, all of whom died during the study, were followed for less than sixty-three days, far too short a period of time for the typical signs of *chronic* mercury poisoning to become apparent.

Incredibly, the researchers concluded that Merthiolate "did not appear to have any deleterious action." Smithburn and his coworkers conveniently ascribed the deaths and all adverse reactions to the meningitis![6]

And Smithburn's patients were evaluated only for evidence of shock or anaphylaxis (a severe allergic reaction) and not for signs of mercury toxicity. There was no control group (placebo) in this so-called research!

Despite the obvious and serious flaws in this study, Eli Lilly readily agreed with Smithburn that the patients who succumbed had "died from meningitis, (and that) thimerosal was safe, and (so they subsequently) brought it to market."[7]

1930: Smithburn and his associates applied thimerosal (Merthiolate) topically to the noses of meningococcal carriers and were successful in eradicating the organism; however, *adverse symptoms were also noted.*[8]

---

4   "A Comparison of the Resistance of Embryonic Tissue and Bacteria to Germicidal Substances." *Proc Soc Exp Biol Med.* 32 (665-667; *Am J Pub Health,* (30) 129-137.

5   Wikipedia, *Encyclopedia Britannica*

6   Geier, D. et al. "A Review of Thimerosal (Merthiolate) and its Ethyl Mercury Breakdown Product..." *J of Toxic and Envir. Health, Part B,* 10; 579-596; 2007.

7   Bryan, Jepson. *Changing the Face of Autism.* p. 215.

8   Geier, Op Cit

1930: Merthiolate was now being marketed as a topical antiseptic for cuts, scratches, and superficial infections. Thimerosal was introduced in multidose vials of diphtheria toxoid vaccine. Its use as a preservative in the pertussis and tetanus vaccines and in the combined DPT shot also started in the early 1930s, but the widespread use of these vaccines in childhood did not occur until the late 1930s.

1931: Powell and Jamieson studied the effects of thimerosal (merthiolate) on animals and found that administering low doses of thimerosal to a variety of animals *caused acute toxicity in all and death in some,* yet they cited the Smithburn study and concluded that "the toleration of such intravenous doses [of thimerosal that Smithburn had used on the seriously ill meningitis patients] indicates a very low order of toxicity of Merthiolate in man."[9]

Their scientifically absurd conclusions regarding the safety of thimerosal have been repeatedly cited since that time as evidence of thimerosal's low potential for toxicity in humans.

1931: Vivian, the oldest of the eleven autistic children described in Dr. Kanner's landmark report, was born in a city that had just launched a campaign to eradicate diphtheria with the *new thimerosal-preserved diphtheria toxoid injection.* Many of the other ten children that Kanner described also had likely contact with mercury.[10]

1932: Morris Kharasch, the inventor of thimerosal, files another patent *that acknowledged the newly discovered toxicity of thimerosal* (Merthiolate). He notes that thimerosal, when "first made," appeared initially to be "entirely bland, both to skin and mucous membranes," but that *it breaks down rather rapidly* to form both ethyl mercury hydroxide and thiosalicylate compounds, and that the ethyl mercury derivative "might mediate adverse reactions in humans." And indeed it does![11]

1935: Kharasch tries again. He applies and receives a third patent for "organo-mercuri-sulfur compounds" (like thimerosal) in which he acknowledges his *continuing failure* to *stabilize thimerosal adequately* and prevent its breakdown into potentially toxic substances (like ethyl mercury). Or as he puts it, "Thimerosal and similar compounds)… without such stabilization tend to break down and form disassociation products…[which] both lose their effectiveness as antiseptic germicides (while) develop(ing) certain medicinally undesirable properties."[12]

1935: Researchers reveal that 50 percent of the dogs injected with various dilutions of serum preserved with thimerosal (Merthiolate in dilutions from 1:40,000 to 1:5,000) had adverse reactions, some of them serious.[13]

1935: Salle and Lazarus find that thimerosal is *35 times more toxic* to embryonic cells than it is to the bacteria that are the intended target.[14]

1937: S.L. Cummins does a study that involves injecting guinea pigs with 1 cc (about 1/5th of a tsp) of various dilutions of thimerosal, ranging from one part in a hundred *to one in ten million.* After just twenty-four hours, *all of the guinea pigs are dead.*[15]

1938: The FDA (Food & Drug Administration) starts mandating the safety testing of products. Thimerosal is "grandfathered in" since it is already in use, so no further safety testing is required (although further testing continues). Thimerosal is now being used as a preservative in all the DPT vaccines given to babies and young children. Also in 1938, Dr. Leo Kanner first becomes aware of the disorder that he would later label as "autism."

1939: Welch of the U.S. FDA does a study comparing the relative toxicities of thimerosal, iodine, phenol, and other preservatives then currently in use and finds *thimerosal to be many orders of magnitude more toxic than the others tested.*[16]

---

9   Powell, H. & Jamieson, W. "Merthiolate as a Germicide." 1931. *Am J of Hygiene* (13) 296 ff.

10   Age of Autism and ageofautism.com

11   Kharasch, 1932. "Stabilized Bactericide and Process of Stabilizing It." U.S. Patent 1,862,896.

12   Kharasch, 1935. "Stabilized Organic Mercuri-sulfur Compounds." US Patent 2,012,820.

13   Sub-committee on Humans Rights and Wellness. p. 34-35.

14   "A Comparison of the Resistance of Embryonic Tissue and Bacteria to Germicidal Substances." *Proc Soc Exp Biol Med* 32: 665-667.

15   "Merthiolate in the Treatment of Tuberculosis." *Lancet*, 962-963.

16   *J. Immunol* (37)525-533.

1940: Welch and his FDA colleague Hunter again measure the toxicity of thimerosal and nine other antibacterial agents and find that *thimerosal is the most toxic of the nine tested substances and almost seven times more toxic to human white cells and guinea pig cells than it is to bacteria.* They conclude, "It becomes obvious that if any antiseptic destroys the function of the leukocyte (white blood cell) much more readily than it kills bacteria there is little hope that it act efficiently as a chemotherapeutic agent."[17]

1943: Leo Kanner publishes his landmark study in the journal *Nervous Child* describing the first eleven cases of autism and names the condition. A number of these children likely had mercury exposure.[18]

1947: The FDA bans the use of mercuric chloride in baby's teething powders as it has been clear for many years that this toxic substance has been responsible for the epidemic of Pink Disease (Acrodynia), a sometimes fatal malady, with many symptoms similar to those noted in autistic children.

1971: Lilly restudies thimerosal and determines that it is "toxic to tissue cells," and that the concentration in vaccines was "100 times higher than the level it considered to be safe, but they continue to market it as non-toxic."[19]

1977: A Russian study showed brain damage in adults, years after exposure to *ethyl* mercury *chloride* (a fungicide). Ethyl mercury makes up half of the thimerosal molecule.[20]

Ten babies at a Toronto hospital died that same year when an antiseptic preserved with thimerosal was dabbed onto their omphaloceles (*an abdominal defect*).[21]

Also in 1977, Parry observed thimerosal induced significant *genetic alterations* in yeast cells at a level of less than one part per billion. This is the same amount that will kill human brain (neuroblastoma) cells (see Table 10.1).[22]

> *"According to Chang at the University of Arkansas, one microgram of thimerosal damages nerve tissue. It takes 70 days to eliminate half of it.... Glioma cells of the brain are destroyed at 0.2 ppm (parts per million) ionic mercury, and only 0.04 ppm of methylmercury.*
> *"Even the most resistant parts of the central nervous system are destroyed at 2.5 ppm. Ten ppm ionic mercury will induce cancer-causing DNA-DNA cross-links. This amount can also cause genetic defects....*
> *"The blood-brain barrier loses its protective selectivity at 1ppm within hours of administration of either ionic form or methylmercury.... One atom of mercury kills brain (cells)."*
>
> — Hal Huggins

1980: The Russians ban the use of thimerosal. All the Scandinavian countries plus England, Austria, and Japan *subsequently* ban this toxic preservative.

1982: The FDA (Food and Drug Administration) also concludes that thimerosal is toxic to cells and that it "caused cell damage, was not effective in killing bacteria or halting their replication" and that thimerosal was "not recognized as being safe or effective." The FDA called for the removal of thimerosal from over-the-counter products, but not from immunizations![23] In the early 1980s, more and more babies were receiving immunizations (DPT with thimerosal) prior to one year of age, and the autism incidence increased slowly in step with the rise in the number of babies immunized.

---

17   *Am J Pub Health* (30) 129-137.
18   Olmsted, Dan and Mark Blaxill. *Age of Autism.*
19   Geier, op cit &http://www.ageofautism.com/2015/01/more-evidence-of-harm-thimerosal-found-to-disrupt-mitochondrial-function-in-cells-from-people-with-autism.html?utm_source=feedburner &utm_medium=email&utm_campaign=Feed percent3A+ageofautism+ percent28AGE+OF+AUTISM percent29
20   Mukhtarova, N.D. 1977. "Late sequelae of nervous system pathology caused by the action of low concentrations of ethyl mercury chloride." *Gig. Tr. Prof. Zabol.* 3:4–7.In 1977.
21   Fagan, D.G., Pritchard, J.S., Clark56754772.son, 56754772.T.W., and Greenwood, M.R. 1977. "Organ mercury levels in infants with omphaloceles treated with organic mercurial antiseptic." *Arch. Dis. Child.* 52:962–964.
22   Parry, J.M. 1977. "The use of yeast cultures for the detection of environmental mutagens using a fluctuation test." *Mutat. Res.* 46:165–176.
23   *Federal Register.* 1982, vol 47, No.2

Table 10.1. Thimerosal Concentrations and Toxic Effects

Thimerosal Concentrations and Toxic Effects
1 ppb mercury = Kills human neuroblastoma cells (Parran et al. *Toxicol Sci* 2005).
2 ppb mercury = U.S. EPA limit for drinking water (http://www.epa.gov/safewater/contaminants/index.html#mcls)
20 ppb mercury = Dendritic cells damaged, calcium channels interrupted (UC-Davis MIND Institute, 2006).
200 ppb mercury = level in liquid the EPA classifies as hazardous waste (http://www.epa.gov/epaoswer/hazwaste/mercury/regs.htm#hazwaste)
600 ppb mercury = Level in a currently licensed Hepatitis B, multi-dose vaccine vial, labeled as "trace." This is administered at birth.
2,000 ppb mercury = 0.50-mL injections of thimerosal-containing vaccines (FDA CBER's definition of "trace").
ppb = parts per billion; ppm= parts per million

1986: The National Childhood Vaccine Injury Act becomes a law. This landmark legislation was formulated to create the basis for a national immunization program that would protect vaccine manufacturers and medical professionals from liability from vaccine injury. It would also establish the means by which those injured or killed by vaccines could be compensated via the Vaccine Injury Compensation Program (VICP), and it hoped to promote safer vaccines by encouraging vaccine research.

1988: The FDA again rules that thimerosal be removed from over-the-counter products, but it gives the industry another *sixteen years* to phase out thimerosal's presence. In 2015, thimerosal is still found in immunizations—influenza vaccines and tetanus (Td) boosters—in the U.S. and in many other immunizations given to children and adults in so-called "Third World" countries around the world.

The mercury-containing conjugate HIB vaccine is introduced and is phased in over the next two years. It is administered at 2, 4, 6, and 18 months of age. Autism incidence starts to rise dramatically.

1990: The CDC (Centers for Disease Control and Prevention) is *mandated* by Congress to track all vaccine-related adverse events and creates the VAERS (Vaccine Adverse Events Reporting System) database, which requires that all adverse events be reported.

1991: The FDA considers banning thimerosal from use in *animal* vaccines; however, it eventually reneges due to industry pressure.

That same year, a Merck vaccine developer (Maurice Hilleman) notes that six-month-old children who received their shots on schedule would get a mercury load up to *87 times higher* than allowed by guidelines for the maximum daily consumption of mercury from fish. Merck is able to and does manufacture thimerosal-free vaccines for Sweden, which has banned thimerosal, but continues to offer only thimerosal-preserved vaccines for American children.[24]

The hepatitis B vaccine is introduced and also contains thimerosal. It is given to babies on day one, at one month, and again at six months of life. It also contains neurotoxic aluminum as an adjuvant.

1997: New Jersey congressman Frank Pallone attaches an amendment to the FDA Modernization Act, which gave the Food and Drug Administration two years to "compile a list of drugs and foods that contain intentionally introduced mercury compounds and [to] provide a quantitative and qualitative analysis of the mercury compounds in the list."[25] The bill was signed into law on November 21, 1997.

---

24   *L.A. Times* article-memo obtained under the FOI Act.
25   21 USC 397 Section 413, 1997

1998: The FDA reviews thimerosal-containing products and finds *more than 30 licensed vaccines contain thimerosal.*[26]

The FDA finally bans thimerosal in over-the-counter products because "it is neither safe nor effective," However it does not enforce that ban. Thimerosal is allowed in over-the-counter products as long as it is not listed as an *active* ingredient.[27]

1999: The FDA and the CDC are startled to discover that the mercury exposure from vaccines exceeds Federal Safety Guidelines by a huge margin, and refer thimerosal to the Center for the Evaluation of Risks to Human Reproduction for further evaluation.

The American Academy of Pediatrics (AAP), the American Academy of Family Practitioners, and the U.S. Public Health Service recommend removal of thimerosal from vaccines "as soon as possible."

With no evidence to support their contention, the AAP assures parents that, "The current levels of thimerosal will not hurt children, but reducing those levels will make safe vaccines even safer." Some parents appropriately wonder how, if thimerosal is so safe, removing it can make vaccines "even safer."

In August 1999, a public workshop is held at Bethesda in the Lister Auditorium by the National Vaccine Advisory Group and the Interagency Working Group on Vaccines to consider thimerosal risk in vaccine use. And based on what was discussed in that conference, *thimerosal was ordered to be removed from the hepatitis B vaccine.*

Vaccine makers Merck and Smith-Kline-Beecham (later Glaxo-Smith-Kline) inform the CDC that thimerosal-free vaccines for hepatitis B and DTaP could be made available almost immediately. *Incredibly, the CDC does not take them up on their offer,* and mercury is still present at high levels in many of these vaccines until 2003, and possibly early 2004 (confirmed by 2003 PDR and by sampling of vaccines by Mark and David Geier in 2003 and by Professor Boyd Haley). It remains at high levels in several vaccines in 2015: influenza shots and tetanus-diphtheria (TD) boosters and others.

2000: A team of scientists measures the mercury levels in newborns and premature infants 48-72 hours after their first hepatitis B vaccination (which is generally injected on their day of birth) and finds that premature infants (average birthweight 748 grams) given this vaccination had much higher toxic levels of mercury than did term newborns (average birth weight 3,588 grams).[28]

It is interesting to note that these researchers were the first and apparently the only scientists to measure the blood levels of mercury before and after a thimerosal-containing vaccination. The CDC seemed to be concerned about this study not because of the potentially toxic effects this mercury load might have on newborns, but rather because they feared that immunization compliance rates would decline if the study's findings got out.[29]

2000: The CDC calls an *illegal secret meeting* to discuss the potentially terrifying consequences of Thomas Verstraeten's CDC-sponsored study and what needed to be done about it. Also present at the meeting are representatives of the American Academy of Pediatrics, the World Health Organization, and various vaccine manufacturers.

Dr. Verstraeten, an epidemiologist, was tasked by the CDC in 1999 to analyze the vaccine-related data on the CDC's own VSD (Vaccine Safety Datalink) files on over 70,000 children.

Verstraeten states at that meeting that his initial analysis of the data demonstrated a clear and convincing link between thimerosal dosage and developmental delays, attention deficit disorder, hyperactivity, tics, and speech delays.

---

26   Parker, S et al. *Pediatrics.* Vol. 114 No. 3 September 2004, pp. 793-804.

27   *Federal Register, Department of Health and Human Services, Food and Drug Administration.* "Status of Certain Additional Over-the-Counter Drug Category II and III Active Ingredients." (April 22, 1998); 63(77):19799-19802. 21 CFR Part 310 [Docket No. 75N-183F, 75N-183D, and 80N-0280.

28   Prevaccination blood levels were 0.04-0.5 μg Hg/L. The preterm infant levels rose to an average value of 7.4 μg Hg/L, whereas the levels in term infants were 2.2 μg Hg/L. These levels are similar to those expected from methyl mercury. (Hg is the symbol for mercury; L=Liter)

29   Stajich, G.V. et al. "Iatrogenic exposure to mercury from hepatitis B vaccination in preterm infants." *J Pediatrics.* 2000 May; 136(5):79-81.

If Verstraeten's study were to be published, it would place in jeopardy the vaccine program itself, as well as the physicians who prescribed it and the governmental authorities and vaccine makers who allowed thimerosal to be used as a vaccine preservative, who failed to calculate the total dosage of thimerosal that babies were receiving, and who thereby were personally and collectively responsible for poisoning millions of children with a known neurotoxin and causing an epidemic of ADHD, autism, and other neurodevelopmental disorders.

The problem needed to be contained and "handled." And it was. What happened during and after that infamous conference will be discussed at some length subsequently.

"Gold be a key for every locke…"

— *English playwright John Lyly, in* Euphues and his England, *1580*

2001: The CDC contracts with an allegedly "independent" private organization, the Institute of Medicine (IOM), to form an Immunization Safety Review Committee (ISRC) to review the data on thimerosal and vaccines as they related to the rising number of autism cases.

The IOM convenes a meeting of scientists to review the data, but *before* any science is discussed or evaluated, Dr. Mary McCormick, chairman of the Immunization Safety Review Committee, states in released transcripts of private conversations [between Dr. McCormick and Kathleen Stratton, Ph.D., the ISRC study director] that the "CDC wants us to declare, well, that these things (thimerosal preserved vaccinations) are pretty safe on a population basis."

In other words, *the CDC told the IOM what it expected the conclusions of this so-called independent committee study to be.* Later in the transcript, Dr. McCormick states, "We are never going to come down that it (autism and other neurodevelopmental disorders) is a true side effect (of the immunizations)."

Dr. Stratton, in the same transcript, states, "[W]e said this before you got here, and I think we said this yesterday, the point of no return, the line we will not cross in public policy is to pull the vaccine, change the schedule. We could say it is time to re-visit this, but we would never recommend that level. Even recommending research is recommendations for policy. We wouldn't say compensate, we wouldn't say pull the vaccine, we wouldn't say stop the program."

In other words, even if the Institute of Medicine found evidence of serious harm from the immunization program, it would not consider stopping or amending the vaccination schedule, or recommend further research or suggest that parents of children harmed by the immunizations be compensated. Unbelievable![30]

The ISRC, nevertheless, did concur with the recommendations of the American Academy of Pediatrics, the American Academy of Family Practice, and other organizations that had previously recommended the *expeditious* removal of thimerosal from vaccines given to pregnant women, infants, and children.[31]

However, that removal has never been officially mandated, nor were existing stocks of thimerosal-containing vaccines discarded. They were simply "used up" over the next several years, and thimerosal remains to this day as the preservative in the multidose influenza vaccines given to babies and pregnant women and in the Td (Tetanus-diphtheria) boosters given to older children.

"I have talked to mothers who asked to see the vaccine inserts as late as 2004 and found thimerosal present as a preservative in infant vaccines being used in certain clinics. Also, in 2002 the influenza vaccine was recommended by the CDC for infants 6 months of age and older."

— *Boyd Haley, Ph. D., Prof. of Chemistry; Univ. of Kentucky*

---

30   *Medscape Medical News.* April 10, 2006; reviewed by Dr. Gary D. Vogin, M.D. www.medscape.com/viewarticle/529583
31   www.nap.edu for complete transcript of the 2001 meeting.

2002: A highly controversial piggyback to the Homeland Security Act exempted drug companies from any liability in lawsuits alleging thimerosal toxicity. This "Eli Lilly Protection Act," as it has been referred to by outraged opponents, was recalled two years later.

In May 2002, the CDC and the American Academy of Pediatrics (AAP) announced their recommendations that all pregnant women and babies aged 6-7 months and older get the thimerosal-preserved influenza vaccine and yearly after that. What happened to the "expeditious removal of thimerosal from vaccines"?

Those CDC and AAP guidelines meant that a baby whose mother received the flu vaccine during the pregnancy would be exposed to three doses of thimerosal-containing immunizations by 18 months of age (before birth and again at 6 and 18 months of age).

2003: Thimerosal is still present in c. 50 percent of the manufactured lots of hepatitis B, DTaP, influenza, and Td vaccines, although it is alleged to have been removed in 2001.[32]

In May of 2003, following a three-year evaluation of mercury toxicity, the U.S. House of Representatives, Government Reform Committee released a report, "Mercury in Medicine—Taking Unnecessary Risks."

The report found, "Mercury is hazardous to humans. Its use in medicinal products is undesirable, unnecessary and should be minimized or eliminated entirely.... The FDA has never required manufacturers to conduct adequate safety testing on thimerosal and ethyl mercury compounds."[33]

2004: The Chiron Corporation, one of only two pharmaceutical companies supplying influenza vaccine to the U.S., is forced to close its Liverpool factory for three months when it is discovered that the "flu" vaccine it had produced that year was contaminated with a bacterium called Serratia marscesens that can cause urinary infections and pneumonia. The vaccine was preserved with thimerosal, which was obviously ineffective in eradicating this potentially harmful bacterium.[34]

Thimerosal is still present at pre-2000 concentrations in some vaccines routinely given to infants and children. The thimerosal-preserved influenza vaccine is recommended by the CDC to be given *yearly* to infants at or older than six months of age as well as to pregnant women despite no evidence that it is effective in this regard.

The Coalition for Mercury-Free Drugs (CoMeD) petitions the FDA to *comply with the law*, follow existing regulations, and provide proof of the safety and efficacy of mercury in drugs.[35]

At the time of filing, mercury was found in at least *45 different prescribed and over-the-counter drugs* (according to the FDA), "including various eye ointments, ear solutions, nasal sprays, vaccines, biologics, and in 'flu' vaccines," which were and are still being administered to millions of pregnant women, babies, children, and the elderly.[36]

The EPA reveals that mercury levels in fetal umbilical cord blood are actually 70 percent higher than levels in the mother's blood, suggesting that even if a mother's blood mercury levels are in the "safe" range, her baby's may not be.[37]

2006: CoMeD files a lawsuit against the FDA in August 2006, alleging that it did not answer the issues raised in the original petition.

In September 2006, the FDA, which had found thimerosal to be ineffective "in killing bacteria or halting their replication," and which twice ruled (1982 and 1988) that it be removed from over-the-counter products because it was

---

32   2003 PDR and verified by Mark and David Geier.
33   http://frwebgate.access.gpo.gov/cgi-bin/multidb.cgi?WAIStemplate=multid b_results.html&WAISqueryRule= percent24WAISqueryString& WAISdb-Name=2003_record+Congressional+Record percent2C+Volume+149 + percent282003 percent29&WAISqueryString= percent22Mercury+In+Medicine+Report percent22&Submit.=Submit&WAISmaxHits=200&WrapperTemplate=crecord_wrapper.html
34   Dyer, Owen. "Factory loss of license halves supply of flu vaccine to US." *BMJ.* 2004 October 16; 329(7471): 876-b.
35   FDA Docket: 2004P-0349, filed on Wednesday, August 4, 2004.
36   http://adventuresinautism.blogspot.com/2006/10/comed-sues-fda-to-force-mercury-out-of.html
37   "Mercury threat to fetus raised: EPA revises risk estimates." *Washington Post.* February 6, 2004.

"not recognized as being safe or effective," replies to CoMeD and *denies the petition to remove mercury from medications, but admits to having done no safety studies on thimerosal.*

In October 2006, CoMeD files an amended complaint in U.S. Federal Court disputing the FDA response it had received in September, which defended the use of mercury in medicine.[38]

The Combating Autism Act, a "landmark piece of bipartisan legislation," was introduced into the senate by members Rick Santorum (R-PA) and Chris Dodd (D-CT). The bill, which was endorsed by every major autism organization in America, authorized $860 million in federal funds over five years for autism screening, research, education, and therapy, and it doubled the funds the NIH received for autism studies.

Opposition to the bill came from a surprising source: the American Academy of Pediatrics.

Why would the AAP oppose this bill?

According to lobbyists for the AAP, the bill provides millions of dollars toward "research on a broad array of environmental factors that have a possible role in autism, including but not limited to vaccines, other biological and pharmaceutical products, and their components (including preservatives)."[39]

What's wrong with researching the environmental causes of autism?

According to the AAP lobbyists, "Any bill that contains any questions about vaccines, we are not going to endorse. There is absolutely no link between thimerosal and autism. Period. To endorse the bill implies that this is an open question, and it is not. The bottom line is that we don't want to look into this. It is inappropriate to waste precious research dollars on something that we know will be disproved."[40]

Or was it that they knew the link would be proved?

The American Academy of Pediatrics got its way. "The revised bill, ultimately approved by the Senate, did not include the provisions that would have specified funding for investigating possible environmental causes."[41]

"The lady doth protest too much, methinks."

— *William Shakespeare,* Hamlet

2007: President Bush vetoes a bill from Congress (FY 2008 HHS Labor-Education Appropriations Bill) that would ban mercury from all childhood influenza ("flu") vaccines, *even though he promised to work to remove mercury from vaccines when he was running for office in 2004.*

2007: Representative Carolyn Mahoney (D-NY) introduces H.R. 2832, the "Comprehensive Comparative Study of Vaccinated and Unvaccinated Populations Act of 2007," which directed "the Secretary of Health and Human Services to conduct or support a comprehensive study comparing total health outcomes, including risk of autism, in vaccinated populations in the United States with such outcomes in unvaccinated populations in the United States, and for other purposes." The bill never became law.

2010: Thimerosal is still present in the Td booster (Tetanus/diphtheria) given to older children and adults and in the influenza vaccination recommended for all individuals, including pregnant women, infants, and children. Many other vaccines contain some thimerosal, as it is used in the manufacturing process, and then removed, but not entirely. The so-called "trace amounts" that remain pose significant hazards (see "Thimerosal Concentrations and Toxic Effects" in Table 10.1). Children in their first five years and vaccinated according to the recommended schedule

---

38   Ibid.
39   Washington meeting January 2006; reported by journalist David Kirby in the *Huffington Post*. March 22, 2006.
40   Ibid.
41   http://en.wikipedia.org/wiki/Combating_Autism_Act

will receive slightly over 50 percent of the mercury they were getting in the 1990s (mostly from the annual influenza vaccinations).

2010: The National Autism Association joins forces with seventy other autism groups to form the Combating Autism Act Reauthorization Coalition (CAARC). It lobbies Congress to reauthorize the Combating Autism Act.

On December 17, 2010, Senator Christopher Dodd drafted legislation that recognizes that autism has become "a national health emergency." The bill requests $2.75 billion over five years toward autism research, and $3.15 billion over six years in autism services funding. This bill will go a long way to helping the families of autistic children cope with their huge therapy costs. However, *the bill allocates not one penny for vaccine safety research,* despite the obvious need for such research.

"The most important research program," as the CAARC points out, "is an examination of the health of unvaccinated children (about 4 percent of the population) to determine the prevalence of autism and other chronic ailments within that group." This would be an easy and not terribly expensive undertaking. However, it was not to be.

Once again, our politicians, under the influence of what can only be described as pernicious lobbying against doing such research by the American Academy of Pediatrics and other powerful groups, have not included any provisions for funding this absolutely vital investigation.

2013: In April, Congressman Bill Posey (R-Fl) was joined once again by Rep. Carolyn Mahoney (D-N.Y.) in introducing H.R. 1757, The Vaccine Safety Study Act, which directs the NIH to conduct a retrospective study of health outcomes, including autism, of vaccinated versus unvaccinated children. Congressman Henry Waxman (D-CA) refused to cosponsor the bill.

2014: Dr. Thomas Insel, Director of the National Institute of Mental Health, the National Institute of Health, and Chairman of the Interagency Coordinating Committee admitted that:

> [A]fter eight years and spending $1.7 billion, the programs developed in the Combatting Autism Act (2006) have failed to determine the causes of the enormous increase of the prevalence of autism, failed to prevent a single case of autism, failed to produce any new biomedical treatment for autism, failed to materially reduce the age of diagnosis of autism, failed to ensure appropriate medical care for the co-occurring health problems faced by many with autism, failed to ensure even basic safety protocols for people with autism who "wander," unfortunately some to their deaths, and overall, failed the families facing autism—most especially the approximately one-third of families with children most severely affected by autism, who literally cannot speak for themselves, and whose severe disabilities portend one of the largest unfunded federal fiscal liabilities of the 21st century.[42]

Conclusion: We have learned that thimerosal is a very toxic substance, that it is unstable, and that it has been inadequately evaluated in regard to its safe use in humans and, particularly, in regard to its potential harm to babies and young children.

We are alarmed to discover that the regulating authorities were "asleep at the switch" in failing to recognize that babies and young children were (and still are) receiving neurotoxic doses of mercury from their routinely administered thimerosal-preserved childhood immunizations.

We are not, however, surprised to learn that the CDC and the American Academy of Pediatrics vehemently oppose doing studies that would compare the health consequences of vaccinated vs. unvaccinated populations. Both of these organizations (and others) were privy to the findings of the secret CDC study that showed quite clearly that thimerosal-preserved immunizations were significantly likely to cause ADHD, autism, language disorders, and a variety of other neuro-developmental harms.

---

42   http://www.ageofautism.com/2014/06/rep-bill-posey-blogs-fix-the-combatting-autismact.html?utm_source=feed burner&utm_medium=email&utm_ campaign=Feed percent3A+ageofautism+ percent28AGE+OF+AUTISM percent29

And there is a great deal of additional evidence supporting the thimerosal/mercury link to autism spectrum disorders that will be presented in the following chapters.

"Every great mistake has a halfway moment, a split second when it can be recalled and perhaps remedied."

— Pearl S. Buck (1892-1973)

DEPARTMENT OF OOPS!

In 1999, Dr. Peter Patriarca, Director of the Division of Viral Products at the FDA, contacted the head of the CDC (Centers for Disease Control) and declared that no one had added up the mercury dosage that babies were receiving as a result of all the newly added immunizations. He wrote, "I am not sure if there will be an easy way out of the potential perception that the FDA, CDC, and immunization policy bodies may have been 'ASLEEP AT THE SWITCH' regarding thimerosal until now."[43]

Dr. Neal Halsey echoed Dr. Patriarca's concerns: "In most vaccine containers, thimerosal is listed as a mercury derivative, (at) a hundredth of a percent. And what I believed, and what everybody else believed, was that it was truly a trace, a biologically insignificant amount. My honest belief is that if the labels had had the mercury content in micrograms, this would have been uncovered years ago. But the fact is, no one did the calculation."[44]

Drs. Patriarca and Halsey were mistaken, however. Our governmental agencies may have been "asleep at the switch," but Merck, one of the many vaccine manufacturers, had done the calculation at least eight years earlier, as was made clear in a 1991 internal memo from Merck, obtained by the L.A. Times under the Freedom of Information Act. The memo from Dr. Maurice Hilleman, a famous Merck scientist and vaccine researcher, pointed out that six-month-old children who received their shots on schedule would get a mercury load up to 87 times higher than allowed by guidelines for the maximum daily consumption of mercury from fish.[45]

According to Elizabeth Mumper, MD, President and CEO, Advocates for Children, Associate Professor of Clinical Pediatrics, University of Virginia School of Medicine: "The vaccine experts who added new vaccines into the routine schedule in the late 80's and early 90's have acknowledged that they did not add up the cumulative doses of mercury to which our children were exposed. The CDC's own data shows an increased risk of 2.48 for autism* in children who received full immunizations by six months compared to a less vaccinated population."[46]

*The risk was much higher before the CDC manipulated the original data (see Vertsraeten study in Chapter 13).

"The safety of the people shall be the highest law."

— Cicero

---

43   FDA internal e-mail written on June 29, 1999, obtained by Rep. Dan Burton
44   Allen, Arthur. "Not-So-Crackpot Autism Theory." *New York Times.* November 10, 2002. Quoting Neal Halsey M.D., Pediatrician and Vaccinologist, Johns Hopkins University, Chairman of the American Academy of Pediatrics committee on infectious diseases from 1995 through June 1999.
45   *L.A. Times*
46   Published in an open letter to President Bush "In Support for a White House Conference on Autism."

DEPARTMENT OF "OH, REALLY?"

March 12, 2010: the Vaccine Court, a special branch of the U.S. Court of Special Claims, ruled that thimerosal is not to blame for autism. The ruling said the parents were arguing that the effects from mercury in vaccines differ from mercury's known effects on the brain.

Dr. Paul Offit of Children's Hospital of Philadelphia agreed with the ruling. He declared that the thimerosal-autism theory had "already had its day in science court and failed to hold up."

— Schafer Autism Report, March 15, 2010

DEPARTMENT OF "MUCH MORE LIKELY"

"It is highly probable that the use of thimerosal as a preservative has caused developmental disorders, including autism, in some children."

— George Wayne Lucier, former senior official at the National Institutes of Health in Environmental Toxicology, and scientific advisor for the EPA.

A three-year investigation by the Government Reform Committee concluded in May of 2003:

"Thimerosal used as a preservative in vaccines is likely related to the autism epidemic.

"This epidemic in all probability may have been prevented or curtailed had the FDA not been asleep at the switch regarding the lack of safety data regarding injected thimerosal and the sharp rise of infant exposure to this known neurotoxin.

"Our public health agencies' failure to act is indicative of institutional malfeasance for self-protection and misplaced protectionism of the pharmaceutical industry."[47]

And there is a lot more evidence linking thimerosal and autism, as we shall see in the following chapters.

"Science is but a perversion of itself unless it has as its ultimate goal the betterment of humanity."

— Nikola Tesla

---

[47]   http://www.chat-hyperacusis.net/post/Pink-Disease-Mercury-Autism-The-Brain-Gut-Ears-1599210?trail=100

Chapter 11
More Evidence Linking Thimerosal and Mercury to Autism

"The right to search for truth implies also a duty.
One must not conceal any part of what one has recognized to be true."

— Albert Einstein
{Engraved in stone on the National Academy of Sciences building in Washington,
D.C., Home to the NIH and the IOM.}

WHAT EVIDENCE EXISTS *That Thimerosal and Mercury Promote Autism?*
A number of convincing lines of evidence implicate thimerosal and mercury (as well as other toxins) as promoters of the autistic state in susceptible individuals.

1. Thimerosal (and mercury itself) are both extremely toxic and, in particular, very neurotoxic. The increased susceptibility to mercury toxicity in males may help explain why autism is much more common in males.

2. Many mercury toxicity symptoms are remarkably similar to those seen in autistic individuals.

3. The physiological effects of mercury also parallel those seen in autistic individuals.

4. The rise in autism cases mirrors the increase in infants' mercury exposure from immunizations.

5. Autistic children have an impaired capacity to detoxify mercury and appear to have an increased body burden of mercury as compared to non-autistic children. Their total body-burden of mercury appears to correlate with the severity of their autism. Autistic children on average are also more sensitive to mercury's toxic effects than are non-autistic children.

6. Thimerosal and mercury are proven to interfere with certain enzymes, which when inhibited promote the autistic state. Likewise, certain genetic variations (mutations/polymorphisms) in particular enzymes (their concentrations or activity) can exacerbate mercury's deleterious effects in this regard.

7. U.S. children, at least up until 2003 and possibly 2004, were being given routine childhood thimerosal-preserved vaccinations, invariably in amounts that far exceeded the allowable upper safe limit established by regulating authorities like the EPA. Thimerosal is still found at high levels in vaccines given to babies and children today in amounts known to cause neurological damage.

8. Animal studies show that thimerosal (a source of ethyl mercury) injected into baby monkeys and rodents in doses comparable to those found in human vaccinations gets into the brain readily, gets con-

verted into inorganic mercury in greater amounts than does methyl mercury, persists longer in the brain than it does in the bloodstream, and that it also causes neurological damage comparable in many ways to that noted in autistic children.

9. There are many studies demonstrating that children who received thimerosal-preserved immunizations have a significantly higher risk of developing autism, ADHD, significant developmental delays, and other neurological disorders, and that the risk increases as the body load of mercury increases. We call these the positive studies.

10. There are epidemiological studies that demonstrate that children who live near mercury-emitting smelters, toxic waste dumps, and other industrial sources of mercury (and other pollutants) have a significantly increased risk of becoming autistic, and the closer they live to the source, the greater the incidence of autism.

11. Autistic children who have their mercury (and other heavy metals if present) removed, via a process known as chelation, often significantly improve their overall functioning.

12. Certain porphyrin compounds that form only when mercury toxicity is present are commonly and more frequently seen in autistic children as compared to their non-autistic peers, and their levels correlate with the degree of autism.

13. The *negative studies* that purport to show no relationship between immunizations, thimerosal, and autism are for the most part fraudulent, poorly done, or highly suspect. There are actually *no valid studies* that refute or disprove the contention that thimerosal or immunizations may promote autism in susceptible individuals.

What Is the Validation for Contention 1?

CONTENTION 1: *Thimerosal and mercury in all its forms are both extremely toxic, in particular, very neurotoxic. The increased susceptibility to mercury toxicity in males may help explain why autism is much more common in males.*

The references for mercury toxicity and specifically neurotoxicity are legion. We have already covered some of thimerosal's toxic effects. See references (Appendix I) for additional studies in this regard. This isn't controversial. What is controversial is whether the amount of mercury in thimerosal-preserved vaccines is sufficient to cause autism and other neurodevelopmental disorders. This will be discussed at length subsequently.

We will list here just a few of the many studies that implicate mercury as a neurotoxin.

In a 1997 study, prenatal exposure to *methyl* mercury *at levels considered to be safe* was shown to relate to *significant cognitive dysfunctions* in the domains of language, attention, and memory in seven-year-old children. These children also exhibited visuo-spatial and motor function deficits, albeit to a lesser degree. All these symptoms are characteristics of autism-affected children (and children with ADHD). When the Vaccine Court suggests that mercury does not promote autistic symptoms in children, it just might want to go back and review this study.[1]

Other research revealed that *prenatal* exposure to *methyl* mercury could result in symptoms ranging from severe neurological impairments like mental retardation, cerebral palsy, and visual and auditory deficits to milder, more subtle changes in functioning, *depending on the timing and dose of the chemical agent*.[2]

---

1   Grandjean, P. et al. "Cognitive deficit in 7-year-old children with prenatal exposure to methylmercury." *Neurotoxicol Teratol*. 1997 Nov-Dec; 19(6):417-28.
2   Mendola, P. et al. "Environmental factors associated with a spectrum of neurodevelopmental deficits." *Ment Retard Dev Disabil Res Rev*. 2002; 8(3):188-97.

New Zealand scientists found that children's test scores correlated inversely with their mothers' hair levels of mercury at the time of their birth.[3]

In another study, investigators showed that low levels of prenatal mercury vapor exposure can alter the levels of nerve growth factor and its receptors resulting in neuronal damage during development.[4]

Mercury from any source is not only implicated as a major cause of autism and a host of other neurological dysfunctions, but it has also been shown to promote Alzheimer's disease, a type of adult onset dementia.[5]

At the NVIC International Vaccine Conference held in Arlington, Virginia in September, 1997, Dr. Hugh Fudenberg, a well-respected and widely published immune-geneticist stated that *if an individual had five or more consecutive flu shots, his chances of getting Alzheimer's would be 10 times higher than if he had one, two, or no shots.* The suspected reason for this association is the presence of neurotoxic mercury (as thimerosal) and aluminum in these vaccines.

Amazingly, the American Academy of Pediatrics recommends that pregnant women get the influenza vaccine and that all babies receive the vaccine yearly, which even today (2015) may contain thimerosal.

A 2009 lab study of neuronal cells exposed to very low (nanomolar) concentrations of thimerosal and other toxic metal salts (including lead acetate and aluminum sulfate) demonstrated that thimerosal induced significant cellular toxicity in human neuronal and fetal cells and that this cellular toxicity was similar to that observed in autism disorder studies.

Thimerosal caused time-dependent mitochondrial damage, reduced oxidation-reduction activity, cellular degeneration, and cell death. Thimerosal was found to be significantly more toxic than the other metal compounds examined.[6]

Why Are Autism and ADHD More Common in Males?

Gender-Selective Toxicity of Thimerosal

It has been well-established that autism, Asperger's syndrome, and ADHD occur more frequently in males than in females. The ratio in mild to moderate autism is about 4:1 in boys to girls and is higher in more severely afflicted individuals.[7]

Mercury exposure in utero and in infancy, as we shall show, promotes autism. A dental study of mercury excretion from dental amalgams in children revealed that *females given the same exposure as males excrete more mercury.*[8]

One of the functions of the metallothionine proteins, it may be remembered, is to detoxify mercury. Impaired metallothionine function as commonly seen in autism offers us an explanation for the predominance of autism and ADHD in males. It has been found that the "female hormones" estrogen and progesterone induce the manufacture of metallothioneins, so females would be expected to have higher levels of metallothioneins than males and thus manifest some enhanced protection in this regard.

---

3   Crump, K.S. et al. "Influence of prenatal mercury exposure upon scholastic and psychological test performance: benchmark analysis of a New Zealand cohort." *Risk Anal.* 1998 Dec; 18(6):701-13. 9972579 PubMed.

4   Soderstrom, S. et al. "The effect of mercury vapour on cholinergic neurons in the fetal brain: studies on the expression of nerve growth factor and its low- and high-affinity receptors." *Brain Res Dev.* 1995 Mar 16; 85(1):96-108.

5   *http://commons.ucalgary.ca/showcase/curtains.php?src =http://apollo.ucalgary.ca/mercury/movies/Lor2_QTS_700kb_QD.move&screenwidth=512&screenh eight=400&curtains=no] Univ of Calgary short film on mercury's effects on neurons and how it promotes Alzheimer's disease 2010.*

6   Geier, D.A., P.G. King, and M.R. Geier. "Mitochondrial dysfunction, impaired oxidative-reduction activity, degeneration, and death in human neuronal and fetal cells induced by low-level exposure to thimerosal and other metal compounds." *Toxicological & Environmental Chemistry.* Vol. 91, No. 4, June 2009, 735-749.

7   Holmes, A.S., Blaxill, M.F., and Haley, B.E. "Reduced levels of mercury in first baby haircuts of autistic children.". *Int J Toxic.* 2003; 22:277-85.

8   Woods, J.S., Bernardo, M.F. et al. "The contribution of dental amalgam to urinary mercury excretion in children." *Environ Health Perspect.* 2007. 115:1527-1531.

Dr. Valerie Hu, a professor of biochemistry and molecular biology at George Washington University, has investigated the RORA gene, whose expression is regulated by the male and female sex hormones. "RORA is involved in several key processes implicated in autism, including brain cell (Purkinje) differentiation; muscle tone and development of the cerebellum; protection of neurons against chemical stress; suppression of inflammation; and regulation of circadian rhythm."[9]

Dr. Hu's research has shown that RORA is decreased or somewhat inactivated (by methylation) in many severely affected autistic individuals of both sexes. One of the functions of RORA is to regulate an enzyme called aromatase which converts testosterone to estrogen. A RORA deficiency or inactivation leads to decreased aromatase activity, and *decreased aromatase activity leads to an elevation of testosterone levels*, which is exactly what has been found in many autistic individuals.

What Dr. Hu and her coworkers also discovered was that *aromatase was indeed deficient in autistics compared to controls*, supporting a mechanism that would help explain why testosterone levels appear to be increased in many autistic children.

In earlier research published in 2009, Dr. Hu and her colleagues found that a deficiency in RORA was seen in both male and female autistics, and in particular, in the most severely affected individuals.

How does this relate to thimerosal? There is good evidence that *the toxicity of thimerosal and mercury, in particular, is enhanced by the "male hormone" testosterone.*[10]

This association was confirmed in a study by Boyd Haley, Professor of Chemistry at the University of Kentucky. He found that:

> Neurons that were pre-incubated with estrogen demonstrated substantial protection against thimerosal-induced neuron death. In contrast, the addition of testosterone caused a very large increase in thimerosal-induced neuron death.

> A low nanomolar level of thimerosal that gave less than 5 percent neuron death in three hours could be increased to 100 percent cell death by the addition of one micromolar level of testosterone.

> Testosterone alone at this level also showed less than 5 percent cell death. The opposing effects of estrogen and testosterone may explain the gender-based four-to-one ratio. Most important, the tremendous enhancement of thimerosal toxicity by testosterone points out the impact of synergistic effects when addressing mercury toxicity.[11]

So children with an inherited or acquired impairment of RORA would be expected to have an excess of testosterone, which in turn would tend to magnify the toxic effects of any mercury or thimerosal exposures. Females, on the other hand, have lower levels of testosterone, higher levels of estrogen, and an increased ability to excrete mercury, and would thus be expected to have a lower incidence of autism.

Further evidence to support this theory comes from a recent mouse study. Donald Branch, a scientist at the University of Toronto, was attempting to assess the maximum tolerated dosage of thimerosal in CD1 mice. He injected a relatively high dose of thimerosal (c. 38-77 mg/kg in a 10 percent DMSO diluent) into seven male and seven female mice, and much to his surprise *all seven of the male mice succumbed but none of the female mice did.*

Dr. Branch concluded that this study, while still "preliminary," due to the "small numbers of mice examined...nevertheless (provides) the first report of gender-selective toxicity of thimerosal and indicate(s) that any future studies of thimerosal toxicity should take into consideration gender-specific differences."[12]

---

9   Christopher Badcock, Ph.D. http://www.psychologytoday .com/blog/the-imprinted-brain/201102/rora-just-the-gene-autism-we-wanted

10   Geier, M., Geier, D. "Testosterone: A Key to Understanding Mercury-Autism Link." *Autism Research Review;* Vol. 19, No. 1, 2005.

11   Boyd Haley http://www.flcv.com/hgsynerg.html

12   Branch, Don R. *Exp Toxicol Pathol. 2009 Mar; 61(2):133-6. Epub 2008 Sep 3; Departments of Medicine and Laboratory Medicine and Pathobiology, University of Toronto, Ontario, Canada.* PMID: 18771903.

And there are additional studies that bolster the theory that elevated levels of testosterone in utero are a risk factor for autism. These studies include:

1. J.T. Manning, et al. "The second to fourth digit ratio in autism."[13] In this study it was found that the ratio of the length of the second finger to the fourth finger was influenced by intra-uterine testosterone levels and that autistic children (and their relatives) tended to have a finger ratio that coincided with elevated testosterone in utero.

2. Bonnie Auyeung, et al. "Fetal testosterone and autistic traits."[14] This study demonstrated that increased levels of testosterone in utero tended to promote autistic-like traits in the child. These findings were confirmed in a more recent article by the same research team.[15]

3. Simon Baron-Cohen, et al. "Elevated fetal steroidogenic activity in autism."[16] In this study, the research team found that babies who later went on to develop autism not only had elevated levels of testosterone in their amniotic fluid (compared to their non-autistic peers), but they also had elevated levels of many other steroidal hormones, like hydrocortisone and progesterone, as well.

And there are still other possible mechanisms that could help explain the male predominance in autistic disorders. Chemists have found that *mercury ions in the body bind readily to homocysteine*. Researchers Christy Bridges and Rudolfs Zalups point out that *homocysteine levels are higher in males than in females*, and suggest that this might account for the increased tissue retention of mercury in males, which would in turn account for the higher incidence for autism in males.[17]

Researchers at the University of Washington found that a variant (CPOX4) in an enzyme (coproporphyrinogen oxidase) in the biochemical pathway that results in the manufacture of heme (the protein in hemoglobin) makes male children in particular more susceptible to the neurotoxic effects of mercury. In this 7-year study of over 500 children who were assessed annually in regard to their neurobehavioral performance and exposure to mercury from dental amalgams "all underlying dose-response associations between mercury exposure and test performance were restricted to boys with the CPOX4 variant, and all of these associations were in the expected direction where increased exposure to mercury decreased performance." There was a "paucity of responses among same-age girls with comparable mercury exposure."[18]

A vitamin D deficiency is found in virtually all autistic children and appears to be one of the factors that promotes autism in susceptible children. Vitamin D is actually a hormone that in addition to its well-known role in enhancing calcium absorption is also vital for immune function and brain development. *Estrogen increases vitamin D in the brain and testosterone does not.* Vitamin D, as has been previously discussed, increases the levels of glutathione in the brain, which in turn assists in the detoxification of mercury and protects against free radical damage.[19]

What Is the Validation for Contention 2?

CONTENTION 2: *Mercury toxicity symptoms may actually be remarkably similar to those seen in autism.*

Sallie Bernard is the executive director and co-founder of "SafeMinds," "a non-profit organization dedicated to investigating the risks of exposure to mercury from medical products. SafeMinds was founded in 2000 and is led by the parents of autistic children.

---

13   *Developmental Medicine and Child Neurology*, 2001, 43, 160-164.

14   *British Journal of Psychology* (2009), 100, 1–22.

15   Auyeung et al. *Molecular Autism* 2010, 1:11 http://www.molecularautism.com/content/1/1/11

16   *Molecular Psychiatry*. Advance online publication 3 June 2014; doi: 10.1038/mp.2014.48.

17   "Mercury bound to homocysteine Molecular and Ionic Mimicry and the Transport of Toxic Metals." *Toxicol Appl Pharmacol*. 2005 May 1:204 (3)L 274-308; also Novembrino, C. et al. "Homocysteine and Mercury Dental Amalgam." Paper presented at Eighth International Conference on Mercury as a Global Pollutant, doi:10.1289/ehp.11235 available via http://dx.doi.org [Online 24 June 2008].

18   Woods JS, et al. Modification of Neurobehavioral Effects of Mercury by a Genetic Polymorphism of Coproporphyrinogen Oxidase in Children, Neurotoxicol Teratol. 2012 Sep; 34(5):513-521.

19   Ref. 69: Garcion, E. et al. "New clues about vitamin D functions in the nervous system." Trends in Endocrinology and Metabolism. April 2002, Vol. 13, Issue 3, 1, p. 100-105.

In 2001, Ms. Bernard and her associates published a review article in the journal *Medical Hypotheses*. In that article, "Autism: a Novel Form of Mercury Poisoning," the authors reported that *all of the major symptoms of autism*—like language deficits, stereotypic behaviors, social withdrawal, low muscle tone, intestinal problems, sleep problems and excessive salivation—*have also been reported in infantile mercury poisoning.*[20]

However, Nelson and Bauman, in a later review, contested the assertion that the symptoms of mercury poisoning were similar to those seen in autism spectrum disorders. They alleged that these were two distinct entities.[21]

In March 12, 2010: the Vaccine Court, a special branch of the U.S. Court of Special Claims, ruled that thimerosal is not to blame for autism. The ruling said the parents were arguing that the effects from mercury in vaccines differ from mercury's known effects on the brain. In so doing, the Vaccine Court and Nelson and Bauman seem to have disregarded the findings of the U.S. Agency for Toxic Substances and Disease Registry, which found that infantile exposure to mercury can manifest as mental impairment, poor coordination, muscle weakness, and an inability to speak, all of which are commonly noted in autistic individuals.[22]

See Appendix IV, Table A for a long list of symptoms common to autism and mercury poisoning with references.

The pronouncements of Nelson and Bauman and the U.S. Court of Special Claims notwithstanding, the toxic effects of mercury in vaccines (and from other sources) may be strikingly similar to the symptoms of autism *if the comparison is made appropriately*. This caveat is critical because the symptoms of mercury toxicity may and often do differ in different individuals due to a number of confounding factors. These include:

- The age at which an individual is exposed to the mercury containing substance: Fetal or neonatal exposure to mercury and thimerosal would be expected to, and often does, cause different symptoms and toxicity manifestations than childhood, adolescent, or adult exposures would be expected to and does.

- The exposed individual's unique genetic susceptibility to mercury's toxic effects (how well that person detoxifies and metabolizes mercury compounds, for example).

- The form of mercury that enters the body (organic: methyl, ethyl, etc., vs. inorganic: mercury in teething powder, amalgam fillings or vapor, for example).

- Whether the exposures are acute or chronic, pulsatile, or continuous.

- How the mercury enters the body (through the skin or mucous membranes, orally, by direct injection [as in vaccinations] or through the lungs [mercury vapor]).

- The total and individual doses of mercury entering the body.

- The stability of the mercury-containing compound that enters the body. Thimerosal, for example, is a highly unstable molecule that, as has been documented, breaks down over time and also when exposed to certain components in the human (and animal) body.

- Other factors that can influence mercury's toxic potential in a given individual: These factors include the presence of other toxins, like lead and aluminum, that can multiply the toxic effects of mercury, or even sex differences (testosterone, the "male hormone" for example, potentiates the toxicity of mercury, while estrogen, the "female hormone," reduces mercury's toxic effects.

---

20   *Med Hypotheses*. 2001, 56(4):462471.
21   Nelson, K.B., Bauman, M.L. "Thimerosal and Autism?" *Pediatrics*. 2003. 111(3):674-9.
22   "Toxicological Profile for mercury." in section 1.6. U.S. Department of Health and Human Services, 1999.

A Brief History of Recent Mercury Poisoning

To better illustrate the importance of understanding the similarities and differences in the physiological effects of exposures to mercury and its various compounds, in varying dosages on human health at different ages, and through different pathways into the human body, we will review a number of historical episodes of documented mercury poisoning:

Pink Disease (also called *Acrodynia* and many other names): Starting in 1885, doctors around the world began to recognize an increasingly common syndrome in babies characterized by puffy, swollen, pink hands and feet (hence the name). Babies who evinced these symptoms frequently were found to have other, often severe, symptoms. These included painful skin eruptions, peeling skin, *light sensitivity*[23], *muscle weakness, clumsiness, digestive problems*, anemia, gum ulcerations, *irritability*, excessive salivation, loss of teeth, *seizures*, enlarged lymph glands, low blood sodium levels, and *hypersensitivity to touch, temperature, water, and UV light.*

Also noted were *head banging, poor muscle tone*, and death in 10-30 percent of the children. *"Some children appeared (to be) unaware of their parents, (didn't) respond to their kisses, (and did) not seem to notice them when they came close or left."*

Obsessions, lack of speech, and strange behaviors were also observed.[24]

The disease was ultimately traced to the use of teething powders containing *mercurous chloride*, a form of *inorganic* mercury. About one in 500 babies so exposed showed symptoms of the disease. The theory that mercury poisoning was a possible cause of this affliction was first proposed in 1922, but it took until 1947 for the FDA to ban the use of mercury salts in teething powders.[25]

Although some of the Pink Disease symptoms are not characteristic of autism, a number that are include: digestive disturbances, light sensitivity, other sensory issues, coordination difficulties, poor muscle tone, poor eye contact, head banging, other self-injurious behaviors, unusual behaviors, unawareness of others, seizures, insomnia, loss of speech, obsessive behaviors, repetitive behaviors, and irritability.[26]

Pink Disease also clearly illustrates the importance of the interrelationship between genetic susceptibility (*in this case to mercurous chloride poisoning*) and the inciting environmental factor (*the mercurous chloride*) that caused the illness. Only one in 500 babies exposed to the mercury-infused teething powder came down with the disease. In this regard, the parallels to autism should be apparent to all.

The causative agent in Pink Disease, mercurous chloride, differs from a suspected toxin in autism, ethyl mercury, structurally and chemically. In the case of Pink Disease, the mercurous chloride entered the body through the mouth and GI tract. In the case of autism, the ethyl mercury was injected. These differences could and should be expected to result in different symptoms in the children so exposed.

An interesting and very germane sidelight to this story is the revelation that *the grandchildren of Pink Disease survivors have a dramatically increased risk of becoming autistic.* These findings came to light as a result of a recent Australian study.

Swinburne University researchers surveyed 522 Australian survivors of Pink Disease and found that 1 in 25 of their 398 *grandchildren* aged 6 to 12 had an autism spectrum disorder. This prevalence was *over six times higher than the one in 160 diagnosed* in the general Australian population at that time.[27]

Study coauthor Associate Professor David Austin stated that, "Since autism was first recognized as a disorder, scientists have been trying to identify its cause. There have been two warring camps: one that attributes autism to genet-

---

23   Symptoms in italics are those also common in autistic children.
24   http://www.whale.to/v/Acrodyniacomp.pdf
25   www.pinkdisease.org
26   "Pink disease or infantile acrodynia: its nature, prevention and cure." Preliminary Report by D. B. Cheek and C. Stanton Hicks, *The Medical Journal of Australia*, Jan 28, 1950; Warkany, J. "Acrodynia—postmortem of a disease." The Fourth Annual Joseph B. Bilderback Lecture, Portland, Oregon, Feb 3, 1966.
27   Shandley K, et al. "Ancestry of pink disease (infantile acrodynia) identified as a risk factor for autism spectrum disorders." *J Toxicol Environ Health A*. 2011; 74 (18): 1185-94.

ics and the other which claims it is caused by an environmental trigger. This study suggests that it may actually be a combination of the two. That is, genetic susceptibility to a trigger [mercury] and then exposure to that trigger."[28]

There is also an interesting recent report of an eleven-month-old Swiss boy who developed signs of both *acrodynia* (Pink Disease) and *autistic regression* four weeks after exposure to mercury from a broken thermometer.

Up until that time, he had been in excellent health and his development had been normal. During a two-week period, he regressed, ceased to laugh or play, slept only 1-2 hours at night, lost his ability to crawl and stand, and developed swollen red hands and feet with skin peeling (desquamation). He sweated excessively, showed stereotypic movements typical of autism (kneading of hands), and repeatedly bit objects and his own hands. He was noted to have poor muscle tone (hypotonia), and was diagnosed as having features consistent with a diagnosis of autism, but he also had many Pink Disease symptoms (puffy red and peeling hands and feet, irritability, hypotonia, etc.) as well.[29]

Mad Hatter Disease: Milliners, in previous centuries, used mercury compounds to turn fur into the felt that was used in the manufacture of hats. They generally worked in poorly ventilated rooms and were thereby exposed to *inorganic* mercury-containing *vapors* and *salts* (*mercurous nitrate*). As a consequence, they often suffered from a variety of neurological symptoms including trembling hands, numbness, and tingling in fingers and toes, vision, speech and hearing defects (in higher dosages), excess salivation, intestinal disturbances, loss of memory, and mental derangement, including pathological shyness (not noted in studies until 1912).

Dr. Joseph Addison Freeman, after reviewing about 100 cases, provided the first recorded study of the occupational hazards associated with mercury exposure in 1858. His observations were published two years later in the Transactions of the Medical Society of New Jersey under the title "Mercurial Disease among Hatters."[30]

This and other published studies did not cause an end to the use of mercury in the felt hat industry, however. It was not until 1941, when mercury was needed for making detonators, that the use of this highly toxic metal in the manufacture of felt hats was discontinued. Apparently, no one was concerned enough about the brain damage being suffered by the hatters to order a halt to this highly dangerous manufacturing process until a military-industrial need arose![31]

In 1995, a more recent description of a thirty-eight-year-old man exposed to toxic levels of *inorganic* mercury was published under the title, "The Neuropsychiatric Sequelae of Mercury Poisoning: The Mad Hatter's Disease Revisited."[32]

The man under study was assessed four years after his mercury exposure and was found to have many physical and psychiatric complaints. These included muscle spasms, tremors, rashes, and also *attention and focus deficits, marked anxiety, and agitation*. The latter symptoms are, of course, characteristic of autism.

Again, the toxin in Mad Hatter's Disease, mercurous nitrate, differs structurally and chemically from that in Pink Disease (mercurous chloride) and autism (ethyl mercury). The route of entry differed again in this disease as the mercury entered the body of the millinery workers via the lungs as well as the GI tract. Also, the age at exposure differed. Only adults were affected. As can be appreciated, the symptoms of Mad Hatter's Disease are not the same as those of Pink Disease or of autism, although there are shared symptoms in all these conditions, and they also differ from those found in Minimata disease sufferers.

Minamata Disease: In 1956, many Japanese citizens and animals living in and around Minamata City in Japan began to experience disturbing neurological symptoms, including muscle weakness, numbness of the hands and feet, difficulty coordinating movements, and problems with vision, hearing, and speech. More severely affected individuals

28   Ibid.

29   Chrysochoou, C. et al. "An 11-month-old boy with Psychomotor Regression and auto-aggressive Behaviour." *Eur J Pediatr* 2003; 162: 559-61.

30   Lewis Carroll's "Mad Hatter" appeared in *The Adventures of Alice in Wonderland* seven years later in 1865.

31   Weiss, Harry B. and Grace M. Weiss. *The Early Hatters of New Jersey*. Trenton NJ: NJ Agricultural Society, 1961.

32   O'Carroll, R.E. et al. *The British J of Psych* 167:95-98 (1995).

suffered from insanity, paralysis, coma, and death. Pet cats and dogs and farm animals also became ill and died at alarming rates.[33]

The cause of this calamity was ultimately traced to the release of mercury-contaminated wastewater that had been discharged by the Chisso Corporation into Minamata Bay since 1932. Fish and shellfish in the Bay became contaminated with the organic waste compound, *methyl mercury*, and when these sea creatures were eaten by the local populace and their pets, they succumbed to the toxic effects of the poison.

Methyl mercury is similar to, but has different physiological properties than the *ethyl* mercury found in thimerosal, just as *methyl* alcohol (methanol), which is extremely poisonous, differs in its toxicity and physiological effects from *ethyl* alcohol (ethanol), which is the alcohol found in all alcoholic beverages.

The Chisso Corporation, a chemical manufacturing company, had previously been cited in 1926 and again in 1943 for releasing toxic substances into the local bay and contaminating the fisheries there, and it continued to discharge mercury-containing waste water into both the Minamata Bay and later the local river until 1968.

The company, *often in apparent collusion with government officials*, continually lied to the public about its culpability in this matter, and also lied about its efforts to remedy the situation after it became clear that the epidemic of mercury poisoning was due entirely to its negligent practices.

By March 2001, over 78 percent of the 2,265 recognized victims of Minamata disease had died, and thousands more had been brain damaged. It wasn't until 2004 that the company was forced to clean up its contamination of the river and bay, by which time it had also paid eighty-six million dollars in damages to over 10,000 suspected victims, but a final compensation agreement for the remaining victims wasn't reached until 2010.

A second outbreak of "Minamata disease" occurred in a different Japanese prefecture in 1965. The poisoning was again due to the discharge of a methyl-mercury-containing effluent by another negligent chemical manufacturer, the Showa-Denko Company, which was later cited for its manufacture of contaminated tryptophan, an essential amino acid, that sickened[34] and killed many of the individuals who had unwittingly purchased this toxic product.[35]

An interesting and relevant sidelight to these tragic epidemics was the observation that many Minamata area mothers, who were seemingly unaffected by the disease, gave birth to babies with an increased incidence of cerebral palsy and other infantile neurological disorders, *including autism*. These children, many of whom were born after the Minamata outbreak and who had never been exposed to contaminated fish, exhibited many of the same symptoms noted in adult Minamata sufferers.

Dr. Masazumi Harada and other investigators who studied these children discovered that their symptoms were also due to mercury poisoning. This was confirmed by lab studies and autopsy analysis performed on two of the children who had died. The surprising and disturbing conclusion the investigators came to was that *the placenta, which would normally be expected to protect the fetus from exposure to toxic chemicals, actually concentrated the mercury in the fetus.*

So, an apparently neurologically unaffected mother with a body burden of *methyl* mercury insufficient to cause acute symptoms in herself was able to pass a portion of her mercury load to her fetus in amounts sufficient to cause serious neurological damage to the fetus that was exposed to this toxin *since conception*.

Thus in Minamata disease, the baby is *methyl*-mercury poisoned *prior to and during the formation of the infant's nervous system*. In contrast, the autistic infant is *ethyl*-mercury poisoned at birth (Hepatitis B vaccine with thimerosal) or shortly before birth[36] and on a regular basis after birth, the neurological damage being done at later stages of nervous system growth and by different compounds.

---

33   Stoller, K.P. "Autism as Minimata disease variant." *Medical Veritas* 3 (2006) 772–780.
34   eosinophilia-myalgia syndrome
35   Wikipedia.
36   From the influenza vaccine or from Rhogam (formerly with Thimerosal as preservative) given to the mother prior to delivery.

We can see that each form of mercury poisoning is unique in its toxic effects, although some symptoms are certainly shared. The manifestations of mercury toxicity differ in different individuals due to their age at exposure to the toxin, the chemical form of the toxin, the length of exposure to the toxin, the dose of each exposure, the route of entry of the toxin and the genetics of the individual so poisoned.

To conclude, as the Vaccine Court did, that the parents were wrong in suggesting that ethyl mercury in thimerosal could be causally linked to autism because "mercury's known effects on the brain" were not the same as the symptoms of autism is preposterous, as there has *never* been a study of the manifestations of *injectable low-dose ethyl*mercury in infants and children, and as can be readily appreciated from the description of the various mercury poisoning side effects seen in Pink Disease, Mad Hatter Disease, and Minamata Disease, there is no one "mercury effect on the brain."[37]

Poisoned Seed: The largest episode of methyl mercury poisoning was caused by contaminated wheat seeds and occurred in Iraq in the early 1970s. After several years of poor harvests, the Iraqi government decided to import wheat seeds from Mexico, which had been sprayed with *methylmercury*, a fungicide. The seed was colored red and farmers were warned that it was only for planting and not for eating.

However, the seed arrived too late for planting and the farmers were hungry, as were their livestock. So many farmers fed the grain to the animals, and seeing no immediate adverse effects, started eating the grain themselves. After several months, the animals and farmers and their families began to show the symptoms of mercury poisoning, similar to those seen in Minamata disease sufferers.

The government reacted immediately and forbade the farmers from possessing any of this poisoned seed under penalty of death. Panicky farmers took the bags of grain and dumped them in roadways, and in streams and fields. The mercury worked its way into the soil and water, and much of the seed was eaten by wild animals and birds.

The end result of this catastrophe was the death of close to 10,000 people, as well as tens of thousands of animals, and brain damage to c. 100,000 Iraqi citizens.

The Pacific Island Studies: Larger and older fish and marine mammals have been found to harbor potentially harmful amounts of *methyl* mercury. Maternal fish consumption is very high in certain parts of the world, and in particular, in the Faroe Islands, the Seychelles, and New Zealand.

Prospective studies were done in all these locations to see whether maternal fish consumption correlated with the mercury load in their offspring, and indeed, it did. Researchers involved in the Faroe Islands[38] (1,000 mother-child evaluations) and New Zealand[39] studies also found that the mercury load correlated with neurodevelopmental harm in the breast-fed children of frequent fish-consuming mothers.

However, the University of Rochester Medical Center researchers in the Seychelles study (700 mother-child evaluations) did not find such an association after following the children in the study for 66 months. Why did this study come to such a diametrically different conclusion regarding the safety of mercury? The answer lies in the study itself. *Sixty percent of the participants dropped out of the study*, a very large number, which renders the results and conclusions from this study suspect. The islanders also consumed smaller and younger fish with less mercury content.

In addition, the researchers investigated only 1784 individuals. The estimated autism rate in the Seychelles at that time was one in 500. That means that only about three children with autism might have been identified in the study group. Furthermore, the researchers excluded children with injuries and illnesses known to be associated with developmental problems. They did this, they allege, in order to parse out "the subtle effects of mercury." But by so doing,

---

37   Harada, Masazumi. *Minamata Disease*. Kumamoto Nichinichi Shinbun Centre & Information Center/Iwanami Shoten Publishers, 1972. p. 68-77.
38   Grandjean, P. et al. "Cognitive deficit in 7-year-old children with prenatal exposure to methylmercury." *Neurotoxicol Teratol.* 1997; 19:417–428. doi: 10.1016/S0892-0362(97)00097.
39   Crump, K.S. et al. "Influence of prenatal mercury exposure upon scholastic and psychological test performance: benchmark analysis of a New Zealand cohort." *Risk Anal.* 1998; 18:701–713. doi: 10.1023/B: RIAN 0000005917.52151.e6.

they distorted the results in favor of a no mercury neuro-developmental harm linkage.[40]

Scientists at the National Research Council (NRC) were aware of the Seychelles Island results when they published their report and recommendations regarding fish consumption and its possible risks in 2000.[41]

"The overall conclusion of that report was that, at levels of exposure in some fish- and marine mammal-consuming communities (including those in the Faroe Islands and New Zealand), subtle but significant adverse effects on neuropsychological development were occurring as a result of *in-utero* exposure."

In their follow up commentary in 2004, the authors responded to the suggestion that the results of the Seychelles Island study might cause them to come to a different conclusion regarding the toxic potential of fish and whale meat consumption.

They did not change their conclusions, however. They stated that, "It has recently been posited that these (Seychelles) findings supercede those of the NRC committee, and that based on the Seychelles findings, there is little or no risk of adverse neurodevelopmental effects at current levels of exposure. In this commentary, members of the NRC committee address the conclusions from the NRC report in light of the recent Seychelles data. We conclude that no evidence has emerged since the publication of the NRC report that alters the findings of that report."[42]

What Evidence Supports Contention 3?

CONTENTION 3: *The physiological effects of mercury also parallel those seen in autistic individuals.*

There are, indeed, many similarities between the neuro-toxic effects of mercury and the neurological abnormalities seen in autism. A 2012 review article by Janet Kern and colleagues found many parallels, including:

(1) Microtubule degeneration, specifically large, long-range axon degeneration with subsequent abortive axonal sprouting (short, thin axons);

(2) Dentritic overgrowth;

(3) Neuroinflammation;

(4) Microglial/astrocytic activation;

(5) Brain immune response activation;

(6) Elevated glial fibrillary acidic protein;

(7) Oxidative stress and lipid peroxidation;

(8) Decreased reduced glutathione levels and elevated oxidized glutathione;

(9) Mitochondrial dysfunction;

(10) Disruption in calcium homeostasis and signaling;

(11) Inhibition of glutamic acid decarboxylase (GAD) activity;

(12) Disruption of GABAergic and glutamatergic homeostasis;

(13) Inhibition of IGF-1 and methionine synthase activity;

40   Myers, G.J. et al. "Prenatal methylmercury exposure from ocean fish consumption in the Seychelles child development study." *Lancet.* 2003; 361:1686–1692. doi: 10.1016/S0140-6736(03)13371-5.
41   National Research Council Toxicological Effects of Methylmercury. Washington, D.C.: National Academy Press, 2000; and Stern, Alan et al. "Do recent data from the Seychelles Islands alter the conclusions of the NRC Report on the toxicological effects of methylmercury?" *Environ Health*; 2004; 3:2; published online Jan 30, 2004. doi: 10.1186/1476-069X-3-2.
42   Stern, Alan; Ibid.

(14) Impairment in methylation;

(15) Vascular endothelial cell dysfunction and pathological changes of the blood vessels;

(16) Decreased cerebral/cerebellar blood flow;

(17) Increased amyloid precursor protein;

(18) Loss of granule and Purkinje neurons in the cerebellum;

(19) Increased pro-inflammatory cytokine levels in the brain (TNF-α, IFN-γ, IL-1β, IL- 8);

(20) Aberrant nuclear factor kappa-light-chain-enhancer of activated B cells (NF-kappa B).

The authors conclude that, "The evidence suggests that mercury may be either causal or contributory in the brain pathology in Autism Spectrum Disorders (ASD), possibly working synergistically with other toxic compounds or pathogens to produce the brain pathology observed in those diagnosed with an ASD.[43]

See Appendix IV, Table A for further references that support this contention.

BAMBOOZLED?

"One of the saddest lessons of history is this: If we've been bamboozled long enough, we tend to reject any evidence of the bamboozle. We're no longer interested in finding out the truth. The bamboozle has captured us. It's simply too painful to acknowledge, even to ourselves, that we've been taken. Once you give a charlatan power over you, you almost never get it back."

— *Carl Sagan*

What Evidence Supports Contention 4?

CONTENTION 4: *The rise in autism cases parallels the increase in infants' mercury exposure from immunizations, at least up to the early 2000s.*

Table 11.1. lists the U.S.A. mandated vaccines, the year added to the schedule, the number of doses given in childhood to age 5, and the cumulative number of vaccines up to that date.

Table 11.1. Adapted from a table at www.fourteenstudies.org

Year Added to USA Schedule	USA Mandated Vaccines for children (0-5yrs)	Doses Given to age 5 in the USA/total doses to date
Early 20th Cent -1940s	Smallpox-(Vaccinia) **Diptheria, Tetanus, Pertussis (DTP)**	1-2/1-2 5/ 6-7
1955	Inactivated Poliovirus (IPV)	4/ 10-11
1971	Measles, Mumps, Rubella (MMR)	2/ 12-13
1972 1985 1990	Smallpox vacc. discontinued **Hemophilus Influenzae type B (Hib)**; 1st marketed in 1985 and universally recommended in 1990	-2/ 10-11 4/ 15
1991	**Hepatitis B (HepB)**	3/ 18

---

43   Kern, J.K. et al. "Evidence of parallels between mercury intoxication and the brain pathology in autism." *Acta Neurobiol Exp (Wars)*. 2012; 72(2):113-53.

Year Added to USA Schedule	USA Mandated Vaccines for children (0-5yrs)	Doses Given to age 5 in the USA/total doses to date
1995	Varicella (chickenpox)	2/ 20
1998	Rotavirus (RV)	3/ 23
2000	Pneumococcal (PCV)	4/ 27 (26 vaccinations by end of year 1)
2004	**Influenza**	7/ 34
2004	Hepatitis A (Hep A)	2/ 36
2006	Meningococcal (high risk groups only)	?/ 36
2014	Total Vaccines to US Children < 5 yr	36 vaccinations by year 5!

Vaccines in bold font have contained thimerosal.

The Influenza & TD booster vaccines still contain thimerosal. There are so-called "trace" amounts of thimerosal in many other childhood vaccines in the U.S., and high amounts in many vaccines administered to babies and children worldwide.

The graph in Figure 11.1. illustrates the correlation between *autism percentages* and *continuing vaccine exposures*. It clearly shows that the rise in California autism prevalence tracks proportionately with the increases in the number and kind of childhood immunizations.

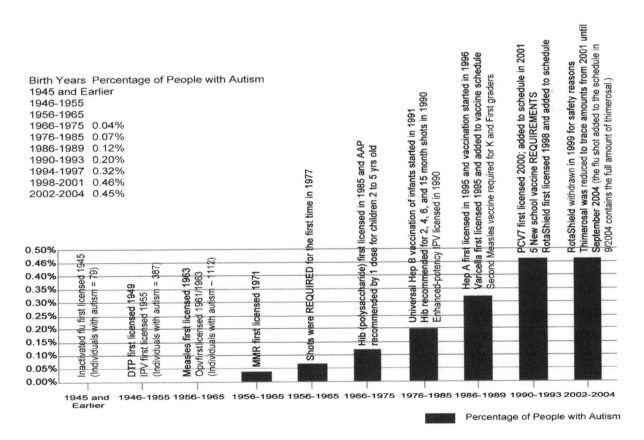

Figure 11.1. Percentage of California individuals with autism by birth year compared to the recommended childhood vaccine schedule

In the graph in Figure 11.1, the vertical bars represent the percentage of people with autism. Note that the slope in the rise of *autism cases parallels the introduction of new vaccines, and in particular, the thimerosal-containing vaccines* (DTP, Hib, AAP, Hep B, Hep A, PCV7). The slight decrease in the percentage of people diagnosed with autism in the 2002-2004 cohort also tracks nicely with the decrease in thimerosal exposure during that same time period.[44]

These findings were reinterpreted in the following graphical analysis (Fig. 2) in which the average cumulative dose of *mercury exposure* in the U.S. from vaccines was compared to the estimated prevalence (per 10,000 population) of children diagnosed with autism-like disorders in California from 1987 until 1998.[45]

It is clear from the graph that *autism prevalence* figures paralleled *cumulative mercury exposure* during that eleven-year period.

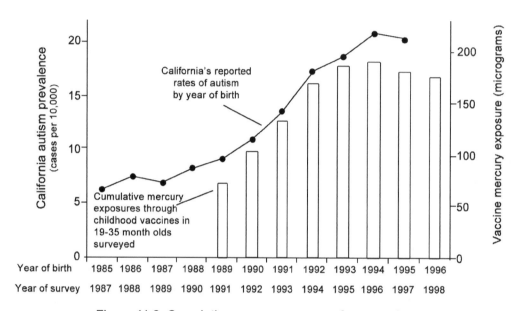

Figure 11.2. Cumulative mercury exposure from vaccines
compared to California childhood autism rates[46]

Even Dr. Verstraeten acknowledged the biological plausibility that mercury causes neurological damage:

> When I saw this (finding a significant relationship between mercury in vaccines and adverse neurodevelopmental outcomes, including autism), and I went back through the literature, I was actually stunned by what I saw, because I thought it is plausible.

> First of all there is the Faeroe study, which I think people have dismissed too easily, and there is a new article in the same Journal that was presented here, the *Journal of Pediatrics*, where they have looked at PCB. They have looked at other contaminants in seafood and they have adjusted for that, and still mercury comes out. That is one point.

> Another point is that in many of the studies with animals, it turned out that there is quite a different result depending on the dose of mercury, depending on the route of exposure and depending on the age at which the animals were exposed.

> Now, I don't know how much you can extrapolate that from animals to humans, but that tells me mercury at one month of age is not the same as mercury at three months, at 12 months, prenatal mercury, later mercury. There is a whole range of plausible outcomes from mercury.[47]

44   http://safeminds.org/mercury/correlation-between-autism-and-vaccines.html
45   Mark Blaxill; Institute of Medicine Presentation; July 16, 2001.
46   Graphical ecological analysis presented by Mark Blaxill to the Institute of Medicine July 16, 2001.
47   Dr. Verstraeten, commenting in Simpsonwood Conference discussions, June 7, 2000.

Chapter 12
Vaccinations, Thimerosal and Mercury

"All great truths begin as blasphemies."
— *George Bernard Shaw*

What Evidence Supports *Contention 5?*

CONTENTION 5: *Autistic children have an impaired capacity to detoxify mercury and appear to have an increased body burden of mercury as compared to non-autistic children. Their total body-burden of mercury appears to correlate with the severity of their autism. The more mercury they have, the more autistic they appear to be.*

Supporting data comes from a number of studies:

1. The Adams (et al.) Study

Children's teeth appear to be a good way to measure the body burden of mercury because teeth represent one of the tissues in the body into which mercury is stored. Jane Adams and associates studied the mercury, lead, and zinc levels in the teeth of young children with autism as compared to those in normally developing children of the same age and found that *the mercury concentration in the teeth of the autistic children, but not the lead or zinc, was significantly higher than that in the non-autistic population.*

The autistic children also had a history of greater exposure to antibiotics during their infancy and early childhood than did the control population. *Antibiotics have been shown to inhibit almost completely the excretion of mercury in rats due to undesirable antibiotic-induced alterations in the balance of gut microbes.* The same mechanism in the autistic children may be one factor that contributed to their higher body-burden of mercury, and a dysfunctional detoxification system is a likely factor as well.[1]

2. The Bradstreet (et al.) Study

Dr. Jeffrey Bradstreet and his research colleagues measured the urinary excretion of mercury after a three-day trial of an oral chelating agent (DMSA) in a group of 221 vaccinated and unvaccinated autistic children and a matched control group of 18 normally developing children. A chelating (KEY-lay-ting) agent like DMSA is able to remove mercury and other metals from the body and to transport them to the kidneys for removal via the urine.

What the research group found was a statistically significant *three-fold excretion* of mercury in the autistic population as a whole as compared to the neurologically normal controls, and the amount of mercury excreted by the *vaccinated autistic* population averaged almost *six times* the level found in the *vaccinated control* population. In the control population, the levels of mercury in the vaccinated and unvaccinated populations was the same. This would

---

1   Adams, J.B. et al. "Mercury, lead and zinc in baby teeth of children with autism vs. controls." *J Toxicol & Environ. Health*; June 2007; 70(12):1046-51.

imply that the *non-autistic children were able to excrete the mercury from the thimerosal in their vaccinations, but the autistic children weren't.* No association was found between urinary cadmium or lead concentrations and autism spectrum disorders.

The authors suggested that, "The observed urinary concentrations of mercury could plausibly have resulted from thimerosal in childhood vaccines, although other environmental sources and thimerosal in Rho (D) immune globulin administered to mothers may be contributory."[2]

3. A Geier (et al.) Study

As was pointed out in Chapter 3, certain kinds of porphyrins (substances used in the manufacture of hemoglobin) when found in elevated amounts in the urine are diagnostic of mercury toxicity.

In one prospective, blinded study by David Geier, these porphyrin toxicity markers were measured in the urine of both autistic and normally functioning children. The researchers found that the (non-chelated) autistic children, compared to the non-autistic control group, were more likely to have *significantly* elevated levels of the abnormal porphyrins associated with mercury toxicity, and the severity of the autism, as measured by standardized CARS (Childhood Autism Rating Scale) scores, paralleled the levels of abnormal porphyrins in their urine. *That is, the more mercury a child had, the more severe was his or her autism.*

These same autistic children also had *significantly lower levels of glutathione*, a protective antioxidant and detoxifying substance, as compared to the neurotypical control group, and *the lower the levels of protective glutathione found, the more severe was their autism.*

As a result of this study, the researchers concluded that, "ASDs (autism spectrum disorders) may result from a combination of genetic/biochemical susceptibilities in the form of a reduced ability to excrete mercury and/or increased environmental exposures at key developmental times."[3]

4-8. Five additional studies that use mercury biomarkers

These studies also confirm the research and conclusions of the Geier et al. study discussed above. All of these research studies demonstrate increased mercury-associated porphyrins in the urine of autistic children compared with controls, and two of them show decreases in the toxicity-marker porphyrins when the affected children were chelated (given a substance that reduced the levels of toxic metals in their system). These studies will be reviewed in more detail later and are:

- Nataf, R. et al. "Porphyrinurea in Childhood Autistic Disorders: Implications for Environmental Toxicity." *Toxicol. Appl. Pharmacol.* 214(2):99-108, 2006.

- Geier, M., Geier, D. "A prospective assessment of porphyrins in autistic disorders: a potential marker for heavy metal exposure." *Neurotox Res.* Aug; 10(1):57-64, 2006.

- Geier, M., Geier, D. "A Prospective Study of Mercury Toxicity Biomarkers in Autistic Spectrum Disorders." *Journal of Toxicology and Environmental Health, Part A*, 70: 1723–1730, 2007.

- Geier, David A., Kern, Janet K., and Geier, Mark R. "A Prospective Blinded Evaluation of Urinary Porphyrins Versus the Clinical Severity of Autism Spectrum Disorders." *Journal of Toxicology and Environmental Health, Part A*, 72: 24, 1585-1591, 2009.

- Kern, J.K. et al. "Toxicity Biomarkers in Autism Spectrum Disorder: A Blinded Study of Urinary Porphyrins." *Pediatrics International* 2010. Accepted Article: "09 June 2010"; doi: 10.1111/j.1442-200X.2010. 03196.x.

---

2   Bradstreet, J. et al. "A Case Controlled Study of Mercury Burden in Children with Autism Spectrum Disorders." *Journal of American Physicians and Surgeons.* Vol. 8. No. 3. Fall 2003.
3   Geier, D. et al. "Biomarkers of environmental toxicity and susceptibility in autism." *Journal of the Neurological Sciences.* DOI: 10.1016/j.jns.2008.08.021.

9. The Holmes (et al.) Study

The human body excretes mercury in urine, stool, finger and toe nails, teeth, and hair. A study was done to determine the levels of mercury in the hair from the first baby haircuts of 95 autistic children as compared to an age and sex matched control group of 45 non-affected children.

Although, as a group, the mothers of the autistic children had a *greater* number of mercury-containing amalgam fillings and a *greater* exposure to a thimerosal-preserved vaccination (Rhogam) during the pregnancy than did the control group's mothers, the hair of the autistic children had *significantly lower levels* of mercury than did the hair of the control group children.

The autistic children's hair mercury levels averaged 0.47 ppm (parts per million) and that of the control group 3.63 ppm. That's *7.7 times* more mercury in the hair of the non-autistic children than was found in the hair of the autistic group.

In addition, the researchers found that *the degree of severity of the child's autism correlated inversely with levels of mercury in their baby hair.* In other words, the less able a child is to excrete mercury (by excreting it into hair, for example) the more likely that mercury is to remain in the child's brain (and elsewhere) where it is more likely to do damage. The less the mercury in the hair, the more severe the autism.

"Within the autistic group, hair mercury levels varied significantly across mildly, moderately, and severely autistic children, with mean group levels of 0.79, 0.46, and 0.21 ppm, respectively.

"Hair mercury levels among controls were significantly correlated with the number of the mothers' amalgam fillings and their fish consumption as well as exposure to mercury through childhood vaccines, correlations that were absent in the autistic group.

"Hair excretion patterns among autistic *infants* were significantly reduced relative to control."

Holmes, et al. state, "These data cast doubt on the efficacy of traditional hair analysis as a measure of total mercury exposure in a subset of the population." In other words, hair analysis will not accurately reflect the body burden of mercury in an autistic child because of that individual's relative inability to excrete this toxic metal.

The researchers suggest that, "In light of the biological plausibility of mercury's role in neurodevelopmental disorders, the present study provides further insight into one possible mechanism by which early mercury exposures could increase the risk of autism."[4]

10. The *corrected* Ip (et al.) study

In 2004, researchers from the University of Hong Kong, Division of Neurodevelopmental Pediatrics published a study that purported to show no statistically significant difference between the mercury levels found in the hair and blood of seven-year-old autistic children as compared to age matched controls.

The researchers concluded their study by stating that, "the results from our cohort study with similar environmental mercury exposure indicate that there is no causal relationship between mercury as an environmental neurotoxin and autism."[5]

That conclusion, however, is clearly unwarranted and incorrect. If autistic children have impaired detoxification mechanisms, as seems to be the case, then the hair results obtained by the Chinese researchers are exactly what one would expect.

Over the years, the seven-year-old non-autistic children would have been excreting mercury efficiently, so their hair levels would be expected to be relatively low. The autistic children may have had, and as it turns out probably

---

4   Holmes, A.S., Blaxill, M.F. et al.. "Reduced levels of mercury in first baby haircuts of autistic children." *Int J Toxicol.* 2003 Jul-Aug; 22(4):277-85.
5   Ip, P. et al. "Mercury exposure in children with autistic spectrum disorder: case-control study." *J Child Neurol.* 2004 Jun; 19(6):431-4.

did have, an elevated body burden of mercury, but due to their *relative inability* to excrete this metal into hair (see Holmes study above), their hair levels were consequently low as well.

But what about the blood levels in the two groups? The autistic children in this study did have elevated *"mean" mercury levels in their blood* as compared to the control group, but as calculated by Ip and his coworkers, the difference did not reach statistical significance [p=0.15].

However, Ip and his fellow researchers were wrong in their calculations due to an embarrassing series of major typographical errors and mathematical miscalculations (in a statistical test called a "*t*-test").

Their multiple mistakes were ultimately discovered thanks to the sharp eyes of a Professor of Epidemiology, Mary Catherine DeSoto, who then notified the *Journal of Child Neurology*. Ip and his fellow researchers admitted their errors in an addendum to the original study published some three years later.[6]

When the errors were remedied, the differences in mean blood mercury levels in the autistic population turned out to be greater than those in the control group by a statistically significant degree (p<0.05, two-tailed; letter to *J Child Neurol* by DeSoto and Hitlan who reanalyzed the "mean" differences between the two groups).

This implies that if the analysis of the mean mercury levels in the two groups is valid, then the autistic children studied by Ip et al. did indeed have an increased body burden of mercury compared to the non-autistic children in this study, and their conclusion should instead have been that "there *does* seem to be a causal relationship between mercury and autism."

However, the story gets even more tangled because yet another statistical analysis of the original and the Desoto/Hitlan corrected data-set by a no longer anonymous online blogger (Dr. John Lawrence Kiely[7]), who calls himself "Epiwonk," suggests that comparing the "mean" blood levels in the autistic and control groups is "inappropriate" and that by reanalyzing the data in another manner one may come to the conclusion that the Ip study results demonstrate neither a significant relationship between thimerosal and autism, nor do they rule out such a relationship. [8]

To further complicate matters, it must be understood that mercury does not remain in the blood for long. Blood *serum* analysis of mercury as a measure of body burden is only accurate for acute or continuous poisonings although *red blood cell* mercury levels may more accurately reflect total body burden of this toxic metal.

The seven-year-old children in this study most likely had their last thimerosal-containing vaccinations when they were five years of age if their physicians followed the generally accepted vaccination protocols. The degree to which other sources of mercury, like fish, contributed to the total body burden of mercury in these children would also be difficult, if not impossible, to assess accurately.

Thus, the blood serum levels of mercury would not necessarily have been expected to differ greatly in the two groups *unless the mercury levels in the autistic children were unusually elevated.* A more rational and appropriate approach to determining mercury body burden would have been to perform a chelated urine challenge test (with DMSA or DMPS for example) in both groups, or an analysis of the porphyrin markers that appear to correlate with mercury levels.

The original Ip study was so flawed that it should never have been published. The retraction of the original article by Ip and his associates helps in some way to ameliorate the damage it caused and still causes in regard to our understanding the true relationship between mercury and autism.

---

6   Ip, P. et al. Erratum to "Mercury exposure in children with autistic spectrum disorder: case-control." *J Child Neurol* 22: 1324, 2007, *and* Desoto, M.C., Hitlan, R.T. "Blood Levels of Mercury Are Related to Diagnosis of Autism: A Reanalysis of an Important Data Set." *J Child Neurol* November 2007. Vol. 22. No. 11 1308-1311.

7   A retired research epidemiologist for the CDC's National Center for Health Statistics, and American editor of the medical journal *Paediatric and Perinatal Epidemiology*.

8   www.epiwonk.com/?p=112

Unfortunately, the original Ip study, which maintains that there is "no causal relationship between mercury…and autism," has been cited by others 83 times, often in an attempt to bolster the argument about just such a lack of an association.[9]

11. The Kern (et al.) Study: Sulfhydryl-reactive metals in autism.

(Kern, J.K. et al. *J Toxicol Environ Health A*. 2007 Apr 15; 70(8):715-21.)

Janet Kern and her colleagues measured the levels of mercury, lead, arsenic, and cadmium in the hair of 45 autistic children aged 1-6 years and compared these levels to those of an equal number of gender, age, and race-matched control children. The toxic metals measured are those that attach to the sulfur-hydrogen part ("sulfhydryl group") of the molecules that contain the amino acids *methionine* or *cysteine* (like glutathione and the metallothioneins, for example).

The researchers found that autistic children had *significantly* less arsenic, cadmium, and lead in their hair than did the control children. Mercury was also lower in the hair of autistic children, but the difference between that group and the control children did not reach statistical significance.

Kern et al. suggest that their study "supports the notion that children with autism may have trouble excreting these metals, resulting in a higher body burden that may contribute to symptoms of autism."

What Evidence Supports Contention 6?

CONTENTION 6: *Thimerosal and mercury are proven to interfere with certain enzymes which, when inhibited, promote the autistic state. Furthermore, certain genetic variations (mutations/polymorphisms) in particular enzymes, their concentrations or activity can exacerbate mercury's deleterious effects in this regard.*

Inhibition of Methionine Synthase

We have previously noted the importance of the transmethylation pathway to everyday health, and have discussed a mechanism by which certain mutations in the methionine synthase enzyme promote some of the features of autism and ADHD.

One of the principal functions of the methionine synthase enzyme is to convert homocysteine to methionine by methylating it (a methyl group is a carbon atom with three hydrogen atoms attached).

One of the places it does this is in the cell membrane in association with the D4 receptor for the neurotransmitter dopamine.

The act of methylating homocysteine then allows certain key membrane substances called phospholipids to receive the methyl group. The end result of all this biochemistry is the creation of a focused, attentive state. If methionine synthase is hampered in its catalytic abilities by mutations or toxic substances, then inattention and hyperactivity, which are characteristics common in both autism and ADHD, result.

Dr. Richard Deth ("Deeth") has shown that mercury, lead, and thimerosal all inhibit this methionine synthase catalyzed reaction *in a dose dependent manner* (the more thimerosal there is, the greater the inhibition).[10]

As Dr. Deth states, "A single vaccination (preserved with thimerosal) produces thimerosal blood levels between 10 and 100 Nm. Our findings clearly demonstrate that thimerosal inhibits PI3-kinase-dependent methionine synthase at concentrations well below these levels, raising the possibility that this inhibition might contribute to the pathology of autism."[11]

---

9   Desoto, M.C. and Hitlan, R.T. "Sorting out the spinning of autism: heavy metals and the question of incidence." *Acta Neurobiol Exp* 2010, 70: 165–176.
10   Deth and Waly, Op.Cit.; *Stajich, G.V., Lopez, G.P., Harry, S.W., & Sexson, W.R. (2000). *J. Pediatr* 136, 679-8.
11   Deth and Waly, Op.Cit.; *Stajich, G.V., Lopez, G.P., Harry, S.W., & Sexson, W.R. (2000). *J. Pediatr* 136, 679-8.

Dr. Deth's findings were confirmed in a more recent study at Northeastern University in which it was shown that *ethanol, lead, mercury, aluminum and thimerosal all inhibited this critical methionine synthase pathway,* which could "lead to neurodevelopmental toxicity."[12]

Other Enzyme Mutations and the Interactions with Toxins Adenosine Deaminase Mutations (Polymorphisms)

Dr. Deth continues: "The risk of developing autism in response to heavy metal or thimerosal exposure may depend upon genetically-transmitted risk factors that interact with methylation events. For example, previous studies showed that adenosine deaminase (ADA) activity is reduced in autistic individuals associated with (an) increased prevalence of a polymorphism (mutation) in the ADA gene that reduces enzyme activity."[13]

"Reduced ADA activity," Dr. Deth states, "will cause elevated adenosine levels that will synergize with impaired methionine synthase activity (see above) to produce higher levels of SAH (s-adenosyl homocysteine), yielding greater inhibition of methylation reactions (since SAH inhibits methylation reactions)."

5'-nucleotidase Mutations

"Increased synthesis of adenosine due to elevated 5'-nucleotidase activity has also been reported in autism."[14]

Adenosyl-succinate Lyase Mutations

Mutations in the adenosylsuccinate (uh-DEN oh-seal SUCK-sin-ate) lyase (LIE-ace) gene are a rare cause of autism.[15]

"These mutations [increase] purine synthesis and limit the availability of 5-methyl-THF (the active form of folic acid). Moreover, increased purine synthesis is common in autism."[16]

"Lower availability of 5-methylTHF (active folic acid) will synergize with the inhibitory effects of metals and thimerosal.

"These examples serve to illustrate how genetic and metabolic abnormalities can predispose to autism. Any impairment in the ability to excrete or detoxify heavy metals will also impose a further increased risk."[17]

What Evidence Supports Contention 7?

CONTENTION 7: *Children in the U.S., at least up until 2003, were being given thimerosal-preserved vaccinations, invariably in amounts that exceeded the allowable upper limit established by regulating authorities, like the EPA (0.1 mcg/kg) and the World Health Organization (0.47 mcg/kg).*[18]

This statement is not controversial and cannot be challenged, as one simply has to do the math to see the correctness of the assertion. The average newborn baby weighs 7.5 lbs (3.4 kg), so the maximum allowable amount of mercury per day for the typical newborn would be 0.34 micrograms (EPA) and 1.7 mcg (WHO).

Immunizations containing thimerosal as a preservative generally contain 25 mcg of mercury. A newborn of average weight in the 1990s receiving a thimerosal-preserved hepatitis B vaccine on his/her first day of life would thus be getting an amount of mercury *73 times higher* than allowed by the Environmental Protection Agency and almost *17 times the maximum* allowed by the less stringent World Health Organization, which still (in 2015) injects infants worldwide with thimerosal-preserved vaccines that are no longer allowed in the U.S.

12   Waly, M. et al. "Activation of Methionine Synthase by Insulin-like Growth Factor-1 and Dopamine: a Target for Neurodevelopmental Toxins and Thimerosal." *Mol Psychiatry.* 2004 Apr 9(4):358-70.
13   Persico, A.M. et al. (2002) *Am. J. Med. Genet.* 96, 784-90 and Stubbs, G., et al; (1982) *J. Am. Acad. Child Psychiatry* 21, 71-4.
14   Page, T. et al. (1997) *Proc. Natl. Acad. Sci. USA* 94, 11601-6.
15   Stone, R.L., et al (1992) *Nat. Genet.* 1, 59-63.
16   Page, T., & Coleman, M. (1998) *Adv. Exp. Med. Biol.* 431, 793-6.
17   Blaxill, M. F. & Haley, B.E. (2003) *Int. J. Toxicol.* 22
18   See "Department of OOPs" at end of Chapter 10.

If a baby were born prematurely (at say 1.5-2 kg) then the toxicity from the mercury given at birth or before ("flu" shot to pregnant woman) would be significantly greater, as would exposing the even tinier developing fetus, which is particularly susceptible to mercury toxicity from the mother, as has been demonstrated in several instances of mass mercury poisoning.[19]

Today's toxicity guidelines don't take into account the cumulative effects of multiple doses of vaccine over time or the possible synergy between neurotoxins like mercury and aluminum, or the diminished detoxification abilities of some babies.

Today (2015), all of the multi-dose influenza vaccines still contain 25 mcg of mercury from thimerosal and are recommended to be given to the pregnant mother *at any time during the pregnancy* and then again to the baby at 6 and 18 months of age and yearly thereafter. (Flu-Zone is given at half dose to children under 3). (See Table 12.1.)

One can reasonably ask: "Is this a wise policy?"

Table 12.1. Mercury (From Thimerosal)[20]

Vaccine	Trade Name	Mercury Concentration	Approval For Thimerosal-Free Vaccine
Seasonal Trivalent Influenza	Fluzone (multi-dose presentation)	0.01 percent (12.5 µg/0.25 mL dose, 25 µg/0.5 mL dose) Children under 3 years of age receive a half-dose of vaccine, i.e., 0.25 mL (12.5 µg mercury/dose.)	
	Fluzone (single-dose presentation)	Free	12/23/2004
	Fluvirin (multi-dose presentation)	0.01 percent (25 µg/0.5 mL dose)	
	Fluvirin (single dose presentation) (Preservative Free)	Trace (<1ug Hg/0.5mL dose)	09/28/01
	Fluarix (single-dose presentation)	Free	Approved 10/19/09, never contained thimerosal
	Afluria (multi-dose presentation)	0.01 percent (24.5 µg/0.5 mL dose)	
	Afluria (single-dose presentation	Free	Approved 11/10/09, never contained thimerosal

What Evidence Supports Contention 8?

CONTENTION 8: *Animal studies (in monkeys and rodents) support the thimerosal-autism link. They show that thimerosal (a source of ethyl mercury) injected into baby monkeys and in rodents gets into the brain readily and lasts longer in the brain than it does in the bloodstream, and significantly longer and in higher concentrations than does methyl mercury, and that it also causes neurological damage.*

1. Human and animal brains contain many types of cells, including neurons, astrocytes, microglial (*MIKE-row-GLEE-ull*) cells and others. Methyl-mercury is the form of organic mercury that has been most studied in terms of its toxicity, and the safety standards established for organic mercury have been based only on the studies done of those exposed to *methyl*-mercury, not *ethyl*-mercury (the kind found in thimerosal).

---

19   http:www.fda.gov/BiologicsBloodVaccines/SafetyAvailability/VaccineSafety/ucm096228.htm
20   Content of currently used Influenza Vaccines 2013 recommended for children under 6 years of age (Adapted from chart on FDA website) http://www.fda.gov/BiologicsBloodVaccines/SafetyAvailability/VaccineSafety/ucm096228.htm

Scientists at the University of Washington, School of Medicine studied the effects of long-term *subclinical methyl-mercury* exposure in macaque monkey brain cells and discovered that the astrocytes *declined* in number while the microglial cells *increased* in population after 18 months of exposure to methyl-mercury. The other cells (neurons, etc.) appeared to be less effected by the exposure.

The researchers also noted that the *organic* methyl mercury in the brain cells of the macaques broke down into *inorganic* form(s) of mercury, and that the cells with highest concentrations of the inorganic forms of mercury were the cells that were the most affected by this toxin, the astrocytes, and the microglial cells.

They concluded that, "The data suggest that the inorganic mercury present in the brains, accumulating after long-term subclinical methyl mercury exposure, may be a proximate toxic form of mercury responsible for the changes within the astrocyte and microglial populations."[21]

2. But what about the toxicity of *ethyl*mercury, the kind found in thimerosal? Researchers Thomas Burbacher and associates compared the total blood and brain mercury levels of infant monkeys exposed to *methyl*mercury or to vaccines containing thimerosal (a source of *ethyl*mercury). These measurements were made over a period of days and weeks, and the brain mercury evaluations were made for both total mercury as well as the inorganic form.

What the researchers found was that while the brain concentration of total mercury was *a third less* for *ethyl*mercury derived from thimerosal as compared to *methyl*mercury, the percentage of *inorganic* mercury in the monkey brains was over *6 times higher* (34 percent vs. 7 percent) in the thimerosal-exposed group compared to the methyl mercury dosed primates.

This means that the thimerosal-exposed monkeys had over twice as much (6 X ⅓) *inorganic* mercury in their brain cells as did the monkeys exposed to methylmercury, and keep in mind, it is the *inorganic* mercury accumulation in particular brain cells that appears to be the proximate cause of the toxicity to those cells, according to the Charleston (et al) study cited above.

The researchers concluded that, "The current study indicates that methylmercury is not a suitable reference for risk assessment from exposure to thimerosal-derived mercury. Knowledge of the toxicokinetics[22] and developmental toxicity of thimerosal is needed to afford a meaningful assessment of the developmental effects of thimerosal-containing vaccines."[23]

3. In another study, Polish researchers injected varying amounts of thimerosal "in a vaccination-like mode" into two varieties of rats on days 7, 9, 11, and 15 after birth in four equal doses and found that the thimerosal was able to get into the rat brain "in significant amounts," and that it remained "there longer than 30 days after the injection."

The rats that received the thimerosal also became *significantly less sensitive to pain* than did the control group of rats. Human and animal brains are capable of producing morphine-like substances known as *endorphins* (from "endogenous morphine") which, like morphine, block pain receptors on cells.

This decreased sensitivity to pain in the rats under study was blocked by Naloxone, an opioid (narcotic) receptor blocker, indicating that thimerosal administration to rats activates the endogenous (from within the body) opioid system. One of the characteristics of many autistic children is a marked decreased sensitivity to pain.[24]

4. These same Polish researchers also did a second study on those unfortunate rats, this time by examining the brains of the rats exposed to thimerosal, and specifically looking at the opioid receptors in three different parts of their brains.

---

21   Charleston, J. et al. "Changes in the number of astrocytes and microglia in the thalamus of the monkey Macaca fascicularis following long-term sub-clinical methylmercury exposure." *Neurotoxicology* 17:127-138, 1996.

22   Toxicokinetics refers to how a toxin is distributed and metabolized in the body, and what damage it does.

23   Burbacher, T. et al. "Comparison of blood and brain mercury levels in infant monkeys exposed to methyl mercury or vaccines containing thimerosal." *Environ Health Perspectives*; 2005 August 113(8): 1015f.

24   Olczak, M. et al. "Neonatal administration of a vaccine preservative, thimerosal, produces lasting impairment of nociception and apparent activation of opioid system in rats." *Brain Res.* 2009 Dec 8; 1301:143-51. Epub 2009 Sep 9.

They found that thimerosal "caused dose-dependent, statistically significant increase(s) in mu opioid receptors (brain receptors for morphine-like compounds) in two parts of the brain (the peri-aqueductal gray matter and the caudate putamen), but decrease(s) in the dentate gyrus," where they noted degenerating neurons and the loss of a synaptic vesicle marker.

These scientists concluded that, "These data document that exposure to thimerosal during early postnatal life produces lasting alterations in the densities of brain opioid receptors along with other neuropathological changes, which may disturb brain development."[25]

5. Researchers at the University of Pittsburgh School of Medicine "examined whether acquisition of neonatal reflexes in (13) newborn rhesus macaques was influenced by receipt of a single (weight adjusted) dose of hepatitis B vaccine containing the preservative thimerosal." They compared this group to four unexposed animals that received saline placebo injections.

"Infants were tested daily for acquisition of nine survival, motor, and sensorimotor reflexes. In exposed animals there was a significant delay in the acquisition of root, snout, and suck reflexes, compared with unexposed animals. No neonatal responses were significantly delayed in unexposed animals." These adverse effects were exacerbated by lower birth weight and/or lower gestational age.[26]

6. However, in a more comprehensive infant macaque study on the safety of the pediatric vaccine schedules, which assessed neurodevelopment, learning, and social behavior and was performed by the same University of Pittsburgh School of Medicine, researchers came to a quite different conclusion. In this follow-up study, they *"found no evidence of an adverse impact of vaccination status on early neurodevelopmental measures, including the acquisition of neonatal reflexes and the development of object permanence."*

"These data," the research team acknowledges, "are in contrast to our previous pilot study in which a delay in the acquisition of the root, suck, and snout survival reflexes were reported for primate infants following exposure to the birth dose of the thimerosal-containing Hep B vaccine…. This discrepancy," they allege, "is most likely due to the larger number of animals in the present study providing more accurate estimates."

Brain volume was not evaluated in this study.

This research was funded by a number of organizations including SafeMinds (which also funded the pilot study) and the National Autism Association.[27]

7. Brazilian scientists were interested in studying the distribution of methyl-, ethyl- or inorganic mercury in rat brain, heart, kidney, liver, and blood following administration of either thimerosal (a source of ethyl mercury) or methyl-mercury. Blood samples were obtained at 6, 12, and 24 hours and 2, 4, and 10 days after exposure.

What the researchers discovered was that:

- Mercury remains longer in the *blood* of rats treated with *methyl*-mercury compared to that of thimerosal-exposed rats.

- Moreover, after 48 hours of the thimerosal treatment, most of the mercury found in blood was *inorganic*.

- Of the total mercury found in the *brain* after thimerosal exposure, 63 percent was in the form of inorganic mercury, with 13.5 percent as ethyl-mercury and 23.7 percent as methyl-mercury.

- In general, mercury in tissues and blood following thimerosal treatment was predominantly found as *inorganic mercury*, but a considerable amount of ethyl-mercury was also found in the liver and brain.

25   Olczak, M. et al. "Neonatal administration of thimerosal causes persistent changes in mu opioid receptors in the rat brain." *Neurochem Res.* 2010 Nov; 35(11):1840-7. Epub 2010 Aug 28.

26   Hewitson L, et al. "Delayed acquisition of neonatal reflexes in newborn primates receiving a thimerosal-containing hepatitis B vaccine: influence of gestational age and birth weight." *J Toxicol Environ Health A.* 2010 Jan; 73 (19): 1298-313.

27   Examination of the Safety of Pediatric Vaccine Schedules in a Non-Human Primate Model: Assessments of Neurodevelopment, Learning, and Social Behavior. Curtis B, et al. *Environ Health Perspect.* 2015 Jun; 123(6): 579–589.

- Taken together, their data demonstrated that "the toxicokinetics of thimerosal is completely different from that of methyl-mercury."[28]

8. Swedish researchers J. Ekstrand and colleagues at Linköping University theorized that, "Individual differences in toxicokinetics may explain susceptibility to mercury" so they fed two genetically different strains of mice and their hybrid offspring the same quantity of oral inorganic mercury chloride and they measured how much of the mercury the animals retained until a steady state was noted after five weeks of measurements, at which time "the organ mercury content was assessed."

What they found were significant differences in the whole body retention and organ concentrations of the mercury in the different mouse strains but not their hybrid progeny. One strain of mouse (A.SW) showed a four-fold increase in whole body and liver retention of mercury and an eleven-fold increase in kidney mercury as compared to the other strain (B10.S).

The scientists concluded that "multiple genetic factors influence the mercury toxico-kinetics in the mouse," and that "the genetically heterogeneous [having different genetic makeup] human population may therefore show a large variation in mercury toxicokinetics." This, of course, is consistent with what has been shown in the studies of mercury retention in autistic children as compared to non-autistic populations as previously cited.[29]

9. In a Japanese mouse study, researchers showed that thimerosal injections induce certain metallothioneins (MT-1 and MT-3) to increase in the cerebellum and cerebrum of the mouse brain, but especially in the cerebellum.

It may be recalled that the metallothionein proteins are found in the brain and throughout the body and perform a variety of functions, including that of detoxifying mercury. The metallothioneins are also inducible proteins, that is to say their concentrations will increase when the organism is exposed to certain toxins like mercury.

The researchers concluded that, "As a result of the present findings, in combination with the brain pathology observed in patients diagnosed with autism, the present study helps to support the possible biological plausibility for how low-dose exposure to mercury from thimerosal-containing vaccines may be associated with autism."[30]

10. Researchers from the University of Pittsburgh and the Thoughtful House for Children, who published the previously cited research on the effects of a single hepatitis B immunization given to newborn macaques, have also "found remarkably similar brain changes to those seen in autism in infant monkeys receiving the vaccine schedule used in the 1990's that contained the mercury-based preservative thimerosal," according to reviewers Dan Olmstead and Mark Blaxill.

The researchers scanned the brains of young monkeys to assess both brain growth and function after the animals received weight-adjusted doses of the MMR and DTaP/HIB immunizations given "at the human equivalent of 12 months" of age.

"Throughout the study period, vaccinated animals showed an increase in total brain volume—a feature of the brain in many young children with autism—when compared with unvaccinated animals. However, a specific part of the brain associated with emotional responses that is thought to be important in autism, the amygdala, did not show abnormalities until after the 12-month vaccines had been given."[31]

The researchers, who scanned the animal brains before and after the MMR/DaPT/HIB injection, found that only after the 12-month equivalent immunizations did "The functional brain scans [show] significant differ-

28   Rodrigues, J.L. et al. "Identification and distribution of mercury species in rat tissues following administration of thimerosal or methylmercury." *Arch Toxicol.* 2010 Apr 13.

29   Ekstrand, J. et al. "Mercury toxicokinetics—dependency on strain and gender." *Toxicol Appl Pharmacol.* 2010 Mar 15; 243(3):283-91. Epub 2009 Sep 2.

30   Minami T, et al. "Induction of metallothionein in mouse cerebellum and cerebrum with low-dose thimerosal injection." *Cell Biol Toxicol.* 2010 Apr; 26(2):143-52. Epub 2009 Apr 9.

31   Ibid.

ences between vaccinated and unvaccinated groups. These functional scans looked at the activity of receptors for morphine-like compounds (opioids) that may play a role in the brain of children affected by autism."[32]

The amygdala of the vaccinated monkeys showed increases in opioid receptors as compared to the monkeys who received placebo injections and whose amygdalas showed declines in opioid binding. These findings are consistent with those of the Polish researchers (Olszac et al.) cited above in regard to thimerosal inducing opioid receptor increases in rat brains.

"The results indicate that multiple vaccine exposures …may have had a significant impact on brain growth and development in ways that are consistent with the published data on autism."[33]

Dr. Kris Turlejski, Editor-in-Chief of the journal *Acta Neurobiologiae Experimentalis*, calls the findings "alarming," because they "support the possibility that there is a link between early immunization and the etiology of autism."[34]

THIMEROSAL FACTS

TRACE AMOUNTS OF MERCURY MAY NOT BE INNOCUOUS

"Although the mercury content in many vaccines on the current schedule has been reduced to "trace amounts," these trace amounts are not regulated by the FDA. Large doses of mercury still remain in some vaccines, including "flu" shots. Other highly toxic substances including aluminum remain as well."[35]

ALUMINUM + THIMEROSAL DOUBLES NEURONAL DEATH

"We have demonstrated the toxicity of thimerosal by using it to kill neurons in culture. At 50 nanomolar thimerosal the neuron killing capacity/rate is about doubled with the addition of levels of aluminum found in vaccines.

"The aluminum alone at this level is not demonstrated to be toxic, so it is enhancing the toxicity of the thimerosal. It likely does this by increasing the rate that thimerosal breaks down releasing ethylmercury, which is the toxic material."—Testimony of Prof Boyd Haley, University of Kentucky

Aluminum's role in promoting autism will be discussed further in Chapter 26.

THIMEROSAL IS ALLERGENIC

A meta-analysis of the MEDLINE database from 1966 to June 2000 for articles relating to testing for allergens related to contact dermatitis (T.R.U.E. Test) revealed that nickel allergy led the way (14.7 percent) followed by thimerosal (5 percent).[36]

THIMEROSAL DEPLETES GLUTATHIONE

Results from a recent study revealed that when certain immune cells (dendritic cells) are exposed to thimerosal at levels readily achieved through vaccinations, glutathione levels are depleted, and this depletion results in a variety of mercury-related immune dysfunctions which may be reversible by increasing glutathione levels in the body.[37]

---

32   Ibid.

33   Ibid. Laura Hewitson, et al. "Influence of pediatric vaccines on amygdala growth and opioid ligand binding in rhesus macaque infants: A pilot study." *Acta Neurobiol Exp* 2010. 70: 147–164.

34   Turlejski, Kris. "Focus on Autism Editorial Comment." *Acta Neurobiol Exp* 2010. 70: 117–118.

35   http://www.chat-hyperacusis.net/post/Pink-Disease-Mercury-Autism-The-Brain-Gut-Ears-1599210?trail=100

36   Krob, H.A. et al. "Prevalence and relevance of contact dermatitis allergens: a meta-analysis of 15 years of published T.R.U.E. test data." *J Am Acad Dermatol.* 2004 Sep; 51(3):349-53.

37   Agrawal, Anshu, et al. "Thimerosal induces TH2 responses via influencing cytokine secretion by human dendritic cells." *Autism Research Review International.* Vol. 20, No. 4, 2006, p. 6.

REMINDER

THIMEROSAL CONCENTRATIONS AND TOXIC EFFECTS

1 ppb mercury = Kills human neuroblastoma cells. (Parran et al., Toxicol Sci 2005)

2 ppb mercury = U.S. EPA limit for drinking water (http://www.epa.gov/safewater/contaminants/index.html#mcls)

20 ppb mercury = Dendritic cells damaged, calcium channels interrupted (UC-Davis MIND Institute, 2006).

200 ppb mercury = level in liquid the EPA classifies as hazardous waste. http://www.epa.gov/epaoswer/hazwaste/mercury/regs.htm#hazwaste

600 ppb mercury = Level in a currently licensed Hepatitis B, multi-dose vaccine vial, labeled as "trace." This is administered at birth.

2,000 ppb mercury = 0.50 mL injections of thimerosal-containing vaccines (FDA CBER's definition of "trace").

25,000 ppb mercury = Concentration of mercury in multi-dose, Hepatitis B vaccine vials, administered at birth from 1990-2000 (and probably until 2004) in the U.S. Not administered at birth in any other developed country.

50,000 ppb mercury = Concentration of mercury in DTaP and Haemophilus B vaccine administered 8 times in the 1990s to children at 2, 4, 6, and 12 to 18 months of age. Current "preservative" level amounts of mercury are currently still found in the influenza, (for pregnant women, babies, children, and adults) and meningococcal and tetanus vaccines (for children 7 and older).

"ppb" = parts per billion.

Chapter 13
The Smoking Gun—The CDC's Secret Study

"Oh what a tangled web we weave when first we practice to deceive."
— *Sir Walter Scott,* Marmion

WHAT EVIDENCE SUPPORTS *Contention 9?*

CONTENTION 9: There are many studies demonstrating that children who received thimerosal-preserved immunizations have a significantly higher risk of developing autism, ADHD, significant developmental delays, and other neurological disorders. We refer to these as the "Positive Studies."

The First Study: Thimerosal VSD Study: Phase I

"Scientific Review of VSD Information"

Thomas Verstraeten, Robert Davis, Frank DeStefano

The unpublished, secret, CDC-sponsored, multiply manipulated, quarantined study that only a select few were allowed to know about—Thimerosal VSD Study Phase I: Thomas Verstraeten, Robert Davis, Frank DeStefano; Study updated: 2/29/00; Presented June 7-8, 2000; Simpsonwood Conv. Ctr., Norcross, GA at a secret CDC sponsored conference entitled "Scientific Review of VSD Information."

The report is dated 2/29/00 and labeled "CONFIDENTIAL...DO NOT COPY OR RELEASE."

We review now the infamous, early Verstraeten (et al.) study that so terrified the CDC, the World Health Organization, the American Academy of Pediatrics, and the vaccine manufacturers that it was suppressed, deviously revised, its data alleged to be "lost," and never published in its original, uncensored state, but it was most definitely "peer reviewed."[1]

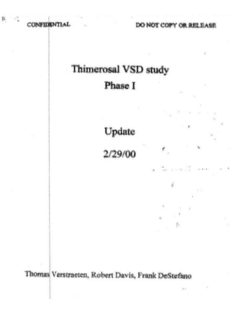

On June 7-8, 2000, a small group of government health leaders, vaccine industry representatives, and representatives from the American Academy of Pediatrics, the World Health Organization, and others were secretly assembled by the Centers for Disease Control and Prevention (the CDC) at the isolated Simpsonwood Convention Center in Norcross, Georgia to discuss some disturbing findings. The public was not invited—making this underpublicized meeting *illegal.*

---

1   http://www.autismhelpforyou.com/EXPERT percent20PAPER percent20- percent20Thimerosal percent20VSD percent20 study001 percent20- percent20Internet percent20File.pdf

~ 137 ~

The official and deliberately unrevealing title of this clandestine conference was "Scientific Review of Vaccine Safety Datalink (VSD) Information." A better name might have been "Uh, Oh; Are We in Trouble?"

According to Dr. Thomas Verstraeten, a CDC visiting epidemiologist, who had at the CDC's request analyzed the data on over 75,000 children in the CDC's own VSD database of *over 2 million children*, thimerosal-preserved vaccines appeared to be *undeniably* linked to dramatic increases in autism, neuro-developmental disorder, and ADHD *in a dose and age-dependent manner.*

That is, the greater the thimerosal exposure, the greater the risk of having a developmental disorder, and likewise, the younger the child so exposed, the greater the risk of harm.

When Verstraeten did his *initial* analysis of the VSD datasets, he was astonished by what he found. Babies who had received more than 25 mcg of mercury as thimerosal in their vaccines by one month of age, as compared to those with no exposure to mercury at that age, had extremely elevated relative risks for:

- ADHD: 11.35 times more likely
- Autism: 7.62 times more likely
- ADD: 6.38 times more likely
- Tics: 5.65 times more likely
- Speech and Language Delay: over twice as likely

And these findings were all statistically significant![2]

This tells us that the CDC is quite able to do a study comparing children who had been injected with thimerosal containing vaccines with those who hadn't received any, and we also now know why they won't do or publish any such study or allow others to access their VSD database to do such a study.

Verstraeten's findings were consistent with those found later by epidemiologists Mark and David Geier (and others). Verstraeten could not explain the reason for this linkage, but affirmed that the data was solid and the results were significant. "I was actually stunned by what I saw," he stated, and he cited other studies that substantiated his findings.

These initial results were so frightening to the CDC that they made Verstraeten rework his data (twice) prior to their hosting this conference. According to investigative reporter Dave Kirby, Verstraeten, by manipulating the data at the CDC's request, was (by February 2000) able to restratify "the kids down to (a) 2.48 relative risk for autism" (down from 7.62).

He did this by eliminating babies who had received hepatitis B immune globulin (generally preserved with thimerosal and containing an aluminum adjuvant)) from the database. Why? Because these babies "were more likely to have high exposures (to mercury) and high outcomes (increased likelihood of becoming autistic)."

Nevertheless, in this, the third analysis of the data, Verstraeten and his colleagues, Robert Davis and Frank DeStefano, still found "increasing risks of neurological developmental disorders with increasing cumulative exposure to thimerosal." And this was unacceptable to the CDC.[3]

"Any relative risk over 2.0 in a court of law is considered causation," Kirby alleges. "Remember, he started with 7.62. He wrote an e-mail to his colleagues, a very famous e-mail called, 'It Just Won't Go Away,' in which Verstraeten decried his inability to make the findings of a significant link between thimerosal-containing vaccinations and autism disappear."[4]

And it wasn't for want of trying. Verstraeten had already eliminated the most susceptible children from the study: those who were born prematurely, those who received the hepatitis B immunization, and those with "neonatal problems." These children have been shown to be at a higher risk for autism.

---

2   SOURCE: Internal CDC report, February 2000 – Obtained through the Freedom of Information Act (FOIA).
3   http://www.ageofautism.com/2011/05/vaccines-and-autism-what-do-epidemiological-studies-really-tellus.html
4   Conference Presentation: David Kirby, reporter, author of *Evidence of Harm.* http://www.whale.to/vaccines/kirby6.html

He also excluded those children who had not received at least two polio immunizations. This group, of course, included those who had not been immunized at all. This devious maneuver further served to weaken the association between thimerosal dose and harmful outcomes.

Verstraeten additionally limited the age of diagnosis of autism, ADHD, and Neurodevelopmental defects to a maximum of five years; this would and did result in the *under-counting* of many of the children who would later be diagnosed with one or more of these conditions.

That is why in his study of 75,000 children, he identified only 62 with autism. That works out to one case of autism for every 1,210 children. The actual incidence of autism at that time was one child in 150-200.

So in presenting his now nefariously manipulated study, Dr. Verstraeten was no longer comparing children who had received thimerosal-containing vaccinations with a control group who hadn't received any thimerosal. Instead, he was comparing full-term, healthier babies, who had received a relatively higher dose of mercury from thimerosal (37.5 mcg or more), with those who received a somewhat lower dose (less than 37.5 mcg)—the control group, assigned a relative risk of 1.

According to Safe Minds, "This would be the same as studying the incidence of lung cancer in two-pack-a-day smokers and three-pack-a-day smokers and not including any non-smokers."[5]

Nevertheless, an alarmed Dr. William Weil, representing the Committee on Environmental Health of the American Academy of Pediatrics, told the assembled participants, "The number of dose related relationships are linear and statistically significant."[6] (i.e., the more thimerosal an infant was exposed to, the more likely that child was to have a neurodevelopmental abnormality or autism or ADHD).

"You can play with this all you want," Dr. Weil added, but concluded, the results of the manipulated data still "are statistically significant...there are just a host of neurodevelopmental data that would suggest that we've got a serious problem. The earlier we go (i.e., the younger and smaller the child), the more serious the problem... to think there isn't some possible problem here is unreal."

And Dr. Richard Johnston, a pediatrician-immunologist from the University of Colorado, echoed similar concerns. "I want my grandson to only receive thimerosal-free vaccines," he told the assemblage, and he added, "(I) favor a recommendation that infants up to two years old not be immunized with thimerosal containing vaccines if suitable alternative preparations are available."[7]

During this meeting, the participants acknowledged that very little was known about the toxicity of ethyl mercury (the form found in thimerosal), except that it was a known neurotoxin and passed readily across the placenta and the blood-brain barrier, and *nothing was known about its excretion.*[8]

Although participants at this clandestine meeting were sworn to secrecy, transcripts of the minutes obtained under the Freedom of Information Act allow us to understand how this already highly "massaged" study, which especially in its earlier and less manipulated comparisons, clearly showed a statistically significant dose-related linkage between thimerosal-containing vaccines and autism, ADHD, and other neuro-developmental disorders, was ultimately corrupted, and intentionally so, by the inclusion of data from a failed HMO noted for its poor record-keeping and by other deceitful statistical maneuvers.

Why would a select group of vaccine manufacturers, the American Academy of Pediatrics, the World Health Organization, other "health officials," and the CDC itself choose to discredit the CDC's own study? Why was Verstraeten trying to make the statistical significance go away? Let's let the participants help us answer those questions.

---

5   http://www.ageofautism.com/2014/01/new-disclosures-on-vaccine-safety-data-link.html?utm_source=feed bur ner&utm_medium=email&utm_campaign=Feed percent3A+ageofautism+ percent28AGE+OF+AUTISM percent29
6   See graphs below, taken directly from this unpublished study, that clearly show the linear relative risk increases in autism, ADHD, and neuro-developmental disorders with increasing doses of thimerosal in the first three months of life.
7   p. 24, 25 and 199 FOIA report
8   p. 15 FOIA report

"We are in a bad position from the standpoint of defending any lawsuits," stated Professor Robert Brent, *Pediatrics* journal editorial board member. "This will be a resource to our very busy plaintiff attorneys in this country," he added.

Translation: "We're going to get sued for malfeasance if this study is published, and we're going to lose!"

Dr. Bob Chen, the then head of *vaccine safety* for the CDC, agreed. However, he seemed not at all concerned about vaccine safety and the dire implications of the data presented by Verstraeten, but was rather more alarmed by the possibility that this data might get out to the general public. "Given the sensitivity of the information," he said, it was good that "we have been able to keep it out of the hands of, let's say, less responsible hands." [sic]

Translation: "The data statistically indicates that many (if not most) autism, ADHD and developmental delay cases are likely induced by immunizations and thimerosal. It's a good thing we won't be letting the public or victims and their families know what is really causing the autism epidemic; they might become very upset and do something irresponsible, like holding us accountable, especially me."

"This study should not have been done at all," was the startling remark made by Dr. John Clements, who acted as a vaccines advisor for the World Health Organization.

Translation: We already know that thimerosal and vaccinations cause autism and other neuro-developmental concerns. Why in the world did we do a study which just proved that?

"The results," Dr. Clements added, "will be taken by others and will be used in ways beyond the control of this group."

Translation: If this information gets out we are all going to be in big legal trouble.

"The research results will have to be handled," concluded Dr. Clements.

And that is what the CDC did. They "handled" it. The relative risk of 1.69 for neuro-developmental disorders, 2.48 for autism and 2.45 for ADHD in this third incarnation of the Verstraeten study was still too high to be publically acknowledged. It was necessary to make any statistical relevance disappear completely.

But, how to do that?

The CDC had already stamped each page of each participant's copy of the Verstraeten study with the words "Confidential" and "Do Not Copy or Release." They subsequently alleged that the study data had been mysteriously and irretrievably *lost*.

However, the study would be reborn anew with new criteria and further statistical manipulations that would serve to nullify Verstraeten's already twice-manipulated findings.

Presumably, they "handled" Verstraeten by getting him a job (one suspects high paying) as "advisor" to vaccine manufacturer Glaxo-Smith-Kline approximately two years prior to the eventual publication in 2003 of his "new, revised and now whitewashed" study.

But how to prevent other independent researchers from accessing the CDCs "secret" VSD database via the Freedom of Information Act (FOIA) and reanalyzing the troublesome data?

That was easy.

The CDC simply quarantined its huge VSD database by transferring it to a private company. This prevented individuals from utilizing the FOIA to gain access to the troubling data, *which the CDC refuses to share,* and it then commissioned the allegedly independent Institute of Medicine (the IOM) to form an Immunization Safety Review Committee (ISRC) to review the manipulated data on thimerosal and vaccines as they related to the rising number of autism cases, and incredibly, *actually instructed it to find that thimerosal-preserved vaccines were safe.*

In 2001, the IOM, which was never shown the *original* Verstraeten study results, hedged; it declared that the link between thimerosal and autism and similar disorders "was biologically plausible," though the evidence neither proved nor negated it.

However, three years later on May 14, 2004 the same Immunization Safety Review Committee of the IOM now concluded "that the body of epidemiological evidence favors rejection of a causal relationship between thimerosal-containing vaccines and autism."

They went on to state that such a relationship was now, miraculously, "not biologically plausible," and that no further studies should be conducted to evaluate it.[9]

Meanwhile, Thomas Verstraeten had time to "rework" his original study, by further "diluting" his initial allegedly lost data with the questionable data of the failed HMO (Harvard Pilgrim, with notoriously poor record-keeping and which was not a part of the VSD database) and through other statistical maneuvers, and finally published his results in 2003, at which time he was working for *vaccine manufacturer* GlaxoSmithKline. The U.S. Congress later cited this as an *ethical violation*, as neither Verstraeten nor the journal *Pediatrics* disclosed this conflict of interest when the study was published.

Verstraeten's "revised" CDC study now showed *no significant association* between thimerosal-preserved vaccines and any of the neurodevelopmental maladies that the original, uncorrupted data had clearly linked to thimerosal-preserved vaccines. Imagine![10]

The three following graphs from the unpublished Verstraeten study presented at the aforementioned June 2000 Simpsonwood Conference show clear *linear* increased relative risks for *neuro-developmental disorders, autism, and ADHD* with increasing exposure to thimerosal at three months of age. These graphs were compiled from data from two of the HMOs contracted with the CDC as part of their Vaccine Safety Database cohort.

Children who were born prematurely (5,728) were *eliminated* from the study, as were children who had not received two polio immunizations (4,574), and also children whose mothers received Hepatitis B immunoglobulin[11] during the pregnancy (192).

Of the 211,693 children who were born into the two evaluated HMOs (NCK and GHC), a total 75,540 children were ultimately eligible for the final analysis of the data. Elimination of those children who were born prematurely, who hadn't received at least two polio immunizations, and those whose mothers received thimerosal-containing immunoglobulin during the pregnancy, would, of course, serve to skew the data to show less risk of developmental disorders and autism.

In addition, most of the children evaluated would have been too young (1-5 years) at the end point of the study to have included all who would eventually be diagnosed with some of the evaluated conditions. Autism and ADHD, for example, are under-diagnosed in children less than five years of age.[12]

It has also been shown that preemies are at increased risk for autism and other developmental disorders.

> *"I sometimes wonder if these people knew that they were being recorded, because when you read the minutes you just can't believe the atrocities: they're shocking. I'm sure they didn't think that the minutes would ever see the light of day. Thank God for the Freedom of Information Act…."*
>
> — *David Kirby referring to the minutes of the infamous June 2000 CDC-sponsored Simpsonwood Convention Center conference[13]*

---

9   www.iom.edu/Reports/2004/Immunization-Safety-Review-Vaccines-and-Autism.aspx
10   Verstraeten, Thomas. "Safety of Thimerosal-Containing Vaccines: A Two-Phased Study of Computerized Health Maintenance Organization Database." *Pediatrics*, November 2003.
11   Which usually had thimerosal as a preservative.
12   Ibid. p. 4.
13   Ibid.

Figures 13.1, 13.2, and 13.3 were taken from the *third* incarnation of the manipulated, unpublished, and quarantined Verstraeten study presented June 7-8, 2000 at the Simpsonwood Convention Center.

Figure 13.1 clearly illustrates the linear increasing risk of neurological developmental disorders with increasing dosages of thimerosal. *NCK and GHC are the two HMOs analyzed.*[14]

Graph 1: Relative risk + 95% C/ of <u>Developmental neurologic disorders</u> after different exposure levels of thimerosal at 3 months of age, NCK & GHC

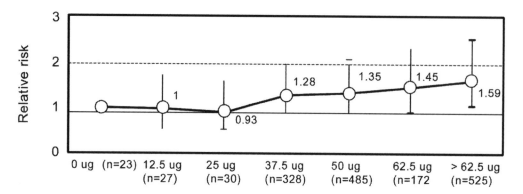

Cumulative mercury exposure (and number of exposed cases (n))

Figure 13.1. Neuro-Developmental Disorders After Different Exposure Levels of Thimerosal at 3 Months of Age

Graph 3: Relative risk + 95% C/ of <u>Autism</u> after different exposure levels of thimerosal at 3 months of age, NCK & GHC

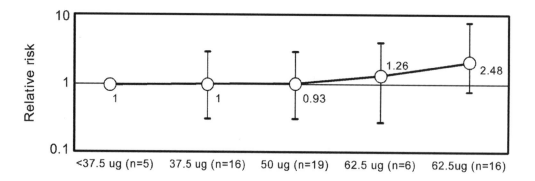

Cumulative mercury exposure (and number of exposed cases (n))

Figure 13.2. Autism After Different Exposure Levels of Thimerosal at 3 Months of Age
Note the linear increase in autism as the cumulative mercury exposure from thimerosal increases.

14   http://www.autismhelpforyou.com/EXPERT percent20PAPER percent20- percent20Thimerosal percent20VSD percent20study001 percent20- percent20Internet percent20File.pdf (p. 14)

Figures 13.2 and 13.3 from the same paper show the linear increase in autism and ADD with increasing exposure to thimerosal in the first three months of life.[15]

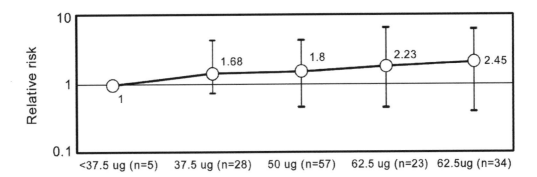

Graph 8: Relative risk + 95% C/ of <u>Attention Deficit Disorder</u> after different exposure levels of thimerosal at 3 months of age, NCK & GHC

Cumulative mercury exposure (and number of exposed cases (n))

Figure 13.3. Attention Deficit Disorder After Different Exposure Levels of Thimerosal at 3 Months of Age
Note the linear increase in risk for attention deficit disorder as the cumulative dose of thimerosal increases.

"Even Verstraeten, in an email following the Simpsonwood meeting, expressed surprise that the data was to be (further) manipulated, stating that one's desire to disprove an unpleasant theory should not interfere with sound scientific methods to evaluate the relationship between thimerosal and neurodevelopmental disorders."

— Mark Geier in a letter to Pediatrics

A LETTER FROM CONGRESSMAN DAVID WELDON, M.D. TO THEN CDC HEAD JULIE GERBERDING

October 31, 2003
Julie L. Gerberding, M.D., M.P.H.
Director, Centers for Disease Control and Prevention
1600 Clifton Road, N.E.
Atlanta, GA 30333

Dr. Julie Gerberding,

I am writing to follow up on our conversation about the article (Verstraeten et. al.) that will be published in the November 2003 issue of *Pediatrics*. I have reviewed the article and have serious reservations about the four-year evolution and conclusions of this study.

Much of what I observed transpired prior to your appointment a year ago as the Director of the Centers for Disease Control and Prevention (CDC). I am very concerned about activities that have

---

15   http://www.autismhelpforyou.com/EXPERT percent20PAPER percent20- percent20Thimerosal percent20VSD percent20study001 percent20- percent20Internet percent20File.pdf (p. 15)

taken place in the National Immunization Program (NIP) in the development of this study, and I believe the issues raised need your personal attention.

I am a strong supporter of childhood vaccinations and know that they have saved us from considerable death and suffering. A key part of our vaccination program is to ensure that we do everything possible to ensure that these vaccines, which are mandatory, are as safe as possible. We must fully disclose adverse events. Anything less than this undermines public confidence.

I have read the upcoming *Pediatrics* study and several earlier versions of this study dating back to February 2000. I have read various e-mails from Dr. Verstraeten and coauthors. I have reviewed the transcripts of a discussion at Simpsonwood, GA between the author, various CDC employees, and vaccine industry representatives. I found a disturbing pattern which merits a thorough, open, timely, and independent review by researchers outside of the CDC, HHS, the vaccine industry, and others with a conflict of interest in vaccine related issues (including many in University settings who may have conflicts).

A review of these documents leaves me very concerned that rather than seeking to understand whether or not some children were exposed to harmful levels of mercury in childhood vaccines in the 1990s, there may have been a selective use of the data to make the associations in the earliest study disappear. While most childhood vaccines now only have trace amounts of mercury from thimerosal containing vaccines (TCVs), it is critical that we know with certainty if children were injured in the 1990s.

Furthermore, the lead author of the article, Dr. Thomas Verstraeten, worked for the CDC until he left over two years ago to work in Belgium for GlaxoSmithKline (GSK), a vaccine manufacturer facing liability over TCVs. In violation of their own standards of conduct, *Pediatrics* failed to disclose that Dr. Verstraeten is employed by GSK and incorrectly identifies him as an employee of the CDC. This revelation undermines this study further.

The first version of the study, produced in February 2000, found a significant association between exposure to thimerosal containing vaccines (TCVs) and autism and neurological developmental delays (NDDs). When comparing children exposed to 62.5 µg of mercury by 3 months of age to those exposed to less than 37.5 µg, the study found a relative risk for autism of 2.48 for those with a higher exposure level. (While not significant in the 95 percent confidence interval for autism, this meets the legal standard of proof exceeding 2.0.) For NDDs (neuro-developmental disorders) the study found a relative risk of 1.59 and a definite upward trend as exposure levels increased.

A June 2000 version of the study applied various data manipulations to reduce the autism association to 1.69 and the authors went outside of the VSD database to secure data from a Massachusetts HMO (Harvard Pilgrim, HP) in order to counter the association found between TCVs (thimerosal-containing vaccines) and speech delay.

At the time that HP's data was brought in, HP was in receivership by the state of Mass., its computer records had been in shambles for years, it had multiple computer systems that could not communicate with one another (*Journal of Law, Ethics and Medicine* Sept. 22, 2000), and it used a health care coding system totally different from the one used across the VSD. There are questions relating to a significant underreporting of Autism in Mass. The HP dataset is only about 15 percent of the HMO dataset used in the February 2000 study. There may also be significant problems with the statistical power of the HP dataset.

In June of 2000 a meeting was held in Simpsonwood, GA, involving the authors of the study, representatives of the CDC, and the vaccine industry. I have reviewed a transcript of this meeting that was obtained through the Freedom of Information Act (FOIA). Comments from Simpsonwood, NJ meeting include: (summary form, not direct quotes):

- We found a statistically significant relationship between exposures and outcomes. There is certainly an under ascertainment of adverse outcomes because some children are just simply not old enough to be diagnosed, the current incidence rates are much lower than we would expect to see (Verstraeten);

- We could exclude the lowest exposure children from our database. Also suggested was removing the children that got the highest exposure levels since they represented an unusually high percentage of the outcomes. (Rhodes)

- The significant association with language delay is quite large. (Verstraeten);

- This information should be kept confidential and considered embargoed;

- We can push and pull this data anyway we want to get the results we want;

- We can alter the exclusion criteria any we way we want, give reasonable justifications for doing so, and get any result we want;

- There was really no need to do this study. We could have predicted the outcomes;

- I will not give TCVs to my grandson until I find out what is going on here.

Another version of the study—after further manipulation—finds no association between TCVs and autism, and no consistency across HMOs between TCVs and NDDs and speech delay.

The final version of the study concludes that "No consistent significant associations were found between TCVs and neurodevelopmental outcomes," and that the lack of consistency argues against an association. In reviewing the study there are data points where children with higher exposures to the neuortoxin mercury had fewer developmental disorders. This demonstrates to me how excessive manipulation of data can lead to absurd results. Such a conclusion is not unexpected from an author with a serious, though undisclosed, conflict of interest.

This study increases speculation of an association between TCVs and neurodevelopmental outcomes. I cannot say it was the author's intent to eliminate the earlier findings of an association.

Nonetheless, the elimination of this association is exactly what happened and the manner in which this was achieved raises speculation. The dialogue at the Simpsonwood meeting clearly indicates how easily the authors could manipulate the data and have reasonable sounding justifications for many of their decisions.

The only way these issues are going to be resolved—and I have only mentioned a few of them—is by making this particular dataset and the entire VSD database open for independent analysis. One such independent researcher, Dr. Mark Geier, has already been approved by the CDC and the various IRBs to access this dataset. They have requested the CDC allow them to access this dataset and your staff indicated to my office that they would make this particular dataset available after the *Pediatrics* study is published.

Earlier this month the CDC had prepared three similar datasets for this researcher to review to allow him to reanalyze CDC study datasets. However when they accessed the datasets—which the researchers paid the CDC to assemble—the datasets were found to have no usable data in them. I request that you personally intervene with those in the CDC who are assembling this dataset to ensure that they provide the complete dataset, in a usable format, to these researchers within two weeks.

The treatment that these well-published researchers have received from the CDC thus far has been abysmal and embarrassing. I would also be curious to know whether Dr. Verstraeten, an outside researcher for more than two years now, was required to go through the same process as Dr. Geier in order to continue accessing the VSD.

You have not been a part of creating this current situation, but you do have an opportunity to help resolve this issue and ensure that confidence and trustworthiness in the CDC and our national vaccination program is fully restored. I would ask that you work with me to ensure that a full, fair, and independent review is made of the VSD database to fully examine this matter. I would like to meet with you at your earliest convenience to move this process forward.

Thank you for your consideration. I look forward to working with you on this urgent matter of great importance to our nation's most precious resource, our children.

Sincerely,

Dave Weldon, M.D., Member of Congress

Conclusion: This unpublished work is without question the most important study done to date in regard to answering the question, "Do vaccines cause autism, ADD, ADHD and neurodevelopmental disorders?"

And the answer from the CDC's initial and subsequent analyses of its own, proprietary VSD data is a clear and unequivocal "Yes!" The VSD database allowed for an accurate and meaningful analysis of outcomes.

Even after two inappropriate attempts by the study authors to reduce the relative risk, their data analysis still showed statistically significant relationships between immunizations, mercury exposure, and increased risks for autism, ADD, ADHD, and neurodevelopmental disorders.

That the CDC intended to hide this data is clear, as were their reasons for their doing so.

They did not want the immunization program to be compromised. They did not want the vaccine manufacturers to face significant losses of income, potential lawsuits, congressional investigations, and massive adverse publicity and embarrassment. They did not want their own institution, the American Academy of Pediatrics, the World Health Organization (WHO still administers numerous thimerosal-preserved vaccines worldwide), pediatricians, and other physicians who administer vaccines to be placed in legal jeopardy as a result of this massive and intentional poisoning of the children of the world.

And the vaccine makers, the World Health Organization, and the American Academy of Pediatrics apparently concurred. They all had the ethical duty to reveal that they now knew that vaccines and thimerosal in a dose dependent manner were likely causative promoters of autism, ADHD, and developmental delay, and they all failed in that imperative.

The CDC had already sinned in burying the Brick Township data that strongly suggested a link between immunizations and the rising tide of autism cases. And they had succeeded for a time in conflating the real rise in autism prevalence by inappropriately altering the states that they analyzed in order to skew the data.

The CDC prevented others from accessing Verstraeten's data files by claiming the data was somehow "lost." But the VSD database was still there for reanalyzing, and that couldn't be allowed. So it became necessary to sell the database to a private company to prevent any Freedom of Information Act access to the data.

It is reasonable to assume that they encouraged Verstraeten to rework the data in such a way as to show no relevant associations between vaccines and neurological harm, which he did. This involved (in part) going outside the VSD database and inserting questionable data from a failed HMO in order to dilute further the statistical relevance of the link between immunizations and autism, ADHD, and developmental delay.

And as we shall soon learn in upcoming chapters, the CDC would continue to sponsor bogus research that purports (but fails) to disprove the association between immunizations, thimerosal, and neuro-developmental disorders like autism.

What should we call those who, in order to support their own nefarious agenda, deliberately lie, manipulate, and hide scientific data, suppress valid criticism and inquiry, and stifle beneficial legislation in order to deceive the public and fellow scientists?

And if the result of this unconscionable deceit is a worldwide epidemic of brain-damaged children with autism, attention deficit disorders, developmental delays, tic and speech disorders, and the need to institutionalize the most severely affected, all at great cost to families and society, only one word comes to mind.

And that word is "CRIMINALS."

"Truth lives on in the midst of deception."

— Friedrich von Schiller

"Conspiracy: a secret plan or agreement to carry out an illegal or harmful act, especially with political motivation." [16]

---

16   http://www.thefreedictionary.com/conspiracy from Collins English Dictionary

Chapter 14
Other Studies that Support the Thimerosal-Autism Link

"The common curse of mankind, folly and ignorance."

— *Shakespeare*, Troilus and Cressida

WHAT OTHER STUDIES *Confirm the Mercury-Autism Link?*

A Second Published Study: (Geier, M.R., Geier, D.A. "Neurodevelopmental disorders after thimerosal-containing vaccines: a brief communication." *Exp Biol Med* (Maywood). 2003 Jun; 228(6):660-4.)

Since 1990, the Centers for Disease Control and Prevention has maintained a compilation of adverse reactions from vaccinations, known as the VAERS (Vaccine Adverse Event Reporting System) database.

U.S. law requires that all adverse reactions following vaccinations be reported to this database, which is monitored by both the CDC and the Food and Drug Administration (FDA) for evidence of any alarming increases in, or unexpected or unusual adverse reactions to vaccines.

VAERS is a voluntary, *passive* reporting system. That means that a doctor, other health care provider, or even a family member must first be made aware that an adverse event occurred after a vaccination and then must determine whether there was a likelihood that that adverse event was related to the immunization, and finally, he or she must take the time to report this information to the CDC's VAERS database.

As one might guess, *significant underreporting* of adverse events occurs. There may also be duplications of reports by various health providers on the same child.[1]

Epidemiologists Mark and David Geier attempted to correct for these duplications. They analyzed VAERS data from 1992 to the year 2000 and compared the adverse reactions reported after children received either thimerosal-containing DTaP (diphtheria, tetanus, and acellular pertussis-whooping cough) vaccines or DTaP vaccine without thimerosal. This series of immunizations is generally given at 2, 4, 6, and 18 months of age.

What they found was highly alarming. Their pioneering study, published in the peer-reviewed journal, *Experimental Biology and Medicine* in 2003, presented the first published epidemiological evidence, "based upon tens of millions of doses of vaccine administered in the United States that (associated) increasing thimerosal from vaccines with neurodevelopmental disorders."

The VAERS database clearly showed *statistically relevant* increases in the relative risk (RR) incidence of autism of 6.0, mental retardation (6.1), and speech disorder (2.2). A relative risk of 6.0 for autism means that the inci-

---

1   http://vaers.hhs.gov/data/index and *Am J Public Health*. 1995 December; 85(12): 1706–1709.

dence of autism in children immunized with thimerosal-containing DTaP vaccines was six times higher than those who received the same series of vaccinations without this toxic preservative or no vaccinations.

These findings parallel those found in the initial, unpublished, and unmanipulated Verstraeten study.

A Third Study: (Geier, D.A., Geier, M.R. "An assessment of the impact of thimerosal on childhood neurodevelopmental disorders." *Pediatric Rehabil.* 2003 Apr-Jun; 6(2):97-102.)

In an attempt to corroborate the findings from their first published study, the Geiers reanalyzed not only the VAERS data, but also studied the data compiled by the U.S. Department of Education Report for the year 2001 (a completely separate database) and found again that "increases in (the) odds ratios of neurodevelopmental disorders from both the VAERS and US Department of Education data closely linearly correlated with increasing doses of mercury from thimerosal-containing childhood vaccines and that for overall odds ratios statistical significance was achieved."

The authors concluded that, "The evidence presented here shows that the occurrence of neurodevelopmental disorders following thimerosal-containing childhood vaccines does not appear to be coincidental."

So we see that analyses of three separate databases (VSD, VAERS, and USDER) all support the link between autism and immunizations and the quantity of mercury therein.

A Fourth Study:[2] (Geier, D.A., Geier, M.R. "Neurodevelopmental Disorders Following Thimerosal-Containing Childhood Immunizations: A Follow-Up Analysis." *International Journal of Toxicology.* Vol. 23, No. 6, 369-376 (2004).

The Geiers published a third report in 2004 comparing the incidence of autism and other neurological disorders following DTaP immunizations both with and without thimerosal and again found significantly increased risk (odds ratios) for autism, mental retardation, speech disorder, personality disorder, and thinking abnormality in the cohort of children who received thimerosal-containing DTaP vaccinations as compared to those who received the thimerosal-free DTaP series.

The Geiers stated that, "The present study provides additional epidemiological evidence supporting previous epidemiological, clinical and experimental evidence that administration of thimerosal-containing vaccines in the United States resulted in a significant number of children developing NDs" (neuro-developmental disorders).

A Fifth Study: Geier, D.A., Geier, M.R. "A comparative evaluation of the effects of MMR immunization and mercury doses from thimerosal-containing childhood vaccines on the population prevalence of autism." *Med Sci Monit.* 2004 Mar; 10(3)

In this study, the Geiers analyzed data from both the CDC's Biological Surveillance Summaries and live birth estimates as well as the U.S. Dept. of Education Data-sets in regard to evaluating the effects of both the MMR immunization and mercury from thimerosal-containing childhood vaccines on the prevalence of autism from the mid to late 1980s to the mid-1990s. Once again, they found "a close correlation between mercury doses from thimerosal—containing childhood vaccines and the prevalence of autism from the late 1980s through the mid-1990s." The correlation was less strong for the MMR vaccine.

So we now add a new database to the three already analyzed in this regard, and all four show the same thing—there is a statistically significant link between thimerosal-containing immunizations and autism prevalence.

A Sixth Study: Geier, D.A., Geier, M.R. "A two-phased population epidemiological study of the safety of thimerosal-containing vaccines: a follow-up analysis." *Med Sci Monit.* 2005 Apr; 11(4):CR160-70. Epub 2005 Mar 24.

---

2   Actually this was their first analysis of the VAERS data which took longer to get published than did numbers 1 and 2 above.

In the first phase of this peer-reviewed study, the Geiers reviewed the VAERS DTaP data from 1997 through 2001, calculating the increased neurodevelopmental risks to children receiving the thimerosal-containing as compared to the thimerosal-free versions of this vaccination series and found, "significantly increased risks for autism, speech disorders, mental retardation, personality disorders, and thinking abnormalities."

In the second phase of this study, the Geiers evaluated a different database, the CDC's own automated and more accurate Vaccine Safety Datalink (VSD) for *cumulative exposures to mercury* from thimerosal-containing vaccines at 1-, 2-, 3-, and 6-months-of-age for infants born from 1992 through 1997 and the eventual risk of developing neurodevelopmental disorders.

They noted, "significant associations between cumulative exposures to thimerosal and…unspecified developmental delay, tics, attention deficit disorder (ADD), language delay, speech delay, and neurodevelopmental delays in general."

This Geier et al. study, using the same VSD database that Verstraeten analyzed in his June 2000 Simpsonwood CDC presentation, supports that study's findings and validates the accuracy of the VAERS database for this type of analysis.

A Seventh Study: Geier, D.A., Geier, M.R. "An evaluation of the effects of thimerosal on neurodevelopmental disorders reported following DTP and Hib vaccines in comparison to DTPH vaccine in the United States." *J Toxicol Environ Health A*. 2006 Aug; 69(15):1481-95.

In this case-controlled study of neuro-developmental disorders, the Geiers again analyzed the VAERS database updated to 31 August, 2004, this time comparing children who received separate thimerosal-containing DTP and HIB (Hemophilus Influenza B) vaccines at 2, 4, 6 and 15-18 months of age or combined as in the Lederle DTPH vaccine.

Those children who received the separate vaccinations would have received 100 mcg more thimerosal over the four vaccination series than the children who got the combined vaccine.

The authors again found, "Significantly increased odds ratios for autism, speech disorders, mental retardation, infantile spasms, and thinking abnormalities…following (the higher mercury) DTP (and separate HIB) vaccines in comparison to DTPH vaccines with minimal bias or systematic error."

An Eighth Study: Geier, D.A., Geier, M.R. A meta-analysis epidemiological assessment of neurodevelopmental disorders following vaccines administered from 1994 through 2000 in the United States. *Neuro Endocrinol Lett*. 2006 Aug; 27(4):401-13.

The Geiers continued their data-mining and performed a meta-analysis of the Vaccine Adverse Event Reporting System database, comparing the neurodevelopment disorders reported following thimerosal-containing Diphtheria/Tetanus/whole-cell-Pertussis (DTP) vaccines and Diphtheria/Tetanus/whole-cell Pertussis/Haemophilus Influenzae Type b (DTPH) vaccines (administered from 1994-1997).

They also compared the thimerosal-containing Diphtheria-Tetanus-acellular-Pertussis (DTaP) vaccines to the thimerosal-free DTaP vaccines (administered from 1997-2000), and once again found that, "significantly increased… risks of autism, speech disorders, mental retardation, personality disorders, thinking abnormalities, ataxia (difficulty coordinating movement), and neuro-developmental disorders in general, with minimal systematic error or confounding, were associated with thimerosal-containing vaccines exposure."

A Ninth Study: Young, H.A. et al. "Thimerosal exposure in infants and neurodevelopmental disorders: an assessment of computerized medical records in the Vaccine Safety." *Datalink Journal of the Neurological Sciences*; Vol. 271, Issues 1-2, 15 August 2008, p. 110-118.

The CDC in conjunction with eight Health Maintenance Organizations (HMOs) started the Vaccine Safety Datalink (VSD) project in 1990 "to monitor immunization safety and address the gaps in scientific knowledge about rare and serious side events following immunization."[3]

---

3   CDC website

Each of the eight HMO sites gathers data on vaccinations given and medical outcomes as well as birth and census data. "The VSD project allows for planned immunization safety studies as well as timely investigations of hypotheses that arise from review of medical literature... (And) since 1990, investigators *from the VSD project* have published more than 75 scientific articles."[4]

In 1988, the National Childhood Vaccine Injury Act of 1986 (Public Law 99-660) created the National Vaccine Injury Compensation Program (NVICP), which is a "no-fault alternative to the traditional tort system for resolving vaccine injury claims that provides compensation to people found to be injured by certain vaccines. The U.S. Court of Federal Claims decides who will be paid."[5]

A *court-appointed* Petitioners Steering Committee, representing children with autism claims pending in the National Vaccine Injury Compensation Program (NVICP), funded a research study of the Vaccine Safety Datalink headed by associate Professor Heather A. Young of the George Washington University School of Public Health and Health Services and assisted by the epidemiological team of Mark and David Geier. (All of these researchers have been consultants in vaccine cases before the NVICP.)

The study evaluated the limited VSD project data[6] (that they were allowed to access) to look for possible associations between thimerosal-containing immunizations and neurodevelopmental harm.

Professor Young and the Geiers evaluated the data on *over a quarter of a million children* with varying mercury exposures who had received their first oral polio vaccination by three months of age between the years 1990 and 1996 and *found consistent significant increased risk (1.7-4.5 times) for autism, autism spectrum disorders, ADHD, tics, and emotional disturbances in those children who had the highest exposures to thimerosal* (100 mcg of mercury).

Professor Young concluded that, "Because of the strong ecological associations found in this study, it is extremely important that additional studies be conducted using this data source, including case-control and cohort studies, which would allow the linking of individual exposure to disease."

The problem, however, according to the aforementioned steering committee, is that the CDC, the HMOs, and the vaccine makers seemed not to be interested in doing any studies of this sort.

In fact, Professor Young and the Geiers are the *only* scientists outside the government who have been given access to the *taxpayer-funded* Vaccine Safety Datalink and then *only after having to face a variety of unnecessary restrictions and unconscionable delays only to find that the CDC limited the data that they could examine.*

To quote Ed Silverman, prize-winning journalist and editor of *Pharmalot*:

> First, the government (CDC) refused to produce the automated data in a way that would have allowed the investigators to link vaccine-mercury exposure to outcome data in individuals. As a result, thimerosal exposure had to be averaged over each birth cohort for the time periods of birth-7 months and birth-13 months, even though the database was set up to permit individual risk assessments.
>
> Second, the government and the HMO's refused to permit access to any data entered after the year 2000, which meant that the maximum follow up period of the neurodevelopmental disorders for some children was only to four years of age. Specifically, for children born in 1997 or later, this restriction to access prevented any examination of true prevalence rates for those later birth cohorts.
>
> Third, only three of the eight HMO's participating in the taxpayer funded database permitted even this limited access (Northern California, Colorado, and Oregon Kaiser plans). Other HMO's blocked access to the data on hundreds of thousands of additional children.[7]

---

4   Ibid.
5   www.hrsa.gov/vaccinecompensation/
6   See Dr. Dave Weldon's letter at the end of Chapter 13.
7   By Ed Silverman for *Pharmalot*. tinyurl.com/56tren] & www.pharmalot.com

Evidently, the hypothesized and likely association between thimerosal and neuro-developmental disorders represents a gap in scientific knowledge that the CDC would actually prefer not to address.

> *"When access to information is restricted, concealed or obstructed, it suggests that there is something that someone wishes to hide."*
>
> *— Anonymous*

A Tenth Study: Gallagher, C.M. et al. "Hepatitis B Vaccination of Male Neonates and Autism." *Annals of Epidemiology*. Vol. 19, No. 9. ABSTRACTS (ACE) September 2009: 651-680.

The previously mentioned Stony Brook University Medical Center study by Gallagher and colleague (see Chapter 9) showed a *threefold rise in autism* spectrum disorders (ASD) in male babies immunized with the thimerosal-containing hepatitis B vaccine in the first month of life compared to children never vaccinated to hepatitis B or those who were vaccinated at a later date. The Hepatitis B vaccine also contained aluminum, which is neurotoxic.

The ramifications of this study explain why Verstraeten was told to eliminate this group of children from his analysis. The CDC presumably didn't want the knowledge that immunizations cause neurodevelopmental harm to be known.

An Eleventh Study: Geier, D.A. and Geier, M.R. "Early Downward Trends in Neurodevelopmental Disorders Following Removal of Thimerosal-Containing Vaccines." *Journal of American Physicians and Surgeons*. Vol. 11. No. 1, Spring 2006.

In this study, epidemiologists David and Mark Geier carried out a two-phase study to evaluate trends in new diagnoses of neurodevelopmental disorders entered into the Vaccine Adverse Event Reporting System (VAERS) database and also the California Dept. of Developmental Services (CDDS) database on a reporting quarter basis from 1994 through 2005.

What they found was significant increasing trends in diagnosis of new neuro-developmental disorders in both databases from 1994 through mid-2002, followed by decreasing trends in newly diagnosed neuro-developmental disorders from mid 2002-2005.

The Geier team concluded that, "The results indicate that the trends in newly diagnosed neuro-developmental disorders correspond directly with the expansion and subsequent contraction of the cumulative mercury dose to which children were exposed from TCVs through the U.S. immunization schedule."

Both databases were in agreement, and the California Department of Developmental Services is the fifth database analyzed by the Geiers that shows the autism risk increases in parallel to mercury exposure from thimerosal-containing vaccines. All these databases lead to the same conclusion!

Critics of this study (and others that the Geiers have published) have suggested that there are a number of problems with the VAERS database and that it was never meant to be used in this manner—i.e., as an analytical tool for epidemiologists. They state that duplicate reports of the same subject may appear multiple times and thus confound the analysis.

The Geiers acknowledge that duplicate reports do occur, and they state in this study that those duplicate reports were screened and eliminated. They further acknowledge "that the potential limitations may include systematic error due to underreporting, erroneous reporting, frequent multiple exposures, multiple outcomes, and lack of precise denominators."[8]

They also contend that both the VAERS Working Group and the FDA analyze and publish epidemiological studies based upon analyses of VAERS data.[9]

---

8   Ibid. p.9
9   Ibid.

The Geiers have potential conflicts of interest, which they allude to at the end of this study.[10] Both have appeared as expert witnesses and consultants in vaccine/biologic cases before the no-fault National Vaccine Injury Compensation Program (NVICP) and in civil litigation.

A Twelfth Study: Desoto, M.C., Hitlan, R.T. "Blood Levels of Mercury Are Related to Diagnosis of Autism: A Reanalysis of an Important Data Set. *J Child Neurol.* November 2007. Vol. 22 No. 11. 1308-1311.

As has been discussed earlier,[11] the reanalysis by Professors Mary Catherine DeSoto and Robert Hitlan of Ip's fallacious study of 2004, which attempted to assess the possible relationship between mercury and autism and was published in the *Journal of Child Neurology*, demonstrated a significant increase in the *mean level of mercury* in autistic children as compared to the non-autistic group. This was true both when recalculating Ip's original data set (which was incorrect due to numerous typographical and mathematical errors) as well as after a *reanalysis of the corrected data.*

There is controversy as to the relevancy of using *mean* mercury levels, as was done in this study, to differentiate differences between the two groups, as has been previously alluded to.

A Thirteenth Study: The Holmes et al. Study: 12 Holmes, A.S. et al. "Reduced levels of mercury in first baby haircuts of autistic children." *Int J Toxicol.* 2003 Jul-Aug; 22(4):277-85.)2003.

This study, which is listed as one of those that supports the hypothesis that autistic children do not excrete mercury as well as their non-autistic cohorts, also provides backing for the contention that thimerosal in vaccines may be a contributing factor to the autism epidemic.

Holmes et al. found that the degree of severity of a child's autism correlated *inversely* with the levels of mercury found in their hair. The implication being that the less mercury a child excreted (in the hair, for example), the greater the amount left in the body, and the more mercury in the body, the greater the harm.

Since newborns and infants tend to be low consumers of fish, the most likely source of most of this presumed mercury burden would be the thimerosal from vaccines and other injections (including Rhogam™ and related immune globulins, which a mother may have received during the pregnancy).

Studies 14 through 20 listed below are the 7 "Porphyrin studies" that provide damning evidence that children with autism have excessive amounts of mercury and that these amounts correlate with the severity of the autism.

A Fourteenth Study: Nataf, R. et al. "Porphyrinurea in Childhood Autistic Disorders: Implications for Environmental Toxicity." *Toxicol. Appl. Pharmacol.* 2006; 214(2):99-108.

Nataf and his research colleagues carried out a retrospective study of urinary porphyrin levels as biomarkers of environmental toxicity. Certain porphyrins (PORE-fer-ins), like coproporphyrin and pre-coproporphyrin, as we have previously discussed, appear to be accurate biomarkers of mercury excess when their levels in the urine are elevated.

The researchers in this study evaluated 269 children with neurodevelopmental and related disorders who were seen at a Paris clinic between 2002 and 2004, and 106 of these children were diagnosed with autism.

Coproporphyrin and precoproporphyrin levels were significantly elevated (p=0.001) in the autistic children relative to the normally developing control groups. Children with Asperger syndrome *did not have elevated porphyrins,* however.

A subgroup of the children with autism were chelated with oral DMSA (DiMercaptoSuccinic Acid), which has been shown to lower mercury and lead levels. Following chelation, there was a significant decrease (P=0.002) in urine porphyrin levels in these children.

---

10   p. 12
11   See Contention 5 in Chapter 12.
12   Ibid.

The researchers concluded that their data "implicate environmental toxicity in childhood autistic disorder."

A Fifteenth Study: Geier, M., Geier, D. "A prospective assessment of porphyrins in autistic disorders: a potential marker for heavy metal exposure." *Neurotox Res.* Aug; 10(1):57-64; 2006.

Mark and David Geier evaluated the urine porphyrin levels of thirty-seven consecutive autistic patients, aged seven years or older, who appeared at the Genetic Centers of America for outpatient genetic evaluations from June 2005 to June 2006. The results were compared to those of a control group of normally developing children who were age, race, and sex-matched.

"An apparent dose-response effect was observed between autism severity and increased urinary coproporphyrins," according to the Geiers. A majority of the patients with autism and autism spectrum disorders who hadn't yet been chelated showed urine porphyrin levels that were *over twice as high* as those found in the control children.

No increase in urine porphyrins was noted in children with Asperger's disorder or in children diagnosed as having pervasive developmental disorder, not otherwise specified (PDD-NOS).

Patients with autism spectrum disorder who had undergone chelation had significantly lower levels of urine coproporphyrins as compared to a similar group of ASD children who had not had any chelation.

The authors concluded that, "Porphyrins should be routinely clinically measured in ASDs, and potential ASD treatments should consider monitoring porphyrin levels. Additional research should be conducted to evaluate the potential role for mercury exposure in some ASDs."

A Sixteenth Study: Geier, M., Geier, D. "A Prospective Study of Mercury Toxicity Biomarkers in Autistic Spectrum Disorders." *Journal of Toxicology and Environmental Health, Part A.* 70: 1723–1730, 2007.

This prospective study compared the urine porphyrin levels of 71 autistic children with those of both normal-developing siblings and an additional control group from the general population. The research was carried out in both the U.S. and France and utilized two different laboratories: LabCorp in the U.S. and Laboratoire Philippe Auguste in France.

What the Geiers found was that the *children with autism spectrum disorders had significant elevations of the biomarkers for mercury*: coproporphyrin, pentacarboxyporphyrin, and precoproporphyrin relative to the controls, and that the coproporphyrin and pentacarboxyporphyrin levels decreased significantly after the children were appropriately chelated.

The Geiers also noted that there was *significant correlation* between urinary porphyrins measured at the two laboratories on each child with ASD.

They concluded that, "The established developmental neurotoxicity attributed to mercury and biochemical/genomic evidence for mercury susceptibility/toxicity in ASDs indicates a causal role for mercury. Urinary porphyrin testing is clinically available, relatively inexpensive, and noninvasive. Porphyrins need to be routinely measured in ASDs to establish if mercury toxicity is a causative factor and to evaluate the effectiveness of chelation therapy."

A Seventeenth Study: Geier, D. et al. "Biomarkers of environmental toxicity and susceptibility in autism." *Journal of the Neurological Sciences.* DOI: 10.1016/j.jns.2008.08.021.

This study has also already been reviewed in Chapter 12, and it, like the Holmes study, demonstrates that autistic children have an elevated body burden of mercury.

In this controlled study, as the reader may recall, the researchers analyzed the urine porphyrin levels in both an autistic and a non-autistic population of children and found that the particular kinds of porphyrins that were representative of mercury toxicity were found at significantly higher levels in the autistics than in the controls.

The authors also found that the presumed degree of mercury burden correlated, as it did in the Holmes study, with the severity of the autism, and was consistent with their findings in Study 15 above.

This study was criticized because the control group was not age and gender matched to the autism group, a legitimate concern.

An Eighteenth Study: Kern, J.K. et al. "Toxicity Biomarkers in Autism Spectrum Disorder: A Blinded Study of Urinary Porphyrins." *Pediatrics International* 2011; 53:147ff; doi: 10.1111/j.1442-200X.2010. 03196.x.

In this double-blind repeat of the aforementioned (seventeenth) study, the researchers once again compared the urinary porphyrin measurements of autistic spectrum disorder children with a typically-developing control population *that was now age and gender matched.*

What the research revealed was that, as with the previous study, the children with ASD had "significantly increased levels of certain mercury-associated porphyrins (pentacarboxyporphyrin, precoproporphyrin,[13] and coproporphyrin) in comparison with the group of normally developing children."

And they again concluded that their "results suggest that the levels of (mercury) toxicity-associated porphyrins are (significantly) higher in children with an ASD diagnosis than (they are in) controls. Although the pattern seen…is characteristic of (mercury) toxicity, the influence of other factors, such as genetics and other metals cannot be completely ruled-out."

Conflicts of Interest: To quote from the study:

> David Geier has been a consultant in cases involving vaccines/biologics before the no-fault National Vaccine Injury Compensation Program and in civil litigation.
>
> Dr. Mark Geier has been an expert witness and consultant in cases involving vaccines/biologics before the no-fault National Vaccine Injury Compensation Program and in civil litigation.
>
> David and Mark Geier have a patent pending for the treatment of autistic disorders.

"Speak truth to power."

— a 1955 Quaker pamphlet

A Nineteenth Study: Geier, David et al. "A Prospective Blinded Evaluation of Urinary Porphyrins versus the Clinical Severity of Autism Spectrum Disorders." *Journal of Toxicology and Environmental Health, Part A*, 72: 24, 1585-1591. 2009.

In this *prospective* blinded study, the researchers measured a variety of urinary porphyrins in 26 autistic children (23 boys, 3 girls, age range 2-13 years) who were diagnosed as being autistic on the basis of a standardized test, the Childhood Autism Rating Scale (CARS). A CARS score above 30 confirms the diagnosis of autism. A score above 39 indicates more severe autism.

Children with known genetically-linked syndromes like fragile X and tuberous sclerosis were excluded from the evaluations in this study. The urine specimens were sent in a blinded fashion to two laboratories—one in the U.S. (Lab Corp.) and one in Europe (Laboratoire Philippe Auguste). Both labs were CLIA-certified to perform the required porphyrin analyses, and both labs came back with comparable results.

---

13   William Walsh, Ph.D., director of the Great Plains Laboratory, questions the validity of the precoproporphyrin-mercury linkage since its structure has never been elucidated. That criticism aside, Walsh's concern does not invalidate the use of pentacarboxyporphyrin and coproporphyrin measurements as surrogate markers for mercury toxicity and, therefore, does not invalidate the conclusions reached by Kern, Geier, Nataf, et al.

The analysis of the study data revealed that:

- There was, "…a significant correlation between the clinical severity of ASD and specific urinary porphyrins."

- Both laboratories demonstrated "roughly equivalent measurements" of the urinary porphyrins. This helps confirm the accuracy of the results.

- "…specific urinary porphyrin elevations were observed regardless of the urinary reference used (i.e., per gram creatinine in the urine, or per liter urine, or per microgram of porphyrins in the urine)."

- The urinary porphyrins that are not associated with mercury toxicity did not correlate with the child's autism severity score.

The researchers concluded that, "this study found that increasingly severe ASD correlated with increasing levels of urinary porphyrins associated with (mercury) body burden," and that, "since the laboratory testing employed in the present study for examining urinary porphyrins is clinically available (covered by many insurance companies in the United States), relatively inexpensive (under $200 per test), and relatively noninvasive, it is recommended that patients diagnosed with an ASD need to be routinely tested for urinary porphyrins to evaluate their present heavy metal body burden."[14]

A Twentieth Study: Austen, David; Shandley, Kerrie Shandley. "An Investigation of Porphynuria in Australian Children with Autism." *Journal of Toxicology and Environmental Health*. 2008; 71(20):2349ff; www.tandfonline.co/doi. full/10.1080/ 15287390802271723

The researchers in this Australian study referenced other studies that had identified atypical urinary porphyrin profiles in children with autism spectrum disorders and wondered whether this association would hold true in the sample of Australian children with autism in their own study. To find out, they conducted an analysis of urinary porphyrin profiles in these children and noted, "a consistent trend in abnormal porphyrin levels" that correlated with mercury toxicity. Their findings were consistent with data "previously reported in the literature."

"The results are suggestive of environmental toxic exposure impairing heme synthesis." They point out that, "three[15] independent studies from three continents have now demonstrated that porphyrinuria is concomitant with ASD, and that mercury may be a likely xenobiotic[16] to produce porphyrin profiles of this nature."[17]

A Twenty-First Study: Youn, S.I. et al. "Porphyrinuria in Korean Children with Autism: Correlation with Oxidative Stress." *J Toxic Env Health A* 2010; 73 (10): 701-10.

Urinary porphyrins were determined in 65 Korean patients with ASD and compared to 9 control patients during the time period June 2007 to September 2008. Also analyzed were urinary organic acids reflective of liver detoxification function and oxidative stress.

Compared to controls, significant increases in the ASD patients' urine were seen for total porphyrins as well as for the abnormal porphyrins (pentacarboxyporphyrin, precoproporphyrin, and coproporphyrin) that are associated with toxic metals like mercury.

The quantity of urinary porphyrins also was found to correlate significantly to oxidative stress and hepatic detoxification markers.

This is the eighth independent study (in four countries) of urinary porphyrins in children with autism and related disorders, and all of them demonstrate that compared to developmentally normal children, autistic children have

---

14   Ibid
15   They refer to Nataf et al. 2006, Geier & Geier 2007, and their own study. There are now at least seven such studies (14-20 above).
16   A "xenobiotic" is a chemical compound that is not normally produced or expected to be present in an organism. In this case, it refers to mercury.
17   Ibid. abstract.

increased levels of mercury as evidenced by increased urinary amounts of the abnormal porphyrins found only in those with elevated levels of mercury.

A Twenty-Second Study: Geier, D.A., Geier, M.R. "A Case Series of Children with Apparent Mercury Toxic Encephalopathies Manifesting with Clinical Symptoms of Regressive Autistic Disorders." *J Toxicol Environ Health A*. 2007 May 15; 70(10):837-51.

In this IRB approved study, the epidemiologic team of Mark and David Geier reviewed a case series of nine patients who presented to the Genetic Centers of America for genetic and developmental evaluation. One of the nine patients had autism due to Rett Syndrome. The other eight, to quote the Geiers:

- Had regressive autism spectrum disorders (ASDs);
- Had elevated levels of androgens (male hormones, like testosterone);
- Excreted significant amounts of mercury post chelation challenge;
- Had biochemical evidence of decreased function in their glutathione pathways;
- Had no known significant mercury exposure except from thimerosal-containing vaccines/Rho(D)-immune globulin preparations; and
- Had alternate causes for their regressive ASDs ruled out.

"There was a significant dose-response relationship between the severity of the regressive ASDs observed and the total mercury dose children received from thimerosal-containing vaccines/Rho (D)-immune globulin preparations.

"Based upon differential diagnoses, 8 of 9 patients examined were exposed to significant mercury from thimerosal-containing biologic/vaccine preparations during their fetal/infant developmental periods, and subsequently, between 12 and 24 mo of age, these previously normally developing children suffered mercury toxic encephalopathies that manifested with clinical symptoms consistent with regressive ASDs."

The Geiers concluded that, "Evidence for mercury intoxication should be considered in the differential diagnosis as contributing to some regressive ASDs."[18]

A Twenty-Third Study: Geier, Mark R., Geier, David A. "A Prospective Study of Thimerosal-Containing Rho(D)-Immune Globulin Administration as a Risk Factor for Autistic Disorders." *The Journal of Maternal-Fetal and Neonatal Medicine*. May 2007; 20(5): 385–390.

In this prospective case study, the Geiers evaluated fifty-three *consecutive* patients with autism spectrum disorders who presented to the Genetic Centers of America for outpatient evaluations. The study's purpose was to evaluate the possible relationship between *prenatal* mercury exposure to thimerosal and autism spectrum disorders.

The prenatal exposure under investigation derived from the then thimerosal-containing injections (Rho(D) immune globulins) given during the pregnancy to the mothers who were Rh negative.

The Rh factor is one of the substances that determines blood type. Rh negative means that the individual does not have the Rh factor.

What the researchers found was that children with autism spectrum disorders were *significantly* more likely (28 percent) to have Rh-negative mothers than were the controls (14 percent). Each autistic spectrum disorder patient's mother "was determined to have been administered a thimerosal-containing vaccine during the pregnancy." Thus the *autistic children were significantly more likely than the non-autistic children to have been exposed to mercury from thimerosal in utero.*

The Geiers suggest that, "The results provide insights into the potential role prenatal mercury exposure may play in some children with ASDs."

---

18   Ibid. abstract.

"We found that more than 53 percent of our mothers of autistic children were rh- negative and received an immunoglobulin preserved with thimerosal during pregnancy. In contrast, only 3 percent of our mothers with normal children were Rh-negative."

— *Stephanie Cave*[19]

A Twenty-Fourth Study: Geier, D.A. et al. "Neurodevelopmental Disorders, Maternal Rh-Negativity, and Rho(D) Immune Globulins: A Multi-Center Assessment." *Neuro Endocrinol Lett* 2008; 29:272-80.

As in the previous study the researchers hypothesized that if "prenatal Rho(D)-immune globulin preparation exposure was a risk factor for neuro-developmental disorders then more children with neuro-developmental disorders would have Rh-negative mothers compared to controls" since their mothers would have likely been given the then thimerosal-containing Rho(D)-immune globulin.

The researchers also hypothesized that "if thimerosal in the Rho(D)-immune globulin preparations was the ingredient associated with neuro-developmental disorders, (then) following the removal of thimerosal from all manufactured Rho(D)-immune globulin preparations from 2002 in the US, the frequency of maternal Rh-negativity among children with neuro-developmental disorders should be similar to control populations."

The researchers evaluated 298 children with neurodevelopmental defects and known Rh status at two participating clinics located in different states. The frequency of Rh negativity was also determined for the control groups at each of the two clinics.

What the researchers demonstrated was that, as in the previous study, there were *significant* and comparable increases in maternal Rh-negativity associated with pre-natal thimerosal exposure among children with neuro-developmental disorders, including autism and attention deficit/hyperactivity disorder as compared to those children in the control groups.

However, children with neuro-developmental disorders born *after 2001* (when thimerosal was no longer in the Rho(D)-immune globulin) had an Rh-negative frequency similar to that of the controls.

The implication that was drawn from this study was that prenatal exposure to thimerosal-containing Rho(D)–immune globulin is associated with some neuro-developmental deficits in children. Although the Rho(D)–immune globulin no longer contains thimerosal, the flu vaccines currently being administered to pregnant women usually do have thimerosal in them as a preservative (in the multi-dose vials).

A Twenty-Fifth Study: Gallagher, C., Goodman, M. "Hepatitis B Triple Series Vaccine and Developmental Disability in US Children Aged 1-9 Years." *Toxicol Environ Chem* 2008; 90:997-1008.

Hepatitis B is a virus that causes chronic hepatitis in many. An immunization to this disease was first made available in 1982, but its use was not mandated until 1990. It was decided that newborn babies should receive this immunization series of three shots starting on the first day of life with follow-up immunizations given at 1 month and 6 months. Prior to 2000, the hepatitis B series was preserved with thimerosal in the multidose vials and contained neurotoxic aluminum as well (and still does).

Researchers Gallagher and Goodman investigated the association between vaccination with the hepatitis B series of three injections given prior to the year 2000 and developmental disability in over 1800 children aged 1-9 years. Developmental disability was assessed by the child needing and receiving early intervention or special education services.

The odds of a child having received early intervention or special education services was found to be *nine times as great for vaccinated boys as for unvaccinated boys (after adjustment* for cofounders).

---

19   http://www.whale.to/vaccine/cave.html

The authors concluded, "This study [an addition to the aforementioned ninth study] found statistically significant evidence to suggest that boys in United States who were vaccinated with the triple series Hepatitis B vaccine, during the time period in which vaccines were manufactured with thimerosal, were more susceptible to developmental disability than were unvaccinated boys."

The study did not look for specific disabilities like autism, but it did demonstrate a likely association between early exposure to thimerosal and aluminum and neurodevelopmental abnormalities in general, most of which are characteristic of autism.

A Twenty-Sixth Study: Geier, D.A. "Blood mercury levels in autism spectrum disorder: is there a threshold level?" *Acta Neurobiologiae Experimentalis*. Vol. 70, No. 2 (2010) p. 177-186.

In this study, *red blood cell* mercury level data were examined from 83 subjects diagnosed with an autism spectrum disorder and compared to the results found in 89 normally developing control children. The data was collected from 2003 to 2007. The analysis was done by Vitamin Diagnostic Labs and found to be consistent with measurements on the same blood samples analyzed by University of Rochester lab technicians.

The researchers found that mean mercury levels (21 µg/L) in the autistic cohort were almost *twice* (1.9x) that of the control group (11 µg/L). The odds of that difference being due to chance was calculated at less than one in ten thousand ($p<0.0001$).

At red blood cell mercury levels greater than 15 µg/L there was over a six-fold (odds ratio 6.4) likelihood of a child being diagnosed with an autism spectrum disorder in comparison to the control group.

Comment: This appears to be a well-done study. The lab results were checked and found to be consistent with those of the University of Rochester lab analyses. Note that these analyses were done on red blood cells and not on whole blood or serum. The results of this study are consistent with and support the contention that mercury poisoning of the brain plays a role as a causative factor in autism.

A Twenty-Seventh Study: Geier, D.A., King, P.G. & Geier, M.R. "Mitochondrial dysfunction, impaired oxidative-reduction activity, degeneration, and death in human neuronal and fetal cells induced by low-level exposure to thimerosal and other metal compounds." *Toxicological & Environmental Chemistry*. Vol. 91, Issue 4, 2009; p. 735-749 DOI:10.1080/02772240802246458.

The researchers in this study were interested in testing a variety of neurotoxic compounds on human cell cultures in order to assess their toxic effects. Lab cultured human neuronal and fetal cells were exposed to thimerosal (a source of *ethyl mercury*), as well as *aluminum* sulfate, *lead* acetate, *methyl mercury* hydroxide, and *mercury chloride*. Damage was measured using standard vitality assays and microscopic digital capture imaging techniques.

The researchers found that thimerosal at low nanomolar concentrations induced *significant* cellular toxicity in human neuronal and fetal cells, and the damage done to those cells included *time-dependent mitochondrial damage, reduced oxidative-reduction activity, cellular degeneration, and cell death.*

The research team found that, "Thimerosal-induced cytoxicity (toxic cellular damage) is similar to that observed in autistic disorder pathophysiologic studies. Thimerosal was found to be significantly more toxic than the other metal compounds examined."

Comment: This was a good study that found that thimerosal causes neuronal cell damage that mirrors that seen in autistic children. It is pertinent to note that thimerosal was more toxic than either methyl mercury or mercury chloride. Further studies need to be done to evaluate any possible additive effects of having two or more toxins present in the cells, like lead and aluminum with mercury, for example.

A Twenty-Eighth Study: Adams, J.B. et al. "The Severity of Autism Is Associated with Toxic Metal Body Burden and Red Blood Cell Glutathione Levels." *Journal of Toxicology* 2009, 2009:7. Article ID 532640

In this paper, James Adams and his colleagues investigated the possible relationship between the severity of autism in 63 children aged 3-8 years with ASD and their body burden of toxic metals including mercury. The investigators also looked for possible correlations between autism severity and the amount of glutathione present in the autistic children's red blood cells.

Urine levels of toxic metal before and after a provoking challenge with DMSA, a heavy metal chelator, were determined and red blood cell (RBC) glutathione levels were also determined prior to the DMSA chelation provocation.

The researchers found, "Multiple positive correlations…between the severity of autism and the urinary excretion of toxic metals (especially mercury and antimony at baseline). Variations in the severity of autism measurements could be explained, in part, by regression analyses (a type of statistical calculation) of urinary excretion of toxic metals before and after DMSA and the level of red blood cell glutathione."

They concluded that, "This study demonstrates a significant positive association between the severity of autism and the relative body burden of toxic metals." That is to say, *the more toxic metals found in the child, the more severe was their autism, and likewise, the lower the levels of red cell glutathione (which plays a vital role in the detoxification of heavy metals) the greater the severity of their autism.*

A Twenty-Ninth Study: Sharpe, M.A., Gist, T.L., Baskin, D.S. "B-Lymphocytes from a Population of Children with Autism Spectrum Disorder and Their Unaffected Siblings Exhibit Hypersensitivity to Thimerosal." *J Toxicol.* 2013; 801517. Epub 2013 Jun 9.

The researchers in this study evaluated the effects of thimerosal on cell proliferation and mitochondrial function from certain immune cells known as B-lymphocytes, which were taken from individuals with autism and their siblings.

They grew the B-cells "with increasing amounts of thimerosal to examine the effects on cellular proliferation," and they performed a variety of assays to assess mitochondrial function as well. They then compared the results to those obtained from a matched control group.

What they found was that "a sub-population of eight individuals (4 ASD, 2 twins, and 2 siblings) from four of the families showed thimerosal hypersensitivity, whereas none of the control individuals displayed this response.

"The thimerosal concentration required to inhibit cell proliferation in these individuals was only 40 percent of controls. Cells hypersensitive to thimerosal also had higher levels of oxidative stress markers…."

Their results suggested to the scientists that "certain individuals with a mild mitochondrial defect may be highly susceptible to mitochondrial specific toxins like the vaccine preservative thimerosal."

This study again demonstrates that autistic individuals appear to be more sensitive to the toxic effects of thimerosal and adds to the large body of evidence implicating this neuro-toxin in the etiology of autism.

A Thirtieth Study: Sajdel-Sulkowska, Elizabeth M. "Oxidative Stress in Autism: Elevated Cerebellar 3-nitrotyrosine Levels." *American Journal of Biochemistry and Biotechnology* 4 (2): 73-84, 2008.

In this study, the autopsied brains of young autistic individuals who had died were analyzed for *an oxidative stress marker for mercury* called 3-nitrotyrosine and also for the trace mineral selenium. The results were compared to those of a control group of non-autistic children, and a "positive correlation between cerebellar 3-nitrotyrosine and mercury levels" was found. Selenium level differences in the two groups were not statistically significant.

"While preliminary," says author Elizabeth Sajdel-Sulkowska, "the results of the present study add elevated oxidative stress markers in the brain to the growing body of data reflecting greater oxidative stress in autism."

This study "shows a potential link between mercury and the autopsied brains of young people with autism. A marker for oxidative stress was 68.9 percent higher in autistic brain issue than controls (a statistically significant result), while mercury levels were 68.2 percent higher."[20]

A Thirty-First Study: Grønsborg, T.K., Schendel, D.E., Parner, E.T. "Recurrence of Autism Spectrum Disorders in Full- and Half-Siblings and Trends over Time: A Population-Based Cohort Study." *JAMA Pediatr*. 2013 Aug 19, 2013.

The purpose of this study was to determine the likelihood of a child becoming autistic if a sibling were autistic. The authors claim that "this is the first population-based study to examine the recurrence risk for autism spectrum disorders (ASDs), including time trends, and the first study to consider the ASDs recurrence risk for full and half-siblings."[21]

Therese Grønsborg's team analyzed the Danish autism database and found an almost seven-fold increase in ASD risk if an older sibling had an ASD diagnosis compared to older siblings with no ASD diagnosis. "In children with the same mother, the adjusted relative recurrence risk of 7.5 in full siblings was significantly higher than the risk of 2.4 in half siblings. In children with the same father, the adjusted relative recurrence risk was 7.4 in full siblings and significant, but no statistically significant increased risk was observed among paternal half siblings, the results also indicate."[22]

"The difference in the recurrence risk between full and half siblings supports the role of genetics in ASDs," say the authors of this study," while the significant recurrence risk in maternal half-siblings may support the role of factors associated with pregnancy and the maternal intrauterine environment in ASDs," they conclude.

So, what does this study have to do with thimerosal, mercury, immunizations, and the risk of becoming autistic?

Further analysis of this CDC-sponsored study by John Gilmore revealed some interesting data, the implications of which put a lie to the conclusions of an earlier Danish study by Madsen, et al.[23] in which it was alleged that autism rates *increased slightly* after thimerosal was removed from Danish vaccines in 1991, suggesting that thimerosal was not a risk factor for autism spectrum disorders.

As can be seen by the graph below taken from John Gilmore's analysis of the data from the Grønsborg study, the prevalence of autism was not only not increasing, but it was actually *declining* during the study period (1995-2000), which supports the contention that thimerosal-preserved vaccines are indeed a major cause of autism.[24]

The graph also illustrates the purported (and factitious) slight rise in autism during that same period as alleged by Madsen et al.[25]

It should be pointed out that both groups of researchers (Madsen et al. and Grønsborg et al.) analyzed exactly the same data from the same time period, yet came up with diametrically opposite results as well as an entirely different number of autism cases.

The earlier study found only 956 cases of autism in Denmark during the 29-year period from 1971 to 2000, but the 2013 Grønsborg team identified 12,698 such cases from 1995-2000, a shorter period of time—a huge discrepancy that can only be explained by the *deliberate falsification and analysis of the data* by Kreesten Madsen's team!

The Madsen study was rejected by several journals because of obvious methodological flaws and is itself a study in statistical manipulation and malfeasance.

20   http://adventuresinautism.blogspot.co.uk/2007/06/no-evidence-of-any-link.html
21   Grønborg, T.K., Ibid.
22   http://www.sciencedaily.com/releases/2013/08/130819162509.htm
23   Madsen, Kreesten M. et al. "Thimerosal and the Occurrence of Autism: Negative Ecological Evidence From Danish Population-Based Data." *Pediatrics*. 2003; 112:3 604-606.
24   http://www.ageofautism.com/2013/09/danish-mercury-study-fabricated-new-study-differentresults.html?utm_source=feedburner&utm_medium=email&u tm _campaign=Feed percent3A+ageofautism+ percent28AGE+OF+AUTISM percent29&utm_content=Yahoo percent21+Mail
25   Madsen op. cit.

It was deviously designed to show the results that the CDC wanted it to show, to whit, that vaccines (and thimerosal) don't cause autism. In reality, it does no such thing! A more detailed critique of the flawed Madsen study will be presented in Chapter 17.

It is reasonable to ask why the CDC would want to sponsor a study whose findings might support the link between vaccines, thimerosal, and autism spectrum disorders. Has there been a change of heart (or conscience) in the CDC hierarchy?

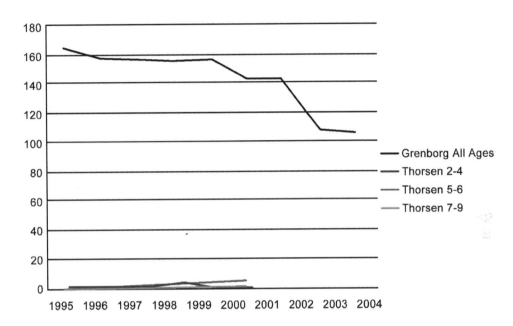

Figure 14.1. The numbers on the vertical axis represent the autism rate percentage X100. The declining upper line shows the decline in autism prevalence after mercury was removed from vaccines. The lower lines represent the flawed data analysis from the 2003 Madsen, et al. study analyzing the same data and coming up with entirely different results. This will be discussed further in Chapter 17.

Is this ethically-challenged institution now prepared to condemn the Madsen study as fraudulent? Is the CDC now willing to admit that mercury is a likely factor in causing autism?

Sadly, no. The CDC just goofed. It was "hoisted by their own petard," as the saying goes. This study was not designed to be relevant to the issue of autism and mercury-containing vaccines, so there was no need to manipulate the data.

What the CDC did not anticipate, we suggest, is that an independent analyst (John Gilmore) would use the Grønsborg study data to counter the claims of Kreesten Madsen's team. And as we have seen, did he ever!

As John Gilmore states, "This study clearly shows a steady decline in the number of Danish children with autism every year from 1995 through 2000."[26]

Comment: The CDC and the Madsen team have a lot of explaining to do! This study should be the final "nail in the coffin" of the thimerosal/vaccine-autism link deniers. Its data clearly support the mercury-autism association.

---

26   Ibid.

Table 14.1. Comparison of Autism Rates 1994-2004[27]

Year	Rate of Autism
1994-95	1.65%
1996-97	1.58%
1998-99	1.56%
2000-01	1.43%
2002-04	1.06%

A Thirty-Second Study: Alabdali, A. et al. "A key role for an impaired detoxification mechanism in the etiology and severity of autism spectrum disorders." *Behavioral and Brain Functions.* 2014, 10:14.

Further evidence that autistic children have higher levels of the toxic metals lead and mercury comes from this small study.

Researchers measured the red blood cell levels of mercury and lead in autistic children and also the plasma levels of glutathione and vitamin E and found that the autistic children had lower levels of glutathione and vitamin E and higher levels of lead and mercury than did the control group.

Not surprisingly, the higher the concentrations of lead and mercury, the more severe were the autism symptoms in these children. The authors concluded that impaired detoxification in autistic children was a likely etiological mechanism for the disorder.

Conclusions: Mercury, like lead and aluminum, is well-established as being neurotoxic. During the 1990s, it was present in vaccines in amounts given to babies and young children that far exceeded those allowed by the Environmental Protection Agency.

We have reviewed many animal studies and over two dozen human studies that emphatically associate mercury exposure to autism. Numerous studies show that the more mercury a child is exposed to or retains, the greater the risk for autism, and the earlier that mercury exposure, the greater the harm.

The analyses in multiple studies of *five different databases* confirm the link between thimerosal-containing vaccines and the prevalence of autism and other neuro-developmental disorders.

Many studies show that children with autism are less able to excrete mercury. One study revealed that children with autism are also more sensitive to thimerosal than are non-autistics. We understand now why autism predominates in males and the role mercury plays in this regard.

Another recent study found significantly more mercury in the brains of autistic children than in controls and greater oxidative biomarkers indicative of mercury toxicity. And a revealing study determined that autism rates declined in Denmark after mercury-containing vaccines were withdrawn.

Mercury from thimerosal and other sources is, therefore, overwhelmingly likely to be a major causative agent in autism. But there is a whole lot more to this story, and there are even more studies pointing to mercury (as well as other agents) as contributors to the worldwide autism epidemic.

"It's easier to fool people than to convince them that they have been fooled."

— Mark Twain

---

27   http://www.ageofautism.com/2013/09/danish-mercury-study-fabricated-new-studydifferentrsults.html?utm_source=feedburner&utm_medium=email&utm _campaign=Feed percent3A+ageofautism+ percent28AGE+OF+AUTISM percent29&utm_content=Yahoo percent21+Mail

SYNERGISTIC TOXICITY

LEAD AND MERCURY

A 1978 study[28] found that a quantity of lead that will kill 1 percent of exposed rats when combined with the amount of mercury that will kill only 1 rat out of 100 didn't just kill 2 percent of the rats, it caused the death of every rat (100 percent)! That's synergistic toxicity!

"What this proves," according to Prof. Boyd Haley, "is that one cannot define a 'safe level of mercury' unless you absolutely know what other toxicants the individual is being exposed to."

ALUMINUM AND MERCURY

Many vaccines contain aluminum. "Experiments were done to determine if aluminum would increase the toxicity of very low levels of thimerosal. The results were unequivocal: the presence of aluminum dramatically increased the rate of neuronal death caused by thimerosal. Therefore, the aluminum and thimerosal combination found in vaccines produces a toxic mixture that cannot be compared to situations where thimerosal alone is the toxic exposure."[29]

TESTOSTERONE AND MERCURY

"Neurons that were pre-incubated with estrogen demonstrated substantial protection against thimerosal-induced neuron death. In contrast, the addition of testosterone caused a very large increase in thimerosal-induced neuron death.

"A low nanomolar level of thimerosal that gave less than 5 percent neuron death in three hours could be increased to 100 percent cell death by the addition of one micromolar level of testosterone.

"Testosterone alone at this level also showed less than 5 percent cell death. The opposing effects of estrogen and testosterone may explain the gender-based four-to-one ratio. Most important, the tremendous enhancement of thimerosal toxicity by testosterone points out the impact of synergistic effects when addressing mercury toxicity."[30]

28   Schubert J et al. *J.of Toxicology and Enviromental Health.* 1978; v4: 763-776.
29   Boyd Haley http://www.flcv.com/hgsynerg.html
30   Boyd Haley http://www.flcv.com/hgsynerg.html

Chapter 15
Airborne Toxins, Chelation Efficacy, and Porphyrin Testing

"Things come apart so quickly when they have been held together with lies."

— *Dorothy Allison,* Bastard out of Carolina

W**HAT** E**VIDENCE** S**UPPORTS** *Contention 10?*

CONTENTION 10: *There are population studies demonstrating that children exposed to airborne toxins from mercury-emitting smelters and other industry sources of mercury have a significantly increased risk of becoming autistic, and the closer they live to these sources, the greater the prevalence of autism.*

The Palmer et al. Studies: Palmer, R.F. et al. "Environmental mercury release, special education rates, and autism disorder: an ecological study of Texas. *Autism Research Review International.* Vol. 19, No. 1, 2005 February. *and* Palmer, R.F. et al. "Proximity to point sources of environmental mercury release as a predictor of autism prevalence." *Health & Place.* doi:10.1016/j.healthplace. 2008.02.001.

In these related studies, Dr. Ray Palmer of the Univ. of Texas Health Science Center and his colleagues not only found a *statistically significant* association between the quantity of industry-released mercury and the incidence of autism, but also demonstrated, apparently for the first time in scientific literature, a *statistically significant* association between autism risk and distance from the mercury source.

In the first study, Raymond Palmer and colleagues used EPA data to assess levels of mercury emissions for each county in Texas. "They then used statistics from the Texas Education Agency to determine the rates of autism and special education services reported by school districts in 254 counties in the state, controlling for multiple economic and demographic factors."[1]

Palmer et al. report, "On average, for each 1,000 pounds of environmentally released mercury, there was a 43 percent increase in the rate of special education services and a 61 percent increase in the rate of autism."

Non-autistic special education numbers did not correlate with mercury release, only the autistic children's numbers did, indicating that "the association between mercury release and school district special education rates was completely accounted for by increased rates of autism."

In their second related study, the researchers measured the mercury-release data from 39 mercury-emitting, coal-fired power plants and 56 other industrial facilities in Texas. Autism rates examined were from 1,040 *Texas school districts.* Their conclusions:

---

1   http://gordonresearch.com/articles_autism/mercury_autism_link_texas.html

1. "For every 1,000 pounds of mercury released by all industrial sources in Texas into the environment in 1998, there was a corresponding 2.6 percent increase in autism rates in Texas school districts in 2002."

2. "For every 1,000 pounds of mercury released by Texas power plants in 1998, there was a corresponding 3.7 percent increase in autism rates in Texas school districts in 2002."

3. "Autism prevalence diminished 1 percent to 2 percent for every 10 miles from the source."

Although these studies don't prove the contention that mercury exposure causes autism in certain individuals, they certainly are consistent with and support that hypothesis.

The DeSoto Study: DeSoto, M.C. "Ockham's Razor[2] and Autism: The Case for Developmental Neurotoxins Contributing to a Disease of Neurodevelopment." *Neurotoxicology.* 2009 doi:10.1016/j.neuro.2009.03.003.

A third recently published and related study, by epidemiologist Mary Catherine DeSoto, evaluated the incidence of autism and its relationship to the distance from "Superfund" toxic waste sites in Minnesota, the state with the highest incidence of autism spectrum disorders. These sites contain not only mercury, but also arsenic, chromium, cadmium, lead, chloroethylenes, and benzene.

What the author of this study found was that, "School children living within a 10- or 20-mile radius of toxic waste sites are nearly twice as likely to have autism compared to children living farther away from such sites. [The findings were highly statistically significant (p=0.0001)]. These data support the widely speculated but controversial idea that exposure to chemical contaminants can increase the risk of developing autism."

What Evidence Supports Contention 11?

CONTENTION 11: Autistic children who have their mercury and other heavy metals removed, via a process known as chelation, often significantly improve their overall functioning.

Chelation (key-LAY-shun) is the technical term for the process whereby a chelating agent (like DMSA or DMPS) is used to chelate ("KEY-late"—chemically remove) undesirable substances (like mercury and lead).

There is a good deal of anecdotal evidence supporting the use of chelating agents in autism spectrum disorders, and just a few studies.

The Nataf (et al.) Study: Nataf, R. et al. "Porphyrinurea in Childhood Autistic Disorders: Implications for Environmental Toxicity." *Toxicol. Appl. Pharmacol.* 2006; 214(2):99-108.

It may be recalled that in this previously reviewed study (see Chapter 14) the researchers found abnormal porphyrin metabolites in children's urine that signified mercury toxicity, and that they had also chelated a subgroup of the children with autism with oral DMSA, a chelating agent that has been shown to lower mercury and lead levels.

Following chelation, there was a significant decrease (P=0.002) in urine porphyrin levels in these children, indicating that DMSA is an effective chelator of mercury. This study was not designed to evaluate any possible clinical benefit from DMSA chelation; however, the following studies did find that chelation could be helpful in ameliorating some of the clinical symptoms of autism.

The Holmes Studies: Holmes, A. "Heavy metal toxicity in autistic spectrum disorders: Mercury toxicity." In Rimland, B. ed. *DAN! (Defeat Autism Now!) Fall 2001 Conference Practitioner Training.* San Diego, CA: Autism Research Institute, 2002.

In 2001, Dr. Amy Holmes reported on a preliminary study that she did at her clinic using DMSA (dimercapto succinic acid) as a chelating agent for mercury and other heavy metals. At the time of her presentation, she had over 500 autistic children and young adults under treatment with DMSA. DMSA is approved by the FDA for removal of lead, and it can also chelate other metals like mercury and antimony.

---

2   The rule of Ockham's Razor states "the simplest explanation is likely the correct one."

Dr. Holmes' protocol was to chelate these patients with DMSA until their urine showed little or no mercury and then to continue therapy with DMSA plus lipoic acid. By mid January-2001, eighty-five patients had completed the protocol with DMSA alone, and they also had had at least an additional four months of DMSA plus lipoic acid. The improvement percentages are listed in Table 15.1.[3]

Table 15.1. Chelation Therapy Success Rates

n = 85		Improvement (percent)			
Age	Number	Marked	Moderate	Slight	None
1-5	40	35	39	15	11
6-12	25	4	28	52	16
13-17	16	0	6	68	26
18+	4	0	0	25	75

As Table 15.1 makes clear, *the younger the child, the better the results.* All 6 of the 1-2 year-old children who had completed the chelation therapy course had returned to normal functioning (became non-autistic) "by parent reports and repeat psychological testing."

Dr. Homes notes that "the rapidity of excretion seems to decrease markedly with each additional year of age. There are several children, mostly in the younger age groups, who have made remarkable progress to the point of being able to be mainstreamed in school, but who are still have [sic] some 'oddities' of behavior—none of these children have completed treatment yet."[4]

At a Defeat Autism Now! Conference in the fall of that year, Dr. Holmes was now able to report on the results of a total of 152 autistic children aged 1-18+ years who had completed her detoxification protocol. The results were consistent with the earlier study.

Overall, 83 percent of the children showed improvement in functioning, and again there was a distinct age gradient. Of the 1-5 year olds, 91 percent had improved in contrast to only 28 percent of those over 18 years of age. The best results were noted in the youngest children and in those who had developed normally and then later regressed.

Dr. Holmes observed that some children's behaviors worsened initially before showing signs of improvement. Some of the children appeared to improve immunologically (decreased auto-antibodies against the central nervous system and loss of IgE mediated allergies) by the end of the chelation process.

Common side effects were diarrhea and fatigue. Abnormal blood counts, liver enzyme elevations, and mineral abnormalities were less commonly noted.

The Cancelled NIMH Study: Kim N. Dietrich, et al. "Effect of Chelation Therapy on the Neuropsychological and Behavioral Development of Lead-Exposed Children after School Entry." DOI: *Pediatrics* 2004; 114; 19.

In September 2006, the National Institute of Mental Health began an IRB-approved, blinded 12-week study of DMSA vs. placebo in a group of 120 autistic children aged 4-10 to see whether DMSA chelation might improve their social and language skills. The study was cancelled in February 2007 because the results of another study on *rodents* showed that DMSA caused cognitive harm in *lead-free* rodents who were chelated with the DMSA, although *DMSA substantially helped the rodents who were lead toxic.* The researchers felt that this raised "red flags" regarding the safety of DMSA.[5]

---

3   http://www.healingarts.org/children/holmes.htm
4   http://www.healing-arts.org/children/holmes.htm
5   Stangle, et al. *Environmental Health Perspectives.* October 2006.

It should be noted that an earlier blinded study of DMSA chelation of 7-year-old children, who as infants had very elevated lead levels, did not show any evidence of neurological harm after three consecutive 26-day courses of DMSA.[6]

It is perhaps just as well that the NIMH study was called off because in order to qualify for this study, the children selected had to have had *low levels of mercury* in their blood or the investigators felt that they could not ethically be given a placebo.

But it is, of course, just those children with an elevated body burden of mercury who would have been the most likely to benefit from chelation. The study had, therefore, been designed to fail.[7]

The First Adams, Baral, et al. Studies: Adams, James B. et al. "Safety and efficacy of oral DMSA therapy for children with autism spectrum disorders: Part A—Medical Results."[8]

Two additional linked studies were published in the October 2009 edition of the journal *BMC Clinical Pharmacology* in which the researchers attempted to ascertain the efficacy of using DMSA as a chelating agent in autistic children.

In the first of the studies, 65 children aged 3-8 years with autism spectrum disorder were given a single round of oral DMSA and their urines collected shortly thereafter. The 49 children excreting *high levels of toxic metals* were then selected (in phase 2 of the study) to receive in a *randomly assigned, double-blind fashion* an additional 6 rounds of either DMSA or placebo. DMSA was found to increase greatly the excretion of lead (by ten times) and, to a lesser extent, a variety of other metals, including mercury.

The initial round of DMSA (given 3 times per day for just 3 days) was shown *significantly* to normalize the red blood cell levels of glutathione "in almost all cases, and greatly improved abnormal platelet counts, suggesting a significant decrease in inflammation."

Dr. Adams and his colleagues concluded that, "Overall, DMSA therapy seems to be reasonably safe, effective in removing several toxic metals (especially lead), dramatically effective in normalizing red blood cell glutathione, and effective in normalizing platelet counts. Only 1 round (3 days) was sufficient to improve glutathione and platelets. Additional rounds increased excretion of toxic metals."

Elevated platelet counts are a marker for inflammation. The normalization of the elevated platelet counts by one round of DMSA therapy in about half the children suggested to the researchers that "some of the inflammation in children with autism is due to toxic metals which are removable by DMSA."

The researchers did not note any adverse effects of the chelation on blood counts (CBCs), zinc levels or liver panels, but they did note that chelation decreased serum potassium and chromium levels and recommended supplementing with these minerals while chelating.[9]

The Second Adams, Baral et al. Study: Adams, J. et al. "Safety and efficacy of oral DMSA therapy for children with autism spectrum disorders: Part B Behavioral results." *BMC Clinical Pharmacology* 2009, 9:17.

In the second part of the study, the children who continued the DMSA therapy (3 days on and 11 days off) *showed benefits in improved language, cognition, and sociability*. These results do need to be confirmed in a larger, blinded study.

One of the authors of this study, Matthew Baral, stated, "Toxic metals are a common problem in autism, and I have personally observed that many of my patients with autism have greatly benefited from DMSA therapy. I hope this data answers the question that many physicians have: whether chelation is safe and effective, and clearly it's both."

---

6   Ibid.
7   "Stalled Chelation Trial for Autism Highlights Dilemma of Alternative Treatments." *Science*. 18 July 2008. Vol. 321. www.sciencemag.org
8   *BMC Clinical Pharmacology*. 2009, 9:17
9   Adams, James B. et al. Ibid. Part A; Medical Results.

Lead author Professor James Adams agreed, "This study shows that DMSA therapy…should be considered as a possible treatment for children with autism who have (a) significant body burden of toxic metals."

Please note that *the researchers appropriately recommend only chelating those children who have an elevated body burden of toxic metals.*[10]

The Egyptian Study: Blaucok-Busch, Eleanor et al. "Efficacy of DMSA Therapy in a Sample of Arab Children with Autistic Spectrum Disorder." *Maedica: A Journal of Clinical Medicine.* Vol. 7. No. 3. 2012.

In this study, 39 confirmed autistic children[11] 3-9 yrs of age were given urine tests for heavy metals both before (baseline) and after a chelation challenge using DMSA as the chelating agent.

The purpose of the study was to see whether treating these children with a *once-a-month* DMSA dose for a period of six months would improve their neurological and social functioning and reduce their toxic metal burden.

What was found was that "The DMSA challenge test increased the urine metal output for a number of potentially toxic metals. Statistically significant differences were noted between the baseline urine and DMSA challenge test regarding the level of cadmium, mercury, and lead ($P=0.006$, $P=0.049$, and $P=0.008$ respectively)."

They "also noted that behavioral effects, typical for ASD (autism spectrum disorders) were reduced with this method of detoxification. A comparison between CARS (Childhood Autism Rating Scale) Subscales and Total Score before and after a 6-month chelation program showed greatest improvements for verbal and nonverbal communication ($P<0.001$), Taste, Smell and Touch (P 0.001) and Relating to People (P 0.005). Other improvements were noted for Adaptation to Change and Improvement."

The researchers also found that, "There was a *significant positive correlation between baseline urine aluminum and body use, taste, smell, touch responses, and total Childhood Autism Rating Scale scores.*"

This indicates," they continued, "that a higher aluminum exposure is associated with increased impairment in these body functions and higher total CARS (score)."

They concluded that, "DMSA chelation increased the urinary output of toxic and neurotoxic metals," and that "detoxification treatment with oral DMSA has (a) beneficial effect on ASD patients."[12]

What Evidence Supports Contention 12?

CONTENTION 12: *Certain porphyrin compounds that form only when mercury toxicity is present are more frequently seen in autistic children as compared to their non-autistic peers.*

The eight studies listed on this page have been previously discussed, and they all confirm that the quantity of certain urinary porphyrin compounds indicative of the presence of mercury is significantly greater in autistics than in controls, and the amount found correlates with the severity of the autism.

- Nataf, R. Lam, A., Lathe, R., Skorupka, C. "Porphyrinurea in Childhood Autistic Disorders: Implications for Environmental Toxicity." *Toxicol. Appl. Pharmacol.* 214(2):99-108, 2006.

- Geier, M., Geier, D. "A prospective assessment of porphyrins in autistic disorders: a potential marker for heavy metal exposure." *Neurotox Res.* Aug; 10(1):57-64, 2006.

- Geier, M., Geier, D. "A Prospective Study of Mercury Toxicity Biomarkers in Autistic Spectrum Disorders." *Journal of Toxicology and Environmental Health, Part A,* 70: 1723–1730, 2007.

---

10   Adams, James B. et al. Ibid. Part B: Behavioral Results and Adams, J.B. et al. "The Severity of Autism Is Partially Explained by Toxic Metal Body Burden and Red Blood Cell Glutathione Levels." *Journal of Toxicology.* 2009, 2009:7. Article ID 532640.

11   Plus 2 with Asperger's Syndrome and 3 with PDD-NOS for a total of 44 children, 84 percent of whom were boys.

12   Ibid.

- Geier, D. et al. "Biomarkers of environmental toxicity and susceptibility in autism." *Journal of the Neurological Sciences.* DOI: 10.1016/j.jns.2008.08.021.

- Geier, David A. et al. "A Prospective Blinded Evaluation of Urinary Porphyrins Versus the Clinical Severity of Autism Spectrum Disorders." *Journal of Toxicology and Environmental Health, Part A.* 72: 24, 1585-1591, 2009.

- Austin, D.W. et al. "An investigation of porphyrinuria in Australian children with autism." *J Toxic Env Hlth.* 71: 1349-51, 2008.

- Kern, J.K. et al. "Toxicity Biomarkers in Autism Spectrum Disorder: A Blinded Study of Urinary Porphyrins. *Pediatrics International.* 2010.

- Youn, S.I. et al. "Porphyrinuria in Korean Children with Autism: Correlation with Oxidative Stress." *J Toxic Env Health.* A2010; 73 (10): 701-10.

"A lie's true power cannot be accurately measured by the number of people who believe in its deception when it is told. It must be measured by the number of people who will go out after hearing it trying to convince others of the truth."

— Dennis Sharpe

Chapter 16
The Flawed "Negative Studies" that Allege to Disprove the Mercury-Vaccine-Autism Linkage

"If you tell a big enough lie and tell it frequently enough, it will be believed."
— Adolf Hitler

FDA "ASLEEP AT THE SWITCH"

"The House Government Reform Committee that studied the history of autism and thimerosal concluded in its final report, 'This epidemic in all probability may have been prevented or curtailed had the FDA not been asleep at the switch regarding a lack of safety data regarding injected thimerosal, a known neurotoxin.' The FDA and other public-health agencies failed to act, the committee added, out of 'institutional malfeasance for self protection' and 'misplaced protectionism of the pharmaceutical industry'."[1]

FDA & WHO "ARBITRARILY" CHANGE TOXIC EXPOSURE LIMIT TO MERCURY

"The EPA, unlike the FDA, has conducted research into mercury's toxicity and health risks. While the EPA sets a limit exposure of mercury at 0.1 micrograms per kg, the FDA in its favoritism towards mercury's use in vaccines raises the stakes to 0.4 microgram/kg.

"The FDA's figure has no valid supporting scientific data and is arbitrary in order to continue sanctioning the use of mercury (thimerosal) in vaccines.

"The World Health Organization (WHO) sets the limit higher; this may account for the WHO's aggressive campaigns to inoculate the world's poorer populations with heavily laced mercury (containing) vaccines from the drug makers."[2]

WHAT KATHLEEN SEBELIUS SAID

HHS Secretary Kathleen Sebelius, in a CBS TV interview on July 30, 2009, told the nation that, "Study after study, scientist after scientist, has determined that there really is no safety risk with thimerosal."

1   www.healthspectator.com
2   Richard Gale and Gary Null, PhD. Progressive Radio Report; 11-12-09; http://www.whale.to/vaccine/gale11.html

WHAT SHE SHOULD HAVE SAID

Given the huge volume of evidence that counters her assertion, a more appropriate statement from Secretary Sebelius might have been, "Study after study of spurious and flawed research that would likely never pass a graduate school examination, [and] scientist after scientist affiliated or with financial ties to the vaccine industry now dominating our academies and health agencies, have determined that there really is no safety risk with thimerosal."[3]

CAN ALL OF THESE "EXPERTS" BE WRONG?

Department of "You Bet!"

"Five large epidemiological studies have been conducted in the United States and in Europe since 2001. These studies have all consistently provided evidence that there is no association between thimerosal-containing vaccines and autism."
— Every Child by Two, a nonprofit entity funded by Wyeth, a vaccine maker

"There are no valid studies that show a link between thimerosal in vaccines and autistic spectrum disorder. A 2004 report from the Institute of Medicine, Vaccines and Autism, concluded that the available evidence is against the existence of a causal relationship between thimerosal-containing vaccines and autism."
— American Academy of Pediatrics

"The implication that vaccinations cause autism is irresponsible and counterproductive. Although several carefully performed scientific studies have searched for a link between autism and the use of thimerosal in vaccines, no such link has been found."
— March of Dimes

"Scientific data overwhelmingly show that there is no connection between vaccines and autism.... We need more research to investigate the actual causes of autism, but it would be a disservice to the health of our children if we let vaccines take the blame for this tragic and complex disease."
— American Medical Association

"Vaccines do not cause autism and we're not afraid of the truth."
— Dr. David Tayloe, President-elect of the AAP

"It's been asked and answered: Vaccines don't cause autism.... Fourteen epidemiological studies have shown that the risk of autism is the same whether children received the MMR vaccine or not, and five have shown that thimerosal-containing vaccines also do not cause autism."
— Dr. Paul Offit, vaccine patent holder

"The weight of evidence is so great that I don't think that there is any room for debate. I think the issue is done. I'm doing this for all the families out there who don't have a child with autism, who have to deal with the issue of 'Do I get a vaccination or do I risk my child's life' because they don't understand what the science is saying."
— Dr. Nancy Minshew, director of the University of Pittsburgh's Center for Excellence in Autism

"A television show that perpetuates the myth that vaccines cause autism is the height of reckless irresponsibility on the part of ABC."
— Dr. Renee Jenkins, current President of the AAP

"Sixteen separate studies have shown no causal association [between vaccines and autism]."
— Dr. Nancy Snyderman, medical correspondent for NBC

---

3   Gale & Null-Ibid

WHAT EVIDENCE SUPPORTS *Contention 13?*

CONTENTION 13: *The studies that purport to show no relationship between immunizations, thimerosal, and autism (we refer to these as the "negative studies") are for the most part fraudulent, deceptive, or highly suspect.*

> *"Lies and secrets, Tessa, they are like a cancer in the soul. They eat away what is good and leave only destruction behind."*
>
> — *Cassandra Clare,* Clockwork Prince

We will now list these studies with appropriate critiques.

The First "Negative" Study (The "Smoking Gun"): Verstraeten, T. et al. "Safety of Thimerosal-Containing Vaccines: A Two-Phased Study of Computerized Health Maintenance Organization Database." *Pediatrics.* 2003 Nov; 112(5):1039-48.

Thomas Verstraeten's infamous CDC study and its later incarnations have the dubious honor of being used (before the original uncorrupted data was "altered") to substantiate the thimerosal-autism-neuro-developmental delay-AD-HD linkage, and as finally published, to refute that connection.

By the time this "reworked" study appeared in the journal *Pediatrics* in 2003, Verstraeten was able to conclude that, "No consistent significant associations were found between TCVs (thimerosal-containing vaccines) and neurodevelopmental outcomes." This is one of the so-called "major studies," whose conclusion is commonly quoted to support the contention that the mercury-autism link is invalid.

Critique: Dr. Verstraeten and all the attendees at the infamous Simpsonwood conference were clearly convinced that there was an autism (and developmental delay/ADHD) linkage to thimerosal-containing vaccines after Verstraeten's analysis of all the original Vaccine Safety Datalink information provided to him by the CDC prior to 2001. He analyzed the records of over 75,000 children in that study, and his *initial* analysis of the data substantiates this assertion, as do the documented minutes of the infamous Simpsonwood Conference, as does Verstraeten's already twice-revised study report from February 2000.

We know concern existed at the Simpsonwood Conference by many of its members that the original findings, which showed a *significant, linear, dose-related thimerosal linkage to neurodevelopmental disorders,* needed to be "contained" and "handled." That is clearly the reason why the meeting was held, why it was unpublicized, and why the attendees were sworn to secrecy.

If this frightening and damaging information got out, then parents of children harmed by the vaccines would have a legitimate right to sue for redress, and the consequences would be dire for the reputations and financial health of the pharmaceutical companies that made the toxic vaccines, for the individuals and institutions who "were asleep at the switch" by allowing toxic amounts of thimerosal to be included in those same vaccines, and even for the existence of the entire vaccination program.

It strains one's credulity to believe that the VSD data Verstraeten initially analyzed was "lost." The data would certainly have been on Verstraeten and the CDC's own computers, as well as those of the HMOs from which the data was derived. This was clearly a ruse to bury the damaging data and allow Verstraeten time to dilute the original information with data from a failed HMO noted for its poor record-keeping, so that when he ultimately published his report it would show "no significant associations between TCVs (thimerosal-containing vaccines) and neurodevelopmental outcomes."[4]

Verstraeten mentioned no conflicts of interest and declared that he was working for the CDC when his "study" was finally published in *Pediatrics* in 2003, but he was actually at that time a *paid employee* ("advisor") of vaccine maker

4   www.fourteenstudies.org

Glaxo-Smith-Kline, and had been for two years prior to its publication. His duplicity came to the attention of Congress, which, as we mentioned, cited him for an ethical violation in this regard.

The CDC influenced Verstraeten et al. to *manipulate the data deliberately* to eliminate the statistical significance that was undeniable in Verstraeten's initial study. They did this in a number of ways. They eliminated the comparisons of thimerosal-injected children to those who had received no thimerosal. They eliminated premature babies. They eliminated babies who received the hepatitis B immunization at birth.

They also lowered the age of the children available for analysis, thereby reducing the number of children diagnosed with neurodevelopmental disorders, and they included the data from the bankrupt "Harvard-Pilgrim" HMO with "notoriously faulty data systems" in their final analysis. "The general drift of their design changes was clear, to reduce the statistical power through conscious manipulation of statistical methods, data classifications, and samples."[5]

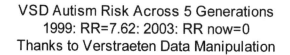

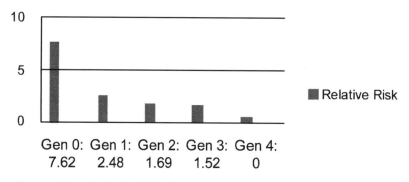

Figure 16.1. Statistical Skullduggery—How to Eliminate Relevance

Figure 16.1 adapted from a David Kirby Lecture Slide; RR = Relative Risk of becoming autistic; Gen 0 = original, Unmanipulated data (1999) RR = 7.62. This is the actual risk. Gen 1-3 Manipulated data (2000) RR = 2.48; 1.69; 1.52 Manipulated risks; Gen 4 = 4th Final *manipulation* (2003) RR = 0. This is what was published.

A re-evaluation of Verstraeten's data by epidemiologist Mark Geier exposed a major error made by Verstraeten in his analysis. As Dr. Geier puts it, "Verstraeten, et al. did not take thimerosal-free DTaP vaccine into account in their study, or if they did, then their paper, as it stands, is replete with inaccurate information."

Why? Because a significant number of the children whom Verstraeten (et al.) apparently assumed had been given the thimerosal-containing DPT shot had actually received the thimerosal-free DTaP immunization. *This error made his conclusions invalid*, even given the corrupted data.

Then CDC director Julie Gerberding acknowledged this in her "explosive" report to the House Appropriations Committee "in which she admits to a startling string of errors in the design and methods used in the CDCs 'landmark' study that found no link between mercury in vaccines and autism, ADHD, speech delays and tics."[6]

Conclusion: This shameful "study" is an embarrassment and an out and out fraud. Its conclusions are invalid. The data were deliberately manipulated to show no linkage between mercury in vaccines and neurodevelopmental disorders. It should never have been published, and having been, it should be retracted. The original study that clearly linked mercury in vaccines with neurodevelopmental disorders should be published in its stead.

---

5   www.fourteenstudies.org

6   Kirby, David. *Evidence of Harm: Mercury in Vaccines and the Autism Epidemic: A Medical Controversy*. New York: St. Martin's Press, 2007.

THE "REVOLVING DOOR" SPINS ON!

In 2006, "five former CDC Directors took the unprecedented move of writing a letter to Dr. Gerberding expressing concern that the agency had lost its way as a result of her attempts to reorganize it. She continued on the same path and as a result the predicted loss of key scientific talent and institutional memory continued. CDC is now a much weaker, less respected and less effective public health agency at a time when we need the opposite."

At the request of the Obama administration on January 20, 2009, Dr. Julie Gerberding, the first woman director of the CDC, resigned her position at that agency.

She took a job as director of the vaccine division at Merck approximately one year later.[7]

A Second "Negative" Study: "The Danish Study"

"For what is a man profited, if he shall gain the whole world and lose his own soul?"

— Attributed to Jesus of Nazareth (c. 5 B.C.—c. 30 A.D.)

A Second "Negative" Study: Madsen, Kreesten M. et al. "Thimerosal and the Occurrence of Autism: Negative Ecological Evidence from Danish Population-Based Data." *Pediatrics.* September 2003.

In this infamous first Danish study, not surprisingly *also initiated by the CDC,* the researchers, *two of whom worked for a Danish vaccine manufacturer,* analyzed the incidence of autism in Danish children between the years 1971 and 2000 and found that the autism rate actually appeared to increase slightly after thimerosal was removed from vaccines in Denmark in 1992.

However, the researchers deceptively computed the incidence of autism in Danish children aged 2 and 10 years from 1971 to 2000 by counting only the autistic children admitted to Danish psychiatric hospitals, but not those diagnosed in outpatient clinics, during the first 25 of those years, and they then added in the autistic children who were diagnosed in Danish outpatient clinics, but only from 1995 through 2000 (after thimerosal had been eliminated from vaccines), and not surprisingly concluded that, "The discontinuation of thimerosal-containing vaccines in Denmark in 1992 was followed by an increase in the incidence of autism. Our ecological data do not support a correlation between thimerosal-containing vaccines and the incidence of autism."

Critique: Children diagnosed as being autistic are rarely hospitalized for this condition, and so data from psychiatric hospitals would be expected to indicate a false-low incidence of autism, which is what Madsen and colleagues found.[8]

During the thirty-year period of surveillance in this study, the researchers documented only 956 cases of autism, with a male to female ration of 3.5 to 1. So the initial incidence data computed by the team of researchers up to 1993 was unusually low.

The criteria for diagnosing autism in Denmark expanded in 1993, and the new, broader criteria in the new diagnostic code allowed certain children who would previously not have been diagnosed with autism now to be so diagnosed. This would, of course, result in a misleading increase in the apparent incidence of autism after 1993.

An even more egregious bit of statistical malfeasance in this study is the inclusion of children diagnosed as being autistic in Danish outpatient clinics, but *only from the years 1995 to 2000* (after thimerosal was removed from the immunizations).

---

7   http://scienceblogs.com/effectmeasure/2009/01/obama_dumps_cdc_director.php?utmsource= sbhomepage& utm_medium=link&utm_content=channellink

8   A quote from this study: "Also, outpatient activities were included in the Danish Psychiatric Central Research Register in 1995, and because many patients with autism in former years have been treated as outpatients this may exaggerate the incidence rates, simply because a number of patients attending the child psychiatric treatment system before 1995 were recorded for the first time, and thereby counted as new cases in the incidence rates."

Since outpatient clinics are where most children in Denmark (and around the world for that matter) get their diagnosis (93 percent get diagnosed there in Denmark), the devious inclusion of this outpatient population, which prior to 1995 had been completely disregarded, deceptively skewed the incidence data upward.

In other words, the researchers admit that they didn't count 93 percent of the children with autism during the time when thimerosal was in the vaccines, but did count them when it wasn't. Therefore, their assertions about a rising trend in autism during the 1990s *have no basis in fact.*

The authors of this study actually acknowledged that reality. They stated that "the proportion of outpatient to inpatient activities was about 4 to 6 times as many outpatients as inpatients," and they added that "this may exaggerate the incidence rates."

"*May* exaggerate the incidence rates"? Are they kidding? There's no "may" about it. The inappropriate, and one suspects, deliberate inclusion of the huge population of children diagnosed with autism in outpatient settings, but only during the post-thimerosal era, invalidates the author's conclusion that there was a rise in autism incidence after thimerosal was removed from the vaccines. Acknowledging one's errors does not negate them.

The First "Nail in the Coffin"

However, *a more serious and damaging aspect of this study* may be what it did not include. A Danish co-author of this study alerted the CDC (in a 2002 e-mail) to missing Danish autism data from 2001 that should have been included in the study.[9]

This data showed a clear *decline* in the incidence and prevalence of autism in 2001 supporting the notion *that the removal of thimerosal from vaccines in Denmark was associated with a decline in autism* and not a rise as the study's authors erroneously suggested.

This information was provided to the editors of the journal *Pediatrics* well *prior to its publication* but was *deliberately not included in the article* itself in 2003. Jose Cordero of the CDC had in fact encouraged *Pediatrics* to overlook the study's deficiencies, and to *expedite* review and publication of this tainted work in a 2002 letter to that journal.[10]

The Coalition for Mercury-Free Drugs (CoMeD) obtained this information through the Freedom of Information Act. CoMeD head Brian Hooker (a Ph.D. biochemist) has demanded that the CDC launch an investigation to determine whether there was *deliberate fraud* in regard to this study. He also wants the journal *Pediatrics* to retract the article.[11]

Conflicts of interest: This study was financed in part by the Stanley Medical Research Institute, an independent charitable organization known to support medicating mentally ill patients against their will.

Two of the seven researchers in this study were employees of Statens Serum Institute, Denmark's largest vaccine manufacturer, and the study was initiated by the U.S. CDC, whose pernicious influence on the Verstraeten study makes the flawed data collection and analysis used in this study more than highly suspicious.

Poul Thorsen, M.D., Ph.D., one of the researchers in this and another CDC-influenced study that purported to exonerate the MMR vaccine as a factor in promoting autism, has been found guilty of illegal activities, including fraud and grand theft (embezzlement). While he was a full-time employee of Aarhus University in Denmark, he is believed by officials at that institution to have forged documents, allegedly from the CDC, in order to obtain the release of two million dollars from the university.

He was also working full-time at Emory University in the U.S. at the same time he was drawing a salary as a full-time employee at Aarhus University. "Double-dipping" was forbidden under his contract with Aarhus. The other

9   See Chapter 14 for a discussion of this more recent research investigation. Grønborg, T.K., Schendel, D.E., Parner, E.T. "Recurrence of Autism Spectrum Disorders in Full- and Half-Siblings and Trends over Time: A Population-Based Cohort Study." *JAMA Pediatr.* Aug 19, 2013.

10   http://www.ageofautism.com/2013/09/danish-mercury-studyfabricatednewstudydifferentresults.htm?utm_source=feedburn er&utm _ medium=email&utm_campaign=Feed percent3A+ageofautism+ percent28AGE+OF+AUTISM percent29& utm_content=Yahoo percent21+Mail

11   http://www.anh-usa.org/cdc-mercury-in-vaccines/

researchers in this study allege that Thorsen's contribution as a reviewer was minimal and that he did not influence any of the data or its analysis and interpretation. A dubious distinction, as it turns out!

The Final "Nail in the Coffin"

And the final "nail in the coffin," as we have previously asserted, comes from a recent study that demonstrated that the Madsen/Thorsen study is a *complete fraud*. In this 2013 study, which we previously discussed, researcher Grønborg analyzed the same data as did Madsen et al. in their study, but came up with diametrically opposite findings.[12]

Grønborg found that autism rates had dramatically *declined* after thimerosal was removed from the vaccines and most definitely had *not increased as Madsen had alleged*. This, of course, supports the hypothesis that mercury causes autism, and puts the lie to the findings of the Madsen study.

Grønborg's team also discovered many more cases of autism (12,698) than did Madsen and colleagues (just 956) in the years 1971-2000. How could Madsen's team have missed all those autism cases? Their data needed rechecking, so Dr. Brian Hooker submitted several Freedom of Information requests to the CDC to obtain both the Madsen datasets and the relevant CDC correspondence. Some of these requests were made over eight years ago, but *the CDC has yet to respond*. What is the CDC hiding, and why?

As John Gilmore points out, "Without this information it is impossible to verify the 2003 study. Replicating the study is also impossible, and a scientific study that cannot be replicated has no scientific value."[13]

Marcellus: "Something is rotten in the state of Denmark."

— *William Shakespeare*

Conclusion: This bogus study and its erroneous conclusions are another shameful example of junk science masquerading as fact, and should certainly be retracted.

That this deceptive work of fiction and the aforementioned corrupt Verstraeten study represent two of the "major" pieces of evidence used by opponents of the thimerosal (mercury)-autism link to prove their case is both distressing, and at the same time, somehow, not surprising.

It is also important to note that these two fraudulent studies were the ones presented by the CDC to the once revered IOM (Institute of Medicine) just prior to the release of their 2004 report, which found that there was not only no association between thimerosal containing vaccines and autism, but also that such a relationship was suddenly now not biologically plausible and so no further research in this regard would be necessary!

A Third "Negative" Study: Fombonne, Eric et al. "Pervasive Developmental Disorders in Montreal, Quebec, Canada: Prevalence and Links with Immunizations." *Pediatrics*. Vol. 118. No. 1 (July 2006) p. e139-e150.

The purpose of this work was to estimate the pervasive developmental disorder (PDD)[14] prevalence in Montreal, Canada, in a survey of 27,000 plus children born from 1987 to 1998 and to see whether the incidence of PDD was influenced by their having received thimerosal-containing vaccinations or the MMR immunization(s).

The researchers calculated the children's cumulative exposure to ethyl mercury by age two at different time periods and found that, "A statistically significant linear increase in pervasive developmental disorder prevalence was noted during the study period. The prevalence of pervasive developmental disorder in thimerosal-free birth cohorts was significantly higher than that in thimerosal-exposed."

---

12   See Chapter 14 for further discussion of this study.
13   http://www.ageofautism.com/2013/09/danish-mercury-study-fabricatednew studydifferentresults.htm?utm_source=feedburner&utm_
medium=email&utm_campaign=Feed percent3A+ageofautism+ percent28AGE+OF+AU TISM percent29& utm_content=Yahoo percent21+Mail
14   Includes autism, Asperger's Syndrome, and PDD-NOS.

They thus concluded that they had "clearly failed to detect an association between either thimerosal exposure or MMR vaccine uptake and pervasive developmental disorders (PDD) rates in Montreal."[15]

Critique: The researchers measured the PDD incidence in only one of the five schoolboard districts in Montreal. They admitted that the data from the other schoolboards, which represented 86 percent of the total school population, should have been evaluated, but alleged that "this information was not available in the survey data that we could obtain." However, a critic of this study, Dr. David Ayoub, M.D., pointed out that such data was "easily obtained" from the Ministry of Education of Quebec, and he obtained it.[16]

Dr. Ayoub analyzed the data from the other school boards that Fombonne and associates had failed to obtain or analyze and found that the PDD rates at the school district analyzed by Fombonne were "significantly higher than (those of) the other four school boards, separately or combined. In some matched birth cohorts, the prevalence of PDD was as much as three times higher.... Therefore, Fombonne's objective to calculate the PDD prevalence in Montreal could not possibly have been accurately estimated by assessment of this particular school board and any conclusions about a relationship between vaccines and PDD rates in Montreal could be seriously flawed."[17]

The school district studied by Fombonne et al. is known as "A Center of Excellence in Autism." It integrates PDD students into its classes at a higher rate than do the other schoolboards, which entices parents of PDD-diagnosed children to want to enroll them in this school district, which in turn results in an overestimate of the true PDD incidence in Montreal. This fact was not taken into account in this study—a major flaw.

Montreal is a conglomerate of native French speakers (43 percent), immigrants whose native language is neither French nor English (37 percent), and English speakers (22 percent).

The school district that Fombonne et al. studied is an English-only district. French speakers and immigrants are forced by Quebec's language law (Bill 101) to attend French-speaking schools. Hence, the ethnic diversity of Montreal is not accurately represented in this study's school population.

This is relevant because foreign born children and children of immigrant parents are reported to have greater thimerosal exposures, which would then, if there is a thimerosal-PDD link, be expected to result in this population having a greater incidence of PDDs. And that is indeed what Dr. Ayoub found.

He analyzed the PDD incidence in the subgroup of the same school population that the Fombonne study encompassed for the years 2003-2004 and "discovered a rate of 106.6 per 10,000 in foreign-born children vs. 67.6 among natives. PDD rates were also significantly higher among (the) children (in that school district) with one or more immigrant parents."

One of the very important assumptions made by Fombonne and his associates was that after 1996 the exposure of Montreal children to thimerosal-containing vaccines was "nil." However, that assumption is absolutely incorrect.

Thirty-three licensed vaccines were still in use in Canada after 1996 (according to Canadian government healthcare documents), and some of these contained thimerosal. Examples include the hepatitis B vaccine, the "Penta" vaccine series, some of the meningococcal vaccines, and all of the influenza vaccines. These are all immunizations which may be given to infants.

The first thimerosal-free hepatitis B vaccine wasn't even licensed in Canada until March 2001. The Penta Vaccine, given at 2, 4, 6, and 18 months of age, still contained 25 mcg of mercury per dose (as thimerosal) in 1997. A Canadian baby in 1997 receiving the full complement of hepatitis B and Penta vaccines would have had a cumulative mercury exposure of *137.5 mcg by 18 months* of age. If that child had also received the influenza and meningococcal vaccines, the cumulative dose would have been even higher.

---

15   Fombonne; Ibid.
16   www.fourteenstudies.org
17   Ibid.

Fombonne's team failed to take into account that certain groups, like the children of immigrants and foreign-adopted children, had higher immunization rates than did native Canadian children. This is because foreign-born children and native-born children under seven years of age with one parent who emigrated from an area where hepatitis B was prevalent had to have the complete hepatitis B series, and immigrant children with no or inadequate vaccine records had to complete the entire Canadian immunization schedule.[18]

A "cumulative exposure" to a vaccine is supposed to be calculated by multiplying three independent variables: *the dose per vaccination, the shot frequency (number) and the coverage rates* (what percentage of the population received the vaccine). Dr. Fombonne and his research colleagues used one standard for defining cumulative exposure to thimerosal and another for evaluating the effects of the MMR vaccination. That's a "no-no."

For ethyl mercury exposure, Dr. Fombonne and his associates considered only the concentration of thimerosal in each vaccine and the vaccine frequency, but *did not consider* the coverage rates.

The standard they used for MMR exposure ignored the dosage and frequency and included only the coverage rates. By so doing, they conveniently disregarded the fact that autism rates increased after the number of MMR shots was increased from one to two after 1996, although the coverage rates, as Fombonne et al. claim, *allegedly* went down minimally at that time. But the researchers are also incorrect in that allegation as well.

Contrary to Fombonne's assertion, the doubling of the MMR vaccine shots actually did result in an *increase* in the cumulative exposure (which Fombonne failed to calculate accurately) to the measles virus from the MMR vaccine, despite the alleged marginal decrease in the coverage rate.

This failure to calculate the cumulative exposure correctly for both the thimerosal and the MMR analysis, and the use of different and incorrect criteria for defining the cumulative exposure to each is scientifically unsound and deceptive, and it totally invalidates the results and their interpretation.

According to Dr. Ayoub, Fombonne's group "ignored the potential impact of mass measles immunization campaigns in Quebec and Montreal that delivered a second dose of measles to a large number of infants and children throughout 1996. The subsequent rise in [pervasive developmental disorder] shortly after that campaign is clearly depicted in their figures and would lead us to believe this observation supports an association between PDD and MMR exposure."[19]

SCIENTIFIC FRAUD?

"[W]e ought to consider whether Fombonne and his coauthors—in complicity with the editors of the journal "Pediatrics" and the directors of the corporation known as the "American Academy of Pediatrics"—have committed an act of scientific fraud for the purpose of altering public perceptions regarding vaccinations."

— *Teresa Binstock, Researcher in Developmental & Behavioral Neuroanatomy*

Competing for Fombonne's most egregious offense is his inappropriately associating the MMR vaccination rates in Quebec, 265 kilometers away from Montreal, with the alleged PDD incidence in Montreal, when the vaccine rates differed in the two cities.

Dr. Edward Yazbak, M.D. reviewed several published vaccine uptake surveys of Montreal MMR vaccine rates and found that in children 24-30 months of age, those rates increased from 85.1 percent in 1983[20] to 88.8 percent in 1996-97[21] and then jumped to 96 percent in 2003-04,[22] which suggests, as Dr. Yazbak confirmed, "that in Montreal

---

18   Ibid.
19   Ayoub Ibid.
20   Baumgarten
21   Valiquette
22   Health Dept. Survey

pervasive developmental disorder prevalence and MMR vaccination rates were in fact increasing in tandem during the study period."

This, of course, is just the opposite of what Dr. Fombonne concluded: "Pervasive developmental disorder rates significantly increased when measles-mumps-rubella vaccination uptake rates significantly decreased."

How can we explain this discrepancy?

Fombonne analyzed the wrong data. As Dr. Yazbak put it in his letter to the journal *Pediatrics* (which the journal declined to publish): "The readers deserve to know why the authors compared developmental data from a specific group of children in Montreal with MMR vaccination data from the city of Quebec, some distance away."

Good question!

Conclusion: Another truly terrible study—an embarrassment. All its conclusions are invalid. As with the previous two studies, this one should never have been published, and having been, should be withdrawn and an apology and retraction issued.

Fombonne et al. did not sample a representative population of children from Montreal, although they could have.

The authors of this study failed to recognize the different subgroups in that population that had differing immunization rates and different incidences of PDD/autism. They, therefore, were unable to calculate accurately the incidence of PDD in the unrepresentative population that they did study.

Their basic assumption about when thimerosal was no longer present in vaccines was incorrect. Their conclusions in this regard are, therefore, invalid.

The researchers used different and incorrect standards in defining the cumulative dosage for the vaccines that contained thimerosal vs. the vaccine for measles, mumps, and rubella (MMR), and their definitions and calculations of cumulative dosage were, therefore, incorrect.

They failed to account for the impact of giving twice as many MMR immunizations on the incidence of PDD in their study population, which, contrary to their assertions, actually demonstrated a likely association between the MMR vaccine and pervasive developmental disorders.

And they analyzed the data from the wrong city (Quebec) in their erroneous determination that MMR vaccination uptake rates had decreased (which they may have in Quebec), but not in Montreal where they actually increased.

Fombonne has appeared on a number of occasions as a paid "expert witness" for the manufacturers of vaccines, although he goes out of his way to assert that he had not been employed by them in any other capacity. Given the quality of his research, that would be understandable.

Collusion?

> *"The Fombonne et al. article appears to be part of a larger collusion wherein some officials seek to enforce the idea that injecting thimerosal does no harm, despite a growing body of evidence that thimerosal injections are injurious."*
>
> — Teresa Binstock, Researcher in Developmental & Behavioral Neuroanatomy

> *"Think of the press as a great keyboard on which the government can play."*
>
> — Joseph Goebbels

A Fourth Negative Study: Schechter, Robert et al. "Continuing Increases in Autism Reported to California's Developmental Services System." Arch Gen Psychiatry. January 2008; p. 19-24.

Many studies regarding autism incidence have used data from the California Department of Developmental Services (DDS), which has been keeping records of children and adults with developmental disabilities, including autism, for decades.

Robert Schechter of the California Department of Public Health and his colleague, J. Grether, analyzed DDS data to determine the time trends in the incidence of autism in children (who were active status DDS clients) from ages 3 to 12 years between January 1, 1995 and March 31, 2007.

What they found was that the incidence (how many subjects in a given time period) of autism *increased for each year of age* throughout the study period, and also that the "estimated prevalence (percentage of subjects) of DDS clients aged 3 to 5 years with autism increased for each quarter from January 1995 through March 2007. Since 2004, the absolute increase and the rate of increase in DDS clients aged 3 to 5 years with autism were higher than those in DDS clients of the same ages with any eligible condition including autism."

The authors declare that, "The exclusion of thimerosal from childhood vaccines in the United States was accelerated from 1999 to 2001," and they conclude by stating, "The DDS data do not show any recent decrease in autism in California despite the exclusion of more than trace levels of thimerosal from nearly all childhood vaccines. The DDS data do not support the hypothesis that exposure to thimerosal during childhood is a primary cause of autism."[23]

Critique: The authors' assumptions about when thimerosal was removed from vaccines are incorrect, as we have documented; therefore, their entire study is based on a flawed premise.

Even in 2014, it is recommended that pregnant women get an influenza immunization and that babies receive an influenza vaccination at age 6 months and 18 months of age and yearly thereafter, and at the time of this writing (2015), most of these immunizations still contain 25 mcg of thimerosal (in the multi-dose vials), not a trace amount at all.

An optimally immunized baby is currently injected with 75 mcg of thimerosal by 18 months of age, and that figure does not include the thimerosal mercury in the other vaccines (3 Hepatitis B, 4 DPT/HIB, and others), which are labeled as "trace."

It may be recalled that the term "trace amount" has not been well-defined and that the amount of thimerosal currently present in "trace amounts" in the hepatitis B vaccine is 600 ppb (parts per billion). That figure is three times the amount that the EPA labels as hazardous waste. Twenty ppb will damage neurons.

Thus, babies at 18 months will generally even today have been exposed to more than 75 mcg of thimerosal—a significant amount, and this starts while they are still in utero. To put that amount into perspective, the CDC has a limit of 0.1 mcg mercury exposure per kilogram of body weight. Thimerosal is about 50 percent ethyl mercury. *A baby would have to weigh 125 kg (275 lb) in order for that amount not to be an overdose.*

And thimerosal was still listed as an ingredient in high amounts in many other vaccines given to babies in the 2003 *Physician's Desk Reference*. Professor Boyd Haley confirms that thimerosal-containing vaccines other than influenza were reported to be administered to babies as late as 2004, and many vaccines had an expiration date of 2005, but none were recalled.

The 2004 California law that would ban the use of mercury-containing vaccines for pregnant women and children under the age of three did not go into effect until December of 2006.

Possible Conflict of Interest: The California Department of Health supported this study, and the lead author, Robert Schechter, works for that institution. His job is to help ensure that children in California are adequately vaccinated.

---

23   Ibid.

The authors admit that they did not have mercury exposure data for the individuals in the study or for the population as a whole for that matter. This is a *major problem* since they had to estimate exposures to mercury in the population as a whole for the various ages and dates evaluated in the study. They state that, "Based on these estimates, children aged 3 to 5 years…reported to the DDS since the first quarter of 2004 are assumed to have reduced exposure compared with children aged 3 to 5 years reported from 1995 through 2003." It isn't entirely clear that that statement is true, as it is based on the flawed assumption that thimerosal was "essentially absent" from infant vaccines after 2002.

Data from the youngest children is unreliable. The CDC waits until a child is 8 years of age before it conducts its autism surveillance studies. The average age of diagnosis of autism varies from one region to another, and in general, the earlier the study, the later the average age of first diagnosis of autism occurs.

This observation was confirmed in a study published in the *Archives of Pediatric and Adolescent Medicine* in 2008 that states, "Shifts in age at diagnosis inflated the observed prevalence of autism in young children in the most recent cohorts (sample group) compared with the oldest cohort," which would in part account for "the apparent increase in autism in recent years."[24]

California data *are not reliable* for the purpose of conducting incidence studies. The reason for this, according to the Institute for Medicine, is that this data does not account for "changes over time in the population size or composition, in diagnostic concepts, in case definitions, or in age of diagnosis."[25]

The California Department of Developmental Services (DDS) agrees and states that analyzing its quarterly reports *may lead to misrepresentations of the incidence of autism* because, "Increases in the number of persons reported from one quarter to the next do not necessarily represent persons who are new to the DDS system."[26]

Safe Minds summarizes these concerns:

The conclusions of this study rely solely on one year of data in one state among the youngest children who presumably received markedly less thimerosal in their vaccines.

Basing such a conclusion on the youngest cohort data is unreliable, partly because the falling age of diagnosis creates an artificial increase (in the apparent incidence of autism).

The IOM said the California data is not reliable for incidence studies, the California Department of Developmental Services cautioned against drawing conclusions from the database, and the authors themselves warned that their findings must be confirmed from later data, something that has not happened—and cannot happen (because entry criteria for DDS services were changed the next year (2008).[27]

The authors of this study could have and should have plotted not only the incidence of autism by age over a period of time but also *changes in the rate of increase*, but they did not. If they had, they would have uncovered evidence that contradicts their conclusions.

Consider the following statistics obtained by Rick Rollens, co-founder of the California M.I.N.D. Institute at UC Davis. He analyzed *the same California DDS database* that Schechter did and made the following observations:

In 1999, DDS released its now famous and historic autism caseload report that documented a 273 percent increase in the number of new cases of autism entering California's developmental (disability) services system from 1987 through 1998.

---

24   Parner, E.T., Schendel, D.E., Thorsen, P. "Autism prevalence trends over time in Denmark: changes in prevalence and age at diagnosis." *Archives of Pediatric and Adolescent Medicine.* 2008 Dec; 162(12):1150-6. Online at: http://www.ncbi.nlm.nih.gov/pubmed/19047542.
25   http://www.ageofautism.com/2011/05/vaccines-and-autism-what-do-epidemiological-studies-really-tell-us.html
26   http://www.dds.ca.gov/Autism/Home.cfm
27   http://www.ageofautism.com/2011/05/vaccines-and-autism-what-do-epidemiological-studies-really-tell-us.html

In 2003, DDS followed up with an updated report that documented a 97 percent increase in the autism caseload over the 48 month period from December 1998 through December 2002.

According to DDS, during the…45 month reporting period from January 2003 through September 2006, there has been a 50 percent increase in the autism caseload. The rate of increase declined by nearly half over the previous reporting period.

Mr. Rollens goes on to add, "During the four year reporting period between October 2002 and October 2006 there has been a large increase in the 10-21 year old population in the system, while the younger, 3-9 year old cohort reflects the substantial, declining rate of increase as noted above. The largest increase has been in the 14-17 year olds (127 percent), while the smallest increase has been in the 22 year olds and older (35 percent)." *These data parallel each cohort's thimerosal exposure from vaccines.* "Reasons for this phenomenon," he explains, "could include the lessening burden of mercury in vaccines slowing the numbers of new young children entering the system, a tightening of eligibility criteria that took effect in July 2003…and Regional Centers responding to the pressure to qualify more older persons with higher functioning autism spectrum conditions."

He concludes: "One thing is for sure, the hidden hordes of adults with autism that needs to be accounted for in order to discredit the existence of an autism epidemic and an increasing incidence of autism, have yet to come forward or be discovered."

Consider also Table 16.1. The data was compiled from the same California DDS statistics that were evaluated in this study and clearly shows a decline in the rate of increase of newly diagnosed autism cases in those populations (the over 22 [35 percent] and the under 5 years [57 percent]) that were exposed during their first 18 months to lower amount of thimerosal from vaccines.

Hence, these data are consistent with the hypothesis that thimerosal and mercury exposure in infancy (and in utero) may be causally related to the epidemic of autism.

> *"Falsehood flies and truth comes limping after, so that when men come to be undeceived it is too late, the jest is over and the tale has had its effect."*
>
> — Jonathan Swift

Joseph, the father of an autistic boy, posted a graph (see Figure 16.1) and information on the "Autism Natural Variation" blog site.[28]

He was interested to see what was happening to the California DDS 18-21 year-old cohort from 1995 through 2007, so he put the data into a graph format.

Note the increasing slope of the graph after 2001 (which represents the group exposed to more thimerosal).

It is noteworthy that this data also again demonstrates that the increase in autism over the years is a real phenomenon and is not just due to increased diagnosis. In the most recent years, the annual caseload growth in the 18-21 year-old cohort (born 1989 or earlier) was roughly 20 percent, or about 20 times the annual population growth in the state. Compare this to the 10 percent annual growth rate for the 3-5 year-olds (born 2004 or earlier) during the same period.

We can thus conclude that the rate of increase in newly diagnosed cases of autism has declined, and *has declined to a greater degree in those with the lowest exposures to thimerosal.*

These findings are significant and are consistent with the observation that *thimerosal and mercury may be causally linked to the incidence of autism.*

---

28   http://autismnaturalvariation.blogspot.com/2007/09/epidem-of-autism-among-18-21-year.html

Table 16.1. Percent Increase in Autism Incidence

# of New Cases		Percent Increase		2006 Cohort		Estimated Max. Thimerosal
Age	2002	2006	from 2002	Year Born	exposure by 18 mo in µgms	
3-5	3932	6188	57%	2001-2003		75 to ?
6-9	5697	----	----	1997-2000		275 or less
10-13	3531	6157	74%	1993-1996		125-237.5*
14-17	1732	3934	127%	1989-1992		125-237.5
18-21	1047	2021	93%	1985-1988		125
22+	3696	4994	35%	1984 and earlier		100 or less

*Some children in the mid-1990s received a combined DPT and Haemophilus influenza vaccination (DPTH), which would have lowered their total thimerosal exposure by 100 µgms. Lowest percent increase in autism incidence is in those children exposed to the lowest amount of thimerosal. Data compiled by Rick Rollens; U.C. Davis M.I.N.D. Institute from California DDS

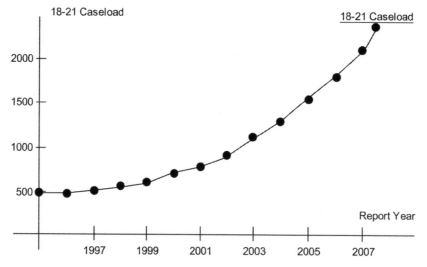

Figure 16.1. Caseload Increase from 1995 to 2007 (This caseload has increased by a factor of 4.4—or 440%).

Therefore, Schechter and Grether are incorrect in their conclusions (which they themselves suggest need to be confirmed). Unfortunately, that confirmation is now not possible since the entry criteria for DDS services was broadly expanded in 2008.[29]

29   In California, entry criteria for DDS services were broadly expanded to include children with PDD-NOS and Asperger's Disorder in January 2008. "Information from these new items will not be comparable to prior information," a DDS statement says. http://www.ageofautism.com/2011/05/vaccines-and-

The apparent rise in autism prevalence the suspect California DDS data suggest, even if valid, does not by any means rule out thimerosal or mercury as causative factors in the autism epidemic, especially *since babies and children are still getting significant amounts of thimerosal in their vaccinations* (53 percent of the average 1999 dosage). [See below]

In fact, the data support that contention and are consistent with the Geier study, which analyzed the VAERS database before and after 2002 and which showed a decrease in the rate of rise of autism in the years after thimerosal exposure from vaccines was in decline.[30]

The apparent increasing incidence of autism and related disorders noted in the California DDS database could also simply indicate that other environmental influences in addition to thimerosal-mercury must also be considered, like, for example, *the increasing presence of neurotoxic aluminum in two newly introduced vaccines* (Pneumococcus and Hepatitis A) and the increasing number of vaccines administered each decade.

Some of these likely additional ASD promoting factors will be discussed in upcoming chapters.

> *"Do not put your faith in what statistics say until you have carefully considered what they do not say."*
>
> — *William W. Watt*

A Fifth Negative Study: "Neuropsychological Performance 10 Years after Immunization in Infancy with Thimerosal-Containing Vaccines." Tozzi, A.E. et al. *Pediatrics*. 2009 Feb; 123(2):475-82.

This *CDC-supported and influenced* Italian study attempted to discern whether two specific groups of 11-year-old children who were enrolled in an efficacy trial (during their infancy) of two different DTaP vaccines, and who would have received either 62.5 or 137.7 mcg of ethyl mercury by the end of their first year of life, faired any differently ten years after those immunizations were given. This study was not designed to determine whether autism rates would differ between the two groups.

Less than 70 percent of the invited subjects agreed to participate in this assessment, leaving a total of only 1,704 children in the study. The children were divided into either the high or low mercury-exposure group and were given a battery of standardized psychological tests to determine their abilities in memorization, learning, executive function, motor skills, visual and spatial functions, and language.

The researchers found that girls who had been exposed to the higher thimerosal dose had *significantly* lower scores on the *finger tapping* and *Boston Naming Test*, but otherwise, the differences in scores between the higher and lower thimerosal dosed groups were not statistically significant.

Only 1 percent of the children in this study had received the then thimerosal and aluminum-containing hepatitis B vaccination at birth. This is in contrast to the U.S. where a majority of babies receive their first hepatitis B vaccination on their day of birth with the second dose being injected at one-month of age.

Only one case of autism was noted in the 1,704 children evaluated, and that child was in the group with the lower thimerosal dosage. At the time of this study, the incidence of autism in the U.S. was 1:150 children, over ten times greater than that found in this study.

The authors of this study concluded that, "Given the large number of statistical comparisons performed, the few (statistically significant) associations found between thimerosal exposure and neuropsychological development might be attributable to chance."

---

autism-what-do-epidemio-logical-studies-really-tell-us.html.

30   Geier, D.A., Geier, M.R. "Early Downward Trends in Neurodevelopmental Disorders Following Removal of Thimerosal-Containing Vaccines." *Journal of American Physicians and Surgeons*. Vol. 11. No. 1. Spring 2006.

Critique: This study is so fraught with limitations that it renders the study virtually meaningless, and the fact that these limitations were recognized and acknowledged by the authors does not make them any the less critical. Consider: "The cumulative intake of thimerosal was relatively low, compared with that in other countries including the United States, where vaccination schedules included more thimerosal-containing vaccines in the first year of life."

That means the researchers were comparing children with comparatively moderate thimerosal exposure to another group of children who had been exposed to a relatively lower dose of thimerosal.

There were an insufficient number of children enrolled in the study. It is legitimate to study children receiving varying dosages of thimerosal, but to be able to appreciate differences in the two dosage groups such as those in this study would take a far greater number of children than were evaluated by Tozzi et al.

Any epidemiologist will confirm that, given an incidence of autism of just 1 in 1,704 children and a study that is limited to only those 1,704 children, who are then divided into higher and lower thimerosal-exposed cohorts, it is a certainty that the study will not result in any statistically significant conclusions regarding the autism prevalence difference (if any) between those groups.

This does not mean that such a difference does not exist. It does mean that this study was so poorly constructed that it was not able to determine that significance. In order to discern statistically significant differences between two such groups of children who had both received thimerosal-containing inoculations during their first year of life, it would have been necessary to study many thousands of children. This means that any conclusions drawn from such a study are invalid.

"There was no comparison group with no exposure to thimerosal." All the children in both groups received all the immunizations normally given, and all the children received at least 62.5 mcg of thimerosal. Babies in the U.S. before 1980 were receiving thimerosal only in the DPT vaccine, and at the time, they were getting just 75 mcg of thimerosal total in their first year of life. The incidence of autism at that time was c. 1-5 cases per 10,000 births.

So the researchers were actually comparing children who received a higher dose of thimerosal (137.5 mcg) to those who received half that amount, and all these children got thimerosal in amounts *significantly lower and significantly later* in the first year of life than did children in the U.S. at that time.

Keep in mind the previously discussed hepatitis B study that showed that babies given the thimerosal-preserved hepatitis B vaccination at birth had a much (3 times) higher risk of getting autism than did those who never had the vaccine or had their initial dose *later* in the first year of life. *The age at which a child is initially poisoned by thimerosal (and aluminum) is a very relevant factor in determining the neurodevelopmental consequences of that exposure.*

This age-associated risk was also clearly demonstrated by Verstraeten before the CDC made him alter his data.

What the researchers could have and should have done is to evaluate the children who had received the full thimerosal-containing vaccine series and compare them to children who had not had any thimerosal in their immunizations and also to children who had never been vaccinated at all. The results then would likely have been significant. But the CDC is apparently afraid to do this kind of study.

The "analysis included only healthy children who were selected during enrollment in the original trial," say Tozzi et al.

"This preselection," they continue, "might have eliminated children who were more likely to become autistic," like low birth weight infants who were largely excluded from this study, and they add, "our study was not powered to detect an association of thimerosal exposure and neuropsychological development in low birth weight infants."

There's no "might" about it! The incidence of autism is very high in low birth weight infants, and 8 percent of autistics are born prematurely.

In a recent study in the journal *Pediatrics*, researchers tracked a group of premature babies born in the early to mid-1980s for 21 years. They found that 5 percent of newborns (one in twenty!) weighing less than 4 pounds, 7 ounces were later diagnosed with an autism spectrum disorder, as were nearly 11 percent (one in ten) of a subgroup born below 3 pounds, 5 ounces.[31]

These findings are consistent with the hypothesis that the earlier the exposure to immunizations and thimerosal and the lower the weight of the baby so inoculated, the greater the incidence of autism. At the time these children were born, they would have been given thimerosal-containing DPT vaccine at least three times during their first year of life. *Omitting this group of vulnerable children from the Tozzi study would tend to skew the results of the study in favor of a finding of no relationship between thimerosal-containing vaccinations and autism.*

"Some families might have declined to participate in the present study," said Tozzi (et al.), "because their children had cognitive developmental problems. This might have reduced the prevalence of adverse neuropsychological conditions and might have made potential differences hard to detect." Indeed!

Dr. Lewis, Editor-in-Chief of *Pediatrics*, the journal in which this study was published, wrote on his blog, "You'll be reassured that the results (of the Tozzi study) show essentially no differences between groups who did or did not get thimerosal in their vaccines—and you'll want to know this information when talking with parents of your patients about the safety and benefits of vaccines."

What is Dr. Lewis talking about? Evidently, he didn't read or understand the study, as Tozzi et al. did not compare groups who "did or did not get thimerosal." They studied two groups of children, both of whom received thimerosal!

Correspondent John Stone certainly disagreed with Dr. Lewis's conclusions, inquiring in his letter to *Pediatrics*, "How it would be possible to draw any useful scientific conclusions from a study with such deficiencies in relation to the issues it purportedly set out to investigate?"

Dr. Vincenzo Miranda, M.D. of Italy concurred: "[T]his study cannot lead to any conclusion," he stated categorically.

However, the Associated Press, after reviewing this article and discussing the results with the lead author and others, declared, "A new study from Italy adds to a mountain of evidence that a mercury-based preservative once used in many vaccines doesn't hurt children, offering more reassurance to parents."[32]

"Mountain of evidence"? Thus far, as we have shown, there is actually no evidence at all supporting that contention, not even a "molehill." The conclusions arrived at by Tozzi and colleagues are invalid because of the inadequate number of children analyzed, the high dropout rate, the exclusion of high risk babies, and because parents of cognitively impaired children may have declined to participate in the study.

This is a CDC-sponsored and influenced study. Why is that a concern? Let's review. The CDC is the same government organization that:

- Sequestered data that showed that the incidence of autism in Brick Township, N.J. skyrocketed after the thimerosal-containing HIB and hepatitis B vaccines were introduced
- Engaged in statistical chicanery in the 1990s to show that autism incidence wasn't increasing when it was
- Refuses to do a study comparing vaccinated and unvaccinated children
- Initiated and hosted the clandestine and illegal Simpsonwood meeting
- Refused to publish the initial, unmanipulated Verstraeten data that clearly showed that thimerosal, autism, and neurodevelopmental disorders were most assuredly linked.

31   Pinto-Martin, J.A. et al. "Prevalence of Autism Spectrum Disorder in Adolescents Born Weighing <2000 Grams." *Pediatrics*. 2011 Nov; 128(5):883-91. Epub 2011 Oct 17. PMID: 22007018.
32   Johnson, Carla. "Study adds to evidence of vaccine safety." Assoc. Press. http://www.google.com/hostednews/ap/article/ALeqM5jp7ZD1RFVm7yOzga-B04Ra4dY

- Encouraged Verstraeten to manipulate the data to decrease the relevant association between vaccines, thimerosal, and neurodevelopmental disorders, including autism and ADHD.

- Claimed the data was subsequently "lost," an unlikely event.

- Prevented others from examining their VSD database.

- "Encouraged" Verstraeten to republish a new and patently false study in the journal *Pediatrics*, which found no significant association between thimerosal and autism, when the original uncorrupted study came to the exact opposite conclusion.

- Demanded that the pharmaceutical industry-influenced Institute of Medicine review the flawed research on the thimerosal-immunization link and find thimerosal-containing vaccinations to be safe.

- Sponsored the bogus Danish study (Madsen, et al.), which was (like the Tozzi Italian study and the Fombonne study and many others) also published in *Pediatrics*, the journal of the American Academy of Pediatrics.

Should we now also be concerned that the journal *Pediatrics* appears to be bolstering its own not so well-hidden agenda by repeatedly publishing tainted, fraudulent, and biased articles that support the contention that thimerosal-containing vaccines are safe, and that has censored criticism of some of those studies?

Should we likewise be suspicious of the American Academy of Pediatrics, publisher of that very same journal? The academy knew of Dr. Verstraeten's original study (which had convincingly demonstrated the link between thimerosal-immunizations and developmental disorders like autism), but it now refuses to endorse "any bill that contains any questions about vaccine" because it alleges that "there is absolutely no link between thimerosal and autism."

Or should we perhaps ignore these facts and rejoice in the delusion that "a mercury-based preservative once used in many vaccines doesn't hurt children"?

> *"It isn't what we don't know that gives us trouble; it's what we know that ain't so."*
>
> *– Will Rogers*

A Sixth "Negative" Study (sometimes called "The Swedish Study"): "Autism and Thimerosal-Containing Vaccines: Lack of Consistent Evidence for an Association." Stehr-Green, Paul. et al. *American Journal of Preventive Medicine*, Vol. 25, Issue 2. p. 101-106. (August 2003)

The authors of yet another CDC designed and sponsored study claim to have compared the prevalence and incidence of autism in California, Sweden, and Denmark with "average exposures" to thimerosal-containing vaccines from the mid-1980s through the late-1990s.

They state that:

> [I]n all three countries, the incidence and prevalence of autism-like disorders began to rise in the 1985–1989 period, and the rate of increase accelerated in the early 1990s.

> However, in contrast to the situation in the United States, where the average thimerosal dose from vaccines increased throughout the 1990s, thimerosal exposures from vaccines in both Sweden and Denmark—already low throughout the 1970s and 1980s—began to decrease in the late 1980s and were eliminated in the early 1990s.

What the researchers alleged to find was that the autism rates in Denmark and in Sweden appeared to increase after thimerosal was eliminated from vaccines in those two countries.

They conclude by stating, "The body of existing data, including the ecologic data presented herein, is not consistent with the hypothesis that increased exposure to thimerosal-containing vaccines is responsible for the apparent increase in the rates of autism in young children being observed worldwide."

Critique: The autism incidence in Sweden at the time this study was done was 1 in 10,000 births or *60 times less* than it was in the U.S. during that same period! The authors neglect to mention this huge discrepancy in their paper. Could this amazingly low autism incidence be related to the significantly lower exposure to thimerosal in the Danish and Swedish populations?

The authors published charts[33] previously compiled by Mark Blaxill (father of an autistic child, founder of Age of Autism, and board member of Safe Minds) "that demonstrated an association between rising autism rates in California and thimerosal exposure in childhood vaccines."

However, as Blaxill asserts, "In their re-use of my charts, the authors err in describing the rates of autism reported therein as rates for the larger class of "autism-like disorders," because, in reality, the rates reported by Blaxill were confined to the category of just (DSM-IV) autism itself.

The consequence of this misclassification is that the authors *underestimated the true incidence of autism in California during the period in question and minimized* "the severity of the situation in California."[34]

The most egregious error made in this report was to replicate the unconscionable mistakes made in the previously discussed "Danish study."

Paul Stehr-Green and colleagues incorrectly assessed the incidence of autism in both Sweden and Denmark for two-thirds of the study period by tabulating the number of autism cases in just inpatient (hospital) settings prior to the removal of thimerosal from the vaccines in those countries. This was the same statistical "error" that the Madsen team made in its flawed Danish study.[35]

To quote from the study: "Prior to 1992, the data in the national register did not include cases diagnosed in one large clinic in Copenhagen (which accounts for approximately 20 percent of cases occurring nationwide). Prior to 1995, the autism cases reported to the national register reflected only cases diagnosed in inpatient settings."

Since (as has been previously discussed) autistic children are generally diagnosed (93 percent of the time in Denmark[36]) in outpatient settings, utilizing only inpatient data results in a serious undercount of the true autism incidence.

The outpatient data was then included only for the period of time following the elimination of thimerosal from vaccines. This, of course, resulted in a *factitious* apparent increase in the rate of autism in that time period.

As Mark Blaxill relates, "Based on these flawed trend assumptions, the authors use the shift in Sweden and Denmark from comparatively low thimerosal exposures to thimerosal-free vaccines in an attempt to falsify the autism-mercury hypothesis. Absent a clear increase in autism rates in Denmark and Sweden, this attempt at falsification fails."

There are also multiple "errors, inconsistencies and misrepresentations" in the rate and exposure assessments, according to Mr. Blaxill. These include:

- Mischaracterizing the autism cohorts in Sweden as birth year cohorts when they are actually *moving average* cohorts of 2-10 year olds.
- Measuring autism case *counts*, not *rates* in Denmark.
- Reporting vaccine compliance rates in Denmark (over 90 percent) that are inconsistent with the mercury exposures in their display.

---

33   See Chapter 12.
34   www.fourteenstudies.org
35   Madsen, K.M. et al. "A population-based study of measles, mumps, and rubella vaccination and autism." *N Engl J Med.* 2002; 347(19):1477-82.
36   Ibid.

- Representing the Danish pertussis (whooping cough) exposures as standard, when they are highly unusual (and, therefore, suspect).

- Acknowledging non-standard and changing diagnostic criteria[37] and incomplete institutional coverage in their Danish case count without attempting to correct these concerns.

- Reporting just the time at diagnosis, and not the year of birth, in their Danish population, which, Blaxill asserts, is a "common mistake."

- Representing, despite these serious flaws and omissions, that their choice of Swedish and Danish sources was based on "high quality records."[38]

There are also major potential conflicts of interest. The CDC not only helped fund this study, and aided in "the preparation and review of this manuscript," but it also helped the researchers "design and conduct their investigation." (Another uh oh!)

This so-called "research" was also supported by the Swedish Institute for Infectious Disease Control and the Danish Statens Serum Institut (Denmark's largest vaccine company).

The researchers could have and should have compared the autism incidence of thimerosal-exposed children to those who had been immunized to only thimerosal-free vaccines and also to those who had never been immunized at all, but they chose not to.

Conclusion: This is yet another flawed study based on false assumptions and questionable data whose conclusions are not supported by the facts (or lack thereof).

It nevertheless remains as one of the so-called "major" studies that are commonly quoted to discredit the autism-mercury link, although on close analysis, it clearly fails in that attempt.

This tainted and clearly biased paper should never have been published, and having been so, should be retracted.

"Torture numbers and they'll confess to anything."

— *Gregg Easterbrook*

A Seventh "Negative" Study (AKA the "British Study"): Heron, John and Jean Golding et al. "Thimerosal Exposure in Infants and Developmental Disorders: A Prospective Cohort Study in the United Kingdom Does Not Support a Causal Association." (September 2004). *Pediatrics*. Vol. 114. No. 3. September 2004. p. 577-583.

The authors of this flawed British study state that "there has been concern that…exposure to mercury may be of some detriment to young children. The aim of this research was to test in a large United Kingdom population-based cohort whether there is any evidence to justify such concerns."

To accomplish their task they assessed population data on over 14,000 children from a longitudinal study on childhood health and development. The children were all born between 1991 and 1992.

"The age at which doses of thimerosal-containing vaccines were administered was recorded, and measures of mercury exposure by 3, 4, and 6 months of age were calculated and compared with a number of measures of childhood cognitive and behavioral development covering the period from 6 to 91 months of age."

And what did these researchers discover? "Contrary to expectation, it was common for the unadjusted results to suggest a beneficial effect of thimerosal exposure." A beneficial effect? From toxic mercury? Yes, Heron and Andrews found that "exposure at 3-months was inversely associated with" a variety of undesirable outcomes later on, like hyperactivity, and conduct and speech problems.

---

37   The new DSM IV autism diagnostic criteria established in 1993 broadened the definition of autism and would have resulted in increased diagnoses of this condition after that point in time.

38   fourteenstudies.org

The researchers' conclude at the end of the *abstract* of this study that, "We could find no convincing evidence that early exposure to thimerosal had any deleterious effect on neurologic or psychological outcome."

But the conclusion to the abstract of this study is incorrect, dishonest, and deliberately misleading because it omits some very key words, which we find at the end of the study itself and which change the abstract conclusion and its import entirely. This is critical because many people only read the abstract and don't evaluate the actual study.

The summation of this study states, "We could find no convincing evidence that early exposure to thimerosal had any deleterious effect on neurologic or psychological outcome when given according to an accelerated schedule."

Oops!

Critique: This devious "study" is so awful that it is hard to know where to begin. But let's start with what the researchers actually did evaluate.

The database used derived from a then ongoing study (The Avon Longitudinal Study of Parents and Children) and from that data set they calculated the cumulative ethyl mercury exposure for each child, which at the time came *solely from either the thimerosal-containing DPT or the DT injections* the children had received up to the age of 6 months.

The British children in this study *did not receive* the (then thimerosal-containing) hepatitis B or HIB (Haemophilus influenza B-a bacterial pathogen) inoculations at that time, so the DT or DPT injection was their only source of injectable mercury ostensibly, and that meant that their cumulative exposure to ethyl mercury would have been 75 mcg for those children who had received all three injections.

Heron and Golding et al. then compared the outcomes of the children who had completed the initial series of three injections by 3, 4, or 6 months of age. If a child had received his or her third dose of the DPT/DT after 6 months of age, that injection was calculated as having been given at 6 months of age.

So what did this study actually accomplish? Did the researchers compare children who were injected with thimerosal to those who had never received thimerosal?

No, but they could and should have.

Did they compare children who had received higher doses of thimerosal to those who had received lower doses of thimerosal?

No, in fact all the children received exactly the same dose of thimerosal.

Did they compare children who were vaccinated with any immunizations at all to those who weren't?

No, but they could and should have.

So what did they compare?

They compared children who had received a 75 mcg cumulative dose of thimerosal with children who received exactly that same dose, and all the children received the same cumulative dose of thimerosal by 6 months of age, and all received the final (3rd) dose within a three-month period of time (between month 3 and month 6 of life). There was thus no real difference between the two groups.

And what did they hope to accomplish?

They allege that they wanted to see whether giving the third dose of thimerosal before a child reached 6 months of age would be a concern. They compared the developmental outcomes of babies who had received exactly the same cumulative dose of thimerosal (75mcg) by 3 months, 4 months, or 6 months of age. The only variable was when these infants received their third dose of thimerosal. This "overmatching" of the two groups is a statistical trick designed to hide relevance, and in that, it succeeded!

What did they find?

Those who received the final dose of DPT (Diphtheria, Pertussis, Tetanus) or DT (Diphtheria/Tetanus) by 3 months of age appeared to fare slightly better in some developmental outcomes than those who received the final dose at 6 months of age.

Did the researchers then actually discover a "beneficial effect" of thimerosal?

No. They simply found that the children who completed their immunization series early (by 3 months of age) appeared to have better developmental outcomes than did those who completed the same series of inoculations at 6 months of age. They could just as well have concluded that the toxic effects of thimerosal are augmented by a brief delay in the completion of the DPT/DT series of three immunizations.

Did this report at least rule out thimerosal as a possible cause of autism or developmental disorders?

No. The study wasn't designed to do that. All the children received exactly the same dose of thimerosal.

The aim of this study, according to the authors, was to see whether there was any justification for the concern that thimerosal exposure might be of some detriment to young children. Did this study clarify that concern?

No.

Then isn't the title of this study deliberately misleading and factually incorrect?

Yes.

And what about the conclusion of the abstract, isn't it also deliberately misleading and factually incorrect?

Yes.

Isn't the total dose of thimerosal (75mcg) that the study babies received by 6 months of age similar to the dose that American babies would have received in the 1950s to early 1980s, before the introduction of the HIB and hepatitis B vaccines (and many others) and prior to the spike in autism incidence?

Yes.

Wasn't the incidence of autism in America in the decades prior to the 1980s about 1-5 per 10,000 births?

Yes.

Wouldn't that imply that in this study, the expected autism and related developmental disorder incidence would have been about 2-7 children out of the c. 13,000 who were ultimately included in this study?

Yes.

Wouldn't that have been an inadequate number from which to draw any conclusions in this study even if the researchers had compared a thimerosal-exposed group of children with a thimerosal-free group (which they didn't)?

Yes.

Did this study identify any children who were autistic?

No.

Was this study a complete waste of time and money?

Pretty much.

Is this one of the so-called "major studies" that are commonly cited as showing no link between thimerosal and autism?

Yes.

Is that why it was published in *Pediatrics,* the journal of the American Academy of Pediatrics?

Probably.

Potential conflicts of interest: Funding for this study was provided by the British version of the American CDC, the Department of Health.

Conclusion: What more can one say? This is junk science at its best! Retract this shameful parody of good research and apologize to all the journal readers who may have been taken in by its deceptive title and inaccurate conclusions.

> *"Get your facts first, and then you can distort them as much as you please."*
>
> — *Mark Twain*

An Eighth "Negative" Study: Thompson, W.W. et al. Vaccine Safety Datalink Team. "Early Thimerosal Exposure and Neuropsychological Outcomes at 7 to 10 Years." *New England Journal of Medicine.* (September 27, 2007) 357(13):1281-92.

This CDC-sponsored and designed study (yes, be very concerned) sought to compare the developmental outcomes of a series of children (from 4 HMOs) between the ages of 7-10 years who had received varying dosages of thimerosal-containing vaccines in infancy and (or) whose mothers had received a thimerosal-containing immune globulin (Rhogam) during the pregnancy with the child under study.

"Of 3648 children selected for recruitment" by the researchers only "1107 (30.3 percent) were tested. Among children who were not tested, 512 did not meet one or more of the eligibility criteria, 1026 could not be located, and 44 had scheduling difficulties; in addition, the mothers of 959 children declined to participate."

Of the 1107 children tested, an additional 60 were excluded for a variety of reasons and thus only "1047 children were included in the final analyses." So *less than 30 percent of the children originally selected for recruitment wound up being evaluated in this study*. This is considered by most epidemiologists to be *an inadequate number from which to draw valid conclusions*.

Children *with a variety of medical concerns at birth* or who were not living with their biological mother were excluded from consideration for inclusion in this research. "Therefore, our findings may have been influenced by selection bias," the authors of this study concede. No kidding!

"Birth dates ranged from January 1, 1993, to March 30, 1997; testing was conducted between June 1, 2003, and April 27, 2004."

Exposure to mercury was calculated based on a variety of medical records and parental interviews, and the researchers then "assessed the association between current neuropsychological performance and exposure to mercury during the prenatal period, the neonatal period (birth to 28 days), and the first 7 months of life."

Importantly, *the researchers disregarded thimerosal exposure after 7 months* because they "hypothesized that the potential effect of such exposure would be small…since most vaccines that are administered after 214 days would typically be given at 12 to 18 months of age, (and therefore) the dose per kilogram would be substantially lower."

The researchers also emphasize that they "did not assess autism spectrum disorders"!

After analyzing their data, they found that "among the 42 neuropsychological outcomes, (they) detected only a few significant associations with exposure to mercury from thimerosal. The detected associations were small and almost equally divided between positive and negative effects."

Critique: There was *inadequate confirmation of the diagnosis' accuracy for the cases analyzed*. Overall, "19 percent of the diagnoses could not be confirmed," and "Of those with a confirmed diagnosis, 39 percent were considered to be transient problems [which is not a description that would normally be applied to autism] and the duration of the problem could not be determined for an additional 35 percent of cases. Thus, only 26 percent of the validation attempts established that problems were long-term in children with a confirmed diagnosis."[39]

There was an insufficient number of unexposed children in the study. According to Safe Minds, "The number of individuals reported to receive no thimerosal exposure during the first 4 months of life was very low, representing only 3.4 percent of infants delivered at term and 5.8 percent of pre-term infants."

"The small number of children with behavioral differences was spread in unspecified distributions across the ten years of information, and attempts at validation provided confirmation of long-term problems in only 20.5 percent of cases. (This) renders analysis of the data base of Andrews and colleagues fraught with uncertainty. In the specific context of autism, any decreased representation in the zero-exposure cohort (i.e., less than a total of 3 cases identified) seems unlikely to be suitable for accurate statistical comparisons."[40]

Furthermore, the analysis of the data in this study is also invalid due to the authors inappropriately utilizing a statistical "trick" called "overmatching." The term refers to the *unnecessary or improper use of matching* in a cohort or case control study.

That means, when comparing two groups in a study, *the two groups should be as alike as possible except for the variable being compared*, in this case, exposure to thimerosal. The same bit of "hanky-panky" was utilized by Heron et al. in the previously analyzed "British Study" in which both groups of children evaluated had been given exactly the same dose of thimerosal.

The greater the difference in exposure to thimerosal between the two groups, the more likely it would be to find a statistically relevant difference in effect, and conversely, the closer the two groups are in their exposure to the variable (thimerosal), the less likely it would be to find a significant difference between the two groups, and that is exactly what occurred with the Thompson, Price, et al. investigation.

The difference between the higher thimerosal exposure group and the lower exposure group in this devious paper was a measly 15 mcg of mercury because of overmatching, although the data allowed for comparing groups of children with much larger thimerosal exposure differences.

Epidemiologists Desoto and Hitlan analyzed this paper and found it to be "flawed" and analytically "unfixable," because "overmatching…is a design flaw."[41]

The article was also lambasted by Brian Hooker and colleagues in a paper published in 2014 in the journal *BioMed Research International*. The reviewers evaluated the 6 CDC sponsored and designed papers (including this one) that alleged to exonerate thimerosal as a contributing factor in causing autism and *found all of them wanting in scientific rigor*. In particular, they questioned the validity of the methodology used in the studies.[42]

Autism was not a diagnosis that was evaluated in this study. This would be a moot point except that this study has often been inappropriately cited by some misinformed or devious individuals as evidence for the safety of thimerosal in their attempt to refute the hypothesized thimerosal-autism link, which this study clearly does not do.

39   http://www.ageofautism.com/2011/05/vaccines-and-autism-what-do-epidemiological-studies-really-tell-us.html
40   Ibid.
41   DeSoto, M.C. and R.T. Hitlan. "Vaccine safety study as an interesting case of "over-matching." *Indecent Advances in Autism Spectrum Disorders*. Vol. I. Fitzgerald, M. Ed., *P.M.F.*, 2013.
42   Vol. 2014 (2014), Article ID 247218, 8 pages. "Methodological Issues and Evidence of Malfeasance in Research Purporting to Show Thimerosal in Vaccines Is Safe." http://www.hindawi.com/journals/bmri/2014/247218/

The researchers disregarded any thimerosal exposure from immunizations in the children who were evaluated in this study after they passed 7 months of age because they hypothesized that since the dose of thimerosal per unit of body weight of the child would decrease as the child got older and gained weight, the effects of that additional mercury would be negligible.

However, that hypothesis is seriously misguided because it ignores the very real evidence that some children do not detoxify mercury well or quickly, and so an ever increasing exposure to thimerosal from additional immunizations after 7 months of age is very likely to add to the total body burden of this toxic metal and cause neurological injury regardless of their body weight.

Indeed, this may be one reason why most cases of regressive autism occur between one and two years of age.

The hypothesis also disregards the possible and likely synergistic (additive) toxicity that may occur between thimerosal-formulated immunizations, aluminum-containing vaccines, and thimerosal-free immunizations, like the MMR. Evidence to support this contention will be presented later in this narrative.

Sally Bernard, *a dissenting member* of the panel of external consultants for this study, objected to the authors' conclusion "that there is no causal association between thimerosal and children's brain function." Her objections to the study include the following:

- The children sampled in the study were those "least likely to exhibit neurological impairments." This was because "children with congenital problems, those from multiple births, those of low birth weight, and those not living with their biological mother were excluded." That bit of statistical flim-flam, as we have seen, eliminated many autistic and developmentally-delayed children who should have been counted in this study.

- "The sample was skewed toward higher socioeconomic status and maternal education—factors that are associated with lower rates of neurobehavioral problems and higher intervention rates and that were not measured."

- The sampling frame included only children enrolled from birth in the health maintenance organization (HMO) and still enrolled after 7 to 10 years, excluding children in higher-mobility families, who tend to have lower academic and behavioral function."[43]

- "Children with neurobehavioral problems may have been less likely to remain with the HMO."

- "Only 30 percent of families selected for recruitment participated, a low rate for scientific research. Among the families selected for recruitment, 26 percent refused to participate. Another 28 percent "could not be located," which included families that did not respond to multiple recruitment attempts (internal documentation from the study contractor, ("Abt Associates")—another form of refusal."[44]

The researchers should have, but did not, evaluate developmental outcomes for children who were fully immunized as compared to those who weren't, and they also could and should have compared the outcomes of those with significant thimerosal exposure vs. those with none.

Without doing these studies, one cannot conclude that "there is no causal association between thimerosal and brain function." The CDC continues to obfuscate and refuses to do the kind of study that would clarify this debate.

Conflicts of Interest: This CDC-sponsored study (another "uh oh!") sets the record for the most conflicts of interest of any study we have mentioned thus far. Most of the researchers were CDC employees. There are documented associations between seven vaccine manufacturers and six study panel members, to whit:

43   Rumberger, R.W. "Student mobility and academic achievement." *Child & adolescent development*. MentalHelp.net. January 23, 2003. (Accessed December 12, 2007 at http://mentalhelp.net/poc/ view_doc.php? type=doc&id=2084&cn=28.)

44   www.fourteenstudies.org

- Dr. William Thompson reports being a former employee of Merck; at the time of this study he was a senior scientist at the CDC's Immunology Safety Office." [He has since become a "whistleblower." See below.]

- Dr. Marcy, receiv(ed) consulting fees from Merck, Sanofi Pasteur, Glaxo-SmithKline, and MedImmune;

- Dr. Jackson, receiv(ed) grant support from Wyeth, Sanofi Pasteur, Glaxo-SmithKline, and Novartis, lecture fees from Sanofi Pasteur, and consulting fees from Wyeth and Abbott and serv(ed) as a consultant to the FDA Vaccines and Related Biological Products Advisory Committee;

- Dr. Lieu, serv(ed) as a consultant to the CDC Advisory Committee on Immunization Practices;

- Dr. Black, receiv(ed) consulting fees from MedImmune, GlaxoSmithKline, Novartis, and Merck and grant support from MedImmune, GlaxoSmithKline, Aventis, Merck, and Novartis;

- Dr. Davis receiv(ed) consulting fees from Merck and grant support from Merck and GlaxoSmith-Kline.

Fraud?

Yes! This is another fraudulent study perpetrated by the highly conflicted Centers for Disease Control and Prevention. How do we know? In 2015, Dr. William Thompson, the lead author of this study (and one of the senior CDC scientists), confessed that he participated in three fraudulent studies sponsored by the CDC, including this one.

> Dr. Thompson says that his superiors at the CDC Developmental Disabilities Branch pressured him to manipulate the study's findings and to bury the links between thimerosal and brain damage. In response to this pressure, the published version downplayed data showing that thimerosal causes 'tics,' a family of grave neurological injuries—including Tourette's Syndrome—that are associated with Autism. Thompson now says that the data actually showed a definitive statistically significant association between thimerosal and tics. "Thimerosal from vaccines cause tics…. I can say tics are four times more prevalent in kids with autism. There is biologic plausibility right now to say that thimerosal causes autism-like features."[45]

Conclusion: This is yet another unethical, CDC-sponsored, fraudulent study that fails totally in its objective to clarify the thimerosal/neurodevelopmental harm debate.

It contains many *fatal flaws*, like biased sampling, overmatching, significant conflicts of interest, inadequate confirmation of the child's diagnosis, the exclusion of over 70 percent of the families that were recruited, the exclusion of premature babies and those with low birthweight or congenital problems, inadequate sample size, the omission of all the data on the potentially relevant immunizations given to the babies after 7 months of age, the failure to compare developmental outcomes of vaccinated and unvaccinated babies, the failure to compare outcomes of highly thimerosal-exposed babies with those who had no or little thimerosal exposure, and most importantly, *the manipulation of data in order to hide the relevant association between thimerosal and neurological damage manifesting as a tic disorder. This deceptive study should be withdrawn.*

Finally, *this study does not include autism in its evaluations of harm*, and so should not be used as evidence that purports to clear thimerosal and mercury as causative agents of autism spectrum disorders. Indeed, the study, when properly analyzed, actually supports the link between thimerosal and autism, according to the CDC's own scientist.

---

45   http://www.ageofautism.com/2015/02/robert-kennedy-jr-cdc-scientist-still-maintains-agency-forced-researchers-to-lie-about-safety-of-mer.html?utm_source=feedburner&utm_medium= email &utm_campaign=Feed percent3A+ageofautism+ percent28AGE+OF+AUTISM percent29

"I think that the government or certain public officials in the government have been too quick to dismiss the concerns of these families (regarding thimerosal and autism) without studying the population that got sick. I think public health officials have been too quick to dismiss the hypothesis as irrational without sufficient studies of causation."

— Dr. Bernadine Healy, former Director of the
National Institutes of Health (NIH)

A Ninth "Negative" Study: The "Second Danish Study." Hviid, Anders et al. "Association between Thimerosal-Containing Vaccine and Autism." *Journal of the American Medical Association*. (October 1, 2003); 290(13):1763f.

In this second Danish study (also sponsored and designed by the CDC), the researchers "evaluated all children born in Denmark from January 1, 1990, until December 31, 1996 (N = 467,450) comparing children vaccinated with a thimerosal-containing vaccine with children vaccinated with a thimerosal-free formulation of the same vaccine," to see whether any relationship existed between thimerosal and the incidence of autism.

In Denmark, according to the researchers, "From 1970 (on), the only thimerosal-containing vaccine in (use) has been the whole-cell pertussis vaccine. In late March 1992, the last batch of thimerosal-containing whole-cell pertussis vaccine was released and distributed from Statens Serum Institut. Only the whole-cell vaccine produced by Statens Serum Institut has been used in Denmark."

"The whole-cell vaccine was administered at 5 weeks, 9 weeks, and 10 months from 1970 and until it was replaced, irrespective of thimerosal content. The thimerosal formulation contained 50 µg of thimerosal (~25 µg of ethylmercury) in the first dose and 100 µg (~50 µg of ethylmercury) in each of the succeeding 2 doses."

During the study, the authors, "identified 440 autism cases and 787 cases of other autistic-spectrum disorders." They found that, "the risk of autism and other autistic-spectrum disorders did not differ significantly between children vaccinated with thimerosal-containing vaccine and children vaccinated with thimerosal-free vaccine."

And they concluded that "the results do not support a causal relationship between childhood vaccination with thimerosal-containing vaccines and development of autistic-spectrum disorders."

Critique: By the year 2000, *over half of the children with autism or ASD were lost from the Danish registry*, and the vast number of those lost cases represented *older* children. This registry data was re-analyzed by epidemiologists at "Safe Minds" who stated that, "Since the relative risk of the Hviid study is based on finding fewer older thimerosal-exposed children than younger unexposed children, the validity of their conclusion exonerating thimerosal in autism is questionable. More likely, the finding is a result of missing records rather than true lower incidence rates among the exposed group."

Sally Bernard, executive director of SafeMinds, puts it more strongly. This "substantial loss of autism case records from the registry...essentially renders the findings of the *JAMA* study by Hviid and colleagues invalid."[46]

"Safe Minds" reanalyzed the Denmark registry data and used an alternative method to avoid the record removal bias. The analysis looked at same-age children, 5-9 year olds, but from different registry years: 1992, when all of the children received thimerosal-containing vaccines, and 2002, when none of the children received vaccines with thimerosal.

After adjusting for the lack of outpatient records in the 1992 registry, the reanalysis showed a *2.3 times higher number of autism cases* among the 1992 thimerosal-exposed group relative to the 2002 non-exposed group.

The analysts then determined an autism incidence rate for the non-thimerosal group of 1 in 1500, while the thimerosal-exposed group had an incidence of 1 in 500, a 3-fold increase."[47]

---

46   fourteenstudies.org
47   Ibid.

In other words, there was actually a significant *increase* in the incidence of autism in those children who received thimerosal-containing vaccines as compared to those who had no exposure to thimerosal. This is the exact opposite of the conclusions of Anders Hviid and associates, and once again clearly demonstrates the association between thimerosal in vaccines and autism.

Also noteworthy is the relatively low incidence of autism (1 in 1,500) found in the Danish non-thimerosal-exposed children as compared to the incidence in the U.S. during the same time period (1 in 150-250).

The Danish children were exposed to much less thimerosal then were their U.S. counterparts, who also received thimerosal-containing HIB and hepatitis B vaccinations during the time period encompassed by this study.

The relatively low incidence of autism in Denmark's children is consistent with their lesser exposure to mercury from thimerosal and supports the hypothesis that immunizations and specifically thimerosal-containing immunizations are causally related to the epidemic of autism.

"Cases and controls as young as 1 year of age were included within the analysis." That is *much too young to have been diagnosed with autism*. Many of these "normal" controls might later have been diagnosed with autism, "and are therefore possibly misclassified."[48]

Potential Conflicts of Interest Not Reported in JAMA: Lyn Redwood, president of Safe Minds, states, "In the Hviid study in *JAMA* we can clearly see how the data was misinterpreted so a conclusion could be drawn to clear thimerosal from any role in autism." This misinterpretation is not surprising given the authors' employment with the manufacturer and promoter of vaccines in Denmark, Statens Serum Institut. This conflict of interest should have been stated by *JAMA*, but it wasn't.[49]

The Danish registry contained only *inpatient*-diagnosed autism cases prior to 1995, and after that time, it also included outpatient-diagnosed cases as well. Since most of the autism cases in Denmark (and everywhere else in the world for that matter) are diagnosed in outpatient settings, this would have resulted in a factitiously apparent increase in the incidence of autism for the study years 1995 and 1996, which was not accounted for in the authors' analysis of the data.

Conclusion: This is yet another shameful, duplicitous study that was cleverly formulated and mis-analyzed to show no linkage between thimerosal and autism when the correct analysis of the data demonstrates just the opposite. The conflicts of interest in this study are probably relevant in that regard (including CDC design and support). As with the majority of the aforementioned "negative studies," this aberration should never have been published, and, having been, should be retracted and discredited.

"Facts are stubborn things, but statistics are more pliable."

— Author Unknown

A Tenth "Negative" Study: The Pichichero Study: Pichichero, Michael et al. "Mercury concentrations and metabolism in infants receiving vaccines containing thiomersal [thimerosal]: A descriptive study." *Lancet*. Vol. 360, Issue 9347, p. 1737-1741. 30 November 2002.

In this study, Dr. Pichichero's team was interested in evaluating the mercury concentration in infants' blood, urine, and stool 3-28 days after they had been given thimerosal-containing vaccines.

Twenty thimerosal-exposed babies were evaluated at age 2 months and another 20 at 6 months of age. They were compared to 21 control babies who had not received any thimerosal-containing vaccines.

---

48   "Methodological Issues and Evidence of Malfeasance in Research Purporting to Show Thimerosal in Vaccines Is Safe." http://www.hindawi.com/journals/bmri/2014/247218/ Ibid.
49   Ibid.

No followup on these babies was done, and no evaluations of neurological or developmental problems, including autism, were undertaken.

The mean mercury doses (exposures from vaccines) in infants exposed to thimerosal were 45.6 µg (range 37·5-62·5 micrograms) for 2 month olds and 111.3 µg (range 87·5-175·0) for 6 month olds.

Concentrations of mercury were found to be low in the urine but high in the stools of the 2 and 6 month olds who had received thimerosal-containing vaccines and, "Only one of 15 blood samples from the control group contained quantifiable mercury. Blood mercury in thimerosal-exposed 2-month-olds ranged from less than 3.75 to 20.55 nmol/L (parts per billion); in 6-month-olds all values were lower than 7.50 nmol/L."

The researchers concluded that, "Administration of vaccines containing thimerosal does not seem to raise blood concentrations of mercury above safe values in infants. Ethylmercury seems to be eliminated from blood rapidly via the stools after parenteral administration of thimerosal in vaccines."

"This study gives comforting reassurance about the safety of ethyl mercury as a preservative in childhood vaccines," Pichichero's team assures us.[50]

But does it?

Critique: This terribly-done study is full of misstatements, lies, omissions, and misinterpretations, and these start in the first sentence: "Thiomersal is a preservative containing small amounts of ethylmercury...." Thimerosal (thiomersal) actually contains a *large amount* of ethyl mercury. Half of the molecule (49.8 percent) is ethyl mercury.

Conflicts of interest: Michael Pichichero declared no conflicts of interest. *He lied.* He is heavily conflicted. His own website declares that he "was a member of the discovery team at the University of Rochester that invented, tested and licensed a Haemophilus influenzae b (Hib) conjugate vaccine (HibTITER®) now universally given to children in the U.S."

In addition, he has received research grants and honoraria from a large number of vaccine manufacturers and pharmaceutical companies. These include Abbott Laboratories, Inc.; Bristol Myers Squibb Company; Eli Lilly & Company; Merck and Co.; Pasteur Merieux Connaught; Pfizer Labs; Roche Laboratories; Roussel-Uclaf; Schering Corporation; Smith-Kline-Beecham Pharmaceuticals; Upjohn Company; and Wyeth-Lederle.

Pichichero, et al. suggested that ethyl mercury, which was rapidly eliminated from the blood, wound up in the stool, but his own figures belie that assertion. The researchers in this study actually demonstrated *slow* stool excretion in many infants. The disappearance of ethyl mercury from the blood does not necessarily mean that it has been excreted and removed from the body. The ethyl mercury could also have been, and undoubtedly was, deposited in a variety of tissues and organs, and as the authors correctly point out, "Organic mercury readily crosses the blood-brain barrier...."

According to chemistry professor Boyd Haley, who analyzed the Pichichero et al. data, "Taking the stool concentration range for mercury from Pichichero et al., we calculated the time required for an infant to excrete the ethylmercury (187.5 mcg) that U.S. infants received by six months of age during the 1990s." Table 16.2 lists these ranges.

Dr. Haley continues: "In the case of maximum excretion, early vaccine exposures are eliminated within the time period of exposure, but for those children with stool concentrations at the low end of the range, the infant elimination rate rises to nearly four years.

"For autistic infants, with evidence of reduced excretion in hair and additional fetal exposures (from maternal amalgam filling, fish consumption and Rho D immunoglobulin injections) these excretion times were likely far longer."[51]

50   Pichichero, Ibid.
51   fourteenstudies.org

Table 16.2.

Stool Hg* concentration ng/gm		Daily Hg excretion mcg/day	Days to excrete 187.5 mcg
Minimum:	23	0.14-0.41	457-1,339 (1.2 - 3.7 yrs)
Maximum:	140	0.84-2.52	74-223

*Hg=mercury

The autism incidence in 2002 was c 1:150. A study, like this one, of just 40 babies who were exposed to thimerosal, would not be expected to yield even one baby who would later go on to develop autism (we'll never know, since none of the babies were followed up to see whether autism or other neuro-developmental problems would manifest).

If we assume (and we do) that most autistic children do not detoxify mercury well or quickly, then even if we accept the data in this study as being meaningful (and we don't), the study would be irrelevant since it may not have included any children with impaired detoxification functions.

Why isn't the data in this study meaningful? Because the blood draws occurred after the likely peak level of mercury was reached. The researchers should have drawn blood samples before the immunizations were given, immediately afterwards, and over several days after they were administered to evaluate how quickly or slowly mercury rises and then falls in each and every child evaluated. This is a standard procedure in a study of this type.

The peak level of mercury in these babies would likely have occurred at 1-3 days after their immunizations, so drawing blood 4 days or more after this peak period, as was done in this study, would have resulted in factitiously lower blood levels of mercury than would otherwise have been obtained if the draws had been done at the appropriate time.

The researchers also assumed that the *methyl* mercury safety standards (which they cited incorrectly) would apply to *ethyl* mercury, with no evidence to support that contention.

In regard to those mercury safety standards, Pichichero and colleagues also erred in their citing a 1994 article by Grandjean, who at that time had suggested that the safe level for *methyl* mercury in blood was 29 parts per billion or less, which was set at 10 times less than the lowest level of mercury (290 ppb) then *thought to cause brain dysfunctions*.

The researchers neglected to mention that Grandjean et al., after doing further research, *retracted that earlier conclusion* when they published their more recent article in 1998 entitled "Cognitive performance of children prenatally exposed to 'safe' levels of methyl- mercury."[52]

Grandjean et al. had now found that neurological dysfunctions could occur in children exposed to mercury in utero who had blood mercury levels of only 58 parts per billion (ppb), or 1/5th of the previously accepted danger level. If we assume a safety margin of 1/10th the danger level, then the upper safe blood level for mercury would be a mere 5.8 parts per billion.

So Pichichero made two mistakes in this regard. He failed to cite the then accepted current standard for mercury blood level safety, and he assumed that *methyl* mercury had the same toxicity as *ethyl* mercury.

As we have noted in the animal studies (previously cited), *ethyl* mercury, the kind found in thimerosal, remains in animal brains a lot longer and in higher concentrations (as inorganic mercury) than does *methyl* mercury.

One of the children in the study whose blood mercury peaked at 20.6 parts per billion had had his blood drawn five days after he received his thimerosal-containing immunizations (he was exposed to 37.5 micrograms of thimerosal).

52   *Environmental Research*, 1998

If the authors are correct in their estimation that the half life[53] of ethyl mercury is about 6-7 days, that would mean that this infant's peak mercury level would have occurred several days earlier and would have been much higher.

According to Michael Bender of the Mercury Policy Project, "Many infants in the 1990s were exposed to 62.5 micrograms of mercury at age 2 months,[54] or nearly double what the study infant received. Therefore, it is probable that the blood levels of some infants given the full regimen of thimerosal vaccines in the 1990s would exceed the 58 ppb threshold for adverse effects."[55]

It is standard protocol in doing a placebo-controlled study to assign the study subjects (babies in this instance) *randomly* to either the study group or the control group, and also to *age and sex-match the controls*. Pichichero and colleagues failed to do either of these things.

Conclusion: This is another truly awful study that fails completely in exonerating thimerosal as a causative factor in promoting autism and other neurodevelopmental disorders. This mockery of good research most assuredly does not give "comforting reassurance about the safety of ethyl mercury as a preservative in childhood vaccines." Instead, it further serves to illustrate how duplicitous or incompetent researchers (pick one or both) can obfuscate reality by means of improper study protocols, misstatements of fact and misinterpretations of data.

> *"Dr. Michael Pichichero, an Eli Lilly-funded researcher and holder of numerous vaccine patents, tried to clear thimerosal as harmful by conducting a blood mercury evaluation after infant vaccination which missed peak blood levels, had a sample size too small to detect susceptible subgroups, and failed to address implications of the findings for long term mercury deposition in the brain.*
>
> *His industry ties were not disclosed by the journal,* The Lancet.*"[56]*

A Negative Review Article: Nelson, Karen et al. "Thimerosal and Autism?" *Pediatrics*. Vol. 111 No. 3 March 2003, p. 674-679.

The purpose of this 2003 review article was to scan the medical literature for what the authors felt were appropriate research studies that related to the known toxic effects of mercury, and to see whether or not these known effects were similar to the symptoms manifested by autistic individuals. Nelson et al. conclude that there is little or no support for those suggesting a thimerosal-autism link and a great deal of evidence suggesting that there is no such linkage.

They do concede that, "Mercury in sufficient dose is neurotoxic and probably more toxic in the immature brain. It is reasonable to ask whether thimerosal in childhood vaccine increases risk of chronic childhood neurologic disability and specifically of autism."

And they go on to state that, "The available data with which to address the question are very limited and largely inferential."

Critique: In doing their evaluation, the authors rejected *all* of the research of epidemiologists Mark and David Geier, because of their use of the VAERS data base, which Nelson, et al. felt was not suitable for statistical analysis, despite the fact the both the CDC and FDA have published research studies based on this database.

They also conveniently ignored the fact that the Geiers have analyzed *five* databases, including the revered VSD base preferred by the CDC, as well as the U.S. Department of Education Report for the year 2001, the CDC's Biological Surveillance Summaries and live birth estimates report, the U.S. Department of Education datasets, and the California Department of Developmental Services (CDDS) database, and *all of these non-manipulated database analyses have yielded exactly the same result*, to whit:

---

53   Half life is the scientific term for the period of time it takes for the concentration of a given substance to be reduced by 50 percent (half).
54   From thimerosal-containing DPT, Hepatitis B, and HIB immunizations.
55   The 14 studies.com
56   http://www.chat-hyperacusis.net/post/Pink-Disease-Mercury-Autism-The-Brain-Gut-Ears-1599210?trail=100

There is a statistically significant causal and dose-dependent relationship between thimerosal exposure and autism and other neurodevelopmental disorders.

Nelson et al. do not, however, reject or even criticize any of the terribly done "negative" studies that we have alluded to above.

This analysis then appears to be highly biased, one-sided, and with a preset agenda that discredits and rejects the thimerosal-autism linkage by selectively and inappropriately criticizing the studies that show an association between thimerosal and autism while not analyzing or criticizing the deceptive and fraudulent studies that yielded negative results, like the Verstraeten study, the Danish studies, etc.

The authors also make the mistake of comparing different kinds of mercury toxicity, finding that the symptoms of these other forms of mercury toxicity are not exactly the same as those seen in autism, and on that basis discounting the thimerosal-autism linkage. We have already discussed why this is not a valid criticism. Various chemical forms of mercury exert their toxic effects in different ways, depending on the dose, route, sensitivity of the individual, age at time of exposure, etc.

It is true that autism's manifestations are not the same as those of Pink Disease, Mad Hatter Syndrome, or Minamata Disease, etc., but then again, these various high dose mercury poisoning conditions are not identical either in their manifestations, and all of these, including autism, share identical features as well as their own unique ones.

There is no one mercury poisoning syndrome, and as the authors correctly point out, "relatively little is known about the impact of ethyl mercury on the nervous system, especially with repeated low-dose exposure."

We have shown that "low dose" ethylmercury exposure inhibits many enzymes, including COMT and methionine synthase, and in conjunction with dysfunctional or inadequate metallothionein proteins in susceptible babies, would be expected to result in a failure to prune brain neurons appropriately, which might then result in an increase in brain volume, and would also adversely affect digestive and immune functioning and negatively impact sensory issues, thinking, speech development, gut biota, and attention (among others).

Virtually, all the features of metallothionein dysfunction are those commonly observed in autistic individuals.

Thus, the Vaccine Court and Karen Nelson et al. got it wrong. Thimerosal's toxic, cell-killing effects, which are more relevant at high doses, may not be the major or primary factors in its promotion of autism, but rather, it is low dose thimerosal's detrimental inhibition of COMT, methionine synthase, and other relevant enzymes in genetically susceptible babies with impaired metallothionein function and impaired ability to detoxify mercury that is likely to result in the manifestations of the condition we know as autism in many of the children so diagnosed.

Conclusion: This is a clearly biased review that is not at all helpful in resolving this debate.

> *"We have seen that mercury, even in concentrations too low to cause cell death can affect multiple neuron cell functions such as membrane transport, calcium regulation, energy production, neurotransmitter control, free radical production, excitotoxicity, enzyme function, DNA stability and repair as well as antioxidant defenses."*
>
> — Dr. Russell Blaylock

An Eleventh "Negative Study": Miles, Judith H. and T. Nicole Takahashi. "Lack of Association between Rh Status, Rh Immune Globulin in Pregnancy and Autism." *American Journal of Medical Genetics*. 2007 Jul 1; 143A (13):1397-407.

The authors of this study analyzed the Rh status of 321 children with autism as well as their mothers to see whether those babies whose mothers had prenatal exposure to a then thimerosal-preserved Rh immune globulin (RhIg: Rho-GAM® and similar brands) had any increased risk for autism spectrum disorders.

What they purported to determine was that neither Rh status nor RhoGAM® posed any increased risk for autism, or more specifically, "that Rh– [negative] status is no higher in mothers of children with autism than in the general population, exposure to antepartum [prior to delivery] RhIg, preserved with thimerosal is no higher for children with autism, and pregnancies are no more likely to be Rh incompatible."[57]

Rh refers to a substance found on the surface of blood cells that helps determine blood type. It is not uncommon for a baby and mother's blood to mix somewhat during the pregnancy, and baby and mother may have different blood types.

If an Rh negative (the Rh factor is absent) mother is exposed to baby's blood that is Rh positive (the Rh factor is present), the mother's immune cells may produce antibodies (immunoglobulins) that are able to "attack" the baby's red blood cells and cause an anemia, which can sometimes be quite severe.

To prevent this occurrence, Rh negative pregnant women in the third trimester of pregnancy may be given the RhoGAM® (or similar) immunoglobulin injection. Prior to 2001, the RhoGAM® injection also commonly contained thimerosal. So any mother receiving this injection would also be exposing her unborn fetus to toxic ethyl mercury, which readily crosses the placenta.

However, Miles and Takahashi conclude that their "findings support the consensus that exposure to ethyl mercury in thimerosal is not the cause of the increased prevalence of autism," and they add that, "These data are important not only for parents in this country but also for the international health community where thimerosal continues to be used to preserve multi-dose vials which in turn makes vaccines affordable."[58]

> *"It is…essential that future vaccine decisions are made by physicians and scientists without even the appearance of conflicts of interest."*
>
> — *Dr. Mark and David Geier*

Critique: In June of 1977, the Coalition for Safe Minds released a review of this study that outlined many of the study's flaws as well as significant conflicts of interest.

The coalition discovered, "an earlier version of the study data, presented by Drs. Miles and Takahashi at a conference in 2005 (which) showed an increased rate of RhIg administration during pregnancy of children later diagnosed with an autism spectrum disorder (ASD) compared to their non-ASD siblings…."

That is to say, the Rh Immunoglobulin injection (RhoGAM® and other similar products referred to as RhIg by the authors) given to pregnant women appeared to be associated with an *increased risk* of autism spectrum disorders in the children of those pregnancies, which is consistent with the research of Mark and David Geier cited earlier.

The 2005 results, presented by the same authors only two years prior to publication of this article, *directly contradict* this study's findings and conclusions.[59]

To help understand the disturbing discrepancies in data, sampling, and the interpretation of results presented by Miles and Takahashi, consider the following:

- The (original) sample was altered so that the majority of multiplex families and nearly half the minority families were removed, representing approximately 1/3 of the original sample.

- The final sample may reflect selection bias related to the exposure variable, RhIg with thimerosal, as 59 percent of the eligible families were lost to follow up or declined to participate, and those excluded are likely to have had greater RhIg exposure.

---

57   Miles et al. Abstract.
58   Ibid.
59   http://www.safe minds org/pressroom/pres_releases/Review_Miles_Takahashi_6-20-07.pdf

- The authors failed to adequately identify the amount of mercury in the RhIg given, invalidating exposure risk calculations. They reported that all RhIg given was the Johnson & Johnson brand RhoGAM®, even though this brand had only half the market share during the period of most study pregnancies.

- The RhIg comparison control group in the journal version consisted of just 27 families, too small for statistical power.

- Between the 2005 and 2007 versions, the control groups changed and major portions of the original autism sample were removed. Calculations based on the original data indicate that children with autism "were 71 percent more likely to have been exposed to RhIg in utero than their non-ASD siblings."[60]

The Best Science Drug Company Money Can Buy?

"This study is just another example of the pharmaceutical industry's corruption of research to suit its own purposes. They back the study designs that give the desired results of no harm."

— National Autism Association President and Parent Wendy Fournier

Conflicts of Interest: Johnson & Johnson was a study sponsor. It manufactures RhoGAM, one of the major brands of Rh immune globulin, and it had and has "a direct financial interest in ongoing legal proceedings regarding thimerosal in Rho D immune globulin therapies and autism."[61]

Dr. Miles has served as an expert witness in RhIg/autism litigation, a conflict of interest not revealed in the article. Conflicts of interest by the study sponsor and lead author could well be associated with the significant concerns noted in this study.

"The authors' clinic is oriented strictly to genetic causality in autism, with no room for environmental contributions like mercury."[62]

There was no discussion or evaluation of the other immunizations each baby received. As we have seen, the cumulative exposure to mercury from thimerosal and other sources is of vital importance in determining the total toxic load that triggers autism in susceptible individuals.

Any study of autism prevalence in children whose mothers may have received Rh immune globulin during that pregnancy, and which ignores the total cumulative toxic mercury load those children were exposed to thereafter, is incapable of reaching the conclusions these authors came to ("ethyl mercury in thimerosal is not the cause of the increased prevalence of autism"), even if the study were valid, and this one certainly isn't.

According to Generation Rescue, "Additional calculations of the data, not done by Miles & Takahashi, show a 71 percent higher rate of Rh immune globulin exposure in children with autism relative to unaffected siblings, in contradiction to their findings but consistent with other studies."[63]

Conclusion: We see clear parallels to the Verstraeten studies here. Researchers do a study that implicates thimerosal as a causative factor in autism. They don't publish that study, but rather alter the data sufficiently to show no significant association between autism and thimerosal, and that's the study that is published!

This is a shamefully done, biased study, probably intentionally fraudulent, and certainly not capable of rendering the conclusions that the authors reached. Thimerosal is most certainly not exonerated as a cause of autism.

---

60   Safeminds.org
61   Ibid.
62   Ibid.
63   fourteenstudies.org

"Definition of Statistics:
The science of producing unreliable facts from reliable figures."

— Evan Esar

A Twelfth "Negative Study": Price, CS. et al. "Prenatal and Infant Exposure to Thimerosal from Vaccines and Immunoglobulins and Risk of Autism." *Pediatrics.* 2010; 126:656-664.

The researchers in this CDC-sponsored study (yes, continue to be very concerned) compared the thimerosal exposures from vaccines and Rho immune globulin in 256 autistic children and 752 matched controls. The authors claim that the study "was designed to examine relationships between prenatal and infant ethylmercury exposure from thimerosal-containing vaccines and/or immunoglobulin preparations and ASD (autism spectrum disorders) and 2 ASD subcategories: autistic disorder (AD) and ASD with regression."

The researchers not only found "no increased risk for any of the three ASD outcomes," but they paradoxically noted a somewhat protective effect from the thimerosal-containing injections!

They concluded that, "prenatal and early-life exposure to ethylmercury from thimerosal-containing vaccines and immunoglobulin preparations was not related to increased risk of ASDs."[64]

Critique: The epidemiologists at Safe Minds reviewed this study and discovered some disturbing facts:[65]

> Planning for this study began in 2001. Over the 9 year study period, the large external panel of consultants providing input to the investigators was reduced to a small subset by study end. The original large panel recommended against the study design ultimately employed, as insufficient to answer the question of early thimerosal exposure and autism rates.

The external consultant panel recommendations were overruled by the CDC and the AHIP (America's Health Insurance Plans), and the study was undertaken using the rejected protocol. That means that this study was from its very onset incapable of clarifying the thimerosal-autism linkage. The protocol was flawed!

Why would the CDC and the medical insurance industry choose to continue this research with a *flawed protocol*?

The likely answer: so the results would not show a cause-effect relationship between thimerosal-preserved injections and autism spectrum disorders.

The study design contained *two primary deficiencies* in the research methodology, which actually allowed for the strange finding of a thimerosal protective effect.

The first deficiency had to do with the factors (variables) that were analyzed. The second concerns the low participation rate leading to sample bias.

The researchers should have and could have compared a thimerosal-exposed group of children with an unexposed group, but chose not to. The CDC, as we have seen, appears to be terrified of this kind of study. Or it could have compared those children who had high exposure to thimerosal to those with lower exposure, but it didn't do this either.

What they did compare were autistic and non-autistic children who had *virtually the same immunizations and thimerosal exposure*, but who completed the series of immunizations at different times (some completed the series on time and some were delayed). This, as the reader may recall from earlier in this chapter, was what Heron and Golding did in their flawed study that compared two groups of children with exactly the same thimerosal exposure.

---

64   Ibid: abstract
65   www.safeminds.org; Schafer Autism Report; Thu, September 16, 2010.

The stratification system used by the researchers would by its design "swing the results to show a lower autism rate among those highly exposed" to thimerosal.[66] This was done using several other statistical "tricks."

The researchers doing this study chose to stratify the children by year of birth and HMO. But the statistician reviewers at Safe Minds state, "The two matching variables compete with the exposure variable to explain differences in the autism outcome."

There was no compelling reason to stratify by year of birth since the nine-year length of the study would have been sufficient time to have diagnosed virtually all the likely autism cases. This stratification scheme did, however, serve to "weaken the signal" that would show a thimerosal-autism link.

The Safe Minds reviewers assert that, "The association between the increased exposure and the increase in ASD can only be detected by removing the birth year variable, which otherwise masks the effect of exposure on outcomes."

There was also a significant sample bias in this study, which could by itself invalidate the results of the study:

> The participation rate in the study was quite low: among the cases, it was 48.1 percent, and among the controls, only 31.7 percent. Controls were more likely than cases to be unable to be located and to refuse participation. The standard for minimal response is 60 percent and higher.

> Moreover, the reported participation rate does not even consider the excessive dropout rate due to the requirement that children enrolled in the study HMOs from birth to 24 months must still have been enrolled in the same HMO at the time of data collection 6-13 years later. Subjects drop out of any long term follow up study, but here, drop out was due to HMO enrollment attrition and resulted in far larger numbers than the typical observational study.[67]

In this study, those who were vaccine-compliant participated at a higher rate than did those who delayed completing the vaccinations series.

> *"The lower the participation rate, the greater the chance for introduction of sampling bias."*[68]

> *"It is the difference between participants and non-participants that determines the amount of bias present."*[69]

Likewise, "participation bias relating to exposure holds true primarily for the controls, since cases are more likely to participate in studies regardless of exposure."[70]

"These simultaneous biases can have the effect of changing the study findings."[71]

"Shifts in participation rates among key groups can dramatically change the results. A similar phenomenon is likely operating in these vaccine studies which purport to show protective effects from mercury exposures."[72]

According to research scientist Brian S. Hooker, Ph.D., "This study is fatally flawed due to a statistical error called overmatching." Overmatching, it may be remembered, occurs when cases and controls are too closely matched to each other. This clever statistical trick actually prevents finding a difference between cases and controls as "all differences (are) matched out case by case."[73]

---

66   www.safeminds.org
67   Ibid.
68   Morton 2005
69   Galena & Tracy, 2007
70   Galena & Tracy, 2007
71   Safe Minds; Ibid.
72   Safe Minds
73   healthimpactnews.com/2013/can-we-trust-the-cdc-claim-that-there-is-no-link-between-vaccines-and-autism/

And it gets worse. Dr. Hooker found that "the study authors hid data regarding the only valid part of the study (i.e., prenatal thimerosal exposure) which showed that children exposed to just 16 micrograms of mercury from thimerosal in utero were almost 9 times (8.73 to be exact) more likely to receive a diagnosis of regressive autism." We know this thanks to a Freedom of Information Act request by Representative Bill Posey on December 18, 2012, which allowed independent analysts, like Dr. Hooker, to review the data. Why wasn't this significant finding published? It certainly contradicted the conclusions made by the authors of this so-called "study."

There are many significant and relevant *conflicts of interest* and concerns in this deceptive work:

- The CDC funded and designed the study and approved the protocol which its own panel of outside consultants had recommended against.

- The CDC's own researchers were key players in this study (David Shay, Eric Weintraub, and Frank DeStefano).

- Cristofer Price, the lead author, as well as researchers Barbara Goodson and Anne Robertson, were employed by Apt Associates, "a contract research organization whose largest clients include vaccine manufacturers and the CDC's National Immunization Program."[74]

- Participants in this study also included members of the "America's Health Insurance Plans," the trade group for the American Health Insurance Industry as well as three HMOs who received "substantial funding from vaccine manufacturers to conduct vaccine licensing research."[75]

- Dr. Michael Marcy received honoraria for speaking for Merck and GlaxoSmith-Kline and grant support for studies on Gardasil and ProQuad from Merck.

- Mr. Lewis received grant support from Medimmune, Sanofi Pasteur, Chiron, Wyeth, Merck, and Glaxo-SmithKline.

- Dr. Bernal received research funding from the CDC, the National Institute of Mental Health, Health Resources and Service Administration, and Autism Speaks.

Conclusion: And yet again, the once prestigious journal *Pediatrics* has demeaned its reputation by publishing another CDC-sponsored, deceitful, and invalid study, which had been previously submitted and rejected by both the *New England Journal of Medicine* and the *Journal of the American Medical Association*.

The study was cleverly designed to show no association between thimerosal and neuro-developmental disorders like autism, and in that it succeeded. The study protocols were known to be improper from the initiation of this "research," but that is exactly what the CDC and insurance industry apparently wanted.

The CDC also "cherry picked" the data it included and deliberately excluded data that ran counter to its desired result. This is an unconscionable act of malfeasance on the part of the CDC and the authors of this deliberate deception.

> The CDC, with the knowledge of the greater risk of autism with prenatal exposures of 16 mcg ethylmercury (as compared to no exposure, in the Abt Associates report dated 12/1/09 and in preliminary results released to CDC as early as May, 2008), recommended the thimerosal-containing seasonal influenza vaccine and the 2009 H1N1 vaccine to pregnant women (with total cumulative exposure of over 50 mcg mercury).[76]

The CDC thus knowingly encouraged the poisoning of unborn children with thimerosal, increasing their risk for the development of autism and autism spectrum disorders.

Dr. DeStefano, M.D., MPH, the CDC's director of immunization safety (there's a laugh!) and a co-author of this study (as well as the infamous Verstraeten study), lied when he stated to Medscape Medical News on September 16, 2010

---

74 www.safeminds.org
75 Safe Minds Ibid.
76 http://www.ashotoftruth.org/price-et-al-2010-pediatrics-126656-study-thimerosal-and-autism-analysis-cdc-documents-obtained-rep

that, "These findings add to the evidence that thimerosal-containing injections during pregnancy or infancy do not increase a child's risk of developing autism." He knew that the data he deliberately excluded from the study proved just the opposite. "In my opinion, further studies are not warranted," he concluded.

Nice try, Dr. DeStefano, but you couldn't be more wrong!

Any conclusions derived from a study with unacceptable protocols, sampling bias, inappropriate and unwarranted statistical manipulations, overmatching, the intentional omission of relevant data, and low participation rates must be considered not only invalid, but deliberately fraudulent!

The weight of evidence presented thus far overwhelmingly supports the contention that thimerosal promotes the autistic state in genetically-susceptible babies, and further uncorrupted studies performed by *independent, non-conflicted* researchers comparing vaccinated and unvaccinated children most certainly are warranted and would be most welcome.

A Thirteenth Negative "Study": Fombonne, Eric et al. "Report regarding mercury levels in the hair and blood of autistic children compared to a control population." Sixth International Meeting for Autism Research; May 3-5, 2007; Seattle Sheraton Hotel, Seattle, WA.

In this report to approximately 900 attendees at the Sixth International Meeting for Autism Research, a meeting that was *closed to the public*, Eric Fombonne presented the results of his study evaluating *whole blood* mercury levels in the hair and blood of 71 autistic children as compared to 75 normally-developing children.

Not surprisingly, he found no significant differences in the mercury levels in the two groups. He concluded that, "there was no correlation between the mercury level and the severity of symptoms and level of functioning of autistic children."

Fombonne further stated that his study findings implied that, "chelation therapies, whereby heavy metals are removed from the body using specific compounds, are not useful in the treatment of autism."

Critique: The *whole blood* or *plasma blood level* of mercury is only relevant for chronic, continuing mercury exposures (from mercury-contaminated food, for example), and is relevant for acute intermittent exposures (from vaccines, for example) only when evaluated shortly after those exposures.

> *"It's too bad that McGill University does not have any toxicologists who could have explained to Dr. Fombonne that his work was a waste of time and money."*
>
> — *Michael Wagnitz, Chemist and Toxicologist; May 7, 2007*

Most of the ethyl-mercury from thimerosal clears the blood in less than ten days and probably reaches peak levels on days 2-3 after exposure. Ethyl mercury may leave the blood and deposit in the brain or other organs, and it may remain there for years in children and adults who do not excrete mercury well.

It is highly likely that *red blood cell* mercury is a more reliable indicator of mercury toxic burden than is *whole blood* or *plasma* mercury based on a study by Berglund and his associates in a 2005 paper. The researchers in that study found that red blood cell mercury levels tended to be significantly higher than mercury measurements made of the whole blood and plasma.[77]

Therefore, random whole blood or plasma mercury levels don't accurately reflect the total body burden of mercury, so they do not mirror brain or organ concentrations of this toxin. The determination of blood levels of mercury months or years after relevant immunizations have been given is consequently *a wasted effort* and unable to address the concern that the mercury in thimerosal may promote autism.

---

77   Berglund, M. et al. "Interindividual variations of human mercury exposure biomarkers: a cross-sectional assessment." *Environ Health*. 2005; 4:20.

The conclusions reached by Fombonne and his colleagues are, therefore, incorrect and additionally so, because, even if we assumed that his measurements of mercury in the hair and blood were relevant, and they aren't, the absence of a known neurotoxin like thimerosal at a given point in time does not mean that the toxin could not have been present at an earlier date and caused significant neurological damage at that time.

Likewise, hair mercury levels, as we have noted previously, do not accurately reflect mercury body burden in autistic children who do not excrete mercury efficiently or rapidly. As previously noted, babies and younger autistic children tend to have low levels of mercury in their hair relative to their peers, and older autistic children tend to have increased hair levels of mercury.[78]

Fombonne failed to do either a chelated urine or stool mercury level on the children or a urine porphyrin evaluation. Any of these tests would have yielded more relevant results.

Dr. Fombonne considers himself an "expert witness" on the subject of autism and mercury. He has appeared on numerous occasions in court hearings testifying against the hypothesized link between both thimerosal and the MMR immunizations and autism. In his testimony, he invariably cites the many fallacious and fraudulent studies, including his own, that we have previously critiqued.

Conclusion: This study, as well as the next, clearly illustrates that the researchers don't understand the toxicology, storage characteristics, appropriate testing modalities, and excretion dynamics of organic mercury compounds and how each may differ in different individuals depending on a number of factors, including genetic predispositions. If they had been more aware of these factors, they would never have used whole blood and hair levels of mercury as determinants of mercury body burden.

None of the conclusions reached in these studies is valid. The proposed thimerosal linkage to autism is by no means disproven, nor are chelating agents able to be written off as effective modalities for toxic metal removal in the many autistic individuals who demonstrate, by means of *appropriate testing*, unacceptably elevated levels of mercury, lead, and/or other chelatable toxins.

> *"Dr. Fombonne refers to the amount of mercury in vaccines as 'trace'.... The concentration of mercury in a multi-dose vaccine vial is 250 times higher than what the United States Environmental Protection Agency (EPA) classifies as hazardous waste."*
>
> — *Michael Wagnitz, Chemist and Toxicologist, May 7, 2007*

A Fourteenth Negative Study: Hertz-Picciotto, I. et al. "Blood mercury concentrations in CHARGE Study children with and without autism." *Environ Health Perspect.* 2010 Jan; 118(1):161-6.

In this study, the researchers measured the *whole blood* mercury concentration in a group of 2-5-year-old children who were divided into an autistic group, including children on the autism spectrum and a control group. Hertz-Picciotto and her colleagues found that there were no significant differences between the mercury levels in the two groups, and that fish consumption and amalgam fillings tended to correlate with increased *whole blood* mercury levels.

The authors apparently encountered pertinent methodological difficulties in their analysis as they noted that there was a *wide variation and skewed distribution of mercury levels in their study*, and further, *non-detectable values of whole blood mercury levels were assigned specific values by the investigators*.

Their unadjusted data, which showed significantly *reduced* concentrations of mercury in the whole blood of autistics and developmentally-delayed children, findings that were inconsistent with previous research studies, made their entire analysis and conclusions highly suspect.

The researchers concluded that, "After accounting for dietary and other differences in [mercury] exposures, total

---

78   Holmes, A.S. et al. "Reduced levels of mercury in first baby haircuts of autistic children." *Int J Toxicol.* 2003 Jul-Aug; 22(4):277-85.

[mercury] in blood was neither elevated nor reduced in CHARGE Study preschoolers with [autism/autism spectrum disorders] compared with unaffected controls, and resembled those of nationally representative samples."[79]

Critique: David Geier and colleagues noted that:

> Hertz-Picciotto and coauthors (2010) observed, in a non-biologically plausible finding, that without adjustment, children diagnosed with an autism spectrum disorder had a significant reduction in their blood mercury levels in comparison to neurotypical controls (32 percent reduction in blood mercury levels), and this same effect was apparent for children diagnosed with developmental disorders (39 percent reduction in blood Hg levels).

> Hertz-Picciotto and others (2010) recognized potential problems in their dataset, and subsequently, attempted to use specialized statistical methods to parse out behaviors associated with an ASD diagnosis that might have an effect on blood Hg levels.

> After the adjustments were made by Hertz-Picciotto and coworkers (2010), a non-significant increase in blood Hg levels among children diagnosed with an ASD in comparison to controls (8 percent increase in blood Hg levels) was observed, but children diagnosed with developmental delay still had a significant reduction in their blood Hg levels in comparison to controls (33 percent reduction in blood Hg levels).

> Considering the consistent finding of non-biologically plausible results by Hertz-Picciotto and colleagues (2010), even after significant adjustments, it is hard to interpret these investigators' findings.

What these critics of the Hertz-Picciotto study are saying is that the data from this study are inconsistent with what we know about children with autism and developmental disorders and that their analysis and conclusions must, therefore, be regarded with great suspicion.

These researchers did not measure hair mercury levels, but erred, as did Fombonne in the aforementioned study, by assuming that *whole blood or plasma mercury* levels not taken shortly after the immunizations were injected would provide relevant data concerning mercury body burden.

Whole blood or plasma levels of mercury, as we have mentioned, do not appropriately reflect ethyl mercury levels in the brain and other organs. Mercury in the blood is found mostly in red cells. The wrong test was done. The conclusions are, therefore, invalid.

We refer the reader to the 2007 study (a reanalysis of the corrected dataset by Ip et al.) by DeSoto and Hitlan (pages 138-139), which showed that the autistic children as compared to the controls had significantly higher levels of mercury in their *red cells* and that red blood cell levels of mercury over 26 nMol/L (5.2 mcg/L) more than tripled the odds of having an autism diagnosis.[80]

These findings were replicated in the Geier et al. 2010 study, which demonstrated significant increases in mercury *red blood cell* levels in autistics as compared to controls ($p < 0.0001$) and that having a level of *red cell* mercury greater than 15 micrograms per liter increased the odds of having an autism diagnosis by a factor of 6.4.[81]

Conclusion: This was a poorly done study with improper protocols. The researchers used the wrong test (whole blood mercury levels) instead of the more appropriate red blood cell mercury levels in attempting to determine mercury body burden.

They measured these levels *months to years* after the last immunizations were given, rendering the results meaningless. Children with autism may have had their thimerosal-induced neurological damage initiated years before the

79   Ibid. Abstract

80   DeSoto, M.C., Hitlan, R.T. (2007) "Blood levels of mercury are related to diagnosis of autism: a reanalysis of an important data set." *J Child Neurol* 22: 1308–1311.

81   Geier, David A. et al. "Blood mercury levels in autism spectrum disorder: Is there a threshold level?" *Acta Neurobiol Exp* 2010, 70: 177–186.

measurements were made. Finding or not finding elevated mercury years later does not and cannot rule out mercury as a precipitating factor in the etiology of autism.

The researchers assumed incorrectly that autistic children metabolized mercury in the same way as non-autistic children. They don't. It isn't surprising that the Hertz-Picciotto team wound up with bizarre and implausible data.

This failed study, therefore, contributes no useful information in regard to the role of the suspected mercury and thimerosal linkage to autism. Its conclusions are meaningless.

"Mercury Free" Vaccines Today Are Not Mercury Free

Thimerosal is still being used in the production of many vaccines that claim to have no or only trace amounts of this ethyl mercury toxin present after it has allegedly been filtered out of the final product.

However mercury binds to the antigenic protein in the vaccines and cannot be completely removed.[82]

Testing of four sample vaccines by Doctors Data Lab revealed that all contained mercury even though two were labeled "mercury free," and all four vials were found to contain aluminum shown to enhance the toxicity of thimerosal and promote neuronal cell death.[83]

A Fifteenth Negative Study: Wright, B. et al. "A Comparison of Urinary Mercury between Children with Autism Spectrum Disorders and Control Children." (2012) *PLoS ONE* 7(2): e29547.doi:10.1371/journal.pone.0029547. Received: September 20, 2011; Published: February 15, 2012.[84]

In this misguided British study, led by Barry Wright, the researchers "set out to test whether mercury concentrations in the urine of children with autism were significantly increased or decreased compared to controls or siblings."

To accomplish this task, blinded urine mercury (and other metals) analyses were carried out on the *morning urines* of 56 autistic children, 42 of their siblings, 121 control children with no symptoms of autism spectrum disorders and 34 non-ASD children who attended special schools.

Wright and colleagues found no significant difference in the mercury levels in the autistic children as compared to any of the other groups. Their conclusion: "This study lends no support for the hypothesis of differences in urinary mercury excretion in children with autism compared to other groups. Some of the results, however, do suggest further research in the area may be warranted to replicate this in a larger group and with clear measurement of potential confounding factors."

Critique:

- The four groups of children participating in this study were neither age nor sex matched. In fact, there were significant differences in both age and gender between the various groups.

- There was *no mention* of the ages of any of the children or when they last received their immunizations, or what immunizations they received, or what the mercury content of those immunizations might have been, or what their intake of fish was or what their exposure to other mercury sources was.

- The analysis of mercury concentration in a random urine sample is not an appropriate way to measure body burden of mercury, even from previous chronic exposure, although chronic continuous exposures will raise mercury levels in those able to excrete mercury. Mercury, as has been mentioned, bonds strongly to fatty tissues, as found in the brain, and to sulfhydryl groups found in proteins throughout the body.

82   Boyd Haley, Ph.D., chemist
83   http://www.whale.to/a/mercury7.html
84   http://www.plosone.org/article/info:doi percent2F10.1371 percent2Fjournal.pone.0029547

- In their study design, the researchers apparently ignored a good deal of research that demonstrates that autistic children have an impaired ability to excrete mercury, even though journal articles supporting that contention were referenced and acknowledged by the authors.

- In that regard, the authors could and should have obtained a *chelated* urine specimen (for toxic metals analysis) on the children, but they didn't.

- Or they could and should also have analyzed the children's urine for porphyrins that reflect mercury burden, but they didn't.

- It is reasonable to assume that an autistic child with a large mercury burden might excrete a much smaller amount of this toxic metal than would a child with good detoxification ability. This could conceivably result in the urine concentrations of mercury in both the autistic and non-autistic groups being equivalent, which would lead the uninformed to the fallacious conclusion that the mercury *burden* in both cohorts was equivalent when it wasn't, and that the *ability to excrete mercury* was similar, when it wasn't.

- Over a long enough period of time, even autistic children with impaired detoxification may eventually be able to rid themselves of much of their mercury load. This does not mean that at an earlier period of their life there did not exist a body burden of mercury sufficient to promote autism.

- The authors quote in support of their fallacious conclusion the many corrupt studies we have reviewed that mislead the reader into concluding that there is no association between immunizations, thimerosal, and autism when the evidence strongly suggests otherwise.

Conclusion: This is another truly terrible study with non-age or sex matched controls, no mention of age of participants, no consideration in study design of the proven disability of most autistic children to detoxify mercury well, no mention of immunization status, or the mercury intake from the children's diet or from thimerosal-containing immunizations they might have received, or the time since their last immunization. The body burden of mercury of each child so examined would have to have been determined to see whether the urine concentrations of mercury measured paralleled the body burden. This wasn't done. The study's conclusion is, therefore, invalid.

So What Have We Learned?

We have analyzed the fifteen commonly cited journal studies and one review article that purport to disprove the link between thimerosal, mercury, and the autism epidemic, and have found *all of them faulty*, and most of them likely to have been intentionally designed and manipulated to negate the thimerosal-autism linkage.

There are thus no credible scientific studies that validate the commonly held belief that "many studies show there is no association between thimerosal-containing vaccines and autism."

And we have reviewed over two-dozen confirmative studies that provide damning evidence that mercury poisoning from thimerosal in immunizations contributes to and is causally related to the worldwide epidemic of autism, ADHD, and other neurodevelopmental disorders that are now manifest, and that that association is most certainly biologically plausible.

> *"The medical establishment has become a major threat to health…. The disabling impact of professional control over medicine has reached the propotions of an epidemic."*
>
> — Ivan Illich, Medical Nemesis (1976)

> *"The great enemy of the truth is very often not the lie…deliberate, contrived, dishonest, but the myth, persistent, persuasive, and unrealistic. Belief in myth allows the comfort of opinion without the discomfort of thought."*
>
> — John F. Kennedy

HOW AND WHY "TO OBFUSCATE THE FALLING AUTISM RATES"

In 2005, when it appeared that autism rates were starting to decrease coincident with the removal of Thimerosal from the vaccines in the routine schedule, the CDC significantly broadened its flu-shot recommendations, so that by age 5 years children exposed to an all-Thimerosal schedule of flu shots would get 53 percent of the mercury children received from all shots in 1999. If this was done on purpose, to obfuscate the falling autism rates, there was a reason.

The WHO (World Health Organization) Strategic Group of Experts (SAGE) met in June of 2001, and stated their objective clearly: "WHO was extremely anxious to preserve the production of vaccines. Industry is expecting clear signals from WHO on the Thiomersal issue, and has been confirmed by informal consultations with some manufacturers during the first half of 2001." At the WHO HQ in Geneva, a meeting was held on May 21 2002.[85]

From the meeting summary more [concerns] were enumerated, such as: (1) Obtaining regulatory approval for the new formulated Thiomersal-reduced or removed vaccines involves complex activities that are costly and time consuming; (2) WHO is concerned about the current situation whereby manufacturers in developed countries have been forced to lower the Thiomersal content of their vaccines; (3) The option of using single dose vaccines is not feasible for WHO... upgrading the infrastructure would result in [a] huge increase in vaccine cost.

The meeting memo went on to state, "In view of the situation, WHO is faced with...support maintenance of Thimerosal as an effective preservative in multidose and possibly also in single dose vaccines."

Lastly, the memo stated, "The actions required from WHO in order to ensure continued availability of these vaccines include the following: ...Develop a strong advocacy campaign to support ongoing use of Thimerosal."[86]

— Dr. Ken Stoller[87]

In other words, the World Health Organization could not afford to use the pricier but safer Thimerosal-free vaccines and thus encouraged support for the continued use of Thimerosal in spite of its known harm to children.

Keep in mind that WHO representatives attended the infamous CDC-sponsored conference in 2000 in Norcross, Georgia where Thomas Verstraeten revealed that thimerosal-containing vaccines likely caused autism, hyperactivity, tics, speech delays, and other developmental abnormalities.

And did the CDC recommend the use of influenza vaccinations (with thimerosal) in pregnant women and babies (shown not to be protective) in order to blunt the decrease in autism incidence that briefly followed the partial phase out of thimerosal?

A scary thought.

---

85   WHO informal meeting on removal of Thiomersal from vaccines and its implications for global vaccine supply.
86   Stoller, K.P. Medical Veritas, 2006; 3: 772-780.
87   Geier, D.A., Geier, M.R. "Early downward trends in neurodevelopmental disorders following removal of Thimerosal containing vaccines." *J Amer Physicians and Surgeons*, 2006; 11(1):8–13.

"TOBACCO SCIENCE?"

There is "a long list of studies on vaccines and neurological disorders in children that are at a minimum fatally flawed but more often complete misrepresentations of the truth.

"Starting in 1999, when the CDC buried strong associations between thimerosal exposure early in life (0 to 1 month), where infants exposed to the highest levels of thimerosal possible were at least 7.6 times more likely to receive an autism diagnosis through this current study, there has been developed a full body of "tobacco science" designed to hide the truth of what has been found behind closed doors.

"It is time for the CDC to come clean. Their own data show that vaccines cause neurodevelopmental disorders in children including autism."

— Brian Hooker, Ph.D.

"I think that the biological case against Thimerosal is so dramatically overwhelming anymore that only a very foolish or a very dishonest person with the credentials to understand this research would say that Thimerosal wasn't most likely the cause of autism."

— Boyd Haley, Ph.D. (2006)

Chapter 17
Why We Need to Be Skeptical About Medical Journal Studies

"I can prove anything by statistics except the truth."

— *George Canning*

"The term "perception management" has firmly entered the public lexicon…
Perception managers are not spin doctors, because they don't spin facts.
They create facts and then sell them to the world as the truth.
And that, to quote the venerable Mark Twain, is the difference between the
lightning bug and lightning.
By using these methods, a major untruth can be established so quickly and
overwhelmingly across the world that no digging by anyone after the fact can
make a dent in public consciousness that it actually isn't true at all.
And that's precisely what makes it so dangerous."

— *David Baldacci, "The Whole Truth"*

THESE SO CALLED *"negative studies" are replete with bias, errors and fraud. How common is this? Should we be losing faith in the integrity of "peer-reviewed" medical journals?*

Expunged Research

In an article published in the *Journal of Medical Ethics*, the study author, Grant Steen, reviewed the PubMed database from the years 2000-2010, looking for every scientific research paper that had been officially expunged from the public record. About 78 records *each year* had been retracted for a total of 788 during the ten-year period of evaluation. A total of 545 of these papers were withdrawn because of a serious error. The remaining retractions were attributed to deliberate fraud: the falsification or fabrication of data.

Mr. Steen discovered that over half of the faked research papers had been written by a lead author who had submitted other fraudulent research articles. Bogus research papers were more likely to have multiple authors, many of whom had additional research papers retracted as well.

Keep in mind that the number of fraudulent or defective studies that Mr. Steen evaluated most likely represents only a small fraction of the papers that should have been withdrawn, but weren't, largely due to a notable lack of critical peer review in the so-called "peer reviewed" journals in which they were published.[1]

---

1   Steen, G. "Retractions in the scientific literature: do authors deliberately commit research fraud?" *J. Med. Ethics*. 2010; doi: 10.1136/jme.2010.038125.

Why Do Researchers Fake Papers?

"It's all about money," says Heidi Stevenson writing for *Gaia Health*. "Get published in a major medical journal and your future is made." According to Richard Horton, an editor of the British medical journal *The Lancet*, "A single paper in *Lancet* and you get your chair and you get your money. It's your passport to success."[2]

Researchers may also "fake" papers by manipulating data and statistical analyses for the purpose of achieving a particular result.

What Is Wrong with the Peer Review Process That Allows All These Manipulated Studies to Be Published?

There is little incentive for peer reviewers to do a thorough job. They are generally unpaid or minimally paid for their work, they are anonymous, and their competence varies from journal to journal.

"Most peer reviewers are doing their own studies," continues Ms. Stevenson. "That's what makes them peers. They want to be able to publish. Therefore, they are not particularly inclined to make more than perfunctory negative comments. Obviously, they don't want to alienate the authors of papers, since they either are or hope to become published themselves."

She adds, "Peer review is a farce. The only kind of review that makes real sense is professional independent reviewers. Yet, for decades we've had peer review trotted out as the be-all and end-all in determining the legitimacy of papers. It's been unquestioned, while a little examination of the concept demonstrates that it's nearly certain to result in fraudulent work being passed as good science."[3]

> *"Trust me, Wilbur. People are very gullible. They'll believe anything they see in print."*
>
> — E.B. White, Charlotte's Web

What About Institutional Review Boards (IRBs) That Must Review Each Study Before It Is Allowed to Proceed? How Can They Have Condoned So Many Poorly Done and Manipulated Studies?

Again, it's all about the money. The for-profit IRBs are paid by the companies and individuals hoping to get FDA approval for their products and studies. If an IRB turns down a research project, the researchers may simply approach another IRB that is less stringent in its criteria. An IRB that is known to be "friendly" is likely to make more money.

One such company, Coast IRB LLC of Colorado Springs, actually approved a fictitious study of a fictitious product made by a fictitious company named Phake Medical Devices. The principal researchers were listed as April Phuls, Timothy Witless, and Alan Ruse. The company's location was alleged to be in Chetesville, Arizona. Coast somehow missed all these not-so-subtle clues.

Congress, aware of possible IRB conflicts of interest and in conjunction with the Department of Health and Human Services, had perpetrated this sting operation, and Coast IRB got "stung." It had actually approved not only this study (without reading the documentation), but it had also approved an earlier research protocol for another non-existent product ("Adhesiabloc") made by another non-existent company (Device Med-Systems) in a previous sting. Congress subpoenaed Coast's CEO, who, instead of admitting guilt, questioned the legality of the Congressional investigation. Amazingly, no legal action was taken against Coast IRB, which met its demise due to the bad publicity.[4]

---

2   http://www.gaia-health.com/articles501/000510-drug-study-corruption.shtml
3   Ibid.
4   http://www.gaia-health.com/articles351/000378-system-sting.shtml

Biased Reporting

Biases are the rule rather than the exception in most research, and good researchers try to acknowledge this in their medical journal.[Ibid.] There are many kinds of bias, and these include design bias, sampling bias, procedural bias, measurement bias, publishing bias, and reporting bias among others.

The prestigious *New England Journal of Medicine,* for example, published (in 2000) a now infamous study on the since withdrawn anti-inflammatory drug *Vioxx,* which noted an increase in myocardial infarctions (heart attacks) in *Vioxx* users, but which also attempted to minimize this concern.

Criticisms about the interpretation of that study were raised in 2001; the drug was withdrawn in 2004 by Merck, but it wasn't until December 2005 that the *NEJM* editors expressed concern about the validity of the original study.

During that five-year hiatus, the journal received over $800,000 for article reprints that Merck used for advertising purposes. The *NEJM* was publicly rebuked for this delay in other medical journals.[5]

If It Looks Like a Medical Journal and Smells…

If it looks like a medical journal, reads like a medical journal, and calls itself a journal, is it a medical journal?

Not necessarily.

Australian doctors who were provided with copies of the *Australasian Journal of Bone and Joint Medicine,* which featured articles boosting Merck products like Fosamax and Vioxx, were likely unaware that it was not only not peer reviewed but was not even a medical journal at all. It was a ruse, a fake, a scam, a deliberately deceptive means of advertising for Merck disguised as a medical journal.[6]

And it was published by *Exerpta Medica,* a respected division of scientific publishing giant Reed Elsevier, which has published other fake medical journals in addition to its catalog of "legitimate" publications like *The Lancet.*

Merck paid *Exerpta Medica* an unknown amount to deceive the medical community. Nowhere in the *Australasian Journal of Bone and Joint Medicine* was there any mention that it was anything other than a valid medical journal. There was no disclosure of company sponsorship whatsoever.

And Merck was not alone…

Between 2000 and 2005, Elsevier/*Excerpta Medica* published six other phony journals, all financed by various undeclared drug companies, which were intended to mislead physicians while promoting those companies' drugs. These so called journals included the *Australasian Journal of General Practice,* the *Australasian Journal of Neurology,* the *Australasian Journal of Cardiology,* the *Australasian Journal of Clinical Pharmacy,* the *Australasian Journal of Cardiovascular Medicine,* and the *Australasian Journal of Bone & Joint [Medicine].*[7]

> *"The* BMJ *reported…that the Murdoch empire's flagship newspaper in Australia has accepted an undisclosed amount of sponsorship money from the drug industry for a series of articles on health policy—and that the idea arose from a meeting between advertising agents."*
>
> *— Journalist Ray Moynihan reporting on the* British Medical Journal *findings "Is journalism the drug industry's new dance partner?"*[8]

---

5   http://en.wikipedia.org/wiki/The_New_England_Journalof_Medicine
6   "Merck published fake journal." *The Scientist—Magazine of the Life Sciences.* http://www.the-scientist.com/blog/display/ 55671/#ixzz 1ZaLivWZO- 30th April 2009
7   "Elsevier published 6 fake journals." *The Scientist—Magazine of the Life Sciences.* http://www.the-scientist.com/blog/ display/55679/#ixzz1ZfVehZgn
8   *BMJ.* Nov 2 2011;343:d6978

Amazing Revelations: Science for Sale?

In her two revealing books,[9] Marcia Angell, M.D. makes some incredible statements. She declares that, "It is simply no longer possible to believe much of the clinical research that is published, or to rely on the judgment of trusted physicians or authoritative medical guidelines. I take no pleasure in this conclusion, which I reached slowly and reluctantly over my two decades as an editor of *The New England Journal of Medicine....* Trials can be rigged in a dozen ways, and it happens all the time."

Richard Smith, a former editor of the equally prestigious *British Medical Journal* and chief executive of the BMJ Publishing Group from 1991 to 2004, agrees with Dr. Angell. He states that, "Sadly I followed the same path and spelt out my disillusionment in my "j'accuse" book *The Trouble with Medical Journals.* I wrote it in 2004, and since then my pessimism has deepened."[10]

And the current editor-in-chief of *The Lancet*, Dr. Richard Horton, affirmed Smith and Angell's assertions. He declared that. "Much of the scientific literature, perhaps half, may simply be untrue. Afflicted by studies with small sample sizes, tiny effects, invalid exploratory analyses, and flagrant conflicts of interest, together with an obsession for pursuing fashionable trends of dubious importance, science has taken a turn towards darkness."[11]

EPA research microbiologist Dr. David L. Lewis (Ph.D.) was dismayed by the corruption he was seeing, and he filed a lawsuit against EPA scientists for covering up problems with chemicals in "organic fertilizers (biosolids) linked to autism."

He also thoroughly investigated and refuted the false charges leveled by "journalist" Brian Deer and others against Dr. Andrew Wakefield, a physician and researcher who had published a study suggesting a possible connection between the MMR vaccine, intestinal inflammation, and regressive autism. That study and the ensuing saga will be discussed in greater detail later in this narrative.

Dr. Lewis recently published his own exposé book *Science for Sale: How the U.S. Government uses powerful corporations and leading universities to support government policies, silence top scientists, jeopardize our health, and protect corporate profits.*[12]

Greek epidemiologist John Ioannidis analyzed a good deal of published scientific literature and concluded that there is *less than a 50 percent chance* that the results of a randomly selected scientific study will be true.[13]

Conflicts of Interest at Universities

"In a [November 2009] report, Daniel R. Levinson, the inspector general of the Department of Health and Human Services, said 90 percent of universities relied solely on the researchers themselves to decide whether the money they made in consulting and other relationships with drug and device makers was relevant to their government-financed research.

"And half of [the] universities do not ask their faculty members to disclose the amount of money or stock they make from drug and device makers, so the potential for extensive conflicts with their government-financed research is often known only to the researchers themselves, the report concluded."[14]

Dr. Arnold Belman, former Editor-in-Chief of the *New England Journal of Medicine* and Harvard Professor of Medicine said, "The medical profession is being bought by the pharmaceutical industry, not only in terms of the practice of medicine, but also in terms of teaching and research. The academic institutions of this country are allowing themselves to be the paid agents of the pharmaceutical industry. I think it's disgraceful."

9   *Drug Companies, Doctors: A Story of Corruption* and *The Truth about Drug Companies: How They Deceive Us and What to Do About It*
10   Alliance for Human Research Protection; http://www.ahrp. org/ cms/ content/view/734/9/
11   http://nsnbc.me/2015/06/19/shocking-report-from-medical-insiders/
12   http://www.ashotoftruth.org/blog/epa-microbiologist-dr-david-lewis-wrote-book-research-misconduct-then-throws-book-brian-deer
13   *PLOS Medicine.* August 20, 2005.
14   http://www.nytimes.com/2009/11/19/health/policy/19nih.html -article by Gardiner Harriss

Conflicts of Interest: Industry, Institutions, and Journals

Conflicts of interest with industry and institutions are extremely common in published research, and studies show that *financial and non-financial bias inappropriately influences study results and conclusions.* This may manifest as data withholding or a tendency to exaggerate or misinterpret the results in favor of the product under study, or even whether a given study gets published or not.

Evidence that the pharmaceutical industry's financial influence can and does bias journal articles is found in many medical journal articles (see references below) and in a PLoS (Public Library of Science) Medicine study entitled "Conflicts of Interest at Medical Journals: The Influence of Industry-Supported Randomized Trials on Journal Impact Factors and Revenue – Cohort Study."[15]

In this review of six prestigious medical journals, the researchers found that up to 75 percent of the published articles (in the *New England Journal of Medicine*, for example) were funded solely or in part by the pharmaceutical industry, and that by selling multiple reprints of a single article to the industry that funded the study, the journal could net upwards of $700,000 (or more).

The study authors concluded that, "Publication of industry-supported trials was associated with an increase in journal impact factors. Sales of reprints may provide a substantial income." And they suggested that "journals disclose financial information in the same way that they require them from their authors, so that readers can assess the potential effect of different types of papers on journals' revenue and impact."

But journals don't do this.

Former *BMJ* editor Richard Smith points out that the money generated by publishing-industry sponsored trials is substantial:

> It's thus very tempting to publish that drug company sponsored trial, and the temptation is increased further by such trials boosting impact factors, as the PloS Medicine paper shows. Such trials are well cited partly because they are important and partly because drug companies have considerable resources to promote the papers, not least by distributing hundreds of thousands of reprints.

> The PloS Medicine authors calculate that the impact factor of the *New England Journal of Medicine* would be reduced by about 15 percent if it declined to publish Drug Company sponsored trials. And high impact factor scores, he points out mean "not only prestige but also more important papers, more subscriptions, and so more money.[16]

"13 percent of the members of FDA advisory committees in the Center for Drug Evaluation and Research (CDER) have a financial interest in the company whose drug is up for committee review."

— Pham-Kanter, G. Milbank Quarterly, 92(3)2014;446f.

Ghostwritten Publications?

To make matters worse, some journal articles and even textbooks are actually "ghost written," and the ghost writer's conflicts of interest are generally not listed in the study's disclosure section. When ghostwritten, credit for the study's authorship often goes to an individual *who may have had nothing to do with the study at all.*

Drug manufacturer Wyeth, for example, provided various medical journals with forty ghostwritten articles that listed distinguished physicians as authors who weren't actually involved in any way in the paper's research or writing. These prominent men had simply allowed their names to be sold for cash, and perhaps they also benefited from the

15   Lundh, Andreas et al. http://www.plosmedicine.org/article/info percent3Adoi percent2F10.1371 percent2Fjournal.pmed.1000354
16   http://www.ahrp.org/cms/content/view/734/9/

pseudo-prestige of having appeared to author a study. Wyeth instigated this deception in a failed attempt to neutralize the evidence that linked its dying cash cow *Prempro* to breast cancer.[17]

According to the Alliance for Human Research Protection,[18] "A letter of complaint by the Project on Government Oversight (POGO) was sent to the director of the National Institutes of Health…documenting $66.8 million in NIH grants that were awarded to a handful of psychiatrists who penned their name to ghostwritten scientific publications." That means that the U.S. taxpayer has paid a great deal of money to psychiatrists for work that they didn't do.

The instances identified in that letter involve ghostwriting by only one company—Scientific Therapeutics Information (STI)—and (promoting) only one drug—GlaxoSmithKline's anti-depressant, *Paxil* (peroxetine).

Duff Wilson of *The New York Times* reports that previously sealed Glaxo-SmithKline documents show that a psychiatry textbook, whose listed authors are psychiatrists, Charles Nemeroff, MD and Alan Schatzberg, MD, was actually ghostwritten by Sally Laden of STI. GSK paid the ghostwriter and the "authors" who penned their names to the book.

"A New Level of Chutzpah?"

The sheer audacity of this fraud prompted former FDA commissioner Dr. David Kessler to exclaim: "To ghostwrite an entire textbook is a new level of chutzpah. I've never heard of that before. It takes your breath away. Surely that is a dubious distinction in academic medicine!"[19]

And the Deceit Goes On…

An editorial in the *British Medical Journal* in 2011 stated that:

> Inappropriate authorship (honorary and ghost authorship) is an important issue for the academic and research community and is a threat to the integrity of scientific publication.

> Our findings suggest that 21 percent of articles published in 2008 in the general medical journals with the highest impact factors had an inappropriate honorary author, and that nearly eight percent of articles published in these journals may have had an unnamed important contributor.

> The highest prevalence of both types of inappropriate authorship occurred in original research articles, compared with editorials and review articles.

> …Both honorary and ghost authorship are unacceptable in scientific publications, and each form of inappropriate authorship has important consequences.

> …Honorary authorship has implications for scientific integrity…. Likewise ghost authorship has important implications and consequences. If unidentified authors are involved in the work and manuscript preparation, readers not only will be unaware of the contributions, perspectives, and affiliations of these individuals, but also may not appreciate the influence or potential underlying agenda these individuals may have on the reporting of material in the article (such as may occur with ghost authors employed by industry).[20]

Suppression of Criticism of Studies

Medical journals often receive comments and criticisms of their published studies, but are under no obligation to print these. Criticism of studies is a valid form of *real* peer review. When a journal refuses to publish *legitimate* criticism, it is engaging in deliberate deception and fraud.

---

17   Associated Press. "Judge orders Wyeth papers unsealed." July 25, 2009.
18   AHRP is a national network of lay people and professionals dedicated to advancing responsible and ethical medical research practices, to ensure that the human rights, dignity, and welfare of human subjects are protected, and to minimize the risks associated with such endeavors.
19   http://www.ahrp.org/cms/content/view/738/150/
20   *BMJ* 2011; 343: d6128

A relevant example of this censorship was provided by Dr. David Ayoub at the Toxic Children, Toxic Lies Rally at the American Academy of Pediatrics (AAP) headquarters in Chicago, Illinois in 2008, at which he highlighted three key epidemiological studies published in the AAP journal *Pediatrics* that purported to show no relationship between vaccines and autism. These were the Madsen, the Verstraeten, and the Fombonne Quebec studies.

According to Dr. Ayoub, who had himself analyzed the Fombonne study data:

> The editor-in-chief (of *Pediatrics*) Dr Jerald Lucey received numerous, substantiated criticisms of each of these studies, but has created an effective roadblock in disallowing any criticisms to be published in the letter to the editor section of the journal. His response to thoughtful and reasonable criticisms has been unprofessional, illogical and insulting. My own letter to Lucey criticizing the Fombonne study was not even allowed to be published on the less publically visible online forum, even though we had obtained a copy of the Fombonne database and vaccine records from several parents proving Fombonne's work fraudulent.[21]

"If we believe absurdities, we will commit atrocities."

— *Voltaire*

Suppression or Delay of Publication of Studies

According to a study published in the *British Medical Journal*, a good deal of drug research, even if sponsored by the federal government, never gets published. In fact "less than half of all NIH-funded clinical drug trials were published in a medical journal within two and a half years of the trial's completion—with fully one-third of trial results remaining unpublished even four years after the trial. Why? Because the drug manufacturers didn't like the data."

Some examples:

- **Avandia Studies:** GlaxoSmithKline knew that its drug Avandia increased the risk of heart attacks and deaths long before the drug had been approved by the FDA, but it hid that information. Of the drug's 42 studies, *only 7 were published*. The other 35 studies, which showed evidence of harm, were only obtained when legal proceedings forced GSK to turn over the data. Where was the FDA?

- **Infuse Study:** An independent analysis by the editor of *Spine Journal* revealed that Medtronic and a group of orthopedic surgeons who were paid millions in royalties from the company to participate in a clinical trial of Medtronic's bone-growth stimulating back surgery product (Infuse) "systematically failed to report serious complications," like unwanted bone growth, which caused the clinical trial to be suspended. However, the results of that unfortunate trial were not published for another *five* years! Where was the FDA?

- **Vytorin Study:** Vytorin was Schering-Plough's attempt to enter the cholesterol-lowering drug market, but it had a problem. The results of its own clinical trial revealed that Vytorin was of *no benefit* in improving artery health. What to do? Schering-Plough elected not to publish the study, and to continue to market the drug. It took a 2008 congressional hearing to put a halt to the advertising campaign. Where was the FDA?

- **Multaq Trial:** Multaq was promoted as a drug to treat cardiac arrhythmias. However, a clinical trial of the drug had to be halted in 2003 because more patients who received the drug were dying than were the control group patients who got the placebo. The study wasn't published for five years (2008), and despite the study failure, the FDA actually approved the drug in 2009 for the treatment of atrial fibrillation, even though it knew that it would likely increase the mortality rate in users! The FDA perhaps forgot that the

---

21   http://www.whale.to/vaccine/ayoub9.html

reason for treating atrial fibrillation is to prevent deaths (from emboli and strokes).

- **Bayer's AG Birth Control Pills:** These pills were shown to cause dangerous blood clots; nevertheless, FDA advisers declared that the benefits of four of Bayer's popular birth control pills outweighed the risks. *The Wall Street Journal* revealed that "three of those advisers had ties to Bayer, serving as consultants, speakers or researchers!" The FDA somehow failed to mention that![22]

Why Do Scientists Agree to Participate in Corrupt Studies?

Scientists are human beings, and they are subject to the same influences as the rest of us. If they wish to keep their jobs and please the governmental or corporate authorities that pay them, many will, of necessity, follow the research direction of their sponsors, even if that means that proper methodological or analytical procedures are compromised in a deliberate effort to manipulate the ultimate results. "Bending" science for personal, financial, legal, or political gain, as we have seen, is not a rare occurrence.

Scientists are also generally aware of what happens when one supports an unpopular position. Whistleblowers often lose their jobs and their reputations. Here are just a few of many examples:

- **Ignatz Semmelweis** (1818-1865) was a Hungarian physician who was condemned by his peers for suggesting that proper handwashing prior to performing gynecological procedures could save lives. That position ultimately cost him his reputation and sanity.

- **Arpad Pusztai**, a renowned scientist, was fired for showing that the process of artificially creating genetically-modified foods is inherently dangerous.

- **Herbert Needleman** was pilloried for his research demonstrating that lead, even at very low blood levels, caused a diminishment of IQ in children. He was ultimately exonerated.

- **Andrew Wakefield** and his colleagues have been maliciously and irresponsibly attacked for alleged ethical violations and the quality of their research regarding the possible relationship between the MMR vaccine, regressive autism, and inflammatory bowel disease, and Wakefield has lost his license to practice medicine as a result. Wakefield's story will be detailed later in this narrative.

In their book, *Bending Science: How Special Interests Corrupt Public Health Research*, authors Tom McGarity and Wendy Wagner state, "There is every reason to believe that…reports of scientific harassment…represent the tip of a much larger iceberg."[23] Attorney Fredrick Anderson agrees and alleges that "well organized campaigns against certain types of research and the researchers that conduct them do appear to be on the rise."[24]

The message: If you want to keep your job, toe the line! Don't make waves!

> *"The thing that bugs me is that the people think the FDA is protecting them. It isn't. What the FDA is doing and what the public thinks it's doing are as different as day and night."*
>
> — *Dr. Herbert Ley, former commissioner of the FDA (1968-9)*

So what's going on with the FDA, the CDC, and the American Academy of Pediatrics (AAP)?

These agencies are heavily conflicted. The FDA receives major funding from drug companies, and many FDA scientists and politicians have expectations that Big Pharma will hire them at top salaries when they leave the Food and Drug Administration. So "Do not bite the hand that will soon feed you" may be the mantra for many at the FDA.

---

22   http://true-conspiracies.com/big-pharma-fda-conspiracy/ and Editorial: Missing clinical trial data; BMJ 2012; 344 doi: 10.1136/bmj.d8158 (Published 3 January 2012)

23   Ibid. 120

24   Anderson, F. "Science Advocacy and Scientific Due Process." *Issues in Science and Technology* 16 (Summer 2000): 71, 74.

CDC officers, like Dr. Jay Lieberman, are often heavily conflicted as well. Lieberman, for example, has affiliations with several major drug companies and serves on the speaker's bureau for three vaccine manufacturers. Dr. Lieberman was not alone in this regard. A report released in 2009 found that the CDC was lax in screening "medical experts" for financial conflicts when they were hired to advise the agency on vaccine safety. Some of these *experts* "were legally barred from considering the issues but did so anyway."[25]

The CDC believes in pushing the agenda of more and more vaccines and has suppressed or manipulated data supporting the vaccine-autism link. This was confirmed by whistleblower and senior CDC scientist William Thompson, who revealed that his bosses at the CDC pressured him into altering the results of studies that he was involved in so as to show no association between immunizations and autism.

"I have a boss who is asking me to lie," confesses Dr. Thompson. "The higher ups wanted to do certain things and I went along with it…in terms of chain in command, I was number four out of the five. Colleen [Boyle] was the Division Chief. Marshalyn [Yeargin-Allsopp] was a Branch Chief. Frank [DeStefano] was a Branch Chief at the time."[26]

As for the AAP, Dr. Ayoub has stated the problem succinctly: "The AAP reports annual revenues of about $70 million, but only 1/4th comes from membership dues. Their website lists extensive corporate donors, none more generous than the vaccine makers. Their journal *Pediatrics* generates about $10,000 per page for a drug ad, translating into $200,000 monthly. Even more money is generated for reprint orders, often 6 figures, that are distributed to pediatricians without of course the criticisms."[27]

Pediatricians make a lot of their money from well-baby and well-child visits during which babies and older children generally receive immunizations. Evidence that questions the safety of immunizations would most certainly have an adverse effect on the revenue stream of these pediatricians.

The Bottom Line

As should now be apparent, the devious immunization and thimerosal studies that we have just reviewed with their improper protocols, mathematical errors, data withholding, data misinterpretation, censorship of criticism, and intentional fraud are, unfortunately, not unique in the field of medical "research."

What is supposed to be "evidence-based medicine," unfortunately, sometimes turns out to be "evidence-biased medicine," and so-called "peer reviewed studies" are too often "poor(ly) reviewed studies." Or as Joseph Mercola, M.D. puts it, "It's become quite clear that instead of evidence-based decision making we now have decision-based evidence making."

Therefore, we must read all journal articles (and textbooks too) with a more skeptical eye, especially those sponsored, designed, or written by individuals, industry, or governmental agencies with significant conflicts of interest.

"We may need to seek them out and destroy them where they live."

(From a Merck internal memo referring to the need to "neutralize" dissent from those doctors who questioned the safety of Vioxx.)

Rout, M. 4/1/09; Vioxx Maker Merck & Co. Drew up Doctor Hit List. Retrieved from http:// aftermathnews.wordpress.com/2009/04/27/vioxx-maker-merck-and-co-drew-up-doctor-hit-list/

---

25   www.nytimes/2009/12/18/health/policy/18cdc.htm l?_r=0

26   http://www.ageofautism.com/2015/02/robert-kennedy-jr-cdc-scientist-still-maintains-agency-forced-researchers-to-lie-about-safety-of-mer.html?utm_source=feedburner&utm_medium=email&utm_campaign=Feed percent3A+ageofautism+ percent28AGE+OF+A UTISM percent29

27   http://www.whale.to/ vaccine/ayoub9.html

Some Relevant References

Als-Nielsen, B. et al. "Association of funding and conclusions in randomized drug trials: a reflection of treatment effect or adverse events?" *JAMA*. 2003. 290: 921–8. DOI:10.1001/jama.290.7.921. PMID 12928469. Research Blogging.

Bloomberg.com "Lilly to Pay $22.5 Million to Settle Zyprexa Suit (Update3)." Retrieved Oct 29, 2009.

Blumenthal, D.; Campbell, E.G.; Anderson, M.S.; Causino, N.; Louis, K.S. "Withholding research results in academic life science. Evidence from a national survey of faculty." 1997. *JAMA* 277: 1224–8. PMID 9103347.

Blumenthal, D. et al. "Participation of life-science faculty in research relationships with industry." *N Engl J Med*. 1996. 335: 1734–9. PMID 8929266.

Blumenthal, D. et al. "Relationships between academic institutions and industry in the life sciences—an industry survey." *N Engl J Med*. 1996. 334: 368–73. PMID 8538709.

Chimonas, Susan; Frosch, Zachary Frosch; Rothman, David J. "From Disclosure to Transparency: The Use of Company Payment Data. *Arch Intern Med*. 2010. DOI:archinternmed.2010.341 35

DeLong, Gayle. "Conflicts of Interest in Vaccine Safety Research." Accountability in Research. 19:65-88. 2012; Copyright © Taylor & Francis Group. LLC ISSN: 0898-9621 DOI: 10.1080108989621.2012.660073

Friedberg, M. et al. "Evaluation of conflict of interest in economic analyses of new drugs used in oncology." *JAMA*. 1999. 282: 1453–7. PMID 10535436. 32

Fugh-Berman, Adriane J. "Ethical considerations of publication planning in the pharmaceutical industry." *Text.Serial.Journal*. Dec 22, 2008. Retrieved Dec 26, 2008.

Ioannidis, John P.A. "Why Most Published Research Findings Are False." http://www.plosmedicine.org/ article/ info:doi/10.1371/journal.pmed.0020124

Laine, C.; Mulrow. C.D. "Exorcising ghosts and unwelcome guests." *Ann Intern Med*. 2005. 143: 611–2. PMID 16230729.

Lexchin, J. et al. "Pharmaceutical industry sponsorship and research outcome and quality: systematic review." *BMJ*. 2003. 326: 1167–70. DOI:10.1136/bmj.326.7400.1167. PMID 12775614. Research Blogging.

Melander, H. et al. "Evidence b(i)ased medicine—selective reporting from studies sponsored by pharmaceutical industry: review of studies in new drug applications." *BMJ*. 2003. 326: 1171–3. DOI:10.1136/bmj.326.7400.1171. PMID 12775615. Research Blogging.

Nieto, A. et al. "Adverse effects of inhaled corticosteroids in funded and nonfunded studies." *Arch Intern Med*. 2007. 167: 2047–53. DOI:10.1001/archinte.167.19.2047. PMID 17954797. Research Blogging.

Papanikolaou, G.N. et al. "Reporting of conflicts of interest in guidelines of preventive and therapeutic interventions." *BMC medical research methodology*. 2001. 1: 3. PMID 11405896.

PLoS Medicine Editors, The. "Making Sense of Non-Financial Competing Interests." *PLoS Medicine*. Vol. 5, No. 9, e199 DOI:10.1371/journal.pmed.0050199 38

Stelfox, H.T. et al. "Conflict of interest in the debate over calcium-channel antagonists." *N Engl J Med*. 2010. 338: 101–6. PMID 9420342. 22 23.0.

Thomas, O. et al. "Industry funding and the reporting quality of large long-term weight loss trials." *Int J Obes* (Lond). 2008. 32 (10): 1531-6. DOI:10.1038/ijo.2008.137. PMID 18711388. PMC PMC2753515. Research Blogging.

Wang, A.T. et al. "Association between industry affiliation and position on cardiovascular risk with rosiglitazone: cross sectional systematic review. *BMJ.* 2010. 340: c1344. DOI:10.1136/bmj.c1344. PMID 20299696. Research Blogging.

Wilson, Duff. "Pfizer Gets Details on Payments to Doctors." *New York Times.* March 31, 2010. http://www.nytimes.com/2010/04/01/business/01payments.html?partner=rss&emc=rss

STRONG WORDS

The politically correct statement would be to say that key individuals from within (the American Academy of Pediatrics/AAP) have gone to great extent to obscure the vaccine-autism connection and by doing so are protecting profits and liability for one of the world's largest and most dangerous industries.

In reality, let me be blunt and politically incorrect. The AAP leadership knows very well that vaccines cause autism. We need not waste any more efforts in trying to educate them, we need to indict them. They may be morally bankrupt, but they are not stupid.

They have lied to legislators, they have lied to journalists, they have lied to pediatricians, and worst of all, they have lied to you and your children.

— Dr. David Ayoub at the the Toxic Children, Toxic Lies Rally ouside the American Academy of Pediatrics Headquarters in Chicago, Illinois in 2008.[28]

---

28   http://www.whale.to/vaccine/ayoub9.html

Chapter 18
Other Sources of Mercury

"The time is always right to do what is right."
— *Martin Luther King, Jr.*

WHAT ARE SOME *Other Sources for Mercury Exposure/Poisoning Besides Immunizations?*
1. Fish

Fish was once considered to be "brain food," but thanks to pollution, we may now consider many fish to be brain-damaging food.

Between 1998 and 2005, scientists from the U.S. Geological Survey scoured the country's streams, rivers, and lakes and collected and tested over 1,000 fish from 291 of those bodies of water and found that *all of the fish had some mercury* and about 25 percent had levels considered to be potentially toxic to humans, according to EPA standards. The fish studied included bass, trout, and catfish.

HEADLINES

*"Fish mercury poisoning warning goes statewide,
W.Va. residents advised to limit eating of sport fish."*

— *Ken Ward Jr.*

Charleston Gazette, *December 14, 2004*
"Mercury levels in Illinois fish exceed federal limits: report."

— *Steve Daniels, April 11, 2006*

"A new report by a local environmental group finds that average mercury levels in fish caught and tested in Illinois between 1984 and 2004 exceeded federal limits by 20 percent."

Crain's, Chicago Daily Business News, *April 11, 2006*

The mercury in these fish is believed to have come from coal-fired power plant emissions and from cement factory dust. The mercury dust from these sources blows in the wind and eventually settles to the earth, enters ground water, streams, and lakes, and is slowly taken up by bacteria and converted into methyl mercury, which gradually becomes incorporated into the cells of small plants and animals, which are, in turn, eaten by larger animals and, ultimately, wind up in the fish that we eat.

The higher up the food chain we go, the greater the amount of mercury we find. Smaller and younger fish usually have less mercury than do larger and older fish.

Blackwater streams on the East Coast and streams that drain mining areas in the West were found to be at particular risk; however, bodies of water in all states have been shown to harbor mercury-contaminated fish, and all but two states have issued warnings regarding the health hazards of eating fish caught in their wild streams, and in particular, they caution consumers about the relatively greater risks to pregnant women and children.

What about salt water fish? They too pose a concern, and as with fresh water fish, the higher up the food chain we go, the greater the risk. In particular, shark, tuna, tile fish, swordfish, and mackerel are cited as often having higher than safe levels of mercury.

The FDA issued this warning in 2004:

> Nearly all fish and shellfish contain traces of mercury. For most people, the risk from mercury by eating fish and shellfish is not a health concern. Yet some fish and shellfish contain higher levels of mercury that may harm an unborn baby or young child's developing nervous system.
>
> The risks from mercury in fish and shellfish depend on the amount of fish and shellfish eaten and the levels of mercury in the fish and shellfish. Therefore, the Food and Drug Administration (FDA) and the Environmental Protection Agency (EPA) are advising women who may become pregnant, pregnant women, nursing mothers, and young children to avoid some types of fish and eat fish and shellfish that are lower in mercury.

No Tuna If You Are Pregnant

In a new study published in January 2011, *Consumer Reports* warns pregnant women to shun canned tuna completely amid test results showing concerning levels of mercury in the fish products.

The magazine's latest investigation of 42 samples from cans and pouches of tuna bought primarily in the New York metropolitan area revealed that even if women of childbearing age eat less tuna than what the U.S. government recommends, they could exceed safe mercury limits. *Consumer Reports* also confirmed that white (albacore) tuna usually contains more mercury than light tuna.

By following the recommendations below for selecting and eating fish or shellfish, women and young children will receive the benefits of eating fish and shellfish and be confident that they have reduced their exposure to the harmful effects of mercury.

- Do not eat shark, swordfish, king mackerel, tuna, or tilefish because they contain high levels of mercury.

- Eat up to 12 ounces (two average meals) a week of a variety of fish and shellfish that are lower in mercury.

- Five of the most commonly eaten fish that are low in mercury are shrimp, canned light tuna, salmon, pollock, and catfish.

- Another commonly eaten fish, albacore ("white") tuna, has more mercury than canned light tuna. So, when choosing your two meals of fish and shellfish, you may eat up to 6 ounces (one average meal) of albacore tuna per week.

- Check local advisories about the safety of fish caught by family and friends in your local lakes, rivers, and coastal areas. If no advice is available, eat up to 6 ounces (one average meal) per week of fish you catch from local waters, but don't consume any other fish during that week."[1]

---

1   http://www.fda.gov/Food/FoodSafety/Product SpecificInformation/Seafood/Foodborne PathogensContaminants/Methylmercury/ucm115662.htm

"Over the past 100 years, there has been a 30-fold increase in mercury deposition, 70 percent of which is from human sources. In fact, there was an exponential peak in mercury occurring in the last 40 years due to major industrialization.

Much of this mercury comes from coal-fired industrial plants and from chlor-alkali plants that use mercury in the process of making chlorine used in plastics, pesticides, PVC pipes, and more."

— *Dr. Mark Hyman*

2. Coal-Fueled Electrical Generating Plants and Toxic Waste Sites

Electricity is generated in the U.S. from a variety of sources, including wind, solar, atomic energy plants, and hydroelectric dams, but perhaps 50 percent or so comes from the burning of coal, and coal contains trace amounts of mercury, which is emitted in the smoke stream from these plants and eventually enters the life cycle of a host of plants and animals. About 48 tons of mercury are released from coal-burning plants in the U.S. annually.

We have seen from the aforementioned Texas study that the risk of autism increases the nearer a child lives to a mercury-emitting source, and this risk also increases proportional to the amount of mercury emitted from that source.[2]

Likewise in Minnesota, investigators found a significant increase in autism in children who lived close to superfund waste sites as compared to those who did not. The researchers found that the autism rate among schoolchildren living within a twenty-mile radius of toxic waste sites was nearly twice that of children living farther away from such sites.[3]

Toxic waste sites are the source of many toxic pollutants, including mercury.

Similarly, a study of San Francisco Bay area children showed a significantly increased risk of becoming autistic in direct relationship to their exposure to hazardous airborne pollutants like mercury.[4]

And a very important study by Ming Xue and associates examined the relationship between population proximity to toxic landfills in New Jersey and the incidence of autism and found a significant correlation. The research team also looked at the relationship between the number of "Superfund" toxic waste sites in the continental U.S. and found that (with the exception of Oregon) there was a statistically significant correlation (p=0.015) between the number of these sites and the rate of autism in each and every one of the other 47 states.[5]

The Environmental Protection Agency (EPA) recognizes that these mercury emissions are a serious concern and has taken steps to address this problem. According to its website, "On March 15, 2005 the EPA issued a rule to permanently cap and reduce mercury emissions from coal-fired power plants."

The Clean Air Mercury Rule was built on the EPA's Clean Air Interstate Rule (CAIR) to reduce significantly emissions from coal-fired power plants—the largest remaining sources of mercury emissions in the country. The goal of these rules regarding mercury was to reduce utility emissions of mercury from 48 tons a year to 15 tons, a reduction of nearly 70 percent.

The Clean Air Mercury Rule establishes "standards of performance" that limit mercury emissions from new and existing coal-fired power plants and creates a market-based cap-and-trade program to reduce nationwide utility emissions of mercury in two distinct phases.

---

2   Palmer, R.F. et al. "Environmental mercury release, special education rates, and autism disorder: an ecological study of Texas." *Health Place*, 12(2):203–9 and Palmer, R.F., Blanchard, S. and Wood, R. 2008. "Proximity to point sources of environmental mercury release as a predictor of autism prevalence." *Health* Place, doi:10.1016/j.healthplace.2008.02.001.

3   DeSoto, M.C. "Ockam's Razor and Autism: The case for developmental neurotoxins contributing to a disease of neurodevelopment." *Neurotoxicology.* 2009. doi:10.1016/j.neuro.2009.03.003]

4   Windham, G.C. et al. "Autism spectrum disorders in relation to distribution of hazardous air pollutants in the San Francisco bay area." *Environ Health Perspect.* 2006. 114(9):1438–44.http://www.state.nj.us/dep/srp/kcs-nj/www.IDEAdata.org www.census.gov

5   Ming, Xue et al. "Autism Spectrum Disorders and Identified Toxic Land Fills: Co-Occurrence Across States." *Environmental Health Insights.* 2008:2.

New coal-fired power plants ("new" means construction starting on or after January 30, 2004) will have to meet stringent new source performance standards in addition to being subject to the caps.

The EPA website goes on to say that, "Mercury is a toxic, persistent pollutant that accumulates in the food chain. Mercury in the air is a global problem…fossil fuel-fired power plants are the largest remaining source of human-generated mercury emissions in the United States."[6]

And the Natural Resources Defense Council agrees, "Mercury is a classic global pollutant." It maintains that "when released from a source in one country the potent metal readily disperses around the world, often falling far from its sources of release and entering distant food supplies. Many populations are further exposed to mercury from a variety of local sources, including industrial emissions, consumer products, and waste disposal. As a result, mercury pollution now endangers people on every continent."[7]

> *"There is no safe level of mercury.*
> *And no one has actually shown that there is a safe level of mercury."*
>
> *— Dr. Lars Friberg (Consultant, World Health Organization)*

3. Dental Amalgams

Dental amalgams are almost 50 percent mercury, and according to Charles Williamson, M.D., co-director of the Toxic Studies Institute in Boca Raton, Florida, "The great majority of the body-burden of mercury—87 percent—comes from dental amalgams, which continuously give off mercury vapor."[8]

It may seem unbelievable to some people that the seemingly solid metal amalgam fillings in people's teeth could be discharging mercury vapor, but it is true. Every time someone bites down on a mercury amalgam filling, mercury vapor is emitted. The vapor is highly toxic and enters the body through the lungs, the oral mucosa (lining), the digestive system, and the nasal passages.

The mercury in fillings is also converted by mouth bacteria into organic methyl mercury, which is also extremely hazardous, and which is able to pass through the oral and intestinal lining and enter the bloodstream.

As evidence that these assertions are true, one has only to measure the amount of mercury in an "old" filling and note the dramatic decrease in mercury concentrations as the years go by. A ten-year-old amalgam may have only 40 percent of the original mercury content left.[9]

So where does the mercury in amalgams go?

Scientists helped answer that question by placing radioactive mercury-containing amalgams in the teeth of sheep and primates (monkeys) and found that after a period of time the radioactive mercury could be detected in *all organs and tissues*, proving that the mercury in amalgams is able to leave the amalgam fillings, is readily absorbed into the body of these mammals, and is also able to cause kidney damage in sheep.[10]

But what about research studies in humans? Do they also confirm that the mercury load in the body is significantly affected by having teeth filled with amalgams?

The answer is yes.

---

6   http://www.epa.gov/camr/basic.htm
7   http://www.nrdc.org/international/china/mercury.pdf
8   Charles Williamson, M.D. interview with *Life Extension* magazine staff
9   Radics, L. et al. "The crystalline components of silver amalgam studied using the electronic x-ray microprobe. *ZWR* 79:1031-1036 (1970) [German]; *and* Gasser, F. "New studies on amalgam." *Quintessenz* 27: 47-53 (1976) [German].
10   BBC interview of Fritz Lorscheider (Professor of medical physiology at the Univ. of Calgary) and Murray Vimy (academic dentist and WHO consultant) transcribed on http://www.fluoridealert.org/BBC-mercury.htm transcribed from *BBC Panorama* July 11, 1994.

The University of Arizona's Department of Molecular and Cellular Biology is headed by Professor Vasken Aposhian. He studied the distribution of mercury in the body of volunteer students and concluded that at least two thirds of the mercury in the bodies of these students came from tooth fillings.[11]

The FDA's own advisory panel on dental amalgam recommended in 2010 that dental amalgams should not be used in young children (especially those under six) and not in pregnant women either, but the FDA has made no official ruling as of May 2013.

Other countries, like the UK and Australia, have issued advisories against using mercury amalgams in children and pregnant women. Denmark forbids the use of amalgams in baby teeth and Sweden has totally banned amalgam fillings since June 2009.[12]

"80 to 85 percent of the industrialized world has (mercury) implanted in their teeth, and it's a situation of timed release poisoning."

— Dr. Murray Vimy

4. High Fructose Corn Syrup

High fructose corn syrup (HFCS) has been the sweetener of choice in recent years, often displacing cane sugar in soda, cakes, cookies, and a host of other products. HFCS is cheaper than sugar and also aids in extending product shelf life. There are two processes used in the manufacture of HFCS, and one of them involves the use of mercury-grade caustic soda.

Renee DuFault and her colleagues conducted a pilot study to determine whether any of this mercury got into the corn syrup, and if so, were the mercury concentrations of any concern. And what they found was that, indeed, *about half* of the tested samples of HFCS had levels of mercury *up to* 0.57 micrograms per gram (one fifth tsp) of corn syrup.

The average intake of HFCS is c 50 grams (10 teaspoonsful) per person per day. That means the average person ingesting this high mercury corn syrup would be ingesting up to 25 micrograms of mercury every day (the amount found in many of the vaccines during the 1990s).

Since many individuals, including children and teens, ingest far more than 50 grams of HFCS per day, their daily load of oral mercury would have been even higher. The authors of this study suggest that "it might be necessary to account for this source of mercury in the diet of children and sensitive populations."[13]

Might be necessary?

In another non-peer reviewed study, according to the *Washington Post*, "the Institute for Agriculture and Trade Policy (IATP), a non-profit watchdog group, found that nearly one in three of 55 brand-name foods (bought off the shelf in the fall of 2008) contained mercury. The chemical was found most commonly in HFCS-containing dairy products, dressings and condiments."[14]

"(My husband) is really concerned that the first ingredient in the Enfamil Gentlease that I bought is high fructose corn syrup.
I never even paid attention to that."

— Internet Blogger

---

11   Ibid.
12   See http://iaomt.org/wp-content/uploads/The-Case-Against-Amalgam.pdf for a well-referenced review entitled "The Case against Amalgam."
13   Dufault, Renee et al. "Mercury from chlor-alkali plants: measured concentrations in food product sugar." *Environmental Health.* 2009, 8:2doi:10.1186/1476-069X-8-2
14   http://www.washingtonpost.com/wpdyn/content/article/2009/01/26/AR2009012601831.html

5. Other Foods

In 2003, a study conducted by scientists at Health Canada found measurable mercury levels in dozens of common foods, including *baby formula*, broccoli, carrots, celery, blueberries, grapes, peas, raisins, raspberries, rice, strawberries, and tomatoes. These foods are considered wholesome and healthful, even though they all contain mercury in trace amounts. Mercury levels in canned mushrooms tested for that study were between 5,100 and 16,000 parts per trillion.[15]

6. Fluorescent Light Bulbs

Fluorescent light bulbs contain mercury, and compact fluorescent bulbs contain mercury in its dangerous organic form (methyl mercury) in amounts ranging from 1.4 to 30 mg (average: 9 mg). "Each year, an estimated 600 million fluorescent lamps are disposed of in US landfills, amounting to 30,000 pounds of mercury waste."[16]

And surprisingly, even *intact compact fluorescent bulbs emit mercury vapor.* "In new lamps, mercury vapor is released gradually in amounts that reach 1.3 mg or 30 percent of the total lamp inventory after four days."[17]

7. Cement Manufacturing Plants

Over *6 tons of mercury* were emitted from America's top 100 cement plants in 2006 alone. New standards would reduce mercury and other harmful emissions from cement plants by 92 percent. "The EPA estimates the new standards would save between \$6.7 and \$18 billion in public health costs every year, dwarfing industry's costs of compliance," according to the Environmental Defense Action Fund.[18]

These new protections were recently (January 2011) under assault in Congress. Rep. John Carter (R-TX) led the attack on the new cement plant pollutions standards, which if successful would not only succeed in nullifying these protections, but would also permanently ban the EPA from ever setting similar public health standards on mercury and toxic air pollution from cement plants in the future.[19]

Could this added mercury burden from foods, dental amalgams, toxic waste sites, mercury-emitting plants, compact fluorescents, and other sources be one of the reasons that autism spectrum disorders continued to rise after thimerosal's presence in immunizations decreased?

8. Other Sources of Mercury

Mercury has been found in *cosmetics* and *skin lightening products* in toxic amounts. The latter are popular among citizens of many Central American and Caribbean countries, and their topical use has been shown to increase dramatically the body burden of this poison.[20]

China uses mercury as a catalyst for the manufacturing of *polyvinyl chloride* (PVC) plastic, which it manufactures using coal. PVC plastic is mostly derived from oil in other countries and that process does not require the use of mercury. According to the Natural Resources Defense Council, "the PVC sector, which accounted for more than 600 tons of the mercury consumed in China in 2004, is projected to use more than 1,000 tons per year by 2010 due to the explosive growth of the PVC sector in China."[21]

Mercury thermometers, now banned in the U.S., and *mercury batteries* are other sources of this toxic metal. Mercury also enters the air from the *burning of bodies in crematoria.*

---

15   http://www.prnewswire.com/news-releases/recent-reports-regarding-mercury-and-high-fructose-corn-syrup-flawed-and-misleading-61356312.html
16   AirCycle Corporation
17   http://www.ageofautism.com/2014/01/soylent-greenwashing-the-compact-fluorescent-mandate-mito-epidemics-and-the-brave-newmercuryapolgism.html?utm_source=feedburner&utm_medium=email&utm_ campaign=Feed percent3A+ageofautism+ percent28AGE+OF+AUTIS M percent29&utm_content=Yahoo percent21+Mail
18   "Environmental Defense Action Fund" takeaction@edf.org
19   Ibid.
20   McKelvey, W. et al. "Population-Based Inorganic Mercury Biomonitoring and the Identification of Skin Care Products as a Source of Exposure in New York City." *Environ Health Perspect.* 2011 February; 119(2): 203–209. Published online 2010 October 5. doi: 10.1289/ehp.1002396.
21   http://www.nrdc.org/international/china/mercury.pdf

How Many Americans Are Thought to Have an Excess Body Burden of Mercury?

A scientific panel was convened by the FDA in December 2010 to re-examine the issue of mercury exposure from amalgam dental fillings. The FDA had previously declared amalgam fillings to be safe in reviews dating back to the 1990s, but since that time, a good deal of published research has shown that mercury is toxic at levels previously thought to be safe. As a consequence, various government agencies have been reducing their allowed reference exposure levels (RELs).

The scientific literature on amalgam fillings was reviewed by G. Mark Richardson, Ph.D., of *SNC Lavallin*, Ottawa, Canada (formerly *Health Canada*), who presented his findings to the scientific panel and the FDA regulators in two parts.

Part 1 is titled: "Updating Exposure: Reexamining Reference Exposure Levels and Critically Evaluating Recent Studies." One of the determinations revealed by that review is that "some 67.2 million Americans would exceed the mercury dose associated with the reference exposure level of 0.3 ug/m^2 (micrograms per meter squared of body surface area) established by the US Environmental Protection Agency in 1995, whereas 122.3 million Americans would exceed the dose associated with the more recent reference exposure level of 0.03 µg/m^2 established by the California Environmental Protection Agency in 2008."

In Part 2 of the review (titled "Cumulative Risk Assessment and Joint Toxicity: Mercury Vapor, Methyl Mercury and Lead"), the more recent scientific articles suggest that, "A large proportion (1/3rd) of the US population, is concurrently exposed to metallic mercury or its vapor, methyl mercury and lead on a daily basis. The weight of available evidence suggests that risks posed by concurrent exposure to combinations of these 3 substances should be assessed as additive."[22]

> *"In February 2004, a new analysis by the Environmental Protection Agency revealed that 'about 630,000 children are born each year at risk for lowered intelligence and learning problems caused by exposure to high levels of mercury in the womb,' nearly double the previous EPA estimate."*[23]

> *"Vaccine manufacturers, pharmaceutical companies, and health authorities have known about multiple dangers associated with vaccines but chose to withhold them from the public. This is scientific fraud, and their complicity suggests that this practice continues to this day."*[24]

> *"Few men have enough virtue to withstand the highest bidder."*
>
> — *George Washington*

---

22   Final Report: International Academy of Oral medicine and Toxicology on Behalf of Funders, including the Parker Hannifin Foundation; REF 10738; submitted November 08, 2010; http://iaomt.org/articles/category_view.asp?intReleaseID=329&catid=30
23   http://www.pbs.org/now/science/mercuryinfish.html
24   Lucija Tomljenovic http://nsnbc.me/2015/06/19/shocking-report-from-medical-insiders/

Chapter 19
Conclusions: Indisputable Evidence Linking Thimerosal and Mercury to Autism

"The weight of this sad time we must obey,
Speak what we feel, not what we ought to say."

— *William Shakespeare*, King Lear

So WHERE ARE *we in this debate? What have we learned, and what can we conclude?*
We know and have known for a long time that mercury is highly toxic and specifically is quite neurotoxic.

We also now know that the manifestations of mercury poisoning depend on many factors, including: the chemical form of mercury; at what age the mercury entered the body and by what route; whether the mercury dose was acute, chronic, or intermittent; genetic differences in individuals exposed to mercury; and the presence of other toxic substances that enhance the toxicity of mercury.

We have found that there is an overlap of symptoms from different sorts of mercury poisoning (Minamata disease, Mad Hatter disease, Pink disease, etc.), but that there are also distinct differences in each of these mercury-induced conditions. Many of the symptoms noted in these toxic syndromes are commonly seen in autistic individuals. These include irritability, seizures, poor coordination, anxiety, sensory sensitivities, muscle weakness, thinking and learning dysfunctions, speech delays, attention deficits, and communication impairments.

We have thus come to appreciate that the various kinds of mercury poisoning do not manifest with exactly the same symptoms as those noted in autistic individuals, but that this fact does not in any way rule out ethyl mercury from thimerosal as being a causative agent that promotes autism.

We have established that thimerosal, which is 50 percent ethyl mercury, inhibits certain enzymes, which when inhibited, can induce the manifestations of autism, and that thimerosal is able to do this at extremely low concentrations in genetically-susceptible individuals.

We have established biochemically why mercury exposure from thimerosal and other sources is more toxic to males than to females, and how this would then provide a rational explanation for the dramatic increase in autism and related disorders noted in males.

We have come to realize that not only has the safety of thimerosal *never been established*, but that the limited research studies that were done point to thimerosal being more toxic to living cells than to bacteria and highly neurotoxic. The initial study of meningococcal meningitis patients who were given thimerosal, which was alleged to have established the safety of this toxin, was a farce.

We have discovered that thimerosal is unstable, that it breaks down spontaneously while in solution, and that its breakdown into ethyl mercury and a thio-salicylate compound occurs rapidly when thimerosal is exposed to living tissues and fluids.

We have discovered that thimerosal is so toxic that the FDA proposed to remove it from all vaccines for animals in 1991, but caved to industry demands and cancelled the ban. We know that when applied topically to the omphaloceles of newborns, it caused many deaths. It has been banned for over eighteen years in Russia and the Scandinavian countries, and its *topical* use as Merthiolate is also banned in the U.S.

We know that the "powers that be" were indeed "asleep at the switch" by failing to realize that during the 1990s children were being injected with toxic amounts of mercury (as thimerosal) that far exceeded the safety levels set by the EPA. And they still are!

We have ascertained that the toxicokinetics (how the poison is "handled" by the body) of methyl mercury are not the same as that of ethyl mercury, the kind found in thimerosal.

We know that there is evidence from animal studies that ethyl mercury from thimerosal breaks down into *inorganic* mercury, which appears to be the precipitating factor in causing specific brain cell injury, and it does this to a much greater degree than does methyl mercury.

We have learned from numerous other animal studies that the amount of thimerosal found in vaccines when given in proportionate doses to animals caused neurological and behavioral abnormalities that parallel those noted in autistic children.

We have ascertained that the safe levels of mercury established by the EPA and other entities were based on studies of *methyl* mercury, which we now realize are not applicable to *ethyl* mercury.

We know that the FDA twice ruled (1982 and 1988) that thimerosal be removed from all over-the-counter products because it was "neither safe nor effective," but didn't enforce that edict until April 1998.[1]

We know that the National Vaccine Advisory Group ordered the immediate removal of thimerosal from the hepatitis B vaccine in 1999, but that it was still present in some batches even in 2004 and is still in the influenza vaccine, the DT booster, and other immunizations as of 2014.

In the year 2000, a study demonstrated toxic levels of mercury in newborns after they received *just one* hepatitis B immunization (which also contains neurotoxic aluminum).

We know that in 1998 there were 30 licensed vaccines that contained thimerosal, and that it is still in U.S. vaccines given to babies and pregnant mothers in 2015. Many other thimerosal-preserved vaccines are also still widely used to this day as the routine vaccinations given to babies in many countries around the world.

We know that while individual vaccines have been tested for safety, albeit insufficiently, the vaccine schedule itself has never been tested in this manner. That is to say, the repeated use of a variety of immunizations given concomitantly and over a period of time to babies has *never* been safety tested.

We know that the CDC has conspired with the American Academy of Pediatrics, the World Health Organization, the vaccine manufacturers, and others to suppress the results of Thomas Verstraeten's original epidemiological study, which showed a statistically significant, clear, and certain dose and age-dependent linkage between thimerosal in vaccines and a host of neurodevelopmental ills, including autism and ADHD.

The presence of these four groups at the June 2000 CDC-sponsored Simpsonwood conference means that all of them were aware that thimerosal in a dose and age dependent manner causes neurodevelopmental disorders, autism, ADHD, speech and language delays, and other harmful effects, and they are all, therefore, complicit in the cover-up of that information.

---

1   Federal Register, Department of Health and Human Services, Food and Drug Administration. Status of Certain Additional Over-the-Counter Drug Category II and III Active Ingredients. April 22, 1998; 63(77):19799-19802. 21 CFR Part 310. [Docket No. 75N-183F, 75N-183D, and 80N-0280.]

We know that the CDC, which attempted to hide the true rise in autism for many years, also intentionally presented specious, corrupt studies to the Institute of Medicine so as to get it to declare thimerosal safe and not a cause of autism or developmental disorders.

We know that all of the studies that allege to show no linkage between thimerosal and autism are fatally flawed, and many of them, undoubtedly, deliberately so.

We know that a good many of these "bogus" studies have been sponsored by the CDC and published in *Pediatrics*, the journal of the American Academy of Pediatrics, an organization that appears to become apoplectic when anyone suggests doing further studies on autism and vaccinations.

"Fraud and falsehood only dread examination. Truth invites it."

— *Dr. Samuel Johnson (1709-1784)*

We know that not one of these highly questionable "negative" studies disproves the thimerosal (mercury)-autism connection. Not one.

We know that the CDC continues to prevent researchers from accessing their own VSD database in order to study the possible different outcomes of vaccinated vs. non-vaccinated babies.

We know that there are over 30 human studies that give strong support to the contention that mercury in thimerosal and from other sources is a cause of the autism epidemic.

Of these many studies, six have examined at least *five different databases* that clearly and repeatedly demonstrate what Verstraeten's *original*, uncorrupted, suppressed, and as yet unpublished study proved, which is that there is an undeniable, statistically significant, dose and age-dependent relationship between thimerosal in vaccines and the incidence of autism, ADD/ADHD, and other neurodevelopmental maladies.

Of these studies, many show that surrogate mercury markers, like certain abnormal porphyrins, are significantly elevated in autistic children, and there are still others that demonstrate that autistic children don't excrete mercury well, most likely on a genetic basis.

We also now know that removing mercury via chelation seems to improve autistic children's symptoms.

We have thus determined that there is extensive, damning evidence demonstrating that the thimerosal-autism linkage is not only "biologically plausible," but overwhelmingly likely.

And we can, therefore, conclude that there is more than sufficient evidence to charge the CDC, the American Academy of Pediatrics, the World Health Organization, the vaccine manufacturers, the Institute of Medicine, the Department of Health and Human Services, and many of their associated scientists, pseudo-scientists, political appointees, shills, and others of deception, corruption, malfeasance, and a heinous and massive cover-up.

We recognize that there has been a quite successful effort on their part to distort the truth, and to disregard, disparage, suppress and denigrate the huge body of evidence that contradicts their views.

They have compounded their treachery by cleverly avoiding *critical* peer review of their own flawed research studies, by unethically manipulating data, and by using improper research protocols that would then allow their "investigators" to arrive at the desired specious conclusions.

They have additionally suppressed criticism of their own faulty research; withheld essential information from independent researchers; deliberately and repeatedly lied to the press, the public, and their peers; pressured media not to report contradictory theories or evidence; put improper pressure on politicians and scientists to support their views; and caused important and essential autism legislation to fail.

By perpetrating all these despicable acts, they must bear the responsibility and guilt of having played a deliberate and major role in further brain-damaging millions of children in the U.S. and around the world and of maliciously corrupting science itself.

Keep in mind that all these acts were done solely for the protection and continuance of their personal reputations, their pocketbooks, the fiscal health of the vaccine manufacturers, and an immunization program that they saw and still see as immutable.

They would argue, we imagine, that this was all done for the public good, that the vaccination program was too vital to have doubts cast about its potential risks, that major organizations and individuals like the vaccine manufacturers, pediatricians, the CDC, the World Health Organization, the American Academy of Pediatrics, and many others would no doubt have had to face the embarrassment and massive financial fallout accruing from the myriad lawsuits that would have undoubtedly been appropriately brought as a result of these organizations and individuals having participated in the *intentional* mercury poisoning of millions of babies.

And a good deal of this thimerosal overdosing might have been prevented or minimized had a simple mathematical calculation regarding the amount of thimerosal in each vaccine been performed in time.

But it wasn't.

And this tragic autism/ADHD epidemic might also have been prevented or minimized had the authorities elected to use only the slightly more expensive, preservative-free single-dose vial vaccines, rather than the thimerosal-preserved multi-dose vials.

But they didn't.

They wanted to save money. But any money they may have saved won't come close to paying for the harm they have perpetrated on society.

The naysayers' concerns are, however, not without merit. Had the CDC acknowledged the validity of Verstraeten's original paper, there would certainly have been widespread financial and social repercussions, but all the organizations, including the vaccine makers, would have survived and persevered. The vaccine manufacturers, let's remember, were protected by government decree (Federal Vaccine Court).

The immunization program would certainly have continued, but without thimerosal and other multi-dose vial preservatives. Most parents would undoubtedly have elected to have their children immunized with the slightly more expensive, but safer, single-dose vial vaccines that didn't and don't require the use of any toxic preservative.

The entire vaccine schedule would have had to have been re-evaluated and appropriate changes would have certainly been made. After a period of disruption, America and the rest of the world would still have been protected from vaccine-preventable diseases and untold hundreds of thousands of children and their families would then also have been spared a life of impaired neurological functioning and its consequences.

But that didn't happen.

The CDC didn't acknowledge the validity or even the existence of the original Verstraeten paper. It deliberately hid that information. If it were not for the Freedom of Information Act, its treachery would most likely have remained a secret until this day. In that regard, we must be forever thankful for the many wonderful and dedicated individuals who exposed this massive cover-up and who took the time to analyze the myriad bogus published studies that purport to show no link between immunizations and autism and point out their weaknesses, errors, manipulations, lies, and distortions.

So the bottom line is an unconscionable crime of worldwide proportions has been committed, and unfortunately, it is continuing to be committed.

And the deceivers are getting away with it.

By convincing almost everyone that there is no immunization link to autism, the perpetrators of this falsehood have at the same time also succeeded in preventing the majority of healthcare providers from properly addressing the environmental risk factors that we know are associated with autism.

If a physician does not believe there is a mercury link to autism, he or she will not look for mercury as a possible autism promoter and won't offer chelation as part of the treatment plan if mercury is indeed present in unacceptable amounts.

And it follows that now almost all research money is being spent on solely searching for the *genetic* factors that might be associated with autism, a worthwhile goal to be sure, but a financially-biased one, as a good deal of that research dollar also needs to be spent supporting studies that evaluate the *environmental links to autism.*

"It is hard not to conclude that this funding disparity is strongly influenced by the fit of genetics to the needs of businesses and politicians."[2]

One of the *big lies* being spread by the powers that be is that we don't know the cause of the autism epidemic. Not true! We actually have a very good idea why this epidemic is taking place, and immunizations containing mercury play a major part in that causality, but mercury is not by any means the only cause.

"…people will believe a big lie sooner than a little one; and if you repeat it frequently enough people will sooner or later believe it."

— Hitler as His Associates Know Him (OSS report, p. 51)

In the following chapters, we will show that other neurotoxic substances, certain immunizations, and the immunization program itself all play a major role in promoting autism, and we'll look at other theories of autism causation as well.

It will become apparent that these disparate hypotheses are not mutually exclusive. The various pieces of this puzzle actually fit together quite nicely, and all in all, they will help us to understand the bigger picture of what autism spectrum disorders actually are, what factors contribute to their existence, and *what we can do to prevent and treat these dreaded maladies.*

CDC Studies Fatally Flawed

"The CDC…should not be conducting any type of vaccine safety study based on their primary mandate of maximizing vaccine uptake.

"Their role is conflicted at best.

"(There is) a long list of studies on vaccines and neurological disorders in children that are at a minimum fatally flawed but more often complete misrepresentations of the truth."

— Dr. Brian Hooker, Ph.D.

---

2   http://www.bioscienceresource.org/commentaries/article.php?id=46

Science Has Spoken

"Of all the remarkable frauds that will one day surround the autism epidemic, perhaps one of the most galling is the simple statement that "science has spoken and vaccines don't cause autism."

Anytime a public health official or other talking head states this, you can be assured that one of two things is true: they have never read the studies they are talking about, or they are lying through their teeth."

— J.B. Handley[3]

"It is to be regretted that the rich and Powerful too often bend the acts of Government to their own selfish purposes."

— Andrew Jackson, 7th President of the U.S.

DEPARTMENT OF SPIN

In which we learn that autism isn't "caused" by vaccines. It is just a "result" of getting them. (And we get a $20 million clue as to why the authorities wish to deny an autism-vaccine link)

Family to Receive $1.5M+ in First-Ever Vaccine-Autism Court Award

Posted by Sharyl Attkisson

The first court award in a vaccine-autism claim is a big one. CBS News has learned the family of Hannah Poling will receive more than $1.5 million dollars for her life care; lost earnings; and pain and suffering for the first year alone.

In addition to the first year, the family will receive more than $500,000 per year to pay for Hannah's care. Those familiar with the case believe the compensation could easily amount to $20 million over the child's lifetime.

Hannah was described as normal, happy and precocious in her first 18 months. Then, in July 2000, she was vaccinated against nine diseases in one doctor's visit: measles, mumps, rubella, polio, varicella, diphtheria, pertussis, tetanus, and Haemophilus influenzae.

Afterward, her health declined rapidly. She developed high fevers, stopped eating, didn't respond when spoken to, began showing signs of autism, and began having screaming fits. In 2002, Hannah's parents filed an autism claim in federal vaccine court. Five years later, the government settled the case before trial and had it sealed. It's taken more than two years for both sides to agree on how much Hannah will be compensated for her injuries.

In acknowledging Hannah's injuries, the government said vaccines aggravated an unknown mitochondrial disorder Hannah had which didn't "cause" her autism, but "resulted" in it.

It's unknown how many other children have similar undiagnosed mitochondrial disorder. All other autism "test cases" have been defeated at trial. Approximately 4,800 are awaiting disposition in federal vaccine court.*

---

3   www.whale.to/vaccine/fourteen_studies.html

[That would make a payout of about $96 billion if each of these children were compensated to the degree that Hannah was. If the hundreds of thousands of children who have autism were to be so compensated, the costs would be even more staggering.]

Posted on the CBS News Website September 9, 2010: 2:42 PM

The authors of a study published in the *Pace Environmental Law Review* found 83 cases of autism among those compensated for vaccine-induced brain damage. They state that their "Preliminary study suggests that the VICP (Vaccine Injury Compensation Program) had been compensating cases of vaccine-induced encephalopathy and residual seizure disorder since the inception of the program."[4]

Department of Spin (continued)

In which we learn that vaccines may cause encephalopathy that manifests as autism, but autism isn't actually caused by vaccines.

This is the response from HRSA (the HHS division that runs the Vaccine Injury Compensation Program) to a request from a journalist (David Kirby) about the Poling case as an admission that vaccines can cause autism:

From: Bowman, David (HRSA) [mailto:DBowman@hrsa.gov]

Sent: Friday, February 20, 2009 5:22 PM

To: 'dkirby@nyc.rr.com'

Subject: HRSA Statement

David,

In response to your most recent inquiry, HRSA has the following statement:

The government has never compensated, nor has it ever been ordered to compensate, any case based on a determination that autism was actually caused by vaccines. We have compensated cases in which children exhibited an encephalopathy, or general brain disease. Encephalopathy may be accompanied by a medical progression of an array of symptoms including autistic behavior, autism, or seizures.

Some children who have been compensated for vaccine injuries may have shown signs of autism before the decision to compensate, or may ultimately end up with autism or autistic symptoms, but we do not track cases on this basis.

Regards,

David Bowman
Office of Communications
Health Resources and Services Administration
301-443-3376

Taken from "Adventures in Autism" by Ginger Taylor[5]

---

4   Holland, Mary et al. "Unanswered Questions from the Vicp: A Review of Compensated Cases of Vaccine-Induced Brain Injury." *Pace Environmental Law Review.* Vol. 28. Issue 2. Winter 2011; Article 6; p. 3.

5   http://us1.campaign-archive.com/?u=73910d58c82511a4d92dcaf7e&id=7643fbd4e3

"When one with honeyed words but evil mind persuades the mob, great woes befall the state."

— *Euripides, Orestes*

Les Incompetants:

An Open Letter to the American Academy of Pediatrics (Aap)[6]
By K. Paul Stoller, M.D.
February 26, 2008

Excerpt

As a pediatrician, who has been a fellow of the AAP for two decades, I find the AAP's approach to the autism epidemic to be deeply disturbing.

Not only have they allowed the myth of better diagnosing (and greater awareness)…to be perpetuated, but when they were put on notice at the CDC's Simpsonwood meeting in 2000, that the mercury in the preservative thimerosal was causing speech delays and learning disabilities, they obfuscated and (hid) that information….

For all the above reasons, I will no longer enable the AAP to be party to the damage that is being done to the world's children by sending in my dues for a third decade. It is a token protest, but it has to begin with someone.[7]

---

6   Edited and abridged by the author
7   Read the full letter at http://www.ageofautism.com/2008/02/aap-fellow-resi.html

Chapter 20
The MMR Connection

"Truth is truth to the end of reckoning."
— *William Shakespeare,* Measure to Measure, *Act 5, scene 1*

WHAT IS THE *MMR?*

The MMR is a vaccine made by several pharmaceutical companies that combines vaccines to the measles, mumps, and rubella ("German measles") viruses. It is a live virus vaccine, meaning that the viruses, although "weakened" (attenuated), are capable of infecting their human host in such a way as to provoke an appropriate immune response without causing the disease itself to manifest.

The first licensed vaccine against measles was approved in the U.S. in 1963. The first vaccine against mumps in the U.S. was licensed in 1967, and the immunization to rubella (German measles) was licensed two years after that (1969).

In 1971, Merck (at that time called Merck Sharp and Dohme) received approval to distribute its M-M-R-II® vaccine[1] (MMR) which combined the mumps and rubella vaccines with the measles vaccine.

Merck's ProQuad® vaccination was approved in 2005 and adds the varicella (chickenpox) virus vaccine to the MMR, making it an MMRV vaccine.

The MMR vaccine does not contain thimerosal and never has. Although separate immunizations for preventing measles, mumps, and rubella were once available, that is no longer true in the U.S. and the UK. Merck stopped making the individual vaccines to measles, mumps, and rubella in 2009. Only the MMR (different brands) or MMRV (ProQuad) immunizations have prevailed. The MMR immunization does not fully protect individuals from the measles, and one measles outbreak in New York in 2011 was traced to a fully vaccinated individual.[2]

What Is Measles?

Measles (also known as rubeola in the U.S.) is a highly contagious viral disease that generally starts as an upper respiratory infection with a fever, cough, a characteristic red rash, nasal congestion, and conjunctivitis. It may progress to cause other symptoms like diarrhea, croup, and pneumonia.

About one out of every thousand measles victims in poverty-stricken countries develops a very serious brain infection called measles encephalitis, which can result in permanent brain damage. According to pediatrician Dr. Robert

---

1 Glaxo-Smith-Kline now makes a similar combination vaccine called Priorix®.
2 *Clin Infect Dis,* (2014); 58(9):1205f.

Mendelsohn, in more affluent countries, like the U.S., where malnutrition is significantly less of a problem, the incidence of measles encephalitis is actually closer to one in every 10,000 to 100,000 children.[3]

Five percent of children in the U.S. who get measles also get pneumonia, and 1-3 children out of every thousand cases in the U.S. will die from this disease. Deaths are more common in infants and malnourished individuals. Vitamin A *deficiency* increases the risk of death and is common in the less fortunate populations of the world, and treating malnourished children infected with measles virus with vitamin A in very high (200,000 units per day orally for a short time) doses cuts measles mortality significantly.

Subacute Sclerosing Pan-Encephalitis is another uncommon, but invariably fatal affliction associated with a chronic measles virus infection of the brain. It is estimated to occur once in every 10,000 cases of measles. Symptoms of brain damage start 7-10 *years after* the initial infection, and death follows 1-3 years after that. Individuals who contract measles infection at a young age are at higher risk for getting SSPE.

In 1995, Danish researcher Anne-Marie Plesner reported *gait disturbances* (ataxia) after the MMR. The study was published in *The Lancet*.[4]

In 1997, evidence discovered by Ring, Barak, and Tischer in Israel suggested a connection between measles infection and autism.[5]

In 2000, Dr. Plesner published a follow-up to her 1995 research paper that confirms her allegation that the MMR not only causes gait disturbances in some children, but also leaves some with "residual cognitive deficits."[6]

Unfortunately, all of the serious side effects caused by a measles infection, including encephalitis, pneumonia, and subacute sclerosing pan encephalitis can also be caused by the immunization itself.

What Is Mumps?

Mumps is another very contagious viral disease that can cause fever and malaise. It commonly infects the parotid glands, which are salivary glands located laterally below the jaw and under the ears, and the disease commonly manifests as painful swelling of those glands. The virus may also infect one or both testes in adolescents and adults, causing not only painful swelling of those organs, but also damage to the testes that may result in reduced fertility or even sterility.

Mumps *meningo*encephalitis, another potential side effect of mumps infection (or certain mumps vaccines), is an infection of the brain that can present as severe headache, stiff neck, nausea, and vomiting. It occurs in less than 2 out of every 100,000 individuals infected with the mumps virus.

About 20 percent of mumps-infected individuals exhibit no symptoms at all, but they may shed the virus and, thereby, infect others.

What Is Rubella?

Rubella, also known as "German Measles" and "Three Day Measles," is a generally mild viral infection that may cause a low grade fever, some generalized discomfort, body and head pains, enlarged lymph nodes, a stuffy nose and a mild pink skin eruption. It commonly causes transient joint pains in adults. In many individuals, it causes no outward symptoms at all.

The real concern with rubella lies in its ability to cause severe damage to a developing fetus. If a pregnant mother with no immunity to rubella acquires the disease during the pregnancy, the fetus is likely to exhibit major side effects, including damage to the brain, the heart, and other organs. Babies born with the congenital rubella syndrome are

---

3   Mendelsohn, R. *How to Raise a Healthy Child in Spite of Your Doctor*. New York, NY: Ballantine Books, 1987. p. 236-237.
4   p. 345-316
5   "Evidence for an infectious aetiology in autism." *Pathophysiology*. 1997; 4:1485-8
6   Plesner, A.M. et al. "Gait disturbance interpreted as cerebellar ataxia after MMR vaccination at 15 months of age: a follow-up study." January 2000; *Acta Paed* 89(1):5.

at risk for low birth weight, deafness, blindness, physical defects, mental retardation, heart problems, anemia, and other concerns.

The three-year rubella epidemic in the U.S., which started in 1962, was estimated to have caused 30,000 still births and severe impairment and disability in another 20,000 children.[7]

In order to prevent these tragic side effects, the rubella vaccine was developed and given to most children in the Americas, and it has been extremely successful in preventing this infection. No endemic cases have been observed in the Americas since February 2009.[8]

How Effective Are MMR Vaccines in Preventing Measles, Mumps, and Rubella?

Initially, one injection of the MMR was recommended at 12-15 months of age, and this promoted about 95-98 percent immunity to the measles and rubella components and about 80-95 percent to the mumps component (depending on which strain was present in the vaccine). That means that a small but significant percentage of the immunized children would still be susceptible to getting these diseases. In order to increase the efficacy to over 99 percent, a second MMR booster was recommended to be given to 4-6 year-old children.

Before the era of immunizations against the measles virus, virtually everyone in the U.S. came down with this disease, and the disease appears to convey lifelong immunity. Since the advent of measles immunizations, the U.S. has seen a dramatic 99 percent drop in the incidence of measles. The MMR vaccination has also significantly reduced the incidence of rubella (German measles) and mumps.

The *single entity* injections of just the measles virus or the mumps or rubella viruses have proven to be very effective with both the measles and rubella virus immunizations protecting 95 percent or more of the recipients for 15 years or more. The *single dose* mumps vaccination protection lasts approximately 10 years. Contrast this to the *combined* MMR, which protects only 90 percent of recipients and requires a booster shot three years later.

There have been serious questions raised regarding the effectiveness of the mumps component of the MMR vaccine. Currently, Merck's attenuated Jerryl Lynn strain of the mumps virus in the MMR II is the only mumps vaccine licensed for use in the U.S. Merck claims that its vaccine is 95 percent effective in preventing mumps, but there are reasons to question that statistic.

In 2010, two virologists and former employees of Merck requested whistleblower status. They stated that they had "witnessed firsthand the improper testing and data falsification in which Merck engaged to artificially inflate the vaccine's efficacy findings." They further asserted that Merck's scheme caused the United States to pay "hundreds of millions of dollars for a vaccine that does not provide adequate immunization."[9]

The U.S. government is a major purchaser of vaccines, including the MMR.

It was alleged that Merck scientists intentionally doctored their efficacy study by testing the mumps vaccine's virus-neutralizing ability only against the *weakened* strain of the mumps virus found in the vaccine itself and not against the wild type strain that actually caused the disease. Oops!

Their scientists also allegedly further subverted the test results by adding animal antibodies of a kind that humans could never produce to the serum being tested. This resulted in a factitious inflation of the efficacy statistics of their vaccine.

Protecting their stockholders and their profits was apparently more important to Merck than protecting children.

On June 25, 2012, one week after this False Claims Act complaint was unsealed, Chatom Primary Care of Alabama sued Merck for falsifying its mumps vaccine efficacy data. Merck countered that the false-claims lawsuit was "factually false" and "without merit."[10]

---

7   Wikipedia
8   Ibid.
9   http://www.courthousenews.com/2012/06/27/47851.htm
10   Ibid.

Does the MMR Vaccine or Any of Its Components Have Any Side Effects?

Absolutely! The most common *listed* side effects from the MMR are fever (5-15 percent) and rash (5 percent), occurring a week or so after the inoculation (from the measles component), and joint pain in about one fourth of the adult women receiving the vaccine secondary to the rubella component.

Only rarely (about one in 35,000) does the MMR vaccine causes a temporary drop in the platelet count.

From 1963 through 1971, at least eighty-four cases of neurologic disorders with onset less than 30 days after live measles-virus vaccination were reported in the United States.

Allergic reactions to the vaccine are alleged to be rare, but potentially severe or even fatal anaphylaxis reactions may and do occur, especially after revaccination.[11]

The Urabe strain of the mumps component found only in certain MMR vaccines (Trivirix, Pluserix, and Immravax) has caused significant brain inflammation in many children, and the story of this unfortunate chapter in vaccine history is worth telling.

And Yet Another Tale of Corporate and Governmental Corruption and Collusion

As has been noted, there have been a number of MMR vaccines on the market, and they all include a live *mumps* virus component. The strain of mumps virus used in Merck's (formerly Merck Sharp and Dohme) MMR II vaccine is called the *Jeryl Lynn* strain.

Merck's vaccine was alleged to be safer but more costly than were others that contained a competing mumps virus variant that had been developed in Japan called the *Urabe* (ooh-RAH-bay) AM-9 strain. This strain was present in the Immravax and Pluserix MMR vaccines in the UK and in the Trivirix MMR vaccine in Canada.

The problem with the Urabe mumps vaccine, and it was a big problem, was that it caused meningitis in a significant number of the children who received the vaccination, while the Jeryl Lynn strain did not. Meningitis is an infection of the meninges, the lining of the brain, and can make those so infected quite ill.

Canada had been using the relatively safer[12] Jeryl Lynn mumps vaccine in its MMR immunization for over 15 years before it first introduced the Trivirix brand of MMR with the Urabe strain of mumps virus in early 1988. However, Trivirix was discontinued in July 1988 (just 6 months later) because of its serious side effects. It caused mumps meningitis in a significant number of children.

Japan, Malaysia, the Philippines, and Australia also had similar adverse experiences with the Urabe mumps vaccine, and all ultimately banned its use.

The pharmaceutical company SmithKlein French-Beecham (currently "Glaxo SmithKline") now had a problem. Its Trivirix vaccine, although cheaper than Merck's MMR II vaccine, was dangerous. It caused serious brain inflammation in many children. What to do? Pull it off the market? No way! There was too much money invested and too much yet to be made. Maybe if it just changed the name, people wouldn't realize it was the same vaccine as Trivirix. Great idea! They would call the rebranded vaccine "Pluserix."

In July 1988, the same month that Canada stopped using the harmful Triverix vaccine, the United Kingdom authorities, under the conscious misdirection of immunization program head Dr. David Salisbury, decided to license Pluserix for general use. Their purpose was ostensibly to save money. If people started using the cheaper Pluserix "jab" (as the British refer to it), Merck might be more inclined to lower its prices. Ah, competition!

Dr. Salisbury was made aware of the dangers of Pluserix. He was privy to the Canadian data that showed the identical vaccine with a different name (Trivirix) caused an unacceptably high rate of meningitis in its recipients, but

---

11   Kalet, A. et al. "Allergic reactions to MMR Vaccine." *Pediatrics.* 1992; 89:168-9.
12   At least it didn't seem to promote meningitis.

he chose to ignore that evidence of harm and actively, but unsuccessfully, attempted to suppress the release of the Canadian data to other members of the allegedly independent[13] Joint Committee on Vaccination and Immunization (the JCVI).

He approved the vaccine *against the advice* of a number of members of the JCVI, including one particular committee member, Dr. Alistair Thores, who later became a "whistleblower."

Dr. Thores, using an assumed name, initially contacted Richard Barrs of Dawbarn's law firm in April 1998, and over the next year or so, he also met with gastroenterologist Dr. Andrew Wakefield. Dr. Thores provided his audience with a lot of confidential information about what had been going on regarding the clandestine JCVI approval process for the troublesome Pluserix vaccine.[14]

He related that many JCVI members, when appropriately informed, had expressed their concerns that the Pluserix MMR was being portrayed as "perfectly safe," when they knew that it was anything but. They worried about their own liability if the British experience were to mirror that of Canada's.

Unfortunately, a smaller but influential number of JCVI members appeared not to care about safety issues at all. Indeed, they attempted to suppress dissemination of the JCVI meeting minutes (where doubts about the vaccine's safety were expressed) by delaying their publication for at least six months, and also by "sanitizing" them when they did finally appear. Committee member worries and concerns were "downplayed" in these "whitewashed" minutes.[15]

The vaccine was ultimately approved despite many committee members' misgivings.

The British Government, ever anxious to get the new Pluserix vaccine licensed, fast-tracked the approval process, and in so doing, circumvented the usual and necessary safety trials. They irresponsibly and inappropriately used data from Merck's Jeryl Lynn mumps vaccine as "proxy" for the safety of the Urabe vaccine. However, the Merck MMR II vaccine caused far less mumps meningitis than did the Pluserix vaccine, so the two versions were not equivalent.

At the same time, the legal department at "SmithKlein French-Beecham" (which later became SmithKlein Beecham and then GlaxoSmithKlein) was concerned about licensing its troublesome vaccine in the UK without legal waivers against potential lawsuits. It knew Pluserix was likely to become a target for legal redress when its propensity to cause meningitis became manifest.

The British government acquiesced, agreeing to "immunize" SmithKlein in regard to any liability accruing from possible adverse reactions from Pluserix, and by so doing, was able to pass the costs of all potential lawsuits on to the British taxpayer.

Not to be outdone, the pharmaceutical company Pasteur Merieux (now Aventis Pasteur) got its Urabe-containing MMR vaccine (Immravax) licensed in the UK in September 1989, again with no mention of its propensity to cause meningitis.

What Happened Next in This Unfortunate Drama?

Just what you'd expect:

- The less expensive Pluserix vaccine (and to a lesser degree, the equally dangerous Immravax) became the MMRs of choice in the UK and soon dominated the market.

- The British authorities, unlike their Canadian counterparts, unconscionably provided no money for *active* surveillance of potential adverse events resulting from these untested and troubled vaccines, so it took a lot longer for the harmful side effects of Pluserix and Immravax to be recognized.

---

13   Many members had ties to the pharmaceutical industry.
14   Wakefield, Andrew. *Callous Disregard: Autism and Vaccines—The Truth Behind a Tragedy.* New York, NY: Skyhorse Publishing, 2010. p. 65-75
15   Ibid.

- An increasing number of anecdotal reports of meningitis following vaccination did come in, however. These events usually occurred about 21 days or more after the Pluserix or Immravax vaccine was given, and were reported in *The Lancet* in July 1989.[16]

- Dr. David Salisbury was ultimately forced to divert a small amount of money to investigate whether there was indeed a statistically relevant connection between Pluserix and the rising incidence of meningitis in the children so vaccinated, and that is indeed what the Public Health Laboratory Service found.

- The license to manufacture and distribute the dangerous Trivirix/Pluserix vaccine was revoked in Malaysia, Singapore, and the Philippines and secretly withdrawn in Australia in 1990.[17]

- In 1992, four years after its unfortunate introduction, the dangers of Pluserix and Immravax could no longer be denied, and they were quickly withdrawn from the market. The UK had to go back to using the allegedly more expensive but somewhat safer MMR II vaccine from Merck.[18]

- Many parents of Pluserix/Trivirix-injured children brought suit against GlaxoSmithKlein. Appearing as an expert witness for Glaxo was Dr. Elizabeth Miller of the Health Protection Agency and one of the safety panel members who had approved the faulty vaccine. When asked about the obvious conflict of interest, she stated, "There can be no conflict of interest when acting as an expert for the courts, because the duty to the courts overrides any other obligation, including to the person from whom the expert receives the instruction or by whom they are paid." Oh, really?

So What Can We Learn from This Unfortunate Episode?

- A few individuals in authority can disproportionately and detrimentally influence policy.

- Essential information and access to it can be, has been, and is easily manipulated or suppressed if it suits those in power.

- Misstatements of fact (lies) are readily utilized by individuals and agencies in authority in order to sway public opinion as well as for self-protection.

- Necessary research regarding the safety of one or more vaccines or vaccine components may be bypassed if the likely outcomes of that research prove to be "inconvenient."

- Vaccine costs trump vaccine safety.

- Vaccines touted as being safe by governmental authorities may not be.

- Vaccine manufacturers in Britain, as in the U.S., are able to be protected against liability for harm done by their products, even when those products are proven to be dangerous.

Sound Familiar?

> *"While it may, in some perverse sense, be understandable that public health officials are reluctant to concede that the MMR vaccination programme has damaged thousands of UK children, (they would all be incriminating themselves), given the evidence both scientific and anecdotal, it is surely high time that some brave soul in medicine had the courage to raise his head above the parapet and admit liability."*
>
> — Bill Welsh, President, Autism Treatment Trust;
> October 24, 2008

---

16   Vol 2. p. 98
17   Wakefield, Andrew. *Callous Disregard*. p. 252.
18   Ibid. p. 253

Chapter 21
The Infamous Wakefield Study

*"Truth is incontrovertible, malice may attack it
and ignorance may deride it, but, in the end, there it is."*

— *Sir Winston Churchill, British statesman,
Prime Minister, and Nobel Prize Winner in Literature*

W**HY HAS THE** *MMR Immunization Been Thought to Be Associated with the Autism Epidemic?*
The first clue came in 1971 when a researcher named Chess reported a number of cases of autism following congenital rubella ("German measles") infection. *It is now thoroughly accepted by all that rubella infection during pregnancy increases the risk of the baby later becoming autistic.* Live (attenuated) rubella virus is in the MMR.[1]

Then in 1975, Rivinus and colleagues reported autism occurring after measles virus-caused brain inflammation.[2]

In 1979, researchers E.Y. Deykin and B. MacMahon associated exposure to measles and mumps virus with autism.[3]

In 1991, Reed Warren and his fellow researchers found that many autistic children had a particular genetic immune defect (a null allele at the complement C4B locus) that could result in their "not be(ing) able to clear certain viruses completely or before the viruses affect the central nervous system."[4]

In 1994, Rutter and colleagues published a paper that suggested a link between immunizations (including the MMR and measles vaccines) and autism.[5]

In 1995, N.P. Thompson et al. published a study in *The Lancet* implicating the measles vaccine as a cause of inflammatory bowel disease, a condition seen in many autistic children. One of the co-authors of this study was Dr. Andrew Wakefield. "Is measles Vaccine a Risk Factor for Inflammatory Bowel Disease?"[6]

And in that same journal edition, a Danish researcher reported the onset of gait disturbances after the MMR.[7]

In 1996, Gupta discovered that mothers of children with autism tended to have elevated levels of antibodies to the rubella virus. Gupta theorized that these antibodies could be transferred to the fetus across the placenta and

---

1   Chess, S. "Autism in Children with Congenital Rubella." *J Autism Dev Disorders*; 1971; 1:33-47. *and* Chess, S. "Follow-up report on Autism in Congenital Rubella." *J. Autism Let Disord.* (1977) 7:79.
2   Rivinus, T.M. et al. "Childhood Organic Neurological Disease Presenting as Psychiatric Disorder." *Arch Dis Child.* 1975; 50: 115-119.
3   "Viral Exposure and Autism." *American J of Epidemiology.* 1979; 109: 628-638.
4   Warren, R.P. et al. "Increased frequency of the null allele at the complement C4B locus in autism." *Clin Exp Immunol*; 83: 438-440, 1991.
5   "Autism and Known Medical Conditions: Myth and Substance." *J Child Psych*; 1994; 35:311-322.
6   1995; 345:1071-74.
7   Plesner, A.M. "Gait Disturbances after Measles, Mumps, Rubella Vaccine." *The Lancet*; 1995; 345:316.

could persist in the baby until the MMR vaccination was given. The combination of the anti-rubella antibody and the rubella virus from the MMR vaccine could form immune complexes that could "confuse" the immune system.[8]

Also in 1996, a clinical immunologist, Dr. Hugh Fudenberg, confirmed what many parents of autistic children had been contending for some time—that there are some autistic children who develop "symptoms (of this condition) within a week or so after immunization with the measles, mumps and rubella (MMR) vaccine." Many of these children, Dr. Fudenberg noted, also had a history of fever and often seizures within a day of getting the MMR vaccination.[9]

A mother of one such child with autism reported that her son had "severe mental impairment after having the MMR injection. He has no speech," she declared, "no understanding of language at all, no concentration, bizarre behavioral problems, and rarely acknowledges anyone. He has become very strong and aggressive. He is having constant tantrums, screaming and flinging himself to the ground and biting anyone who tries to restrain him. He is very frustrated and agitated most of the time. Our son was once a bright, happy, normal child who could speak and love everyone."[10]

However, it was Rosemary Kessick, the inspired and determined British mother of another autistic boy, who provided the motivation for researchers to look more closely at the suspected link between autism, intestinal problems, and the MMR vaccination. Mrs. Kessick's son, William, like so many other children, also became autistic within days of receiving his MMR shot at 15 months of age.

Prior to his receiving that vaccination, William had been a happy, healthy baby whose developmental abilities were ahead of those of his peers. He had a multiword vocabulary, pointed, made good eye contact, liked to play peek-a-boo, had normal bowel movements, slept well, and understood language clearly.

After the MMR shot, everything changed. William developed digestive problems characterized by more frequent, loose, smelly, abnormally-colored stools. He slept fitfully, didn't look well, began banging his head, and soon lost all language and social interaction.

None of the doctors that Mrs. Kessick brought her son to were able to help William, but a local pediatrician told her that he knew of a number of children whose symptoms and presentation were similar to those of William's. At his suggestion, Mrs. Kessick contacted the parents of those children, and she became convinced that a common symptom pattern was indeed becoming apparent.

Mrs. Kessick was determined to help her child even though William's own doctors seemed unable to, so she experimented with her son's diet and eliminated certain allergenic foods and was subsequently delighted to discover that the removal of wheat and dairy products resulted in a markedly beneficial effect on the quality of his sleep and his behavior, although he continued to have diarrhea.

William was started in a speech therapy program, but his condition again deteriorated after a few months and he began "throwing tantrums and screaming nonstop." Mrs. Kessick was told that William was "severely damaged" and would need to be "institutionalized for life."

Not accepting that prognosis, Mrs. Kessick continued to look for possible causes for William's condition. She read up on vitamins and their deficiency symptoms and convinced her doctor to start William on daily vitamin B12 injections, which rapidly reversed his tantrums and screaming, but not his diarrhea.

She continued her research and got a local doctor to start William on a probiotic (beneficial gut bacteria) treatment program (which had been shown to be beneficial for patients with Crohn's disease), and that indeed stopped his

8   Gupta, S. et a. "Dysregulated immune system in children with autism. Beneficial effects of intravenous immune globulin on autistic characteristics." *J Autism Develop Dis* 26:439-452, 1996.

9   Fudenberg, H. "Dialyzable lymphocyte extract in infantile onset autism: a pilot study." *Biotherapy* 9:144, 1996.

10   Dawbarn's Solicitors Fact Sheet. "Mumps, measles, and rubella MMR) vaccines and measles rubella (MR) vaccines." Dawbarn's Solicitors. Bank House. King's Staithe Square. King's Lynn, Norfolk, Great Britain PE30 1RD.

diarrhea, but William still had autistic symptoms, and Mrs. Kessick wanted to know why all his problems seemed to start after the MMR "jab."[11]

The Crohn's Disease Clue

Crohn's disease is the name given to a frequently severe, chronic inflammatory process of unknown origin that involves the last part of the small intestine (the terminal ileum) and sometimes other parts of the intestinal tract as well. It is characterized by abdominal pains, diarrhea (sometimes bloody), weight loss, loss of appetite, delayed puberty, and malaise.

This sometimes fatal, debilitating malady is seen in all age groups, but it is more common in adults. As with autism, the incidence of Crohn's disease is increasing dramatically, and that means there is (are) an environmental culprit(s) that play a role in the etiology of this "intestinal scourge." Many scientists have suspected that a microbe (a bacteria, virus, or parasite) might be to blame, and one of the viruses under suspicion is the measles virus.

In 1993, the Inflammatory Bowel Disease Study Group at the Royal Free Hospital in London, led by research gastroenterologist Dr. Andrew Wakefield, discovered that measles virus DNA was present in virtually every sample of Crohn's disease tissue examined but was rarely found in control tissue samples. The group theorized that Crohn's disease might be promoted or caused by a persistent infection with the measles virus.[12]

Evidence to support this theory came from Sweden where an epidemiological study of 93 cases of Crohn's disease "showed a high rate of early life (measles) infections either prenatal in the mother or postnatal in the child."[13]

The British and Swedish researchers then got together and examined the medical histories of over 25,000 babies delivered at a large Swedish hospital. They uncovered just four cases where the mother had measles during the pregnancy, and to their surprise, three of those four babies went on to develop Crohn's disease later in life.[14]

The Measles Vaccine Connection to Crohn's Disease

Andrew Wakefield and his colleagues at the Royal Free Hospital also reviewed the clinical trial groups that had been under study for the original measles vaccine administered in 1964 and found that *those who had received the measles vaccination had three times the risk of developing Crohn's disease compared to the unvaccinated controls.*[15]

Mrs. Kessick, the daughter of a physician father and nurse mother, had learned from her own reading that vitamin B12 was absorbed mainly in the terminal ileum, the last part of the small intestine and the usual target for Crohn's disease inflammation. She also knew that probiotics benefited patients with Crohn's disease. Her son had improved on both the B12 and probiotics, and his chronic intestinal symptoms started a short time after the MMR shot.

She had heard about the research that Dr. Wakefield and others had been doing that implicated measles as a possible cause of Crohn's disease, and she reasoned that William, then age seven, might have an early form of this malady, so Mrs. Kessick contacted Dr. Wakefield on May 17, 1995 to ask for his advice and assistance, and he agreed to help.

Dr. Wakefield was at that time a highly respected researcher and gastro-intestinal surgeon at the Royal Free Hospital. While there, he had been awarded a coveted research fellowship and had later studied small bowel transplant surgery in Toronto. He subsequently returned to the Royal Free Hospital where he founded the Inflammatory Bowel Disease Study Group, a prestigious collaboration of researchers and clinicians, who discussed interesting patients, promoted and published new research (primarily on the causes and mechanisms of inflammatory bowel disease),

---

11   Olmstead, Dan and Mark Blaxill. *The Age of Autism: Mercury, Medicine, and a Man-Made Epidemic.* New York, NY: St. Martin's Press, 2010. p. 261 ff

12   Wakefield, A.J. et al. "Evidence of Persistent Measles Virus Infection in Crohn's Disease." *J Med Virol.* 1993, 39(4): 345-53.

13   Anders, Ekbom et al. "Prenatal Risk Factors for Inflammatory Bowel Disease: A Case-control Study." *Amer. Journal of Epidemiology,* 1990, 132(6); 1111-9.

14   Anders, Ekbom et al .and Andrew Wakefield. "Crohn's Disease after In-Utero Measles Virus Exposure." *The Lancet,* 1996, 348(9026): 515-7.

15   Thompson, N.P. et al. (including Andrew Wakefield). "Is Measles Vaccination a Risk Factor for Inflammatory Bowel Disease?" *The Lancet,* 1995, 345 (8957): 1071-4.

and discussed practical approaches to clinical problems. He was rapidly promoted to senior lecturer in 1993 and then to reader (equivalent to associate professor) in 1997.

Dr. Wakefield was impressed with Mrs. Kessick's drive, intelligence, scholarship, and determination. He decided to refer her son William to Dr. John Walker-Smith, a renowned pediatric gastroenterologist and author of the standard textbook (not ghostwritten) on children's intestinal diseases. Dr. Walker-Smith was about to bring his pediatric gastroenterology practice to the Royal Free Hospital where he would join Wakefield and colleagues in the Irritable Bowel Disease Study Group.

John Walker-Smith not only examined William Kessick, but he investigated 11 other similar cases of children whose symptoms mirrored those of William's. Nine of the children had autism, one had childhood disintegrative disorder, and two had neurological damage secondary to encephalitis. All 12 had bowel symptoms. Ten had regressed shortly after being given the MMR immunization. One had regressed after having a measles infection, and the last regressed after an ear infection.

Both Walker-Smith and Wakefield felt that these cases *might* represent a new syndrome and that they needed to be investigated further. The two men along with their colleagues at the IBD Study Group then proposed doing two investigative studies.

One of these was to be a *case control study*, in which the affected children's findings would be compared to those of a matched control group. Such studies must be correctly designed, which takes time, and they also require strict ethical controls as they involve the parallel examination of otherwise healthy control children. The need to acquire funding for such studies often also delays their start.

In order to evaluate these 12 children more expeditiously, the IBD Study Group decided *first* to carry out a less rigorous (and less expensive) type of investigation known as a *case series study*. Such studies evaluate a series of patients with a similar diagnosis and do not require or employ strict inclusion or exclusion criteria. In this particular instance, that would mean there would be no requirement that the children all had to have been exposed to the MMR vaccine or diagnosed with autism or childhood disintegrative disorder.

Case series studies often lead to the discovery of a new feature of a disease or the formulation of a new hypothesis. They may include an age-matched control group, but this is not a requirement. In this instance, the IBD Study Group did include 19 age-matched children as controls: 5 children for microscopic examination of tissues and 14 for measurement of a urine marker of vitamin B12 sufficiency or deficiency (methyl-malonic acid).

The proposed case series study was "approved by the Ethical Practices Committee of the Royal Free Hospital NHS Trust, and parents gave informed consent."[16]

The study "was supported by the Special Trustees of Royal Free Hampstead NHS Trust and the Children's Medical Charity." That is to say, they provided the funds necessary to perform this case series study.

Dr. Mike Thompson, a pediatric gastroenterologist who worked with Dr. Walker-Smith, suggested that the proposed study should also include a lumbar puncture (LP) evaluation of each of the children in order to rule out a possible mitochondrial disorder that could account for their neurological deterioration.

Such a protocol was approved and then in use at Britain's Birmingham Children's Hospital, and some researchers in the U.S. at that time were also advocating the use of lumbar puncture as part of the diagnostic workup for autism; however, doing an LP as part of the workup for autism was by no means universally practiced at that time (although it was part of the protocol of most providers for childhood disintegrative disorder), and the inclusion of the lumbar puncture on eight of the twelve children included in the *Lancet* study became a major point of contention in a subsequent investigation and criticism of that research.

---

16   Wakefield, Andrew; Murch, Simon et al. "Ileal-lymphoid Nodular Hyperplasia, Non-specific Colitis and Pervasive Developmental Disorder in Children." *The Lancet*, 1998, 351(9103):837-41.

Lumbar punctures in experienced hands are considered to be safe evaluative procedures. Virtually every experienced pediatrician has performed dozens of these procedures, which involve injecting a numbing substance into the lower (lumbar) spine and then inserting a sterile needle in the space between two adjacent vertebrae in order to withdraw a small sample of the fluid that surrounds the spinal cord.

Mitochondria are the tiny energy factories found in cells. Genetic or acquired disorders of the mitochondria can present in a variety of ways, including developmental delays and mental deterioration.

Although lumbar puncture was performed on eight of the twelve children in the *Lancet* study, the procedure was "abandoned" in early 1997 because "In the small number of children who had this investigation…[there was no] evidence of a mitochondrial disorder."[17]

If the lumbar punctures had been part of a research protocol, as the GMC[18] later alleged, all the children in the study would have needed to have the procedure performed, but that's not what happened. The procedure was discontinued when it failed to "yield any useful clinical information…that might have provided insights into diagnosis and possible treatment."[19] In other words, the lumbar puncture evaluation was done to benefit the children and not the research study.

Ironically, recent research has shown that mitochondrial disorders are actually quite commonly seen in children with autism spectrum disorders.[20]

All twelve affected children evaluated in this study also received diagnostic colonoscopies, a procedure where a guided tube is inserted into the colon and the tissues evaluated. In most cases, the tube can be inserted sufficiently to view the terminal ileum as well. Using this device, tiny samples of tissue are able to be taken (biopsied) for microscopic analysis. Dr. Simon Murch, an experienced colleague of Dr. Walker-Smith, performed the colonoscopies, and he was able to view the terminal ileum in 11 of the 12 children under study.

Biopsies were taken from selected sites and compared to those of seven consecutive children who already had had colonoscopies performed for other reasons (the control group: four with normal colonoscopies, 3 with ulcerative colitis but normal terminal ileums).[21]

What Dr. Murch noted in the intestines of the 12 children in the study was a non-specific inflammation of the colon and significant lymph node enlargement in the terminal ileum, a finding that doctors call *lymphoid nodular hyperplasia* (LNH). This appeared to be a new syndrome possibly associated with the MMR vaccination.

Lymph nodes are collections of immune cells called lymphocytes that act as sentinels of the immune system. Lymph nodes are found throughout the body, but they are found in particularly large numbers in the intestinal tract. When they enlarge (hypertrophy), they can form visible nodules (bumps) that make the lining of the intestine look like a cobblestone street.[22] The cause of this enlargement is usually an infectious agent, but it is often unknown.

So the suspicions of Mrs. Kessick and the parents of the other 11 affected children were correct. The children did show evidence of chronic intestinal inflammation, and they also had urine markers that demonstrated a relative deficiency of vitamin B12.

Because the children now had *confirmed* bowel involvement, they were then able to be treated with *mesalazine*, a standard prescription remedy for intestinal inflammation, and *all the children, including William, appeared to improve* after being placed on this medication.

---

17   Wakefield, Andrew. *Callous Disregard*. p. 157.
18   General Medical Council
19   Ibid. p. 148
20   Oliveira, G. et al *Devel. Medicine & Child Neurol.* 2005; 47:185-189; *and* Weissman, J. et al. *PLoS ONE.* 2008; 3(11):e3815
21   Wakefield, Andrew. *Callous Disregard*. p. 11.
22   See the photograph in Chapter 3.

The IBD Study Group wrote up its findings as an "early report," and its case series study was eventually published in *The Lancet* in February 1998 with the rather technical title: "Ileal-lymphoid Nodular Hyperplasia, Non-specific Colitis and Pervasive Developmental Disorder in Children."[23]

Report Findings:

1. Patchy (found in some spots and not in others), chronic (long standing) colonic (large intestine), non-specific (not characteristic of one particular disease or condition), inflammation in 11 of the 12 children. This was the first report to demonstrate intestinal inflammation in autistic children, and the first to show worsening of that inflammation in autistic children after receiving a second measles vaccination.

2. Reactive ileal lymphoid nodular hyperplasia (many large stimulated lymph nodes in the ileum—the last part of the small intestine) in 7 of the 12 children.

3. No focal neurological abnormalities in any of the children.

4. Normal MRI (magnetic resonance imaging) and EEG tests in all the children.

5. All 12 children tested negative for the Fragile X gene.

6. Significantly elevated urinary methylmalonic acid (a marker of B12 deficiency) compared with age matched controls ($p=0{\cdot}003$) in all of the children. This was *the first report to associate vitamin B12 deficiency with autism.*

7. Low hemoglobin in four children (a sign of anemia).

8. Low serum IgA levels (antibody class produced by and protecting the intestinal lining) in four children.

9. The parents or the child's physician had linked the onset of behavioral problems with the measles, mumps, and rubella vaccination in eight (66 percent) of the children, and "In these eight children the average interval from exposure to first behavioural symptoms was 6.3 days (range 1-14)."[24]

10. Five of the twelve children had had *an early adverse reaction to the MMR immunization* (rash, fever, delirium; and, in three cases, convulsions).

11. "One child (child four) had received monovalent measles vaccine at 15 months, after which his development slowed (confirmed by professional assessors). No association was made with the vaccine at that time. He received a (second) dose of measles, mumps, and rubella vaccine at age 4-5 years, the day after which his mother described a striking deterioration in his behaviour that she did link with the immunisation."[25]

12. "Child nine received measles, mumps, and rubella vaccine at 16 months. At 18 months he developed recurrent antibiotic resistant otitis media (a middle ear infection) and the first behavioural symptoms, including disinterest in his sibling and lack of play."

13. This was the first study to demonstrate an *abnormal lactate to pyruvate ratio* in autistic children, an indication of a possible mitochondrial disorder. The mitochondria are the energy-making organelles found in almost all cells.

In the "Discussion" section of the report, the researchers describe, "a pattern of colitis (inflamed large intestine) and ileal-lymphoid nodular hyperplasia in children with developmental disorders. *Intestinal and behavioural pathologies may have occurred together by chance, reflecting a selection bias in a self-referred group;* however, the uniformity of the intestinal pathological changes and the fact that previous studies have found intestinal dysfunction in children with autistic-spectrum disorders suggests that the connection is real and reflects a unique disease process."[26] Note that the authors don't maintain that the connection has been proven—the evidence just "suggested" that there was a connection.

---

23   Wakefield, Andrew; Murch, Simon et al. "Ileal-lymphoid Nodular Hyperplasia, Non-specific Colitis and Pervasive Developmental Disorder in Children." *The Lancet*, 1998, 351(9103):837-41.

24   Ibid.

25   Ibid.

26   Ibid.

They go on to point out that, "Disintegrative psychosis (AKA "childhood disintegrative disorder"—is similar to autism and diagnosed in one of the 12 children) is typically described as occurring in children after at least 2-3 years of apparently normal development. Disintegrative psychosis is recognized as a sequel to measles encephalitis, although in most cases no cause is ever identified."[27]

The researchers then cite a number of referenced studies that:

- Support the link between an intestinal disease (Celiac Disease/Gluten allergy) and abnormal behaviors.[28]

- Demonstrate low levels of a protective intestinal enzyme (alpha-1 antitrypsin) in children with autism that might make them more prone to having an inflamed intestine.[29]

- Demonstrate impaired intestinal permeability in 43 percent of children with autism who had no intestinal symptoms.[30]

- Implicate the production of abnormal small opioid proteins (morphine-like peptides) noted in autistic children and secondary to impaired digestion that can adversely affect cognitive function.[31]

An addendum to the study notes that, "Up to Jan 28, a further 40 patients have been assessed; 39 with the syndrome."

Did These Researchers *Claim* or *Prove* That the MMR Vaccine Caused Autism and Intestinal Inflammation in These Children?

No. They clearly state that "intestinal and behavioural pathologies may have occurred together by chance, reflecting a selection bias in a self-referred group" and they "did not prove an association between measles, mumps, and rubella vaccine and the syndrome described."

They then go on to add that, "Virological studies are underway that may help to resolve this issue." These virological studies were part of a proposed *second* case series study of another 25 affected children initiated by the law firm Dawbarn's Solicitors and supported by funds from the Legal Aid Board. This study was to look for the presence of measles virus in the tissues biopsied during the colonoscopy procedures on the children.

So How Do We Explain the Following Statements By These "Experts"?

"This flawed study concluded that the rise in autism was related to giving the combination vaccine of measles-mumps-rubella (MMR)."

— Art Brown, spokesperson for the American Academy of Pediatrics and the Immunization Action Coalition

"(This is a) study claiming a causal relationship between…(MMR) vaccine and autism spectrum disorders."

— Sir Michael Rutter, expert prosecution witness who also has represented MMR vaccine manufacturers

---

27   Wakefield, Ibid. *and* Rutter, M.; Taylor, E.; Hersor, L. in *Child and Adolescent Psychiatry*. 3rd ed.. London: Blackwells Scientific Publications: 581-82.

28   Asperger, H. "Die Psychopathologie des coeliakakranken kindes." *Ann Paediatr* 1961; 197: 146-151. PubMed.

29   Walker-Smith, J.A.; Andrews, J. "Alpha-1 antitrypsin, autism and coeliac disease." *Lancet* 1972; ii: 883-884. PubMed.

30   D'Eufemia, P.; Celli, M.; Finocchiaro, R. et al. "Abnormal intestinal permeability in children with autism." *Acta Paediatrica* 1996; 85: 1076-1079. PubMed.

31   Panksepp, J. "A neurochemical theory of autism." *Trends Neurosci* 1979; 2: 174-177. CrossRef | PubMed and Reichelt, K.L.; Hole, K.; Hamberger, A, et al. "Biologically active peptide-containing fractions in schizophrenia and childhood autism." *Adv Biochem Psychopharmacol* 1993; 28: 627-643. PubMed *and* Shattock, P. et al. "Role of neuropeptides in autism and their relationships with classical neurotransmitters." *Brain Dysfunction* 1991; 3: 328-345. PubMed.

"Recent reports (referring to this study) claim...that a new phenotype of autism associated with developmental regression and gastro-intestinal symptoms has emerged as a consequence of measles-mumps-rubella vaccination."

— Prof. Eric Fombonne, expert witness on behalf of the vaccine manufacturers

...and this non-expert?

"The dynamite in The Lancet *was the claim that their [the autistic children] conditions could be linked to the MMR vaccine, which had been given to all 12 children."*

— Brian Deer, The Sunday Times, *February 8, 2009*

Answer

Only three possibilities exist for these misinformed statements (we're assuming that these so-called "experts" and the one "non-expert" have at least average intelligence):

1. They didn't read the Wakefield study.

2. They read the study but conveniently or inadvertently skipped or forgot the part that said no association between the MMR vaccine and the syndrome described was proven.

3. They intentionally chose to distort the truth.

Why Is There So Much Controversy Regarding This Study?

That's a good question.

This seemingly well-done case series study has generated more controversy than virtually any other study in recent times, and it was eventually rejected and withdrawn by *The Lancet*, the medical journal that initially published it.

The senior researchers in this study, Drs. Andrew Wakefield, John Walker-Smith, and Simon Murch, have all since been embroiled in a legal, political, and ethical battle that has cost some of them their jobs and medical licenses and which has unfairly damaged the reputations of all of them.

It is a "battle," if you will, that is still being fought to this day, and the repercussions of this conflict are very pertinent not only to our understanding of the nature and causes of autism, but also to our discovering the extent to which malevolent authorities will go in order to disparage good research and honorable and competent researchers for the purpose of protecting their own self-interests and what they presumably perceive to be the greater good.

The details of the controversy surrounding this study are extensively discussed and thoroughly referenced in Dr. Wakefield's book *Callous Disregard*. In it, Dr. Wakefield successfully rebuts the self-serving newspaper and medical establishment distortions, lies, omissions, and obfuscations that have hounded him and his colleagues to this day.

We will review key points of their odyssey in the next chapter, and by so doing, I hope to demonstrate that Dr. Wakefield and his colleagues are honorable and ethical men who have been subjected to unfair and unfounded malicious attacks, that their findings have been replicated in other independent studies that were published in reputable, peer-reviewed journals, and that these discoveries were and are meaningful, scientifically sound, and very relevant to our understanding of the causes and consequences of autism.

We will also be reminded yet again about the lengths to which unscrupulous individuals will go in order to distort reality for their own self-serving purposes.

Chapter 22
The Controversy Surrounding the Wakefield Study

*"Lives of great men all remind us greatness takes no easy way.
All the heroes of tomorrow are the heretics of today."*

— *Yip Harburg*

S O, What Happened *Next?*

A great deal, but first some background....

In May 1995, Dr. Wakefield met with Mrs. Kessick and other parents of children with regressive autism. He referred young William Kessick, as had been mentioned, to Professor John Walker-Smith, renowned pediatric gastroenterologist, for an evaluation of the child's intestinal symptoms.

The following month, a second of the children with regressive autism and GI symptoms was referred to Professor Walker-Smith.

In September 1995, Dr. Walker-Smith joined Andrew Wakefield at the Royal Free Hospital where they applied for and were granted ethics committee approval (#162-95) for biopsy research in the children with regressive autism and GI symptoms undergoing colonoscopy. This was the ethics committee approval that the researchers would need in order to perform intestinal biopsies on those who were to later become the "Lancet 12" children.

In December 1995, the *British Sunday Times Magazine* published an article entitled "A Shot in the Dark," which outlined the research that had previously been done by Andrew Wakefield and others linking the measles vaccine to inflammatory bowel disease. The article also mentioned Dr. Reed Warren's work in the U.S. that had looked at the possible association between the MMR vaccination and autism.[1]

In the following month, January 1996, attorney Richard Barr, whose firm represented parents of children with autism and inflammatory bowel disease (among other concerns), contacted Dr. Wakefield to ask him to act as an expert witness in possible future litigation involving allegations of a possible link *between vaccines and Crohn's Disease* (Note: not autism, Crohn's disease). Dr. Wakefield agreed to do this. (Note also that Wakefield's involvement with attorney Barr occurred 3-4 months *after* Wakefield and Walker-Smith had already decided to do the formal case series study on the affected children.)

Over the next nine months (January–September 1996), protocols for the proposed study were finalized; in July 1996, the first of the children with intestinal complaints and developmental disorder was evaluated as part of the study.

---

1   Roberts, Y. Sunday Times. December 17, 1995; p. 17-23 and Kirby, David. *Evidence of Harm: Mercury in Vaccines and the Autism Epidemic: A Medical Controversy.* New York: St. Martin's Press, 2007. p. 258.

In August 1996, Dr. Wakefield also agreed to accept funding from the Legal Aid Board to support a *second* and newly proposed investigation into whether the measles virus was present in colon tissue biopsies taken from a *different cohort* of 25 developmentally-disabled children with gut issues matched with a control group. Remember, Wakefield had good reason to be suspicious of a measles-Crohn's disease connection.

The two case series studies would overlap. Information about the *second* proposed viral study was reported to the British public in an article published on November 27, 1996 in the newspaper *The Independent.*[2]

In September 1996, Wakefield and his colleagues again sought ethics committee approval for the procedures to be performed in this proposed *second* viral study, and that permission was granted (#172-96) in January 1997. The last of the *Lancet* 12 children was evaluated that same month, and it was also in January 1997 that Dr. Wakefield informed his senior colleagues verbally and in writing about his potential involvement with the Dawbarn's law firm.

On December 12, 1996, Professor John Walker-Smith, in association with pathologist Dr. Paul Dhillon, presented the results of their investigation of 7 of the 12 children, who were eventually to be included in the *Lancet* study, to colleagues at the Royal Free Hospital. Their findings, including the children's medical histories, are identical to those published 26 months later in *The Lancet.*

Between February and July of 1997, the research paper for the first study was written and submitted to *The Lancet* for publication.

In March 1997, attorney Barr wrote a letter to Richard Horton, then editor of *The Lancet,* in which he mentioned Dr. Wakefield's involvement with the firm in regard to possible future MMR litigation and also noted that the (second) study would be funded by the Legal Aid Board. Dr. Horton offered no objection in this regard.

The first study, it will be recalled, was ultimately published in February 1998, and was supported (funded) by the Special Trustees of Royal Free Hampstead NHS Trust and the Children's Medical Charity (and *not* by the Legal Aid Board as was later alleged).

Dr. Wakefield's superior at the Royal Free Hospital at that time was virologist and medical school dean, Dr. Arie Zuckerman. Dr. Zuckerman was being pressured by British Authorities to discourage research that might link the MMR vaccine with intestinal diseases like Crohn's or with autism. The Department of Health stood to be sued if such a link could be established.

Dr. Zuckerman tried to dissuade Dr. Wakefield by suggesting that the money from the Legal Aid Board (a "government-funded legal assistance program") for the *second* proposed study might represent a conflict of interest in that the plaintiffs and their attorneys stood to gain if a link was shown to exist between the MMR "jab" and developmental disorders like autism or with inflammatory conditions like Crohn's disease.

This argument was, of course, pure sophistry, as the Royal Free Hospital had no ethical problem accepting research money from pharmaceutical companies that also stood to gain from positive outcomes of their own sponsored research.

Dr. Wakefield tried to reassure his superior by asserting that the research would be conducted honorably, ethically, and without bias (which it was). The children's intestinal tissue biopsy analysis was to be performed by a pathologist over whom he had no influence and who had no financial or other ties to the pharmaceutical industry.

In October 1996, Dr. Zuckerman, still looking for a way to halt Dr. Wakefield's investigations, contacted Dr. Mac Armstrong, chairman of the ethics committee of the British Medical Association, requesting his opinion in this regard and listing his concern that the proposed research "could lead to a case against the government for damages."[3]

2   Langdon-Down, G. p. 25.
3   Wakefield, Andrew. *Callous Disregard.* p. 53.

When the response from Dr. Armstrong eventually arrived over five months later (March 26, 1997), it was not at all what Dr. Zuckerman had hoped for.

The three-page reply found the proposed research to be entirely ethical and appropriate, and noted that it was "quite logical for the Legal Aid Board…to fund research on relevant issues in law," and that, "funding of research by special interest groups is commonplace, and as long as the findings, or uses to which the data is put, are not influenced by the wishes of the funders, this should not be problematic," and furthermore, "to delay or decline to conduct research which appears to be in the public interest on the grounds that it may embarrass the government or a particular health facility does not appear to be a sound moral argument."[4]

In May of 1997 (nine months before Wakefield's infamous *Lancet* paper was published), the UK's Joint Committee on Vaccinations and Immunizations reviewed many parental reports about serious developmental and communications problems that started shortly after the MMR vaccination was given to their children. The JCVI dismissed all these reports as "anecdotal" and not worthy of follow-up.

While awaiting Dr. Zuckerman's approval of the *second* viral study, the case series report on the 12 children in the ill-fated first study was completed and sent to *The Lancet* in July 1997. That study was, as we know, finally published in February 1998, and prior to its publication, the Legal Aid Board-funded measles virus detection case series study was also approved by the reluctant Dr. Zuckerman and finally started in October 1997.

On February 28, 1998, Drs. Zuckerman and Wakefield held a press conference to discuss the just-published "Lancet 12" article. At that conference, Dr. Wakefield also recommended that until more was known about any potential links between the MMR, inflammatory bowel disease, and developmental disorders, it would (in his opinion) be preferable for children to receive three separate monovalent (just one disease virus per vaccine) vaccines for the measles, mumps, and rubella viruses instead of the combined MMR vaccine, and that they should be given one year apart.

It is important to note that Dr. Wakefield was *not* recommending that children not be vaccinated against these diseases. He was simply proposing what he reasonably felt was a less risky alternative: use the single virus vaccines, not the MMR combined vaccine.

All of these monovalent vaccines were available in the UK at the time Dr. Wakefield made his recommendations. However, just six months later (in August 1998) the UK's Department of Health, *for no rational reason* and despite "unprecedented demand," withdrew the licenses for single vaccines.[5]

Wakefield was unfairly blamed for the decrease in the number of British children getting measles immunizations and for the subsequent rise in measles cases, but the true villains in that regard were the authorities that had irresponsibly withdrawn the popular monovalent vaccines that Wakefield had recommended giving in lieu of the MMR. Merck continued manufacturing them until 2009.

And Dr. Wakefield had made his recommendations regarding his preference for single virus vaccines only after comprehensively reviewing "all safety studies performed on measles, MR (measles, rubella) and MMR vaccines and re-vaccination policies" which he had then compiled into a report that ran some 250 pages.

He found the so-called safety studies to be worthy of derision in that they "appear(ed) to reflect sequential assumptions about measles vaccine safety, MMR safety and latterly, two dose vaccine safety, where each assumption has potentially compounded the dangers inherent in the first."[6]

Wakefield had previously informed all his co-authors and also Dr. Zuckerman of his feelings in this regard in a letter sent to each individual *five weeks prior* to the publication of the "Lancet 12" article.[7]

---

4   Ibid.
5   Wakefield, Andrew. *Callous Disregard*. p. 263.
6   Letter to co-authors and to Dr. Zuckerman; *Callous Disregard*. p. 84-85.
7   Ibid.

In that letter, he goes on to say that he understands parents' frustrations when they have their claims of possible vaccine harm dismissed "out of hand," and when "loss of trust in regulatory authorities" inevitably occurs, he continues, "vaccination compliance… is affected."[8]

Wakefield placed the blame for "this volatile state of affairs" on the "shoulders of the policy makers," that is, the JCVI (Joint Committee on Vaccinations and Immunizations) and the Department of Health. He asserted that since *the safety of the MMR had never been satisfactorily proven*, "all claims of adverse events should have been thoroughly investigated," but the JCVI and the Department of Health had "failed to honour this obligation."[9]

He ended this letter to his coauthors by stating that he appreciated that they might not support him in this regard, and that he completely respected their right to hold that position.[10]

What Was the Response to the Controversial Lancet Article and the Press Briefing?

The response was widespread, explosive, and immediate. News reports broadcast all over the world informed the public about the *possible* link between the MMR vaccination, autism, and intestinal inflammation.

The initial news reports generally underemphasized or neglected to mention Dr. Wakefield's recommendation to continue measles (and rubella and mumps) immunizations via single virus (monovalent) vaccinations in lieu of the MMR. Misinterpretations and misstatements of fact regarding the case series study began to circulate and then escalate.

Dr. Rouse, a public health doctor from the west of England, immediately wrote to *The Lancet*, mistakenly suggesting that some of the children investigated by "Wakefield et al. came to [his] attention because of the activities of [the Society for Autistically Handicapped]." Rouse maintained that "parents referred in this way would suffer from recall bias," and he bemoaned the fact that "Wakefield et al. do not identify the manner in which the 12 children were referred."[11]

These statements were all incorrect. The children had been appropriately "referred through the normal channels" (from their own doctors) "on the merit of their symptoms" and the paper so stated (the children were "self referred"). They were not "recruited" as some have alleged.

Dr. Wakefield had never been contacted by, and indeed was unaware (at that time) of the existence of, the Society for Autistically Handicapped, and he made this expressly clear in his rebuttal letter to Rouse's allegations, which was also published in a later edition of *The Lancet*.

Richard Horton, then editor of *The Lancet*, had also come under attack after the "Lancet 12" article was published. The former president of the UK's Academy of Medical Services telephoned Horton and excoriated him for publishing an article that raised questions about the safety of the MMR. Horton was later asked by another individual whether he thought he would ever be forgiven for having published "that article." He also stated that there were many personal attacks made against him.[12]

In his "mea culpa" book, *Second Opinion*, published in 2003, Horton describes his actions relevant to the Wakefield et al. paper as being "embarrassingly naïve."

In that book, Horton makes a number of misstatements. He alleges, for example, that the single (monovalent) vaccines were not available in the UK at the time when Dr. Wakefield recommended their use. They were.

He maintains that other researchers have "convincingly refuted any association between the vaccine and autism." They haven't.

---

8   Ibid.
9   Ibid.
10   Ibid.
11   Ibid. p.102.
12   Ibid. p.104.

He states that "not one person or group has confirmed the original findings in the *Lancet* paper." They have.[13, 14]

Horton also made a number of factually incorrect statements at the General Medical Council (GMC) hearing held to investigate claims of fraud and impropriety by Drs. Wakefield, Walker-Smith, and Murch in regard to the *Lancet* study.

He alleged, for example, that he was "unaware of any potential litigation surrounding the MMR vaccine" *going back to 1997*, and further that he was "not aware of any other relationship between Dr. Wakefield and Dawbarn's and Richard Barr."

But Dawbarn's attorney Richard Barr had *written and faxed* Horton a detailed letter (on April 3, 1997) outlining the firm's intent to litigate for potential damages to certain children who experienced the sudden onset of *intestinal complaints* following their exposure to the MMR or MR vaccines. Barr requested Horton's retrospective permission to quote four specific *Lancet* references in a fact sheet for parents that the firm had been distributing. Horton initially refused to give that permission.

A footnote from one of those references states, "There is convincing evidence of a link between (measles) vaccination and inflammatory bowel disease.... We are working with Dr. Andrew Wakefield...[who] is investigating this condition."

We know that Horton definitely received and read Barr's letter and facsimile because he responded to that letter and related mailings not once, but *three times*: on April 8, 1997, on April 23, 1997, and still again on June 12, 1997. So when testifying before the GMC, Horton was either lying or exhibiting a remarkable degree of selective amnesia.[15]

In a meeting held in February 2004 with some of the other coauthors of the Wakefield study (but not Wakefield himself), Horton misinformed the group that the *Lancet* study was funded by the Legal Aid Board in order to support litigation by parents of children presumably harmed by the MMR vaccine.

Horton had been given that bit of disinformation by a soon to be famous (infamous?) news reporter who had himself *illegally* been given access to the *confidential* medical records of the children in the "Lancet 12" study by an agency, the North London Special Health Authority, that had oversight over the Royal Free Hospital, and that action opened the flood gates for what was to come.[16]

> *"The only things that are infinite are the universe and human stupidity, and I am not entirely sure about the former."*
>
> — *Albert Einstein*

A Deer in the Headlights and the Headlines

Brian Deer is a freelance journalist and a would-be muckraker who cleverly invents his own "muck" when none appears to exist. He soon became the darling of the medical establishment that sought to discredit Dr. Wakefield, his colleagues, and especially, that inconvenient case series study.

And Deer was the journalist who was surreptitiously and illegally given access to those *confidential* children's outpatient medical records. Deer reviewed those files and other information that he had been given and then promptly and wrongly accused Wakefield of having received money from the Legal Aid Board to fund the study that had been published in *The Lancet*. This, of course, was not true. The *Lancet* study was financed by the Special Trustees of Royal Free Hampstead NHS (National Health Service) Trust and the Children's Medical Charity, and this information was clearly stated in the published report.

---

13   Ibid.
14   I will document these last two assertions subsequently.
15   Wakefield, Andrew. *Callous Disregard*. p. 117-131.
16   Ibid. p. 105.

The Legal Aid Board funds, as previously mentioned, were to fund the *second* case series study whose purpose was to look for the presence of measles virus in the diseased intestines of a new cohort of affected children.

Deer also asserted that Dr. Wakefield had not informed his colleagues at the Royal Free Hospital that he was "helping investigate a claim on behalf of autistic children." That allegation was also false. Dr. Wakefield's senior colleagues at the Royal Free Hospital had been so informed at least *one year* prior to the article's publication. Those informed included coauthor Dr. John Walker-Smith, Dr. Arie Zuckerman, the CEO of the Royal Free Hospital, and even the general public via a report in the national press.[17]

And Dr. Wakefield has documented that the editorial board of *The Lancet* was also fully aware that he "was working as an expert on MMR litigation well in advance of the paper's publication."[18]

Undeterred by the facts, Deer continued his malicious attacks, further alleging that Wakefield had:

- "Contrived an MMR problem in order to sue the vaccine manufacturers."

He hadn't. A *possible* link between autism, inflammatory bowel disease, and the MMR was not realized until the study results had been analyzed, and even then, the authors of the study were careful to state that the link had by no means been proven. The first study was also initiated prior to Wakefield's contact with attorney Barr or his later commitment to act as an expert witness on behalf of the autistic children, and then only in regard to their GI complaints. In addition, Dr. Wakefield "played no active part in the interpretation of (the) clinical findings in these children."[19]

- Stated that the paper concluded "that (the autistic children's) conditions could be linked to the MMR vaccine."

False! No such claim was made by any of the authors and a simple reading of the text confirms that assertion.

- Did not have ethics committee approval.

Another lie! Ethical practices committee approval (162-95) was given to Dr. Walker-Smith for "detailed systemic analysis of children's intestinal biopsies" on September 5, 1995.[20]

- Done testing on the children that was "inappropriate, invasive and unethical."

Untrue. The parents were appropriately informed about all procedures performed on their children. They also gave their *signed, informed consent* for each and every procedure. There were no complaints from the parents of the children under study at any time before, during, or after the study was completed. An institutional review board reviewed all the study protocols and approved them prior to the studies being initiated, and the reader may recall that the second proposed Wakefield study, which utilized virtually the same medical evaluative procedures as were used in the first study, was also approved by a second ethics committee.

The tests done were most certainly appropriate and germane in regard not only to satisfying the study's aims, but more importantly, to fostering a better understanding of the nature of the pathology underlying each child's symptoms. The purpose of the first study was primarily to find out what might be causing the children's intestinal symptoms and regression and, if possible, to do something to improve their condition.

Not only were the children not harmed by the diagnostic procedures (simple blood draws, urine tests, lumbar punctures (in some), colonoscopies, and biopsies of diseased intestinal tissues), but they actually benefited greatly by having finally been correctly diagnosed in regard to their intestinal and other medical concerns, which then allowed for appropriate and beneficial therapies, like mesalazine, to be instituted.

The appropriateness of these procedures was later confirmed by an appeals court decision that exonerated Professor John Walker-Smith of any wrongdoing in regard to his participation in the Lancet 12 Study.

- Was the only one of the 13 authors who "prepared the data used" in the study.[21]

---

17   Ibid. p. 17-21.
18   Ibid. p. 17 and 22.
19   Ibid. 107.
20   Ibid. p. 18 and 21.
21   Ibid. p. 188.

Another falsehood! The opposite is true. The other 12 authors "prepared all of the data that appeared in *The Lancet*."[22] Wakefield, who is not a clinician, asserts that his job was simply to put "their completed data in tables and narrative form," and he adds, "All authors were provided with drafts of the paper for the purpose of checking their data and making amendments as necessary prior to submission."[23]

- Falsified the medical records on the children in the study, and he "fixed" data and misreported clinical findings.

Again, a lie! This is perhaps the most serious charge levied against Dr. Wakefield and his fellow researchers, and it is this accusation that ultimately contributed to *The Lancet* ultimately retracting the paper.[24]

Brian Deer, as has been mentioned, had illegally been given access to the study children's personal *outpatient* medical records, records that Wakefield and colleagues *had not had access to*, and he focused on what he incorrectly deemed to be significant differences in what these records seemed to state and what Wakefield et al. actually reported in their study. He erroneously concluded that Wakefield must have "fixed" the data for his own nefarious purposes.

Deer's false accusations of "manipulating patient data," which initially appeared in the *Sunday Times,* were also mirrored *two years later* in a *British Medical Journal* editorial accusing Wakefield of malfeasance.[25, 26]

These charges of fraud were later *investigated and refuted* by research microbiologist and whistleblower David Lewis and also by the *BMJ*'s own investigator, King's College Hospital gastroenterologist Ingvar Byarnason, who said the forms he was asked to review *didn't support the charges that Wakefield deliberately misinterpreted the records.* "The data are subjective," he stated. "It's different to say it's deliberate falsification."[27]

And Dr. Wakefield himself had already informed both Brian Deer and Dr. Fiona Godlee, editor of the *BMJ*, prior to publication of the defamatory articles, that the allegations of data manipulation were untrue, and he provided both with relevant information that corroborated his assertions.

Dr. Wakefield maintained that any perceived differences between the prior medical records of the children and what was published in the article were illusory or negligible or not germane, and he directed attention to a presentation previously alluded to that was made to the Inflammatory Bowel Disease Study Group on December 20, 1996 by Professor John Walker-Smith in association with Dr. Paul Dhillon, the senior pathologist at the Royal Free Hospital, who analyzed the biopsy slides in a blinded fashion (not knowing which child he was evaluating by name and not being provided with any of their medical information).

At that presentation (made over *two years prior* to the publication of the Lancet 12 study) the case histories of 7 of the 12 children who were later included in the Lancet 12 study, were detailed, and these case histories (and biopsy interpretations) were *exactly identical* to those described in the *Lancet* article for each child so evaluated.[28]

Therefore, Dr. Wakefield could not have "fixed" the data on the children as Brian Deer asserted. He had not originated the data, and the data were not changed.

It is important to note that Dr. Wakefield had nothing to do with the aforementioned Walker-Smith presentation or with the information gleaned by the presenters that was taken from the children's *available* medical records at that time. That means that he did not and could not have falsified or altered any data in at least 7 of the 12 children in the beleaguered Lancet 12 study.

---

22   Ibid. p. 188.

23   Ibid. p. 188-9.

24   Full retraction of the 1998 paper. *The Lancet*. February 2, 2010.

25   Deer, Brian. "MMR doctor Andrew Wakefield fixed data on autism." *The Sunday Times*. February 8, 2009

26   Deer, B. "How the case against the MMR vaccine was fixed." *BMJ* 2011; 342:c5347 doi: 10.1136/bmj.c5347 2. *and* Godlee, F.; Smith, J.; Marcovitch, H. "Wakefield's article linking MMR vaccine and autism was fraudulent." *BMJ* 342:doi:10.1136/bmj.c74523.

27   http://childhealthsafety.wordpress.com/2011/11/14/bmj-editor-head-first-in-brown-stuff/

28   "Enterocolitis and Disintegrative Disorder following MMR: a report of the first seven Cases." 20 Dec 1996; Presentation by J. Walker-Smith.

For the 1998 *Lancet* article to have been fabricated, a "conspiracy to commit fraud" by at least those three individuals (if not others) would have had to exist, and to what end? Neither Professor Walker-Smith nor Dr. Dhillon stood to gain in any way thereby. They were not part of any proposed litigation, and their preliminary report to the Inflammatory Disease Study Group at the Royal Free Hospital in 1996 was simply for the elucidation of their fellow colleagues.

Freelance "journalist" Brian Deer compounded his unfounded attacks on Dr. Wakefield's integrity by distorting the information he gleaned from the medical records of the children in the *Lancet* study. He did this by *omitting essential facts* when they proved to be inconvenient and *misinterpreting* still others. All his assertions about fraud and deceit on the part of Drs. Wakefield, Simon Murch, John Walker-Smith, and their colleagues are totally false and without merit.

The reader is encouraged to read Dr. Wakefield's excellent book, *Callous Disregard*, and in particular Chapter 12 ("Deer") for proof of Dr. Wakefield's assertions in this regard. The book and all chapters are heavily referenced. Dr. Wakefield meticulously catalogs each of Deer's accusations against him, and with appropriate facts and references, he successfully counters each allegation. For further proof that Brian Deer got it wrong, see:

http://www.ageofautism.com/2015/03/sorry-senator-feinstein-wakefield-is-not-a-fraud.html

Independent investigator and former EPA scientist, Dr. David Lewis, also takes Brian Deer's so-called "investigation" of Dr. Wakefield to task in his book, *Science for Sale.*[29]

Dr. Wakefield, understandably upset by the defamatory editorials in *The Sunday Times* and *British Medical Journal*, later filed a formal complaint to the Press Complaints Commission in this regard.[30] The Press Complaints Commission ordered Deer's articles removed from *The Sunday Times* website, but failed to enforce its edict.[31]

What's in a Name? Apparently, a Lot.

Brian Deer wasn't satisfied with just reporting his biased and distorted version of the facts regarding Dr. Wakefield, his fellow researchers, and the ill-fated *Lancet* article in *The Sunday Times*.

Deer also decided to file a complaint with the General Medical Council in February 2004, and the GMC, apparently eager to discredit Wakefield's research, then filed charges against Drs. Wakefield, Murch, and Walker-Smith, alleging that "the research reported…in *The Lancet* was substantially different from that for which approval was granted by the Ethical Practices Subcommittee in that it related to…children with a diagnosis of autism and not disintegrative disorder." [32]

The GMC further asserted that the alleged misrepresentation of the children's diagnoses[33] was "inappropriate, not in the best interests of patients, not in accordance with…professional ethical obligations, likely to bring the medical profession into disrepute, and fell seriously below the standard of conduct expected of a registered medical professional."[34]

Now *childhood disintegrative disorder* (CDD), as we have mentioned (see Chapter 1), is essentially identical to *regressive autism* except that it is usually defined as manifesting after 24 months, a somewhat arbitrarily defined date that not all experts agree on.

Children with regressive autism are alleged to differ from those with CDD in that they regress *prior to* 24 months in most cases. However, in both conditions, the child appears to develop normally for a period of time and then regresses and becomes autistic, and it is likely that these two disorders are actually the same condition, and it has been so deemed by the formulators of the DSM 5 criteria since May 2013.

---

29   http://www.ashotoftruth.org/blog/epa-microbiologist-dr-david-lewis-wrote-book-research-misconduct-then-throws-book-brian-deer
30   *Callous Disregard.* p. 22 & 211
31   Ibid.
32   Incredibly, the citation by the GMC incorrectly listed the wrong subcommittee approval and actually confused the study in question (the first study) with the second study. This malfeasance ultimately cost both Wakefield and Walker-Smith their licenses.
33   Labeling the children as having CDD and not autism in the ethics panel approval proposal.
34   Kirby, David. *Evidence of Harm.* p. 133.

Because the 12 children in the *Lancet* study had normal or near-normal early development followed by later regression and were, therefore, not classically autistic (having the problem since birth) as defined by Kanner, Wakefield's *colleagues in the Department of Child Psychiatry* at the Royal Free Hospital suggested that the 12 children were more typical of CDD than of classical Kanner autism, despite their mostly being younger than two years of age when the regression occurred.

During an ethics committee review for approval of the intestinal biopsies proposed to be performed in the first study, the children were described as having CDD on the basis of the aforementioned recommendation from the Department of Child Psychiatry. However, when the article was eventually published, their diagnosis was changed to "autism" for 11 of the 12 children so included.

It is important to note that *regressive* autism was not universally recognized at that time as being a variant of classical autism, and scientists even today are not certain "about the extent to which…CDD differs from regressive autism."[35]

Indeed, reviewers Malhotra and Gupta, in their article "Childhood Disintegrative Disorders" published in 1999 in the journal *Autism and Developmental Disorders*, note that the disorder has been described as occurring in children from 1.2 years to 9 years of age, and they concluded that CDD "may be a late variant of autism."[36]

Hendry, in a later article, agreed with Malhotra and Gupta. She concluded, after a rigorous review of the literature, that "CDD should not…be considered distinct from autistic disorder."[37]

So if the specious charges made against Wakefield, Murch, and Walker-Smith sound like malicious nitpicking by the GMC, you'd be correct, and even more so because the diagnosis of the children's developmental disorder was not even relevant to getting ethics committee approval for the study. The same ethics committee approval would have been forthcoming for this study regardless of whether the children had been diagnosed as being autistic or as having CDD.

Why?

Because the children were being evaluated because of their intestinal symptoms, and their workup, including the colonoscopies and the other procedures, would have been the same regardless of the name given to their developmental disorder.

So How Did the GMC Come to Investigate Wakefield, Walker-Smith, and Murch, and What Did They Find?

Brian Deer, who not only reported "news," but also excelled at creating it, met with *Lancet* editor Richard Horton on the morning of February 18, 2004 and suggested to Horton that Wakefield's involvement in the *Lancet* study was influenced by his need to support MMR litigation.

Deer also falsely declared that the *Lancet* study hadn't received proper ethics committee approval and that the approval that was given was actually for another study. Although none of these allegations was correct, Horton, who had been under intense criticism for having allowed the study to be published in the first place, apparently allowed himself to accept Deer's false representations as fact.

As a consequence of that presentation, Horton then met with the other senior authors of the *Lancet* paper that same afternoon. Dr. Wakefield was not invited to this session. Horton, reiterating what Deer had told him, informed the others that he believed that Wakefield had used Legal Aid Board funds to underwrite the *Lancet* study, the implication being that Wakefield had an undeclared conflict of interest that compromised the study.

Two days later, Horton publically declared the *Lancet* paper to be "fatally flawed." This malicious and incorrect allegation was then published in a story written by Deer in *The Sunday Times* within days of Horton's announcement.

---

35   ICD-10 http://www.who.int/ classifications/icd/en/bluebook.pdf
36   Vol. 29. p. 491-498.
37   *Clinical Psychology Review.* 2000; 20:77-90.

The story's headline ("head*lie*" would be a more appropriate term) read "Revealed: MMR Research Scandal," and three days later (on February 25th), Deer filed the aforementioned complaint with the UK's General Medical Council (GMC).

On March 6, *The Lancet* issued "a retraction of an interpretation made in the original article" by 13 of the article's 16 authors, who had been misadvised that their study was likely biased by Wakefield's association with the Dawbarn's law firm.

Their so-called retraction read: "We wish to make it clear that in this paper no causal link was established between MMR vaccine and autism as the data were insufficient." That statement was correct and had been so stated in the published report.

"However," they added, "the possibility of such a link was raised and consequent events have had major implications for public health." The retractors were presumably referring to the concern that many parents were refusing to let their children get the MMR vaccination.

They then issued their retraction: "In view of this, we consider now is the appropriate time that we should together formally retract the interpretation placed upon these findings in the paper, according to precedent."

This was an odd statement to make since the paper did not mention any interpretation of the findings, and what precedent were they referring to?

What these retractors were presumably stating was that they were rejecting even the *possibility* of there being an association between the MMR vaccine and autism and intestinal inflammation with absolutely no basis at all to support that absurd assertion.

In light of the evidence from their very own study, which clearly suggested that such an interpretation was not only possible but very plausible, their retraction was not only scientifically unsound but certainly illogical as well. As Dr. Wakefield so aptly put it, "You can't retract a possibility."

The General Medical Council, ever eager to go forward with its case against Wakefield and his two learned colleagues, seemed unsure as to how to proceed. They met with Horton, who counseled them in this regard and who, ultimately, appeared as a prosecution witness.

However, more than three years were to pass before the proceedings against Drs. Wakefield, Walker-Smith, and Murch were to commence on July 16, 2007, and when they did, they continued for a record-setting two and a half more years.

Nineteen months into the proceedings, on February 8, 2009, Deer published additional false claims against Dr. Wakefield in *The Sunday Times*. His headline read, "MMR doctor Andrew Wakefield fixed data on autism."

Making a Mountain Out of a "No-Hill"

"The courts do not consider that the engagement of someone to act as an expert witness in litigation has the effect that that person is then biased. Indeed, if this were the legal position, no paid professional could ever at any time give evidence to a court."

— Barrister Robert Hantusch in a letter to the Times on
February 24, 2004

On January 28, 2010, the GMC finally issued findings "on facts." Dr. Wakefield was found guilty of professional misconduct for not disclosing in the *Lancet* article that he "was a medical expert involved in assessing the merits of litigation against the manufacturers of MMR on behalf of plaintiff children possibly damaged by the vaccine."

In so ruling, the GMC chose to ignore the fact that the *Lancet* study was well underway before Dr. Wakefield had agreed to become involved as an "expert" in possible MMR litigation and that Wakefield was not the practitioner who examined the children in the study or wrote up their histories, or did the colonoscopies or biopsies, or who interpreted the slides (which was done in a blinded fashion), or did the lab work.

In so doing, the GMC also ignored *The Lancet's* own ethical guidelines at the time the story was published. These stated that it was *up to the author of the study* to decide whether he or she had any conflicts of interest that might cause "embarrassment" to the author.

Dr. Wakefield rightly felt that the first study, supported by a non-judicial agency and initiated before he had agreed to serve as an expert witness for the Dawbarn's law firm, did not so qualify, and indeed, it didn't.

He also understood that the conclusions of the *Lancet 12* study only suggested, but did not establish, any proven causal association between the MMR vaccine and either autism or inflammatory bowel disease, and this was clearly stated in that study. *There was, thus, no way that the study conclusions could be used in a court of law to support the MMR litigants' need to prove such an association.*

The GMC also disregarded the evidence that Wakefield's involvement with the Dawbarn's law firm had been openly and appropriately provided to his senior coauthors, to Richard Horton, the editor of *The Lancet*, and also to medical school dean Arie Zuckerman long before the paper was published.

So the GMC and Richard Horton were incorrect. Wakefield told the truth when he asserted that he had no conflicts of interest!

However, it is worthwhile noting that Richard Horton didn't seem at all concerned that Dr. Michael Pichichero had lied when he declared no conflicts of interest in his 2002 study in *The Lancet*, which purported to clear thimerosal of causing mercury toxicity. (See the Tenth "Negative" Study in Chapter 16.)[38]

Pichichero was heavily conflicted. His institution had received research grants from numerous vaccine manufacturers. Apparently if you support the contention that vaccines don't cause autism, your conflicts of interest can be ignored.

And the GMC's unfounded accusations against Dr. Wakefield continued.

Dr. Wakefield had on one occasion asked a group of children who were attending his son's birthday party to donate some blood to be analyzed as part of the control group for the proposed study. The children and their parents all agreed to this. The blood was drawn and the children received a small monetary compensation for their participation. The GMC castigated Wakefield for doing these tests as if the blood draws, which are minimally painful and perfectly safe and relevant procedures, were somehow equivalent to child abuse.

"Framed!"

Dr. Wakefield and his colleagues were also falsely accused of not having ethics committee approval for the *Lancet* study, but the GMC had *deliberately "erred"* in applying the *wrong* ethics committee approval to the *Lancet* study.

The Lancet 12 case series fell under ethics committee approval 162-95 with a start date of September 5, 1995, and this was so listed in the published study. The approval manifested as a short letter allowing Professor Walker-Smith to obtain additional biopsy samples from the intestines of the children undergoing colonoscopies (which didn't require ethics committee approval) as part of their bowel disease workup.

Ethics committee approval 172-96 with a start date of 18 December, 1996 was obtained by Wakefield and his fellow researchers for the *second* proposed study of 25 children with gastrointestinal symptoms and developmental delays.

---

38   Pichichero, Michael. et al. *The Lancet*. Vol. 360, Issue 9347. p. 1737-1741, 30 November 2002.

Incredibly, the GMC deviously and erroneously decided, with no rational reason for so doing, that the EC 172-96 approval actually applied to the *first* case series study of the 12 Lancet children, and by so doing, they were then able to conclude that 7 of the 12 Lancet children in that study had been prematurely admitted to the study (prior to December 18, 1996), which meant that Wakefield and colleagues would then have been guilty of an ethical violation.

What sophistry!

> *"The reliance on the 1996 ethical approval as the exclusive means of framing the facts points to the presence of an ideological agenda in the hands of the GMC, prosecution and panel, and shows how in the end the 3 doctors were framed according to this agenda."*
>
> — *Martin Hewitt*[39]

Wakefield was additionally charged with showing a "callous disregard" for the study children's welfare by requiring some of them to undergo a lumbar puncture (LP), which the GMC felt was an unnecessary procedure.

In their irrational and biased ruling, the GMC chose to ignore the evidence that not only was medical opinion divided in regard to the necessity of having to do a lumbar puncture as part of the evaluation of children with autism, but also that medical opinion was virtually unanimous in asserting the necessity of doing an L.P. for children diagnosed as having childhood disintegrative disorder (CDD), the very diagnosis that the Royal Free Hospital psychiatrists had suggested was most appropriate for the children in the *Lancet* study.

Just five days after the GMC issued its ruling, the *Lancet* issued a full retraction of "that paper."

So What Happened to Drs. Wakefield, Murch, and Walker-Smith?

Professor Simon Murch, who had performed the colonoscopies and intestinal biopsies on the children, was found to have "misled the Royal Free's ethics committee, acted contrary to the clinical interests of children, and failed in his duties as a responsible consultant." However, the panel noted that Murch's involvement with the project was "subsidiary to and more limited" than Wakefield and Walker-Smith's, that he had shown insight into his conduct, and had "demonstrated errors of judgment but had acted in good faith." He was acquitted of serious professional misconduct. He continues his practice of medicine in Britain.

Dr. Andrew Wakefield and Professor John Walker-Smith both lost their medical licenses. As a result, their reputations have been inexorably tarnished in the eyes of a majority of the public and the media.

As of this writing, Dr. Wakefield has not been legally or professionally exonerated, although those who have examined the facts regarding his ordeal know him to be an honest, ethical, and brilliant researcher who has been greatly wronged.

Thankfully, Professor John Walker-Smith successfully appealed his case, and on March 7, 2012, "the High Court ruled that a decision to strike him off over the MMR controversy was unlawful."[40]

The appeals judge, Mr. Justice Mitting, ruled that the decision to "strike off" (cancel Dr. Walker-Smith's license to practice medicine) could not stand. The judge added that the disciplinary panel relied on "inadequate and superficial reasoning," which led them "in a number of instances, (to) a wrong conclusion…. It would be a misfortune if this were to happen again," he added. He further highlighted the disciplinary panel's incompetence by expressing the hope that in the future such cases be "chaired by someone with judicial experience."[41]

In his ruling, Judge Mitting concluded that, "The children reported in the 1998 *Lancet* paper were very ill and did warrant serious clinical investigation and the investigations conducted were entirely appropriate for the children's

39   http://www.ageofautism.com/2010/04/how-the-gmc-framed-doctors-wakefield-walkersmith-and-murch-.html?cid=6a00d8357f3f2969e201348004b89f970c

40   http://www.independent.co.uk/life-style/health-and-families/health-news/mmr-doctor-john-walkersmith-wins-high-court-appeal-7543114.html

41   Ibid.

needs," and thus, "the allegations of fraud based on this misconstruction, propagated by journalist Brian Deer, politician Evan Harris, the Murdoch press and the *British Medical Journal* (and rubberstamped by the GMC) [were] therefore also unfounded."[42]

Since the incompetent and highly conflicted disciplinary panel of the GMC ruled incorrectly in the case of Professor John Walker-Smith as a result of "inadequate and superficial reasoning," does it not follow that it also erred in its investigation and condemnation of Dr. Andrew Wakefield?

Dr. Wakefield, still living under the shadow of the court's biased and irrational ruling, has long since moved his family to the United States to continue his research into inflammatory bowel diseases and autism.

It is our belief that he will be completely vindicated one day—hopefully soon.

"Some rise by sin, and some by virtue fall."

— *William Shakespeare,* Measure for Measure

Duplicity "R" Us: The Real Conflicts of Interest!

The Sunday Times

The Sunday Times published all of Brian Deer's misrepresentations which purported to uncover fraud and conflict of interest in regard to that ill-fated *Lancet* study, and by so doing, helped to discredit the work of Dr. Wakefield and his competent team of researchers.

What the *Times* didn't mention was that *Deer was commissioned to investigate Wakefield by* The Sunday Times *editor Paul Nuki.* Furthermore, Nuki's father, Professor George Nuki, was a member of the Committee on Safety in Medicines when the troublesome and later withdrawn Pluserix MMR vaccine was introduced to the British population.

The *Times* also failed to note that Deer was reporting on stories *that he himself had created and perpetrated.* As Melanie Phillips of the *Spectator* so aptly put it, "Since when has a reputable paper published a story by a reporter who is actually part of that story himself—without saying so—and who uses information arising from the disciplinary hearing which he himself has instigated and which is investigating allegations he himself made in the first place?"[43]

And *The Sunday Times* has other significant conflicts of interest. The Chief Executive Officer of News International, which owns *The Sunday Times*, was (at the time) James Murdoch, who also sat on the Board of GlaxoSmithKline (GSK), a manufacturer of the MMR vaccine and potential litigation defendant. Mr. Murdoch functioned on the Board to oversee, "external issues that might have the potential for serious impact upon the group's business and reputation."[44]

Like potential MMR litigation? Here are some more:

Reuters

On May 24, 2010, Kate Kelland, Health and Science Correspondent for Reuters, reported that Dr. Wakefield, whose "claims of links between vaccination and autism triggered a scientific storm before being widely discredited, was struck off the medical register Monday for professional misconduct." Her story expanded on the findings of the fitness to practice panel.

However, she neglected to report that her boss, Thomas H. Glocer, Chief Executive Officer of the Thomson Reuters Corporation, just happened to be a medical director at Merck, the manufacturer of the MMR II vaccine.[45]

42　Natl. Autism Assoc news release. March 7, 2012. http://us.mg201.mail.yahoo.com/neo/launch?.partner= sbc
43　February 11, 2009. http://www.spectator.co.uk/ melaniephillips/3346281/the-witchhunt-against-andrew-wakefield.thtml
44　Tryhorn, Chris. "James Murdoch takes GlaxoSmithKline role." *The Guardian.* Monday, February 2, 2009
45　http://adventuresinautism.blogspot.com/2010/08/did-anyone-know-that-ceo-of-reuters-was.html

The Daily Mirror

Daily Mirror reporter Miriam Stoppard, who has also written about the allegedly flawed Lancet 12 study and has encouraged parents to give their children the MMR jab, failed to mention that she is married to Sir Christopher Hogg, Chairman of GlaxoSmith Kline.[46]

The Committee on Safety in Medicines (CSM)

The CSM in the United Kingdom is a committee that advises the Medicines and Healthcare-products Regulation Agency (MHRA, and formerly the Medicines Control Agency).

In 2004, "fifteen of the 36 members (42 percent) of the CSM (had) declared personal or non-personal links with companies cited in a class action being brought by parents who believed that MMR had harmed their children.

"Six committee members had personal shareholdings and/or held consultancy posts with MMR manufacturer GlaxoSmithKline and nine have (or had) a past or present association, such as receiving research funding from companies involved. Two members (had) declared interests in both categories."[47]

The British Medical Journal

The British Medical Journal, under the editorial control of Fiona Godlee, Jane Smith, and Harvey Marcovitch, ultimately published Brian Deer's false allegations against Dr. Wakefield, including his mistaken assertions that Wakefield had an unstated conflict of interest because of his potential involvement with MMR litigation.[48]

And Godlee et al. published these accusations of fraud despite *never having actually been shown the children's medical records* that formed the basis of the 1998 *Lancet* paper. There was no "peer review" of these defamatory allegations. Indeed, there was no review at all.

Interestingly, Marcovitch had previously and correctly criticized the American Medical Association and its journal *JAMA* for not disclosing "potential financial conflicts (such as their income from industry sources) as they expect their authors to (do)."

That charge is highly ironic in light of the fact that Fiona Godlee and her co-editors, Marcovitch and Smith, *failed to disclose* their own relevant financial conflicts. The *BMJ*, like most medical journals, receives *significant advertising and sponsorship revenue* from pharmaceutical companies, including MMR manufacturers Glaxo-SmithKline (GSK) and Merck. Oops!

And to add to their sins of omission, *The British Medical Journal* also failed to disclose another of its major business partnerships with Merck through Merck's "information" subsidiary, Univadis. Oops! Oops!

When these undeclared conflicts of interest were brought to the attention of the *BMJ* editors, they published a *partial online* "mea culpa," which conveniently didn't mention their financially-lucrative association with Univadis and *which wasn't linked to the article itself.* That means that online readers of the article would still most likely be unaware of the journal's significant conflicts of interest in this regard, unless they fortuitously happened upon the disclosure statement elsewhere on the website.

But the *BMJ*'s biggest sin of omission (Oops! Oops! Oops!) was its failure to mention that it had itself paid self-described "journalist" Deer to investigate and report on the "hit piece" it had published. Did this represent another serious conflict of interest? You bet. In spades! Why?

46   http://www.mirror.co.uk/lifestyle/sex-relationships/why-mmr-jab-is-a-must-for-school-262690
47   http://www.whale.to/vaccine/walker78.html
48   *BMJ* 2011; 342: c7452doi:10.1136/bmj.c7452.

The *BMJ* is solely owned by the British Medical Association, a trade union to which virtually all of the United Kingdom's doctors belong. If it were shown that vaccines were a causative factor in promoting autism and chronic intestinal disorders, that news would cause serious medico-legal concerns to be raised that would most certainly have adversely affected the British medical establishment. The safety of immunizations would also certainly have been questioned. Immunization rates would have fallen. Those eventualities could not be allowed to happen.

It was, therefore, not sufficient for Wakefield, Murch, and Walker-Smith to be found guilty of ethical violations by a heavily-conflicted investigative body with contempt for facts and fair play.

The findings of the Wakefield *Lancet* study itself had to be thoroughly discredited and retracted, even if that meant intentionally distorting facts, omitting relevant information, lying, and further besmirching the good names of reputable researchers. And who better to perform these unsavory tasks than the man who had already demonstrated his willingness to compromise journalistic ethics for personal fame and gain?

Brian Deer

And that brings us back to Brian Deer, the so-called "independent journalist," who wished to shine again in his own spotlight. It was Deer who had *illegally and unethically* reviewed the personal and confidential medical records of the autistic children in the Wakefield study. And it was Deer who had *lied* (by misrepresenting who he was and why he was asking questions) to the parents of one of those autistic children.

For years, Deer somehow neglected to mention (and actually denied) that it was he who had formally complained to the GMC about what he perceived to be the misdeeds of the senior authors of that infamous *Lancet* study. *He had filed that complaint on the instructions of the then Minister of Health.*

And it was years before his involvement became public and was finally acknowledged in the *BMJ*, the conflicted journal that had also failed to mention that it had funded Deer's more recent "investigations."

Nevertheless, when the editors of that now tainted journal published Deer's mistaken assertions that Wakefield had fraudulently altered the *Lancet* study's children's medical records, they somehow neglected to mention that Deer had "accepted hospitality" at a conference held November 2010 which was sponsored by the pharmaceutical industry (including MMR manufacturer GlaxoSmithKline).

Deceit has its rewards.

However, it wasn't the *British Medical Journal* that *initially* assisted Deer's investigation of the Lancet 12 children's medical records. It was the Association of the British Pharmaceutical Industry through its "front group," Medico-Legal Investigations (MLI).

According to J.B. Handley (www.ageofautism.com), MLI "specialize(s) in getting medical doctors prosecuted by the General Medical Council," and it "assisted" Deer (at no cost) in his Wakefield "witch-hunt" prior to Deer's publishing his allegations in *The Sunday Times* in 2004.

Brian Deer was also supported in his investigation by British Parliamentarian, Dr. Evan Harris, an active member of the British Medical Association and a Glaxo-Wellcome fellow who accompanied Deer to the Wakefield/GMC hearings on a number of occasions. Harris's pediatrician father was a member of the Committee on Safety in Medicines during the years (1990-1992) when it was becoming obvious to all that the Pluserix vaccine was dangerous and needed to be withdrawn. Harris later defended the MMR before Parliament. "On the safety of MMR," he said (despite knowing that the Pluserix MMR had been withdrawn because of safety concerns), "the evidence and scientific consensus are overwhelming. There is a lot of good research that fails to find any significant safety problem with MMR."[49]

---

49   See also: http://www.youtube.com/watch ?v=id _AxZ3zHAc

LIAR, LIAR: Part I

CNN INTERVIEW JANUARY 6, 2011

KIRAN CHETRY (CNN reporter): "Did you have a financial interest in doing this investigation, Brian?"

BRIAN DEER: (Evading the question) "I've been an investigative reporter working for The Sunday Times *of London since the early 1980s. The point you have to remember about this whole issue is, firstly, that the—it's not me saying this. It is the editors of the* BMJ, *a prestigious international medical journal that very extensively peer-reviewed and individually checked the facts which [were] put forward in our investigation this week."[50]*

FACT: Alaistair Brett, legal manager, Sunday Times*: "Mr. Deer should not represent himself as a* Sunday Times *journalist. He is not a member of staff, does not have a regular salary from us, is not on our pension scheme and pays his own tax as a freelance."[51] And the* BMJ *did not extensively peer-review Deer's "facts."*

FACT: There was no peer review at all.

FACT: Mr. Deer attended Andy Wakefield's GMC hearings for 160 days between 2007 and 2010.

JANE BRYANT (Journalist): "Brian, who is paying you for your attendance at the Hearing day after day?"

BRIAN DEER: "The Sunday Times and Channel 4."

FACT: Both The Sunday Times *and Channel 4 denied paying Deer for these services.[52]*

JANE BRYANT: (Interviewing Brian Deer outside the GMC hearing in 2008) "Are you the complainant in this case?"

BRIAN DEER: (Angrily) "No! I've not complained! I've got letters from the GMC saying I'm not the complainant…."

FACT: Transcript from a court document: "Well before the programme [British spelling] was broadcast Mr. Deer had made a complaint to the GMC about the Claimant [Andy Wakefield]."

JANE BRYANT: "You are not prepared to discuss your finances?"

BRIAN DEER: "I've told you who's paying me! I've told you I've never been paid by the drugs companies! I'm not in any way connected with drugs companies!"

FACT: "Before a single word had been written by him, Deer had consulted with and been given free advice and assistance by Association of the British Pharmaceutical Industry company Medico-Legal Investigations Limited, whose specialty was getting doctors on charges before the GMC."[53]

ANDERSON COOPER (Interviewing Dr. Wakefield: 2011): "According to (Deer), he's received no funding from any parties that have interests in this (the MMR/Wakefield study) over the last three years."

FACT: Mr. Cooper didn't go back far enough. The first hit piece by Deer was published in 2004, 7 years prior to the interview, and Deer was conflicted then.* His most recent attack on Wakefield was in 2010 and was paid for by the British Medical Journal *a wholly owned subsidiary of the British Medical Association, whose members (virtually all the MDs in Britain) would definitely be adversely affected by an officially accepted autism & intestinal inflammation link to the MMR vaccine. So Deer lied again; the BMJ definitely had "an interest in this."*

*See "Deer" p 307.

---

50   http://transcripts.cnn.com/TRANSCRIPTS/1101/06/ltm.03.html Aired January 6, 2011 - 08:00 ET

51   www.ageofautism.com

52   J.B. Handley www.ageofautism.com

53   Source reported by J.B. Handley of Operation Rescue; Keeping Anderson Cooper Honest. "Is Brian Deer the Fraud?"

The General Medical Council (GMC)

When the GMC first empanelled its jury (the Fitness to Practice Panel) in the hearings regarding the accusations against Drs.Wakefield, Murch, and Walker-Smith, it appointed Professor Denis McDevitt as chairman of that panel.

When it was later disclosed by outside campaigners that McDevitt had significant conflicts of interest, he was ultimately dismissed from the panel. McDevitt had been a member of the Joint Committee for Vaccination and Immunology, which had irresponsibly approved and licensed the faulty MMR vaccines containing the Urabe strain of mumps virus (we refer again to the Pluserix scandal), which were ultimately withdrawn because they frequently caused meningitis in those who had received those inoculations.

McDevitt was replaced by Dr. Surendra Kumar, whose significant conflicts of interest included relationships with a number of drug companies as well as his ownership of shares in MMR manufacturer and potential litigant GlaxoSmithKline.

Dr. Kumar "would not answer questions about his shareholdings in Glaxo SmithKline, and said *there was no such thing as vaccine damage* and that any parents who claimed that their children had suffered such would be treated with scorn and contempt."[54]

However, the clearly biased and conflicted Dr. Kumar was not dismissed as a panelist.[55]

So the GMC, which had falsely charged Dr. Wakefield with an alleged conflict of interest in regard to his prospective role in MMR litigation, had duplicitously not done any of its own due diligence on either McDevitt or Kumar in regard to their evident conflicts of interest, and it had dismissed or disregarded Dr. Kumar's obvious conflicts.

"There ain't nothin' more powerful than the odor of mendacity."

— *Tennessee Williams,* Cat on a Hot Tin Roof

The Lancet

Although *The Lancet* initially published the "Wakefield 12" study, the journal and its editor, Richard Horton, had come under intense fire from the British Medical establishment for having published that controversial paper, as Horton himself readily relates in his book *Second Opinion: Doctors, Diseases and Decisions in Modern Medicine.* Horton needed to find some way to resolve that conflict, and Brian Deer's witch hunt proved to be the ideal venue from which to proceed against Wakefield.

The Lancet is owned by Reed-Elsevier. Its CEO, Sir Crispin Davis, joined Glaxo's board in 2003, shortly before Deer's first article was published in 2004 in *The Sunday Times.* GlaxoSmithKline manufactured (and still does) an MMR vaccine that was the subject of many lawsuits in Great Britain. Horton never revealed this serious conflict of interest either.

AN INTERESTING SEQUENCE OF EVENTS

1) July 2003: Lancet *proprietor & Reed Elsevier CEO, Crispin Davis, becomes a non-executive director of MMR manufacturer GlaxoSmithKline.*

2) October 2003: The Legal Services Commission at the government's request denies MMR-damaged children the funding necessary to continue their litigation. The parents appeal the decision.

3) February 20, 2004. "The Lancet *throws Andrew Wakefield to the wolves for tenuous reasons. He*

---

54   http://adventuresinautism.blogspot.com/2010/08/did-anyone-know-that-ceo-of-reuters-was.html

55   http://www.medical veritas.com /images /00211.pdf

is dragged through the mud by the BBC and Sunday Times *for four days."*

4) February 27, 2004. Judge Sir Nigel Davis, Crispin's brother, dismisses the litigants' right to appeal for restitution of funding for reasons he has as yet not revealed.

5) June 2004. "Crispin Davis is knighted by the Blair government."

Apparently, knighthood is now being bestowed in Britain for deeds that protect the treasuries of the pharmaceutical companies and British government from potentially costly litigation.

What was once awarded for bravery is now awarded for knavery![56]

The British Government

In Great Britain, the Legal Aid Board was established to help fund litigation in the interest of its citizens. Since early in the 1990s, about 2000 parents of alleged MMR vaccine-damaged children have been seeking legal redress for the harm done to their offspring. Many of these were children who had suffered adverse side effects from the faulty Pluserix/Trivirix vaccines, but the group also included children whose deafness, autism, and intestinal concerns were believed to be related to their having received other MMR brands as well.

The Legal Aid Board was prepared to help fund this litigation. However, in 2004, after almost ten years of preparation, and "only months away from its most important hearing in court," the legal aid was suddenly withdrawn which "brought about the complete collapse of the cases."[57]

As has been mentioned, the High Court judge who ruled against the defendants' access to the legal aid funding was Sir Nigel Davis, brother of Sir Crispin Davis, non-executive director of MMR defendant GlaxoSmithKline and Chief Executive Officer of Reed Elsevier, the company that owns *The Lancet* and many other major medical journals.

Sir Crispin, as mentioned, was appointed to that Glaxo post in July 2003, just three months before the Legal Services Commission was to rule negatively on the MMR children's funding and just eight months before Brother Nigel, in secret hearings, rejected appeals against the Legal Services Commission's disputed decision without providing any reason for so doing. Nigel also neglected to mention his brother's involvement with defendant Glaxo-SmithKline. Any perceived conflicts here?

And the British Government's conflict of interest? It had already assumed all liability for damages done by the Glaxo-SmithKline MMR vaccine (and others?), but in actuality, it had no intention of recompensing any plaintiff for any reason, ever.

The best way to accomplish that goal was to prevent the complainants from being able to go to trial by cutting off their funding. A senior Legal Services Commission official admitted that *the decision to stop legal aid* "came from the government."[58]

In Britain, according to Martin Walker, "No claim has ever been successful against a pharmaceutical company. The New Labour government," he continues, "has supported the industry in a complete refusal to admit to the notion of adverse reactions being admitted or actionable."

So the British government, the media, the pharmaceutical companies, the medical journals, and a host of others were all significantly conflicted, and they succeeded in defending the questionable reputation and safety of the MMR vaccines while also insulating the pharmaceutical companies and the British government against costly litigation. These tasks were accomplished not only by their preventing any damaging MMR litigation from reaching the courts (by the cancellation of litigation funding), but also by maliciously demonizing the *Lancet* study and its authors.

---

56   Adapted from the John Stone blog: http://www.whale.to/vaccine/mmr_judge.html
57   http://www.whale.to/vaccine/walker78.html
58   Mary Wiggen, parent of an autistic child at an open court hearing.

The British Government also irrationally blamed Wakefield and that troublesome study for the dramatic decrease in the number of children getting the MMR vaccine; however, it may be recalled that Dr. Wakefield was careful to stress the importance of continuing to have children immunized, albeit with separate single entity vaccines for measles, mumps, and rubella, until such time that further safety testing justified the continued use of the combined MMR vaccines.

As we now know, all of the single dose vaccines were available when he made that recommendation, and they were in great demand, but they were withdrawn six months later *for no rational reason* by the British Government; therefore, the government, not Wakefield, was actually to blame for the rise in measles seen in that country following publication of the *Lancet* article.

In 1988, the Joint Committee on Vaccination and Immunization stated,

"FOR CHILDREN WHOSE PARENTS REFUSE MMR VACCINE,

SINGLE ANTIGEN MEASLES WILL BE AVAILABLE."

"Considering that the New Labour government would ultimately have been found responsible for compensation pay outs against the British company involved in the claims [GlaxoSmithKline], this move [cancellation of funding] was seen by many to be a defense by the government of its own interests."

— Martin Walker[59]

The BBC and the Cambridge Evening News *Withdrew Their Allegation that Dr. Andrew Wakefield Had Any Conflict of Interest*

In an article published on June 20, we referred to allegations printed in *The Sunday Times* relating to Dr. Andrew Wakefield. The allegations related to two studies conducted by Dr. Wakefield into the link between the MMR vaccination and the onset of autism. *The Sunday Times* alleged that the nature of the funding of one of the studies could potentially have affected the outcome. We have been informed that defamation proceedings have been commenced against *The Sunday Times* in connection with this article.

We would like to make it clear that there was in fact no conflict of interest nor was Dr. Wakefield personally paid to undertake the study as was alleged.

Furthermore we wish to clarify that the studies were carried out under proper ethical authorization.

Finally we accept that the subjects of the studies were selected through appropriate NHS referrals.

We apologise to Dr. Wakefield for any distress caused and at his request have paid an appropriate sum to selected charities.[60]

The British Public is finally beginning to learn the Truth about the Safety of Vaccines.
On October 24, 2010 *The Sunday Times* reported that the UK health authority, the MHRA, was forced to disclose adverse vaccine reaction statistics after a Freedom of Information Act inquiry from a reporter.

---

59   www.whale.to/vaccine/walker78.html

60   http://www.ldonline.org/xarbb/printtopic/13107?theme=print and http://www.cambridge-news.co.uk/news/region_wide/2005/07/16/ 9508081d-0052-4f6d-8679-28f63e6ac5c3.lpf

The British public was shocked to learn that 40 children had died after routine immunizations including the MMR and 2,100 had suffered serious side effects in the preceding seven years. Two of the vaccinated children had permanent brain damage, 1,500 suffered neurological reactions that included 11 cases of brain inflammation and 13 cases of epilepsy and coma.

In September of that year, the government of the UK was compelled by a court to pay damages to a mother whose son was left with severe brain damage after an MMR vaccination, and it was reported that another 500 cases were making their way through the British court system.

Like the VAERS system in the U.S., this is a passive reporting system and is very likely to vastly under-report the true incidence of serious side effects from vaccines. If a doctor does not believe a symptom is due to the vaccine, he won't report it. There is thus a good likelihood that the incidence of adverse reactions is much higher than these numbers might indicate.

Liar, Liar (Part II)

Select Committee on Science and Technology: Minutes of Evidence

Examination of Witnesses (Questions 84 - 85) Monday, March 1, 2004

Mr. Crispin Davis, CEO Reed Elsevier & Non-Executive Director of GlaxoSmithKline

Q84 Mr. Key: Mr Davis, your company owns The Lancet. *Do you think that scientific publishers have a responsibility towards society to ensure that the research they publish is authenticated and not affected by conflict of interest?*

Mr Davis: We absolutely have a responsibility to ensure that what we publish is peer reviewed, accurate, reflects best practice. In the issue of The Lancet *we do have a policy where people who submit their articles have to declare any conflict of interest.... Dr Wakefield said there was no conflict of interest, and in fact three months later in written form repeated that there was no conflict of interest. In all fairness, I do not hold our editor to blame in that instance.... I do not think he or* The Lancet *were at fault at all. We were in our opinion badly misled.*

Q85 Mr. Key: Thank you for explaining that. Is there any evidence that pharmaceutical companies are paying authors to produce papers to promote their products?

Mr Davis: Not that I am aware of, certainly not with our journals.[61]

Oh, Really? How About In Your Pretend Journals?

"Between 2000 and 2005, Elsevier/Excerpta Medica published six phony "medical journals," all financed by various undisclosed drug companies (like Merck) which were intended to mislead physicians while promoting those companies' drugs. These fraudulent journals included the Australasian Journal of General Practice, *the* Australasian Journal of Neurology, *the* Australasian Journal of Cardiology, *the* Australasian Journal of Clinical Pharmacy, *the* Australasian Journal of Cardiovascular Medicine, *and the* Australasian Journal of Bone & Joint [Medicine]." *None were peer-reviewed.*[62]

And Speaking Of Conflicts Of Interest (and double standards)...

Michael Pichichero denied any conflicts of interest in his 2002 Lancet *study that alleged to validate the safety of thimerosal. He lied. He was heavily conflicted. He has had ties to at least 13 pharmaceutical companies, including those that manufacture vaccines, and he was part of the team at the University of Rochester that developed the HIB vaccines (many of which contained thimerosal). The* Lancet *did not seem to have any concerns regarding his dishonesty or his conflicts of interest. Apparently, if you are conflicted and deny it, but you support the immunization program, your sins of omission can be forgiven. Hmmm!*[63]

---

61   http://www.publications.parliament.uk/pa/cm200304/cmselect/cmsctech/399/4030107.htm

62   "Elsevier published 6 fake journals." *The Scientist-Magazine of the Life Sciences*, http://www.the-scientist.com/blog/ display/55679/#ixzz1ZfVehZgn

63   Pichichero, Michael et al. "Mercury concentrations and metabolism in infants receiving vaccines containing thiomersal (thimerosal): A descriptive study." *The Lancet*. Vol. 360, Issue 9347. p. 1737-41. 30 November 2002.

Final Thoughts

Andrew Wakefield

"Let me make it absolutely clear that, at its heart, the GMC hearing has been about the protection of MMR vaccination policy. The case has been driven by an agenda to crush dissent that in my opinion serves the government and the pharmaceutical industry—not the welfare of children. It's important to note that there has never been a complaint against any of the doctors by any parent involved in this case—only universal parental support and gratitude.

"My colleagues, Professors Walker-Smith and Murch, are outstanding pediatricians and pediatric gastroenterologists. They have led the field of pediatric gastroenterology for decades, devoting their lives to caring for sick children. Our only 'crime' in this matter has been to listen to the concerns of parents, act according to the demands of our professional training, and provide appropriate care to this neglected population of children. It is unthinkable that at the end of an unimpeachable career, Professor Walker-Smith would even consider unethical experimentation on children under his care.

"In the course of our work, we discovered and treated a new intestinal disease syndrome in children with autism, alleviating suffering in affected children around the world. This should be cause for celebration. Instead, we have been vilified in the press, and demonized by a wasteful PR campaign by the Department of Health. The aim of this negative publicity was to discredit my criticism of vaccine safety research.

"As long as a question mark remains over vaccine safety; as long as a safety-first vaccine policy is subordinate to profit and self-interest; as long as the benefits of vaccines are threatened by those who have compromised public confidence by denial of vaccine damage, and as long as these children need help, I will continue my work."

Chapter 23
The "Positive" Studies—Research that Supports the MMR Connection to Autism

"Few men are willing to brave the disapproval of their fellows, the censure of their colleagues, the wrath of their society. Moral courage is a rarer commodity than bravery in battle or great intelligence. Yet it is the one essential vital quality for those who seek to change a world which yields most painfully to change."

— *Robert F. Kennedy*

WHAT ADDITIONAL STUDIES *Support the Findings of the Wakefield Group?*
It may be recalled that in the 1998 Lancet 12 study, the Wakefield team found that the 12 autistic children who were evaluated for chronic intestinal symptoms had a high incidence of a non-specific inflammatory bowel disease associated with numerous enlarged lymph nodes (LNH) in the small intestine (terminal ileum), and many of these children appeared to regress shortly after their MMR vaccination.

It was alleged by former *Lancet* editor Richard Horton and others that no additional studies supported these associations, but that allegation was incorrect.

We have previously cited research studies published prior to 1998 that showed:

- Congenital rubella infection increases the risk of a baby becoming autistic, and it is, therefore, not much of a stretch to assume that the live, albeit attenuated, rubella virus in the MMR could do the same thing if administered during the pregnancy.

- Mothers of autistic children tend to have increased levels of antibodies to the rubella virus.

- Autism has been reported to occur after measles-virus caused brain inflammation.

- Early exposure to measles and mumps viruses appear to increase the risk of a child becoming autistic.

- Many autistic children have a particular genetic immune defect that impairs their ability to clear certain viruses completely or before they affect the brain.

- As early as 1994, a link between the MMR or measles vaccination and autism was suggested.

- In 1995, a study implicated the measles vaccine as a cause of inflammatory bowel disease and gait disturbances.

- In 1996, researcher Hugh Fudenberg confirmed that some autistic children develop autistic symptoms "within a week or so after immunization with the measles, mumps and rubella (MMR) vaccine." Many of these children also had a history of fever and seizures within a day of getting the MMR vaccination. (See Chapter 21 for references).

- Additional research by a pediatric immunologist, James Oleske (which began in 1995), led him to the discovery that autistic children, who had regressed after being given the MMR vaccine, had unusually elevated titers of measles antibody compared to what normally would be expected. This data was presented as an abstract ("Elevated Rubeola Titers in Autistic Children") at a National Institute of Health meeting on September 23, 1997.[1]

Since the Lancet 12 article appeared in 1998, many more relevant studies that support Dr. Wakefield's findings have been published in peer-reviewed medical journals.

"All great truths begin as blasphemies."

— George Bernard Shaw

The Studies that Support the Lancet 12 Study

Studies 1, 2, and 3

Yazbak, F.E. "Autism: Is There a Vaccine Connection? Part I, II & III: Vaccination after Delivery." Presented at the American Acad. of Pediatrics in 1999.[2]

Dr F. Edward Yazbak is a practicing Board Certified pediatrician, the former Pediatric Director of Child Development Study at Brown University, and the former Director of Pediatrics at the Woonsocket Hospital in Rhode Island. He is also the grandfather of an autistic child. Since 1998, the year the Lancet 12 study was published, he has devoted his time to researching the causes of regressive autism.

In 1999, Dr. Yazbak published two studies that strongly suggested a link between the MMR vaccination and autism. In the first study, he looked at the offspring of 25 mothers who had received the MMR live virus vaccination shortly after delivery and who had *breast-fed* their babies. These offspring later received the MMR vaccine, and what Dr. Yazbak discovered was that the incidence of autism was incredibly high in those babies; an astounding 80 percent of the mothers so vaccinated had babies who later developed autism.[3]

In the second study, Dr. Yazbak looked at the consequences of immunizing mothers with the MMR just *prior* to conception and again *during* their pregnancy. Six of the seven mothers evaluated (86 percent) gave birth to children who later became autistic, and the child of the seventh mother had developmental delays.[4]

A third follow-up study was done the following year (2000) in which Dr. Yazbak evaluated the consequences of immunizing a mother *around conception, during pregnancy, or at delivery*. Every one of the 22 mothers (100 percent) so evaluated "had at least one child develop autism in connection with or following their own MMR vaccination…. In many instances, the children's autistic manifestations reportedly started or worsened after their first MMR vaccine."

Yikes!

Dr. Yazbak concluded that giving MMR or rubella vaccines to mothers just before, during, or right after a pregnancy "may not be wise or safe." (There's an understatement!) He also encouraged further *unbiased* research in this area.[5]

These three studies were presented at a special session of the American Academy of Pediatrics in 2001 and were published online as well.[6]

---

1   Miller, Neil Z. *Vaccine Safety Manual.* 2nd ed. p.156.
2   www.thinktwice.com/Yazbak 1.pdf
3   Yazbak, F.E. "Autism: Is There a Vaccine Connection? Part I: Vaccination After delivery." 1999. www.thinktwice.com/Yazbak 1.pdf
4   Yazbak, F.E. "Autism: Is there a Vaccine Connection? Part II: Vaccination Around Pregnancy." www.thinktwice.com/Yazbak 2.pdf
5   Yazbak, F.E. "Autism: Is There a Vaccine Connection? Part III: Vaccination Around Pregnancy, the Sequel." www.thinktwice.com/Yazbak 3.pdf
6   http://www.vaccinationnews.com/about-dr-f-edward-yazbak

Comment: None of these case series studies was published in a peer-reviewed journal, although they were ostensibly peer-reviewed.[7]

The participants, who completed detailed questionnaires, were recruited via e-mail or other advertisements. Recruitment, unfortunately, tends to skew the results in favor of families with medical concerns, as they might be more likely to want to participate in the study than would those with no medical issues. And there was no control group.

Despite all these issues, the studies do have some validity, as they point to a potentially serious concern, and Dr. Yazbak's call to have further unbiased research done in this regard is certainly appropriate. Unfortunately, no such further studies have been done to our knowledge.

These three studies most certainly support Dr. Wakefield's findings of a *possible* association between the MMR vaccine and autism.

Study 4

Kawashima, H. et al. "Detection and Sequencing of Measles Virus from Peripheral Mononuclear Cells from Patients with Inflammatory Bowel Disease and Autism." *Digestive Diseases and Sciences*. 2000.

In an independent Japanese study, published in 2000 in the journal *Digestive Diseases and Sciences*, the researchers found measles virus in *some* of the autistic children studied as well as in some of the patients with ulcerative colitis that "were consistent with being vaccine strains."

And "the results were concordant with the exposure history of the patients." They had all been given the MMR vaccine.

Hiroshi Kawashima and colleagues asserted that, "Persistence of measles virus was confirmed in peripheral blood mononuclear cells (a type of immune cell) in *some* patients with chronic intestinal inflammation."

Possible conflicts of interest: None

Comment: The finding of measles virus in the gut wall of these children does not *prove* that the measles virus causes autism or ulcerative colitis, but does *support* the contention that the measles virus from the MMR vaccine *may* play a role in causing intestinal inflammation in those with ulcerative colitis and autism, and these findings do support and are consistent with those of the Lancet 12 study. The study also proves that the live virus found on the measles vaccine can persist and replicate in the gut of certain individuals.

Study 5

Walker, Stephen et al. "Persistent Ileal Measles Virus in a Large Cohort of Regressive Autistic Children with Ileocolitis and Lymphonodular Hyperplasia: Revisitation of an Earlier Study." International Meeting for Autism Research. May 2007.

And further support for the Lancet 12 study comes from another investigation presented initially as a poster display at the 2007 International Meeting for Autism Research (IMFAR). This study approved by the Institutional Review Board (IRB) was begun in 2003 by four scientists at Wake Forest University Baptist Medical Center.

The objective of the study was to examine the biopsy tissue obtained from the ileum (last part of the small intestine) of a proposed large group of children (over 275) with regressive autism who had all been referred to a pediatric intestinal specialist because of chronic intestinal symptoms that warranted further evaluation.

The biopsied tissue was examined for the presence of the measles virus. If the measles virus was found, it was then further analyzed to see whether the virus variety present came from the MMR vaccine or from the wild strain of the measles virus.

---

7   Ibid.

At the time of the poster presentation, the researchers had collected medical data (histories, vaccination data, and other studies) on over 275 children and had obtained biopsy tissue samples on 82 of those children. Of the 82 biopsy samples analyzed, 70 of them (85 percent) showed the presence of measles virus RNA.

Lead author Stephen Walker later commented, "Of the handful of results we have in so far (6 total), all are vaccine strain and none are wild measles."[8]

The scientists concluded that the "Preliminary results from this large cohort of pediatric autistic patients with chronic GI symptoms confirm earlier findings of measles virus RNA in the terminal ileum and support an association between measles virus and ileocolitis *[ILL-ee-oh-coh-LIGHT-us]*/LNH."[9] As well as in:

- Inflammation of the large intestine (colon) and ileum (last part of small intestine)
- Lymphoid-Nodular Hyperplasia: numerous enlarged lymph nodes in the gut wall.

Possible Conflicts of Interest: None

Comment: Once again, we see independent evidence for the *presence* of measles virus in the intestines of children with intestinal symptoms, intestinal inflammation, and regressive autism. This preliminary study lacks a control group of non-autistic children, and needs an appropriate control to rule out cross-contamination. The authors hoped to address these concerns as the study continued. This research was supported by grants from the Autism Research Institute, The National Autism Association, and individual donors.

Study 6

Uhlmann, V. et al. "Potential viral pathogenic mechanism for new variant inflammatory bowel disease." *Mol Pathol.* April, 2002; 55(2):84-90.

Another relevant earlier study published in the peer-reviewed journal *Molecular Biology* did have an appropriate control group. The researchers in this investigation compared intestinal biopsy results of 91 children with regressive autism, LNH, and enterocolitis (inflammation of the intestine) with a control group of 70 non-autistic children.

The latter group included "19 children with normal ileal biopsies, 13 children with mild non-specific chronic inflammatory changes, three children with ileal lymphonodular hyperplasia (LNH) investigated for abdominal pain, eight children with Crohn's disease, one child with ulcerative colitis, and 26 children who had undergone appendicectomy for abdominal pain including appendicitis."

Specialized antibody tests were performed looking for the presence of the measles virus in the biopsied tissue. The investigators found that 75 of the 91 patients (82 percent) with developmental delay, LNH, and enterocolitis were positive for measles virus in their intestinal tissue compared to just 5 of 70 control patients (7 percent).

The authors concluded that, "The data confirm an *association* between the presence of measles virus and gut pathology in children with developmental disorder."

Possible Conflicts of Interest: Three of the ten investigators in this study were Andrew Wakefield, Simon Murch, and John Walker-Smith, all of whom co-authored the 1998 *Lancet* study. Dr. Wakefield had previously agreed to testify on behalf of children alleged to have been harmed by the MMR vaccine (although he never did). The lead author of this study was V. Uhlmann, who had no stated conflicts of interest.

Comment: At first glance, this appears to be a good study with no evidence of manipulation of data and, like the previous two studies, supports the earlier findings of the Wakefield group. However, Dr. O'Leary's lab, which analyzed the biopsy tissue for the presence of measles virus, came under fire by some critics who questioned the accuracy of

8   www.dailymail.co.uk/news/article-338051/Scientists-fear-MMR-link-autism.html (Jan 26, 2011)
9   Lymphonodular hyperplasia

the lab results on a number of grounds. The criticisms appear to have validity and are quite technical.[10]

For whatever it is worth, O'Leary's lab was vindicated in a later study sponsored by the CDC and the American Academy of Pediatrics, which utilized the O'Leary lab and two others in a blinded fashion to analyze intestinal biopsies from 38 children. The results from all three labs were in total agreement in their analyses.[11]

In any event, the finding of LNH in the gut of developmentally-delayed children with gut issues does support the Wakefield group's findings in the earlier Lancet 12 study.

Study 7

Wakefield, A.J. et al. "Enterocolitis in children with developmental disorder." *American Journal of Gastroenterology* 2000; 95: 2285-2295. Retraction in: *Am J Gastroenterology*. 2010 May; 105(5):1214. Comment in *Am J Gastroenterology*. 2000 Sep; 95(9):2154-6.; *and in* Histopathology. 2007 May; 50(6):794. PMID: 11007230.

Andrew Wakefield and his colleagues continued to do additional investigational studies in the years following the publication of the Lancet 12 study. In one of those earlier studies, Drs. Wakefield, Murch, Walker-Smith, and others evaluated sixty affected children via visual examination (ileo-colonoscopy) of their lower bowel (colon) and distal small intestine (ileum).

Intestinal biopsies were taken, as in the 1998 *Lancet* study. Fifty of the sixty children were autistic; five had Asperger's syndrome, two had disintegrative disorder, and the remaining three had ADHD, dyslexia, and schizophrenia respectively. All had chronic intestinal complaints.

Biopsy samples from the affected children were compared to samples taken from 37 developmentally-normal children who were being investigated for possible inflammatory bowel disease. Comparisons were also made with 22 clinically-normal children with no intestinal symptoms and with 20 children with ulcerative colitis.

Three pathologists independently reviewed the tissue slides in a blinded fashion (not knowing the history or the name of the child whose tissues they were examining) and graded the severity of the lympho-nodular hyperplasia (LNH) seen, if any.

They diagnosed LNH in 93 percent of the affected children and in only 14.3 percent of the controls. They also found that, "Scores of frequency and severity of inflammation were significantly greater in both affected children and those with ulcerative colitis, compared with controls." The probability that these differences were due to chance was calculated at less than one in a thousand (p<0.001).

The authors concluded that, "A new variant of inflammatory bowel disease is present in this group of children with developmental disorders."

Comment: This well-done study was retracted in May 2010 by the *American Journal of Gastroenterology* for political reasons. The *British Medical Journal* had that same year accused Dr. Wakefield of altering the data on the children of the 1998 *Lancet* study. That accusation, as we have seen, was false. There was and is no evidence of any data altering in this or any other study associated with Dr. Wakefield.

Dr. Wakefield is not a clinician. He is a gastroenterological surgeon and researcher. The histories taken on the children were obtained by *other* respected clinicians with *no conflicts of interest* and obtained from information provided by their parents and the children's medical records that were made available to the researchers.

Biopsy evaluations in this study were carried out by three *independent* pathologists in *a rigorous and blinded manner* to eliminate bias in their interpretations. There is no reason not to accept the data from this study as factual and relevant.

---

10   www.badscience.net/wp-content/uploads/erp_mmr.pdf.
11   *PLoS One*; Sept 4, 2008; 3(9)

Study 8

Krigsman, Arthur et al. "Clinical Presentation and Histologic Findings at Ileocolonoscopy in Children with Autistic Spectrum Disorder and Chronic Gastrointestinal Symptoms." *Autism Insights*. 2010:2 1–11.

In a more recent peer-reviewed case series study, the medical records of 143 *consecutive* patients with autism spectrum disorders and chronic intestinal complaints were reviewed.

All of the patients "underwent subsequent diagnostic ileocolonoscopy (Ill-ee-oh-coal-un-OS-cuh-pee) and biopsy for suspected bowel inflammation disorders."

All of the patients were referred either by their primary care physicians or by their parents. None were recruited.

The children so evaluated suffered from chronic intestinal symptoms. Constipation was noted in 36 percent, and a majority had abdominal pain and diarrhea. Altogether, 73 percent had numerous, enlarged lymph nodes in the wall of the colon and/or ileum and had inflammation in the colon and/or ileum as well (LNH). *Significant association was found between intestinal inflammation and the finding of LNH and the onset of developmental disorder in these children.*

Possible Conflicts of Interest: Arthur Krigsman, Asst. Professor of Pediatrics, NYU School of Medicine, Carol Stott, and Dr. Andrew Wakefield, who was not an author of this study, were all on the staff of the Thoughtful House for Children in Austin, Texas at the time this article was published. Marvin Boris and Alan Goldblatt were not so affiliated. At the time, Dr. Wakefield was also an editor of *Autism Insights*. Both Krigsman and Stott have been retained by "claimant solicitors in vaccine related litigation" and Arthur Krigsman has also been "retained by claimants in the U.S. omnibus Autism proceeding."

Comment: Although at least two of the researchers were friends with and coworkers of Dr. Wakefield, and although the same two clinicians had appeared as claimant expert witnesses in vaccine-related litigation, there is no reason to believe this study has been falsified in any way.

The medical records of these children were derived from *outside physicians with no conflicts* and *were not altered*. They represented *consecutive* referrals. *The children were not recruited, nor preselected.* The data presented can be readily verified. The *blinded* pathological findings derived from biopsies of affected intestinal tissue corresponded quite nicely with the visual observations.

Conclusion: Children who have both autism *and* evidence of chronic intestinal symptoms (pain, constipation, diarrhea, etc.) have a high likelihood of also having non-specific intestinal inflammation and multiple enlarged intestinal lymph nodes, which is exactly what Dr. Wakefield's team has also repeatedly found.

Study 9

Furlano R, et al. "Colonic CD8 and T cell filtration with epithelial damage in children with autism." *J Pediatr* 2001; 138(3): 366-72. PMID: 11241044.

And in yet another study, scientists evaluated 21 *consecutively referred* children with *both autism and bowel symptoms*. This group was compared in a *blinded fashion* to four other groups of children:

- 8 with normal intestines (ileum and colon)
- 10 with numerous enlarged intestinal lymph nodes (lymphoid nodular hyperplasia) but normal development
- 15 with Crohn's disease of the intestine (an inflammatory intestinal disease)
- 14 with ulcerative colitis of the intestine (also an inflammatory disease)

The comparative evaluations included an examination of the colon (large intestine) and ileum (last part of the small intestine) of all the children via direct observation of the intestinal lining (ileo-colonoscopy), a microscopic review of the intestinal biopsy samples obtained during the procedure, a chemical analysis of the biopsied tissues and a measurement of the thickness of the foundation layer of the intestinal wall (the basement membrane).

The researchers found that *100 percent of the autistic children* had mild inflammatory bowel disease (colitis) characterized by an infiltration of increased numbers of lymphocytes, a type of immune cell, in the colon wall.

They also had statistically significant thicker basement membranes and increased numbers of certain other immune cells (gamma-delta cells and CD8 lymphocytes) as compared to all the other groups except those with ulcerative colitis.

The research team confirmed the existence of "a distinct lymphocytic colitis (colon inflammation with increased numbers of lymphocytes-an immune cell) in autistic spectrum disorders in which the epithelium (intestinal lining) appears particularly affected. This is consistent with increasing evidence for gut epithelial (gut lining) dysfunction in autism."

Comment: This appears to be a well-done study. The use of blinded evaluations in these children eliminated the possibility of bias error. The study again supports the contention that autistic children with intestinal complaints appear to have a nonspecific form of intestinal inflammation as suggested by Wakefield's team in the now retracted *Lancet* study. Drs. Wakefield, Walker-Smith, and Murch all participated in this study, although none was the lead investigator.

Study 10

Torrente, F. et al. "Small intestinal enteropathy with epithelial IgG and complement deposition in children with regressive autism." *Molecular Psychiatry* (2002) 7, 375;382. DOI: 10.1038 sjmp4001077.

In a 2002 study of 25 children with regressive autism, biopsies of the *first section* of their small intestines (the duodenum) were compared with similar biopsies from children with celiac disease and cerebral palsy with mental retardation, and with a normally developing control group.

Many abnormalities were noted in the autistic children compared to the other groups. These included increased numbers of lymphocytes infiltrating certain intestinal cell layers and paralleling what was noted in the colons and ilea of autistic children in the aforementioned studies.

The researchers also noted *increased immune-globulin G antibody deposition* in 23 of the 25 autistic children evaluated, suggesting that this might represent an *auto-immune* phenomenon.

Comment: This study is consistent with Dr. Wakefield's finding that the intestinal tract of autistic children with GI complaints is often inflamed. The inflammation found in these children's upper intestinal tract (duodenums) was similar to that found by other investigators in autistic children's lower intestines (ileum and colon—see above). Drs. Wakefield, Murch, and Walker-Smith were also co-authors of this study, albeit not the lead authors.

Study 11

Singh, V.K.; Jensen, R.L. "Elevated levels of measles antibodies in children with autism." *Pediatr Neurol.* 2003 Apr; 28(4):292-4.

In a study published in the journal *Pediatric Neurology* in 2003, Dr. Vijendra Singh and his colleague R.L. Jensen of the Department of Biology at Utah State University measured antibodies to measles, mumps, and rubella virus in a series of autistic children. They compared those levels to those of a control group of non-autistic children and also to the autistic children's siblings.

The researchers found that, "The level of measles antibodies, but not mumps or rubella antibodies, was significantly higher in autistic children as compared with normal children (P = 0.003) or siblings of autistic children (P <or= 0.0001)."

One particular anti-measles antibody was found in 83 percent of the autistic children but not in either control group and was also directed against a particular protein in the autistic cohort. Singh and Jensen concluded that "autistic children have a hyperimmune response to measles virus, which in the absence of a wild type of measles infection might be a sign of an abnormal immune reaction to the vaccine strain or virus reactivation."

These findings also support the Lancet 12 study's *suggestion* of an association between the MMR vaccination and autism.

Study 12

Balzola, F. et al. "Panenteric IBD-like disease in a patient with regressive autism shown for the first time by the wireless capsule enteroscopy: another piece in the jigsaw of this gut-brain syndrome?" *Am J Gastroenter*. 2005; 100(4):979–81.

In another small study published in 2005 in the *American Journal of Gastroenterology*, small bowel disease was reported in a symptomatic patient with regressive autism. These findings are consistent with and support those of the Lancet 12 study.

Study 13

Gonzalez, L. et al. "Endoscopic and Histological Characteristics of the Digestive Mucosa in Autistic Children with Gastro-Intestinal Symptoms." *Arch Venez Pueric Pediatr*. 2005; 69:19-25.

In a 2005 Venezuelan study, 45 children with autism spectrum disorders were compared with "57 developmentally normal controls presenting for gastrointestinal assessment." Chronic inflammation and lymphonodular hyperplasia (LNH) in the colon and ileum was found in every one of the autistic children compared with 67 percent of the control group (a statistically significant difference), "reflecting a high background rate of infectious enterocolitis in Venezuelan children."

Study 14

Ashwood, P. et al. "Intestinal lymphocyte populations in children with regressive autism: evidence for extensive mucosal immunopathology." *Journal of Clinical Immunology*, November 2003; 23:504-517.

The immune cell known as the lymphocyte exists in a variety of subtypes differentiated one from the other by analysis of their surface markers. A study was published in the *Journal of Immunology* in 2003 that compared the lymphocyte populations of autistic children with intestinal inflammation with those of developmentally-normal children with inflamed intestines and with another group of developmentally-normal children without intestinal inflammation.

The researchers found that certain lymphocyte subtypes in the autistic children differed significantly from those of the two control groups. They concluded that, "The data provide further evidence of a pan-enteric (throughout the intestine) mucosal (intestine lining) immuno-pathology (abnormal or excessive immune reaction) in children with regressive autism that is apparently distinct from other inflammatory bowel diseases."

Comment: This is another well-done study that included both John Walker-Smith and Andrew Wakefield as co-authors, and it also supports the findings of the Lancet 12 research.

Study 15

"GI Symptoms in Autism Spectrum Disorders (ASD): An Autism Treatment Network Study." http://imfar.confex. com/imfar/2010/webprogram/Paper6817. html.

In 2010 at the International Society for Autism Research meeting in Philadelphia, a study was presented by the Autism Treatment Network, which confirmed Dr. Wakefield's assertion that autistic children often have chronic intestinal complaints.

This study analyzed data on over 1,100 autistic children aged 2-18 years from 15 treatment and research centers in the United States and Canada.

Forty-five percent of these children had *chronic intestinal symptoms*, including abdominal pain (59 percent), diarrhea (43 percent), nausea (31 percent), and bloating (26 percent). The prevalence of these symptoms *increased* with age and reached 51 percent in children 7 years of age or older (p<0.0001).

Of the children with intestinal complaints, 70 percent also had sleep problems as opposed to just 30 percent of the autistic children with no abdominal complaints.

Study 16

Singh, Vijendra K. et al. "Abnormal Measles-Mumps-Rubella Antibodies and CNS Autoimmunity in Children with Autism." *J Biomed Sci*. 2002; 9:359–364.

Myelin is the name given to the insulating substance that surrounds nerves. It has been observed that antibodies to a protein found in myelin (myelin basic protein) are noted frequently in autistic children, as are elevated levels of measles antibodies.

In 2002, Dr. Singh and his associates in the Department of Biology at Utah State University conducted a study of auto-antibodies to both myelin basic protein and to measles, mumps, and rubella viruses in serum obtained from 125 autistic and 92 control children.

The researchers found a significant increase in the level of MMR antibodies in the autistic children as compared to controls, and in particular, they noted the presence "of an unusual MMR antibody in 75 of the 125 autistic (60 percent) sera but not in any of the control sera." Further analysis of this unusual antibody revealed it to be immuno-positive for a particular protein (hemagglutinin) "which is *unique* to the measles subunit of the MMR vaccine." None of the control children's sera had this unique antibody.

The scientists also found that "over 90 percent of MMR antibody-positive autistic sera were also positive for myelin basic protein auto-antibodies, suggesting a strong association between [the] MMR [immunization] and central nervous system auto-immunity in autism."

These findings suggested "that an inappropriate antibody response to MMR, specifically the measles component thereof, might be related to the pathogenesis of autism."

Comment: Once again, good research links the MMR vaccination and, in particular, the measles component to autism and suggests a potential mechanism whereby the MMR vaccine might *promote the autistic state*.

Study 17

Bradstreet, J.J. et al. "Detection of measles virus genomic RNA in cerebrospinal fluid of three children with regressive autism: a report of three cases." *Journal of American Physicians and Surgeons*. 2004; 9(2):38-45.

It has been reported that MMR-induced brain inflammation (encephalopathy) can present as autistic regression. In order to investigate this suggested association, Dr. Jeff Bradstreet and his colleagues investigated three autistic children with a history of intestinal complaints who had had visual examinations (colonoscopies) and biopsies of their inflamed intestines (colon and/or ileum).

Numerous, enlarged, nodular lymph nodes (LNH) were found in all the children and measles virus genetic material (RNA) was detected from each of their *intestinal* biopsies.

All three of the autistic children underwent spinal taps to determine whether measles virus could also be detected in their *cerebro-spinal fluid* (CSF), and indeed, the measles virus fusion *gene* was detected in all three of them, but not in any of the three control children who had spinal fluid removed from their indwelling shunts for hydrocephalus.

All the autistic children, but none of the controls, had auto-antibodies to myelin basic protein in their *sera*, and two of the three also had anti-measles and anti-myelin basic protein antibodies in their *spinal fluid*.

None of the autistic or control children had a history of having had the measles. All the children in both groups had been immunized with the MMR vaccine. The research team concluded that, "Findings are consistent with both a measles virus etiology for the autism encephalopathy and active viral replication in these children. They further indicate the possibility of a virally driven cerebral immunopathology in some cases of regressive autism."

Comment: This small study again supports the association of measles virus and autism and implicates that virus as a possible causative agent in this disorder. Dr. Wakefield is listed as a co-author of this study. These results are also consistent with those of the Utah State University study mentioned above.

Study 18

Wakefield, A.J. et al. "The Significance of Ileo-Colonic Lymphoid Nodular Hyperplasia in Children with Autism Spectrum Disorder." *European Journal of Gastroenterology & Hepatology*, August 2005. Source: Thoughtful House Center for Children, Austin, Texas 78746, USA.

Dr. Wakefield was the lead author of another research study published in the *European Journal of Gastroenterology and Hepatology* in 2005. In this study, 148 *consecutive* children (86 percent male) with autism and gastro-intestinal symptoms were evaluated by visual examination of their intestinal tracts (ileo-colonoscopy). Biopsies were taken and the visual and microscopic results were compared to those of a group of 30 control children (83 percent male) with normal development and intestinal symptoms.

What the investigators in this study found was that the *presence* of lympho-nodular hyperplasia (LNH) was *significantly* greater in the autistic population in both the ileum and colon than it was in the control group. And the *severity* of the LNH was also *significantly* greater in the autistic population.

Conclusion: "Ileo-colonic LNH is a characteristic pathological finding in children with ASD (autism spectrum disorders) and gastrointestinal symptoms, and is associated with mucosal inflammation. Differences in age at colonoscopy and diet do not account for these changes. The data support the hypothesis that LNH is a significant pathological finding in ASD children."

Comment: A well-done study that again corroborates the findings of the Lancet 12 and other similar studies, which found that autistic children *with* intestinal complaints have a high prevalence of intestinal inflammation and associated enlarged and numerous gut lymph nodes (LNH).

Study 19

Schultz, Stephen T. et al. "Acetaminophen (paracetamol) use, measles-mumps-rubella vaccination, and autistic disorder." *Autism*. Vol. 12, No. 3, 293-307 (2008).

It is quite common for babies to become irritable and run a fever after receiving the MMR inoculation. Parents often treat those symptoms with pain and fever reducers like acetaminophen/paracetamol (Tylenol® or other brands) or with ibuprofen (Advil® etc.). Many doctors have recommended giving acetaminophen or ibuprofen prophylactically to babies prior to their MMR vaccination.

Scientists at the University of California, San Diego and San Diego State University were curious to know whether taking these medications in association with the MMR vaccine contributed in any way to the likelihood of a child becoming autistic.

This preliminary investigation involved having parents complete an online parental survey. Information was collected over a six-month period from mid-July 2005 until the end of January 2006. This was a "case control" study that compared the data collected on 83 autistic children with that of 80 control children.

The researchers found that, "Acetaminophen use after MMR vaccination was *significantly* associated with autistic disorder when considering children 5 years of age or less (odds ratio 6), [12] after limiting cases to children with regression in development (odds ratio 4), and when considering only children who had post-vaccination sequelae (odds ratio 8). [13]

In doing this analysis, the researchers adjusted for age, gender, the mother's ethnicity, and the presence of illness concurrent with measles-mumps-rubella vaccination.

While the use of ibuprofen in association with the MMR was *not* associated with autistic disorder, the use of acetaminophen after the MMR immunization most definitely was.

Comment: This intriguing study is yet another that supports the Lancet 12 finding of an association between the MMR immunization and the likelihood of a child becoming autistic and, in particular, the association between a child having post-vaccination sequelae, and that child becoming autistic subsequently (Odds ratio 8!).

The study also suggests that acetaminophen, in particular, as a pain reliever and fever reducer may play a synergistic role in promoting the autistic state when used after a child receives his or her MMR vaccination.

A possible mechanism for such synergy may be related to how acetaminophen is metabolized in the body. Acetaminophen is mainly broken down in the liver and its elimination involves the utilization of large amounts of the antioxidant-detoxifier glutathione. Glutathione depletion may help promote the autistic state by reducing the body's capacity to detoxify heavy metals and other toxins and by reducing its ability to combat free radicals. Other mechanisms may also be involved and need to be investigated.

It would be interesting to see whether the use of acetaminophen in conjunction with other immunizations, like the DPT shot for example, or just prescribed for pain or fever in the first years of life would also increase a child's risk of becoming autistic.

In any case, these study results strongly suggest that giving a baby or child acetaminophen before or after the MMR inoculation is unwise.

The relation of acetaminophen (Tylenol and other brands) to autism will be discussed at greater length in a subsequent chapter of this book.

Study 20: Madsen Study Rebuttal

Goldman, G.S.; Yazbak, F.E. "An Investigation of the Association between MMR Vaccination and Autism in Denmark." *Journal of American Physicians and Surgeons.* Vol. 9, No. 3, Fall 2004.

The reader may recall our critique of the faulty Danish study** by Dr. Kreesten Madsen, et al. (see Chapter 17) that purported to show an increase in the incidence of autism after thimerosal-containing vaccines were discontinued in Denmark, but which actually showed the opposite when all the data was correctly analyzed. [14]

Dr. Madsen also published another equally questionable study that alleged that the autism incidence in Denmark did not increase after the MMR was added to the childhood immunization schedule in 1987. This study will be reviewed in more detail in the next chapter. [15]

Dr. Yazbak and his research associate, Dr. Goldman (Co-Founder and President of Medical Veritas International

---

12   "Odds ratio" in this instance refers to the ratio of the odds of exposure to acetaminophen in the (autistic) cases to the odds of exposure to acetaminophen in the controls. An odds ratio of 6, for example, means children who took acetaminophen after their MMR shot were 6 times more likely to become autistic than were the control children who did not take acetaminophen.

13   "Sequelae" (seh-KWELL-ee) means side effects.

14   Madsen, Kreesten et al. "Thimerosal and the Occurrence of Autism: Negative Ecological Evidence from Danish Population-Based Data." *Pediatrics.* Sept 2003.

15   Madsen, Kreesten M. et al. "A Population-Based Study of Measles, Mumps, and Rubella Vaccination and Autism." *N Engl J Med.* Nov 7, 2002; 347:1477-1482.

and Editor-in-Chief of the journal *Medical Veritas*), reviewed the Danish registry data in order to determine the *true* prevalence of autism by age category in that country from 1990 to 1992.

Those were the years that preceded the reclassification of autism in Denmark. The diagnostic criteria that defined autism were broadened in 1993, and after 1995, an additional large cohort of autism cases from outpatient clinics was also included in the prevalence statistics.

Neither of the Madsen studies accounted for these confounding variables, which thus made their conclusions invalid. Drs. Yazbak and Goldman performed a statistical calculation known as linear regression analysis on the data from that two-year period in order to assess more accurately the autism prevalence for the year 2000 free of ascertainment bias.

And they found that the prevalence of autism for every 100,000 Danish children aged 5-9 years *had increased almost nine times* from a mean of 8 in the pre-MMR-licensure era (1980-1986) to 71 in the year 2000 (post-MMR) and leveled off during 2001-2002. *The dramatic increase in autism prevalence found by these researchers contradicts the conclusions of Madsen et al. and more accurately reflects the true prevalence of autism in Denmark during those years.*

Goldman and Yazbak then did another statistical analysis and calculated the relative risk of getting autism at 8.5. [16] After adjusting for better diagnostic awareness, the relative risk was calculated at 4.7, and for all individuals under age 15 at 4.1. So the risk of getting autism was four to five times higher for a child who received the MMR vaccine than it was for a child who hadn't.

Comment: This is a good study that supports the Lancet 12 finding of a *possible* cause-effect association between the MMR and the risk of becoming autistic and counters the findings of the widely publicized, albeit faulty, study of Madsen et al.[17]

Conclusion: We have confirmed that the findings of Dr. Wakefield and his associates in that much maligned Lancet 12 study have been corroborated by a whole host of other relevant studies.

However, there have also been a number of epidemiological and other investigations that purport to disprove any association between the MMR vaccine and measles. Do they really do that?

We will discuss these "negative" studies in Chapter 25, but first, we will review some of the possible mechanisms whereby the MMR inoculation and the measles vaccine in particular might promote the autistic state.

Another Story of a Good Scientist Who Was Irresponsibly Attacked

As discussed in a blog by Dan Olmsted:

> Clear evidence of pediatric lead poisoning emerged by 1904—yet lead actually became ubiquitous after that, powering the rise of the automobile and peaking in the environment in the 1970s. It was then that a courageous, much-vilified scientist named Herb Needleman showed a dose response between lead exposure and IQ—enough "proof" to get the feds to finally face up to the truth. Needleman got the lead out because he demonstrated the reality of subclinical toxicity.

At the Institute of Medicine's two-day Autism and the Environment Workshop in Washington in April 2008, Philip Landrigan, Chair of Community and Preventive Medicine, Mount Sinai School of Medicine, gave a presentation on Environmental Toxicants and Neurodevelopment.

In that talk, he emphasized "the concept that relatively low-dose exposure to lead or other toxic chemicals...may cause harmful effects to health that are not evident with a standard clinical examination.... The underlying premise

---

16   The "relative risk" (AKA "risk ratio") is the ratio of the risk in the exposed individual divided by the risk in the unexposed. For example, a relative risk of 8.5 in this study means that exposure to the MMR vaccine increased the risk (likelihood) of getting autism by a factor of 8.5 relative to those with no exposure.

17   Ibid.

is that there exists a continuum of toxicity, in which clinically apparent symptoms of lead have their asymptomatic, subclinical counterparts."

"The lead industry did their best to pillory Herb Needleman (who showed the subclinical effect). They had a couple of scientists who were in their pay, although they didn't acknowledge they were in the industry's pay until later, who came forward and charged Herb Needleman with scientific fraud. His case was hung up at the NIH for four years while that terribly painful process cranked through. He was eventually completely vindicated and has won a whole series of prestigious awards since that time.

"There was great resistance to learning the results of research or to translating these research results into public policy," Landrigan continued. "I think today one of the reasons we have 80,000 chemicals in commerce, of which fewer than 20 percent have been properly tested, reflects the same legacy of special interests not caring to know about the toxicity of chemicals. I honestly think as a society we need to get beyond that. "We're flying blind if we allow kids to...be exposed to chemicals of untested toxicity."[18]

For further studies that support the MMR-Autism linkage see: http://www.whale.to/vaccine/thrower6.html.

Dr. Andrew Wakefield testified on June 19, 2002 at a special meeting of the House Committee on Government Reform,

Representative Daniel Burton of Indiana, Chairman.

"The sum of the research by my group and our collaborators, taken together with additional work by independent physicians and scientists in the United States, has now confirmed the following facts:

Children with regressive autism and intestinal symptoms have a novel and characteristic inflammatory disease of their intestine.

This disease is not found in developmentally normal control children.

This disease is entirely consistent with a viral cause.

This disease may be the source of toxic damage to the brain.

Measles virus has been identified in the diseased intestine in the majority of children with regressive autism studied, precisely where it would be expected if it were the cause of the intestinal disease.

These children, who suffer the same pattern of regressive autism and intestinal inflammation, come from many countries, including the U.S. and Ireland, where they have been investigated and biopsied independently.

The measles virus in the diseased intestine of autistic children is from the vaccine.

Children with regressive autism appear to have an abnormal immune response to measles virus.

These findings are entirely consistent with parental reports that their normally developing child regressed into autism following exposure to MMR vaccine."[19]

---

18   http://www.chat-hyperacusis.net/post/Pink-Disease-Mercury-Autism-The-Brain-Gut-Ears-1599210?trail=100

19   http://www.whale.to/vaccine/yazbak1.html

Chapter 24
How the MMR Vaccine May Promote Autism

"Truth is treason in the Empire of Lies."

— Ron Paul

B<small>Y</small> **W**<small>HAT</small> **M**<small>ECHANISMS</small> *Could the MMR Vaccination Promote Autism?*

Mechanism 1:

The weakened (attenuated) measles virus, a component of the MMR vaccine, could promote autism by lowering vitamin A levels.

Evidence for this theory was put forth by Dr. Mary Megson, an autism researcher and physician. Dr. Megson conducted a study of 60 children with autism and found that 56 (93 percent) had at least one parent who suffered from night blindness.

This startling finding, she suggested, was likely due to a primary dietary deficiency of vitamin A, or a genetic defect or disconnect in the G-alpha proteins associated with the vitamin A receptor, or to a possible untreated hypothyroid (insufficient thyroid hormone) state, which would impair the liver's ability to metabolize dietary beta-carotene into vitamin A.[1]

"G (alpha) proteins," Dr. Megson explains, "are cellular proteins that upgrade or downgrade signals in sensory organs that regulate touch, taste, smell, hearing and vision. They are found all over the body in high concentration (particularly) in the gut and in the brain and turn on or off multiple metabolic pathways including those for metabolism and cell growth."

Impaired G alpha protein function can interfere with vitamin A signaling and function.

If a vitamin A deficient mother breastfed her child, the baby would be likely also to become vitamin A deficient, but there are other mechanisms by which vitamin A deficiency or dysfunction can and does occur.

Vitamin A is well-known as the vitamin that prevents night blindness, but this remarkable nutrient also plays an important role in immune function as well as in sensory perception, language processing, and attention, and the latter three concerns are all characteristic of autistic individuals.

Dr. Megson cites literature that confirms the pertussis toxin from the pertussis inoculation (in the DPT shot and to a lesser extend the DTaP shot) can separate the G-alpha protein from the retinoid (vitamin A) receptor, thus

---

1   Megson, M. "Is autism a G alpha protein defect reversible with natural vitamin A?" *J.Med Hypo*. March 2000.

preventing the vitamin A signal's incorporation into the cell.[2]

She theorizes that "Natural (cis-and not synthetic trans-vitamin A palmitate) vitamin A may reconnect the retinoid receptors critical for vision, sensory perception, language processing and attention."

Dr. Megson relates the case of a patient Dr. Rimland had referred to her, a 14-week-old, bottle-fed baby who "had stopped making eye contact, began to stare at lights and fans, stopped cooing and laughing, and no longer turned to sound after early normal development." The alert reader will note that these are common symptoms in many autistic individuals.

The baby's mother also had night blindness and irritable bowel syndrome. There are inherited genetic defects in the G-alpha protein that make certain individuals more likely to have night blindness, which is not always due to a shortage of vitamin A.

Normally, when a vitamin A molecule lands on a normally-functioning Vitamin A (retinoid) receptor, the G-alpha protein signal is "amplified ten million times from stimulation by the time it exits the G protein coil, providing night vision in conditions of very low light."[3] However, defective G-alpha protein receptors are unable to magnify the signal effectively, so the result is night blindness.

Dr. Megson instructed the baby's mother to add cod liver oil to the baby's formula. Cod liver oil contains the natural ("cis") form of vitamin A. After the baby awoke from its nap, "he was back to normal, smiling, laughing, turning to sound, and tracking objects."[4] The baby was kept on fish oil supplementation and continued to do well thereafter.

Vitamin A, also known as retinoic acid, functions physiologically only when it is able to attach to a retinoid receptor on the cell's surface, which in turn is connected to an adjacent G-alpha protein molecule.

If the G-alpha protein is abnormal or if the G protein is separated from the receptor (due perhaps to the pertussis toxin from the DPT shot), the function of vitamin A will be understandably impaired, and only the *natural* cis-form of vitamin A found in fish oil appears to be able to bypass the G-alpha protein block and re-establish vitamin A function.

How does all this relate to the MMR vaccination? It turns out that *vitamin A is consumed rapidly when measles virus is present.*[5]

It is, therefore, likely that the live measles virus in the MMR vaccine may also possess this property and will promote a decrease in optimal levels of this necessary nutrient in certain susceptible babies.

Dr. Megson speculates that vitamin A, which in high doses has been shown to protect against viral infections, may incorporate itself into viral particles, which in some manner inhibits their growth and replication, or perhaps the mechanism has to do with the immune-enhancing properties of vitamin A.

Vitamin A has been shown to stimulate the production of immune cells like T and B lymphocytes and natural killer cells, and daily mega-dose injections of up to 400,000 units of vitamin A for 2-3 days can dramatically shorten the course of measles infection and help prevent fatalities associated with the disease.[6]

---

2   Farvel, Z.; Bourne, H.R.; Iiri, T. "The Expanding Spectrum of G Protein Diseases." *N Engl J Med* 1999; 340: 1014, 1018.
3   Ibid.
4   Ibid.
5   Sporn, M.; Roberts, A.; Goodman, D. *The Retinoids: Biology, Chemistry and Medicine.* Raven Press, 1994. p. 331.
6   http://www.megson.com/readings/MedicalHypothesis.pdf

Can We Now Provide a Reason Why Autism Regression Often Occurs in the Second Year of Life and Frequently After the MMR Immunization?

Possibly.

A decline in vitamin A from the MMR immunization in association with disconnected or dysfunctional G-alpha proteins (perhaps from the pertussis toxin in the DPT vaccine) would thus be expected to promote autistic symptoms in older susceptible babies.

This proposed measles vaccine-induced deficiency of vitamin A combined with a decline in vitamin A signaling ability, due to the hypothesized G-alpha protein disruption, could make the measles virus from the MMR a potentially more troublesome entity, allowing it to persist for prolonged periods of time in the gut and brain of susceptible individuals, which is exactly what Dr. Wakefield and other researchers have discovered.

This could explain why autistic children often regress in their second year of life. A subset of autistic children might possess a defective G-alpha protein or vitamin A receptor or be borderline deficient in vitamin A, and when they get the MMR shot during their second year of life, the vitamin A level plummets and a chronic viral infection with the measles component of the MMR ensues.

Unhampered by sufficient vitamin A to inhibit its spread, the measles virus is now able to invade the intestinal tract, causing GI symptoms and enlarged gut lymph nodes. An inflamed leaky gut can prevent optimal digestion and assimilation of nutrients, and at the same time, it allows entry of potentially harmful molecules, which can initiate or aggravate autistic symptoms.

The immune system attempts to rid itself of the persistent measles virus by producing antibodies that in some children cross-react with certain brain proteins, like myelin basic protein.

These auto-antibodies directed against brain proteins may provide another explanation as to why autism symptoms commonly appear in the second year of life in addition to the hypothesized (MMR derived) measles virus-induced vitamin A deficiency.

Keep in mind that the MMR is generally given at 12-15 months of age and a booster DPaP is commonly given at 18 months, the classical age at which autistic regression is commonly seen.

> *"G protein defects cause severe loss of rod function in most autistic children. They lose night vision and shading on objects in the daylight and 3D vision, seeing only colour and shape except for a box in the middle of their visual field. They try to make sense of the world around them by lining up toys, sorting by color. Their avoidance of eye contact is an attempt to get light to land off center in the retina where they have some rod function. Mother's touch feels like sandpaper on their skin. Common sounds become like nails scraped on a blackboard."*
>
> *Testimony of Dr. Mary Megson at Government Reform Committee on Autism April 6, 2000.[7]*

Mechanism 2:

The measles virus vaccination could promote autism in some children by inducing autoimmune reactions that could negatively affect brain function.

Several animal studies have demonstrated that antibodies to myelin basic protein occur after measles virus infection of the brain. Myelin basic protein (MBP) is found in the substance that insulates nerve fibers and is "absolutely essential for higher brain functions."[8]

---

7   Realmuto, G.; Purple, R.; Knoblock, W. "Electroretinograms in four autistic probands and six first degree relatives." *Can J Psy.* 1989; 34; 435-9.

8   Ter Meulen, V. et al. "Measles virus induced auto-immune reactions against brain antigen." Intervirology 1993; 35 (1-4):86-94 and Liebert, U.G. et al.

In a 1993 study, Dr. Vijendra K. Singh and fellow researchers found that *58 percent* (19 of 33) of the autistic children evaluated had antibodies to *myelin basic protein* (MBP) in their sera. These results were significantly different (p ≤ 0.0001)[9] from the age matched control group of children with mental retardation and Down syndrome plus a second control group of healthy non-autistic adults (only *9 percent* positive for MBP). The study results suggested that "anti MBP antibodies are associated with the development of autistic behavior."[10]

In a study published in 1998, Dr. Singh's research team investigated the incidence of antibodies to myelin basic protein, neuron-axon-filament protein (NAFP) and human herpes-6 virus in autistic children as compared to a control population.

Neurons are nerve cells that possess extensions called axons. Inside these axons are thread-like protein filaments. Antibodies directed against the protein (NAFP) in these filaments would likely be expected to interfere with the transmission of signaling in those neurons.

There are two closely related human herpes 6 viruses that have been found to have infected most humans. The generally benign baby-disease known as roseola, characterized by high fever for several days followed by a short-lived pink rash, is caused by these related viruses.

What the researchers discovered was that:

- Antibody titers (amounts) to measles virus and Herpes-6 virus were higher in autistics than in controls, but the differences did not reach statistical significance.

- 90 percent of the autistic children with measles antibodies in their sera also had antibodies directed against myelin basic protein, and 73 percent of this group also had antibodies directed against neuron axon filament protein (NAFP).

- 84 percent of the autistic children with herpes-6 virus antibodies in their sera also had antibodies directed against myelin basic protein, and 72 percent of this group also had antibodies directed against neuron axon filament protein.

The results suggested that "a virus-induced autoimmune response may play a causal role in autism."[11]

In a later study, significant elevations of an antibody to the measles virus were observed in autistic children by Dr. Singh and his colleagues in the Department of Biology and Biotechnology at Utah State University, as compared to non-autistic children (p≤0.003) and the siblings of the autistic children (p≤0.0001).

The researchers also discovered that this antibody was directed against a measles virus protein that was found in 83 percent of the autistic children studied but not at all in the non-autistic children or in the autistic children's siblings. Furthermore, the researchers found no elevation of antibodies to either mumps or rubella virus in the autistic children as compared to the control children.

The authors concluded "autistic children have a hyperimmune response to the measles virus, which in the absence of a wild-type of measles infection might be a sign of an abnormal immune reaction to the vaccine strain or virus reactivation."[12]

In another report, Dr. Singh states that he had "recently summarized laboratory data of approximately 400 cases (autistic and controls) and found that up to 85 percent of autistic children have autoantibodies to specific brain structures, in particular (to) myelin basic protein. These autoantibodies are present quite frequently in autistic children (65-85 percent), but only rarely in normal children."

"Characterization of measles virus-induced cellular autoimmune reactions against myelin basic protein in Lewis rats." *J Neuroimmunology.* 1990 Sept-Oct; 29 (103):139-147.

9   p≤0.0001 means that there was less than one chance in 10,000 that this difference would occur by chance. See also http://www.whale.to/vaccine/thrower6.html for other studies by Dr. Singh in this regard.

10   Singh, V.K. et al. "Antibodies to myelin basic protein in children with autistic behavior." *Brain Behav. Immunol.* 1993 March; 7(1): 97-103.

11   Singh, V.K. et al. "Serological association of measles virus and human herpes virus-6 with brain autoantibodies in autism." *Clin. Immunol. Immunopathol.* 1998 Oct. 89 (1):105-8.

12   Singh, V.K. et al. "Elevated levels of measles antibodies in children with autism." *Pediatric Neurology.* 2003 Apr; 28(4):292-4.

He continues, "Accordingly, I postulated that autism involves a specific autoimmune response to myelin basic protein." This "immune assault," he asserts, "impairs myelin development in the developing brain, thereby modifying the nerve cell function of the brain. "Ultimately," he concludes, "this results in autism."[13]

In a related investigation, scientists at Johns Hopkins and the Kennedy Krieger Institute found that antibodies against fetal brain were more common in mothers of autistic children than in mothers of unaffected children.[14]

A number of other studies have also found an association between maternal antibodies directed against fetal brain. It is not clear in these studies what relationship, if any, prior exposure to the measles virus plays. The studies include:

- Braunschweig, D.A. et al. "Increased prevalence of maternal auto antibodies against fetal brain in autism." Intl Meeting of Autism Research. Montreal, Canada, 2006.

- Cabanli, M. et al. "Brain-specific autoantibodies in the plasma of subjects with autism spectrum disorder." *Ann. N.Y. Acad. of Sci.* 1107: 92-103.

Mechanism 3:

In some children, the measles component of the MMR immunization appears to induce abnormal overgrowth of the lymphoid follicles (collections of immune cells) that line the intestinal tract and, through auto-immune and other mechanisms, promote the autistic state. The overgrowth of lymph follicles in the gut lining is known as lympho-nodular hyperplasia (LNH). It is not clear whether LNH promotes or contributes to autism manifestations or is just a result of having autism (or both).

LNH "is not a disease; it is an exuberant immunological response," says Dr. Arthur Krigsman, a physician and research scientist at the Thoughtful House Center for Children in Austin, Texas. Krigsman has specialized in the evaluation and treatment of autistic children for many years and has personally done hundreds of examinations (endoscopies) of the digestive tracts in these children.

Lymph nodes, it may be recalled, are collections of specialized immune cells known as lymphocytes. Lympho-nodular hyperplasia (LNH) may manifest in children and adults in any number of locations from the soft palate to the esophagus, the stomach, and both the small and large intestines. It is found in both autistic and non-autistic individuals, but more frequently in the former.

1998: Dr. Andrew Wakefield and his colleagues at the Royal Free Hospital in London first noted the association between autistic regression after an MMR vaccination and the presence of inflammatory bowel disease associated with numerous, enlarged intestinal lymph nodes, a condition known as lympho-nodular hyperplasia (LNH).[15]

2000: Drs. Wakefield, Anthony, and others confirmed the 1998 *Lancet* article findings in a study published two years later. They noted that LNH was seen in over 95 percent of the autistic children with intestinal symptoms vs. only 14 percent of the controls.[16]

2001: Buie and others found LNH of the ileum in 15 of 89 autistic children, but not all of these had autistic regression after getting their MMR vaccinations, which may account for the lower incidence.[17]

2002: Arthur Krigsman reported that 90 percent of his autistic patients with chronic intestinal complaints had LNH.[18]

2003: A paper by Dr. Ashwood and colleagues reported that intestinal biopsies of 52 children with chronic intestinal symptoms and autistic regression revealed "a novel lymphocytic enterocolitis (LNH) with autoimmune features."[19]

---

13   http://www.whale.to/v/singh.html
14   Singer, H.S. et al. "Antibodies against fetal brain in sera of mothers of autistic children." *J of NeuroImmunology;* 294 (2008): 165-172.
15   Wakefield, et al. *The Lancet;* 28 Feb 1998.
16   Wakefield, Anthony, et al. *Amer. Jrnl. Gastroenterolog.* Sept. 2000 95(9):2285ff
17   Paper presented by Dr. Timothy Buie to the Oasis Conf. on Autism, Portland, Oregon, 2001.
18   Presentation by Dr. Krigsman to the U.S. Congressional Committee on Govt. Reform; June 2002. "Hearing on the Status of Research into Vaccine Safety and Autism." Washington, D.C.
19   Ashwood, Murch, et al. *J of Clin. Imm.* Nov 2003; 23 (6):504ff.

2004: Dr. Ashwood and colleagues published another paper in which they noted that autistic children with intestinal symptoms exhibited an abnormal pattern of cytokine (inflammatory molecules in this case) production from their intestinal immune cells characteristic of a viral intestinal infection.[20]

2005: Dr. Jyonouchi and his research group found significant numbers of children with regressive autism and intestinal complaints also had LNH.[21]

2005: The team of Wakefield, Ashwood, et al. evaluated 148 consecutive children with regressive autism and chronic intestinal symptoms and found that both the frequency and severity of LNH was significantly greater in autistic children than it was in controls.[22]

2005: Researchers led by Dr. Gonzalez found LNH throughout the intestinal tract of 68 autistic children with persistent intestinal symptoms. LNH was discovered in 8 of 68 duodenums and in 36 of 68 colons (53 percent).[23]

2007: In an excellent review article published in the journal *Medical Veritas* (2007:1522ff), Dr. Krigsman outlined the abnormalities that he has noted in both autistic and non-autistic children. Some of the lesions that he has observed, like LNH, are much more common in autistic children than in non-autistic youngsters. Other lesions, he notes, may occur at about the same rates in both populations.

Mechanism 4:

The MMR (measles, mumps, and rubella) immunization may disrupt the balance between two amino acids: glycine and glutamate (glutamic acid), and this imbalance may damage neurons and promote autism.

Homeostasis, in biological terms, is defined as the "ability or tendency of an organism or cell to maintain its internal equilibrium by adjusting its physiological processes."[24]

A New Jersey-based think tank, The Center for Modeling Optimal Outcomes™ LLC, focuses largely on analyzing neuroscientific principles in business. This organization's members are statisticians, not scientists, but they have engaged scientists in their work. In 2009, they turned their attention to studying factors that might influence the probability of a child becoming autistic.

In November 2009, the center's Life Sciences group issued a press release outlining a "scientifically verifiable model for the highly probable causal path of autism, which they believe is created by an imbalance between a pair of neurotransmitter amino acids called glutamic acid (or "glutamate") and glycine."

Glutamate is an excitatory amino acid, which, in excess, can harm brain neurons. Glycine is a major inhibitory neurotransmitter of the brain stem and spinal cord, but in the forebrain, it acts on a type of glutamate receptor (called an NMDA receptor) where it promotes the excitatory actions of glutamate. Thus glycine acts as both an inhibitory (calming) and excitatory (stimulating) neurotransmitter.

Excessive excitatory neuronal stimulation has been shown to injure or kill neurons.

The center decided to investigate these relationships based on the concern of many parents of autistic children who felt that vaccines in some way contributed to the causality of the condition. The center discovered that the "stabilizer (hydrolyzed gelatin) in the MMR and certain other vaccines is 21 percent glycine."

They further allege that, "based on readily verifiable science, the use of that form of glycine triggers an imbalance between the amino acid neurotransmitters responsible for the absorption rate of certain classes of cells throughout the body. It is that wide spread disruption that apparently results in the systemic problems that

20   Ashwood, Anthony, et al. *J. Clin. Imm.* 24 (6) 2004.
21   Jyonouchi, Geng, et al. *Neuro-psychobiology.* Feb. 2005; 51(2): 77ff.
22   Europ. *J. of Gastroenterology and Hepatology.* 2005; 17 (8).
23   Gonzalez, Lopez, et al. G.E.M; *Suplemento Especial de Pediatria.* No. 1, 2005; ppc41ff.
24   www.thefreedictionary.com; homeostasis

encompass the mind and the body characterized in today's classic autism."

According to the center's founder, William McFaul, "The use of our model indicates each of the disorders within autism spectrum disorder (ASD) is attributable to disruptions in homeostasis."

"Through the application of their model it became apparent that autism is an outcome of several variables that, when the homeostatic relationship of each one is disrupted, a 'perfect storm' scenario results in autism."

They further allege that "The application of this mode identified several of the variables that account for why boys have a 4 to 1 ration of instances over girls, as well as why not every boy is affected."[25]

A number of other studies point to imbalances in the excitatory and inhibitory neurotransmitters in autistic individuals.

A Japanese study published in 2006 found significantly increased levels of the excitatory neurotransmitter glutamate (AKA glutamic acid) in adult patients with autism as compared with normal controls. However, serum levels of other amino acids, including glycine, were equivalent in both groups. The results suggested that "an abnormality in glutamatergic neurotransmission may play a role in the pathophysiology of autism."[26]

Both glutamate and glycine act on a particular neuronal cell receptor known as the NMDA receptor. When this receptor is stimulated, calcium ions rush into the cell and activate it. An excess of calcium ions entering a cell may damage or kill the cell. This can occur if there is an imbalance between the excitatory neurotransmitters (glutamate and glycine, for example) and the "calming" neurotransmitters, like GABA (gamma amino butyric acid). There is reason to believe that excess glutamate stimulation and insufficient GABA calming play a role in the pathology of autism.[27]

Blocking the NMDA receptor improves autistic functioning.[28] Since glycine is also required for activation of this receptor, it is hypothesized that glycine site antagonists may also improve functioning in autism. It is, therefore, appropriate to test glycine site antagonists as a possible new approach for the management of autism.

However, other research suggests that testing glutamate receptor stimulators (agonists) may well prove to be beneficial for autistic individuals, and that autism is a disorder characterized by low glutamate functioning in the brain.

This suggestion is based on neuroanatomical and neuroimaging studies that "indicate aberrations in brain regions that are rich in glutamate neurons and…[also that] similarities [have been observed] between symptoms produced by N-methyl-D-aspartate (NMDA) antagonists in healthy subjects and those seen in autism."[29]

What is clear is that further research into the mechanisms of excitatory-inhibitory brain homeostasis needs to be carried out with an eye on evaluating new therapies that may positively influence brain functioning in autism. It might also be appropriate to find a substitute for the high-glycine, hydrolyzed-gelatin stabilizer component of the MMR vaccine. Hydrolyzed gelatin may also induce autistic symptoms via its ability to inhibit the enzyme DPP IV. This will be discussed further (See Mechanism 7 below).

Mechanism 5:

The use of acetaminophen (Tylenol, etc., but not ibuprofen) in conjunction with the MMR has been shown to increase significantly the risk of becoming autistic.

Pediatricians often recommend using acetaminophen for fever prevention or treatment in association with the MMR

---

25   autisminnb.blogspot.com/2009_11_01_archive.html

26   Shinohe, Atsuko et al. "Increased serum levels of glutamate in adult patients with autism." *Progress in Neuro-Psychopharmacology and Biological Psychiatry.* 30(8) Dec 2006; p.1472ff.

27   Ghanizade, A. "Targeting of glycine site on NMDA receptor as a possible new strategy for autism treatment." *Neurochem Res.* 2011 May; 36(5):922-3.

28   Ibid.

29   Carlsson, M.L. "Hypothesis: is infantile autism a hypoglutamatergic disorder? Relevance of glutamate-serotonin interactions for pharmacotherapy." *J Neural Transm.* 1998; 105(4-5):525-35.

(and other) vaccines. However, the findings from two recent studies suggest that giving acetaminophen in conjunction with the MMR may be very unwise thing because the combination of acetaminophen usage in close proximity to the MMR vaccination appears to increase significantly the risk of the child becoming autistic.

This finding was first discovered by the research team headed by Steven T. Schultz and reported in 2008 in the journal *Autism* (see Study 19 in Chapter 24 for a previous discussion of this article), and the association was confirmed by Stephanie Seneff and colleagues in a study published in 2012 (see below).

It should be noted that ibuprofen given for fever prophylaxis or therapy in conjunction with the MMR did not increase the autism risk.[30]

In a study published in the February 24, 2014 issue of *JAMA Pediatrics*, researchers found that women who took acetaminophen for fever during pregnancy had a 13-35 percent higher risk of having a child with attention deficit hyperactivity disorder, adding weight to the concern about exposing babies to acetaminophen both before and after conception.

Mechanism 6:

Ethylmercury (from thimerosal) may inhibit the clearance of the measles virus from the brain.[31]

Evidence for this assertion comes from two recent journal articles. The first is a study by Johns Hopkins scientists published in 2010. This study found that all forms of mercury promoted the release of certain inflammatory substances called cytokines, but only *ethyl* mercury, the kind found in thimerosal, and not *inorganic* mercury or *methyl* mercury, *decreased interferon gamma production*.[32]

Interferon gamma is one of several interferons (antiviral substances) produced by certain immune cells. The inhibition of its release by ethyl mercury is relevant because it was found in a later study at Case Western University School of Medicine that adequate levels of interferon gamma are "necessary and sufficient" for the clearance of measles virus from brain tissue.[33]

Thus, babies with impaired ethyl mercury detoxification and elimination abilities (typical of children with autism) may have retained sufficient brain *ethyl* mercury (from their immunizations) to inhibit the production of interferon gamma, which then prevents them from being able to clear the measles virus from their brains.

This could explain the finding of live measles virus in the spinal fluid of babies with autism and the tendency for autistic children to have elevated levels of anti-measles virus antibodies that persist for years after their immunizations.

Keep in mind that even in 2015, babies may get ethyl mercury from thimerosal in utero (mother's influenza vaccine) and again at six months and yearly thereafter, and the "trace" amounts found in other vaccines may not be harmless.

Autistic children, as we have noted, are also more likely than are neurotypical children to have antibodies directed against myelin basic protein and other brain substances. Autoimmune reactions like these also have been shown to be induced by mercury.

Dr. Renee Gardner's team at the Johns Hopkins Bloomberg School of Public Health found that small doses of mercury (as mercury chloride) could "affect immune function in human cells by dysregulation of cytokine signaling pathways, with the potential to influence diverse health outcomes such as susceptibility to infectious disease or risk of autoimmunity."[34]

---

30   Schultz, Stephen T. et al "Acetaminophen (paracetamol) use, measles-mumps-rubella vaccination, and autistic disorder." *Autism*. Vol. 12, No. 3, 293-307 (2008); *and* Seneff, S. et al. "Empirical Data Confirm Autism Symptoms Related to Aluminum and Acetaminophen Exposure. *Entropy*. 2012; 14(11): 2227-53.

31   Thank you, Teresa Conrick, for discovering this association.

32   Gardner, R.M. et al. "Differential immunotoxic effects of inorganic and organic mercury species in vitro." *Toxicol Lett*. 2010 Oct -905; 198(2):182. doi: 10.1016/j.toxlet.2010.06. 015. (Epub 2010 Jun 26).

33   Stubblefield, Park S.R. et al. "T cell-, interleukin-12-, and gamma interferon-driven viral clearance in measles virus-infected brain tissue." *J Virol*. 2011 Apr; 85(7):3664-76. doi: 10.1128/JVI.01496-10. Epub 2011 Jan 26.

34   *Environ Health Perspect*. 2009 December; 117(12): 1932–1938.

"Clinical and scientific data is steadily accumulating that the live measles virus in MMR can cause brain, gut and immune system damage in a subset of vulnerable children."

— Dr. Peter Fletcher, former Chief Science Officer at Britain's Dept. of Health and former Medical Assessor to the Committee on Safety of Medicines; February 5, 2006[35]

Mechanism 7:

The Gelatin Connection

Dr. Shaw at the Great Plains Laboratory has found that the MMR vaccine is a potent inhibitor of DPP IV (dipeptidyl peptidase IV [four]), the digestive enzyme that breaks down morphine-like peptides that derive from the partial digestion of casein from dairy products and gliadin or gluten from wheat or other gluten-containing grains.[36]

Dr. Shaw theorizes that the hydrolyzed gelatin component present in the MMR vaccine may be the key factor that inhibits this enzyme. He points out that hydrolyzed gelatin, which is also found in the DPT, varicella (chicken-pox), and other single component vaccines, readily inhibits DPP IV.

If the morphine-like peptides derived from dairy and glutinous grains are not completely broken down by DPP IV, they can cause adverse systemic and neurological effects. Two of these morphine-like peptides, gliadorphin and casomorphin, are able to enter the brain and adversely impact speech and auditory integration functioning. These are areas of concern in autism. These peptides can also adversely impact the GI tract and the immune system.[37]

The process of hydrolyzing gelatin releases small bio-active peptides (tiny proteins) that can also inhibit DPP IV.

The morphine-like peptides from casein and gluten (and perhaps other foods) are also addictive to some degree. Children with autism may crave dairy and gluten-containing foods and show withdrawal reactions that can last for days or weeks when these foods are eliminated from the diet.[38]

It is not known if the gelatin in Jell-O or similar products or in medicine capsules has the potential to promote adverse reactions in autistic individuals. Further research into this area needs to be carried out. The reader is referred to Chapter 30 for a more detailed discussion of these peptides and their effects.

Mechanism 8:

Enzyme Mutations and the Virus Connection

It has been hypothesized by virologist researcher Dr. Judy Mikovitz that defects in a particular enzyme pathway (endonuclease L, also known as RNase L) "may in part be an explanation for the increased risk of autism in black males following MMR vaccination."[39]

Dr. Mikovitz is referring to Brian Hooker's reanalysis of a fraudulent CDC study that alleged to show no link between MMR vaccine and autism, but that (when inappropriately eliminated data was reincluded and reassessed) actually showed a threefold risk for autism in the African American children who were immunized with MMR vaccine earlier in life (before 36 months) as compared to those given the vaccine at a later age (after 36 months). This study will be analyzed later in this narrative. (See Chapter 25.)

---

35   http://www.bmj.com/cgi/eletters/340/apr15_2/c1127#235356

36   http://www.biologicaltreatments.com/book/ch6.asp

37   Cade, R. et al. "Autism and schizophrenia: intestinal disorder." *Nutritional Neuroscience.* 3: Feb 2000, *and* Sun, Z. and Cade, R. "A peptide found in schizophrenia causes behavioral changes in rats." *Autism* 3: 85-96, 1999, *and* Sun, Z. et al. "Beta-casomorphin induces Fos-like reactivity in discrete brain regions relevant to schizophrenia and autism." *Autism* 3: 67-84, 1999

38   http://www.biological treatments.com/book/ch6.asp

39   Personal communication to Sayer Ji from Dr. Mikovitz, forwarded to the author.

The RNase L pathway results in the activation of an enzyme that degrades the viral RNA in a cell and, thereby, protects against viral infection. A genetic mutation or acquired deficiency or abnormality in this enzyme might, therefore, promote the prolonged presence of the viral components of the MMR in cells, thereby offering a possible explanation for why some individuals might experience a prolonged measles viral residence in their intestinal (or other) cells, which in turn would likely promote a chronic inflammatory state and elevated measles antibody levels.

Certain retroviral contaminants (human endogenous retrovirus K fragments) found in many vaccines manufactured using WI-38 fetal cell line, including the MMRII, might likewise be more likely to cause harm in children with a mutated or deficient endonuclease L enzyme. Failure to degrade the viral RNA might well promote adverse immunologic and mutagenic side effects.

Mechanism 9:

The Aborted Human Fetal Cell-Retrovirus Connection

A landmark study by Theresa Deisher and colleagues, published in the September 2014 issue of the *Journal of Public Health and Epidemiology*, revealed that the introduction and widespread use of *vaccines utilizing aborted fetal cells*, including the *MMRII, Hepatitis A & B, polio, and chickenpox* (Varivax) vaccines, was directly related to subsequent dramatic increases in the prevalence of autism. The authors evaluated only autism and not other autism spectrum disorders.[40]

The researchers found that sudden large jumps in autism rates corresponded temporally to increases in exposure to the *fetal and retroviral contaminants* found in these immunizations after their introduction in the U.S., the United Kingdom, Denmark, and Australia. The presence of human DNA, presumably from the aborted fetal tissue, and mRNA viruses was confirmed in both the MMRII and HAVRIX (Hepatitis A) vaccines.[41]

As the authors point out, "human fetal DNA fragments are inducers of autoimmune reactions, while both DNA fragments and retroviruses are known to potentiate genomic insertions and mutations (Yolken et al., 2000; Kurth 1998; U.S. Food and Drug Administration 2011)."[42]

"Recent evidence has shown," the authors continue, "that human endogenous retroviral transcripts are elevated in the brains of patients with schizophrenia or bipolar disorder (Frank et al., 2005), in peripheral blood mononuclear leucocytes of patients with autism spectrum (Freimanis et al., 2010) as well as associated with several autoimmune diseases (Tai et al., 2008)."

The 2014 study focused on three specific times when the autism rates spiked.

The first was in 1980 in the United States and followed approval and introduction of the new MMR II and rubella (MuruvaxII) vaccines the previous year. For the first time, these vaccines contained *human fetal cells* (*WI-38 cell line in all, except Pentacel,*[43] *which utilizes another cell line*), which were used to propagate the viruses in the vaccine instead of the animal cells that had been used previously.

The second change point occurred in 1988, coincident with the recommendation that a second MMR immunization be added to the vaccine schedule for infants. This rise in autism prevalence had been noted by the EPA in an earlier study published in 2010, but the authors had not associated that rise with the change in the vaccine schedule.

The United Kingdom also noted a dramatic rise in autism rates in 1988-1989, and again this "followed a switch in cells used in the MMR vaccines from animal cell lines to cell lines from aborted babies in 1988."[44]

Western Australia, likewise, noted an increase in autism rates in 1990 after a fetal cell line-derived MMR was

---

40   Deisher, T.A. et al. "Impact of environmental factors on the prevalence of autistic disorder after 1979." *J Pub Jlth & Epidem*. Sept 2014; 6(9):271f.
41   Ibid. p. 273.
42   Ibid. p. 271 ff.
43   Pentacel polioviruses are grown on the MRC-5 human fetal cell line.
44   http://www.inquisitr.com/1579092/study-shows-link-between-autism-and-vaccines-using-cells-lines-from-aborted-babies/

recommended to be given to all children.[45]

In 1995, the human fetal cell-derived chickenpox vaccine (Varivax) was added to the vaccine schedule for babies in the U.S., and again, there was a jump in the prevalence of autism the following year. The prevalence of autism also increased shortly after fetal cell-containing vaccines were introduced into the immunization schedule in Denmark.

An additional startling finding to come out of this study was the discovery that "Varicella and Hepatitis A immunization coverage was significantly related to autistic disorder cases." In other words, the greater the coverage rate was for each of these vaccines, the greater the prevalence of autism cases.[46]

Theresa Deisher and her research associates expressed concern that the recently introduced Pentacel vaccine, which contains poliovirus derived from aborted human fetal cells, and which is administered to babies at 2, 4, and 6 months of age, might soon increase the likelihood of regressive autism starting at a much younger age.[47]

In doing this study, the researchers were careful to exclude changes in the criteria for diagnosing autism or paternal age as factors that influenced their findings. Their disturbing conclusion was that, "rising autistic disorder prevalence is directly related to vaccines manufactured utilizing human fetal cells."[48]

Mechanism 10:

The viral inhibition of GAD, the enzyme that converts glutamate to GABA, may promote autism.

Viral infections have been shown to interfere with the conversion of glutamate, an excitatory neurotransmitter, to GABA, a calming neurotransmitter. It may be that one or more of the live viruses in the MMR vaccine have this same effect on the infant brain. A deficiency of GABA and an excess of glutamate promote many of the symptoms seen in autistic individuals.

Everything in the body must be in balance. Too little or too much of a given neurotransmitter will result in adverse symptoms. In the body, glutamate is necessary for many essential brain functions like learning, attention, and processing new information. While high levels are associated with superior memory, excess glutamate increases the risk for seizures, brain inflammation, and cell death.

Excess glutamate may also manifest as insomnia, hyperactivity, obsessive-compulsive disorders, rocking, pacing, body spinning, hand flapping, and echolalia. Ideally, the body converts excess glutamate to the calming neurotransmitter GABA by way of the two enzymes abbreviated GAD (Glutamic acid decarboxylase exists as GAD 65 and GAD 67). *GAD deficiency has been confirmed in autistics.*[49]

GABA is vital for the acquisition and comprehension of speech, and a deficiency also may promote anxiety, aggression, decreased eye contact, attention deficits, and impaired bowel transit.

The rubella virus, found in the MMR vaccine has been shown to decrease the activity of the GAD enzyme *by as much as 50 percent.* Other viruses have also been shown to interfere with this enzyme. If one or more of the live viruses in the MMR vaccine inhibits the GAD enzymes, an increase in autism symptoms would be expected.[50]

Mechanism 11:

A Particular Genetic Immune Defect

We have previously referred to a study by Reed Warren who found that many autistic children had a particular genetic immune defect (a null allele at the complement C4B locus) that could result in their "not be(ing) able to clear certain viruses completely or before the viruses affect the central nervous system." This genetic defect suggests a

45   Ibid.
46   Ibid.
47   Deisher, Op Cit.
48   Ibid.
49   Casanova, Manuel F. ed. *Recent Developments in Autism Research.* Nova Biomedical Books, 2005. p. 128. (Chapter on Gabaergic dysfunction in autism)
50   http://www.holistic help.net/blog/how-to-increase-gaba-and-balance-glutamate/

mechanism whereby the live viruses in the MMR vaccine might adversely affect the central nervous system, and by so doing, promote the autistic state.[51]

Conclusion: We have shown that at least 11 possible mechanisms exist whereby the MMR vaccine might promote or augment the autistic condition. Further research in this regard is certainly desirable.

We have provided strong evidence from 20 peer-reviewed studies that support the findings of the Lancet 12 study by Dr. Andrew Wakefield and colleagues. In the next chapter, we will show that none of the "negative" studies that allege to disprove that association are successful in doing so.

And *none* of these "negative" studies replicate the cohort of children that Dr. Wakefield's group investigated: children who *both regressed and developed chronic inflammatory intestinal complaints after* receiving the MMR vaccine.

> *"The proper authority saw to it that the proper belief should be induced,*
> *and the people believed properly."*
>
> — *Charles Fort*

---

51   Warren, R.P. et al. "Increased frequency of the null allele at the complement C4B locus in autism." *Clin Exp Immunol* 83: 438-440, 1991.

Chapter 25
The Flawed "Negative" MMR Studies

"The studies cited in support of 'no vaccine-autism association' are not flawed because they are epidemiological; they are almost invariably flawed because their aims, design, analytic procedures or conclusions have been inappropriate, and in some instances, plain wrong."

— *Coalition for Safe Minds*[1]

"You can fool some of the people all of the time...."

— *Abraham Lincoln*

WHAT ARE THE *studies and reports that allegedly show no autism/MMR vaccine link?*

Negative Study 1: A Precursor to the "First Finnish MMR study": Peltola, Patja, et al. "No evidence for measles, mumps, and rubella-associated inflammatory bowel disease or autism in a 14-year prospective study." *The Lancet*, 1998, May 2; 1327-1334.

In this fourteen-year *Merck-sponsored*, prospective Finnish "report" started in 1982, Peltola, Patja et al. reviewed the *passively* submitted adverse events data on the Finnish children who had been immunized with the Merck MMR vaccine, the only one utilized in Finland, and alleged to find no association between the MMR vaccine and either inflammatory bowel disease or autism.

"By the end of 1996," the authors maintain, "about three million vaccine doses had been delivered by the Institute (and only) 31 children developed gastrointestinal symptoms after vaccination." Of those with GI symptoms, 55 percent had for the most part only brief episodes of diarrhea. There was no mention of Crohn's disease or ulcerative colitis in any of the children, and *no child in this study of over 1.8 million children was reported to have developed autism. Not one.*

The authors of this study concluded that, "Over a decade's effort to detect all severe adverse events associated with MMR vaccine could find no data supporting the hypothesis that it would cause pervasive developmental disorder or inflammatory bowel disease."[2]

Comment: Isn't it interesting that this brief *report*, based on a fourteen-year study sponsored by Merck, the maker of the MMR vaccine utilized in Finland, was rushed to publication just a few months after the infamous Wakefield

---

1   http://www.safeminds.org/news/documents/Vaccines percent20and percent20Autism. percent20Epidemiology percent20Rebuttal.pdf
2   Ibid.

(Lancet 12) paper was published in that same journal. The powers that be (and *The Lancet*) couldn't wait to reassure the public about the safety of the MMR vaccine. But did this "study" actually vindicate the MMR vaccination? Did it challenge the Wakefield Lancet 12 study findings?

No. It most certainly did not!

In fact, the conclusions (and title) of the study are preposterous. How could the researchers claim that no association was found between the MMR and autism (or pervasive developmental disorder) and inflammatory bowel disease, when *autism was never evaluated in the study* and *virtually all inflammatory bowel disease would have been missed as a result of the study's inclusion criteria*?

Prior to 1996 when the study ended, no one, except the CDC, suspected a connection between vaccinations and autism, and the CDC kept its suspicions well-hidden.[3]

No Finnish health care provider would, therefore, have reported autism to the health authority as a possible side effect of the MMR since this association was unknown during the fourteen-year length of this study.

Professor Peltola even stated in a later interview (BBC Radio-4 on January 13, 2001) that the research *wasn't designed to pick up cases of autism*. Therefore, *Peltola knew that the study's title was a lie*, and this implies *deliberate deception* on the part of the researchers!

Not discovering even one associated case of autism in the 1.8 million children evaluated would have been an unbelievable finding if it were true, especially since Finland has a very high incidence of autism (1 out of every 100 children in 1992).[4, 5]

The study additionally arrived at its erroneous conclusions because it relied inappropriately on *passive* surveillance reporting, which means it relied on the reliability of health providers to report possible vaccine-related side effects to the health authority.

This passive reporting is notoriously inaccurate, however, and misses up to *95 percent* of actual vaccine-related side effects, primarily because the health providers so tasked don't associate them with the vaccination or because they do not wish to take the time to (or don't care to) report the side effects.

This was confirmed in a 1995 *Lancet* study in which British researchers found that *passive* surveillance of vaccine reactions is unreliable and only *active* surveillance could be counted on to provide meaningful data.[6]

The authors also erred in only tracking the children who had symptoms that occurred within a twenty-one-day time period after the immunization. By so doing, they successfully avoided including conditions like autism, irritable bowel disease, Crohn's disease, and ulcerative colitis that often have an insidious onset that may not become obvious clinically for many weeks or months after the inciting cause, in this case the MMR vaccine.

If a child evaluated in this study started to regress developmentally or showed signs of speech impairment or adverse changes in his behavior or intestinal symptoms three or more weeks after the MMR shot, the researchers would not have included that child in their statistics. How convenient for Merck!

Despite its many fatal flaws, this 1998 report was nevertheless praised in early 2001 by the UK's Department of Health as demonstrating that the MMR was safe. However, by the end of that same year, the British Medical Research Council reluctantly admitted that Peltola, Patja et al.'s paper "did not examine the relationship of MMR and autistic

---

3   We refer to the CDC's knowledge about the dramatic rise in autism in Brick Township, New Jersey in the late 1980s after the thimerosal-preserved HIB vaccine was introduced—this was data it never published.

4   Dr. Edward Yazbak reports that he contacted the authorities in Finland to find out the incidence of autism there. On November 11, 2002, a spokesperson for autismiliitto.fi informed him that she did not have accurate figures but that "we are estimated to have 10,000 autistic people in Finland and about 40,000 people with Asperger's syndrome." That would make the incidence of ASD in Finland at that time to have been 1 in 100 children. http://www.whale.to/a/yazbak.html

5   http://www.whale.to/a/yazbak.html

6   *Lancet*; 1995 Mar4; 345(8949):567-9.

spectrum disorders...and does not therefore provide useful evidence on this point."

Other Concerns:

- The study's findings often conflict with known incidence data. For example, the study lists the incidence of fever occurring after the MMR at 0.01 percent (1 out of 10,000 children), whereas the pediatric *Red Book*, a publication of the American Academy of Pediatrics, lists the incidence of fever after Merck's MMR as being 5-15 percent (500 to 1500 children out of every 10,000). Additionally, the incidence of rash following the MMR is 5 percent according to the *Red Book*, but Peltola's group found the incidence of rash to be 8 times higher. These discrepancies and others make the accuracy of the reported surveillance data highly suspect!

- Less than 200 children who exhibited side effects within 21 days after the MMR were followed for the length of the study. The remaining 1.8 million children were not followed at all. It is entirely possible that many of these untracked children developed autism and inflammatory bowel disease that was related to the MMR but would thereby not have been included in the study's findings, thereby rendering them inaccurate.

- Merck partially funded this study.

Conclusions: We once again discover another highly deceptive, biased, deeply flawed study based on incomplete and inaccurate data and reaching deceptive, erroneous, and patently false conclusions. One could easily make a case for this study being an example of deliberate fraud.

Negative Study 2: Gillberg, C.; Heijbel, H. "MMR and Autism." *Autism*; 1998 2: 423-424.

This study appeared as a commentary in the journal *Autism* in July 1998, and like the previous study, it also appears to have been rushed to publication to counter the findings in the infamous Lancet 12 study.

Gillberg and Heijbel analyzed the autism incidence in children born between the years 1975 and 1985 in just two cities in Sweden and found a total of only 55 autistic children.

The authors allege that MMR coverage increased in the 1980s in Sweden. They found that of the 55 children diagnosed with autism, 62 percent (34 children) were born prior to the increase in MMR vaccine coverage and just 38 percent (21 children) were born after the increase in MMR coverage.

They concluded that since the incidence of autism was less in the children born in the early 1980s than in the pre-1980 era, it demonstrated that the increase in MMR coverage was not accompanied by a rise in autism prevalence as would be expected if the MMR were a causative factor in promoting autism.

Comment: And again, we encounter another deliberately deceptive study, designed not to enlighten, but rather to reach the conclusions the authors intended.

- The number of children analyzed is insufficient to draw any conclusions.
- The study was cleverly designed to skew the statistics improperly.
- Children born in the years 1982-1985 would have been 3 years old or less by the end of the study, an insufficient period of time to have all the potentially autistic children diagnosed as such. This would serve to lessen the number of children counted as being autistic in the "after 1980" group.
- Children in the pre-1980 group, on the other hand, would have been 5-9 years old when the study ended, thus increasing the likelihood that they would be appropriately diagnosed as being autistic. As has been pointed out before, many autistic children aren't diagnosed until well after the age of four, especially in the era when this study was done (1970s and 1980s). Therefore, we would expect more children in the pre-1980 group than in the post-1980 group to be diagnosed with autism, based solely on how the study was designed and irrespective of any possible influence of the MMR on autism.

- The study also makes no attempt to address the findings of the Wakefield-Lancet study, which analyzed children who both regressed and had chronic intestinal complaints after their MMR. There was no such comparable group in this study.

Conclusion: The conclusions reached by the researchers are not warranted. This study was not designed to counter the findings of the Wakefield-Lancet 12 study, but it was deliberately designed to reach an erroneous result. In that, it succeeded.

"If a million people say a foolish thing, it is still a foolish thing."

— Anatole France

Negative Study 3: Taylor, B., Miller, E., Farrington, C.P.; *Lancet.* 1999; 353: 2026-2029. "Autism and MMR Vaccine: No Evidence for a Causal Association."

Professor Brent Taylor and colleagues performed an epidemiological study (funded by the Medicines Control Agency) to determine whether the MMR vaccine might be causally related to autism. They identified 498 cases of autism in children born since 1979, of which 31 percent were "atypical" and 38 percent Asperger's syndrome cases.

The authors noted a steady yearly increase in cases but no sudden "step up" in the trend line after the MMR was introduced. No difference existed in age of diagnosis between the cases vaccinated before or after 18 months of age and those never vaccinated.

They found "no temporal association between onset of autism within 1-2 years of vaccination with MMR." Additionally, "developmental regression was not clustered in the months after vaccination."

They concluded that their analyses "do not support a causal association between MMR vaccine and autism." They end their study with the hope that their results "will help restore confidence in the MMR vaccine."

Comment: This study has been re-analyzed by qualified members of the Allergy Induced Autism (AIA) organization, "a membership based medical research charity." It found so many serious flaws in the study that it called for the resignation of the study authors. To whit:

- The authors noted a *25 percent rise* in the number of children diagnosed with autism since the introduction of the MMR. This would support the notion that the MMR vaccine promoted autism.

- "The data underlying the key graphs are fundamentally incorrect," the AIA alleges *because the authors ignored a large group of children who should have been included in this study*. These were children who had previously received the measles vaccine but not the mumps or rubella vaccines. These children subsequently were given the MMR vaccine in the second year of life, but they were not counted in this study.[7]

- "Had the children vaccinated in the 'catch up' campaign been properly accounted for, as well as having been diagnosed by 60 months of age (as per the study's criterion), the *relevant* starting year of birth should have been 1986."[8]

- "Figure 1 in the study clearly shows a significant rise in cases between those born in 1986 over those born in 1985." The AIA analysts conclude that, "This has been (either) a totally inept analysis of the data or a deliberate attempt to cover the truth. There is a step up (rise)," they continue, "and the conclusions in relation to the first hypothesis are without doubt invalid."[9]

- "With regards to the age of diagnosis of autism in relation to the MMR," the AIA critics point out that, "most children have been vaccinated with MMR by 15 months, and subsequent time of diagnosis rela-

---

7   www.whale.to/vaccines/aia.html
8   Ibid.
9   Ibid.

tive to parental concern is an unknown variable."[10]

- They further allege that *the authors fail* to "declare the relative numbers of vaccinated to unvaccinated children. Thus the second analysis is not only totally meaningless in any scientific sense, but it also bears no relation to the second hypothesis, and certainly does not exclude exposure to vaccine as having a causal relationship to autism."[11]

- "It is not surprising," they note, "that the study finds no significant relationship between timing of diagnosis considering the wide variation of age at which the diagnosis is completed."[12]

- "The third analysis looked at the first expression of parental concern about their child's behavior in relation to any potential temporal relationship to MMR vaccination. What was identified was actually a significant statistical cluster of first parental concerns within 6 months of MMR vaccination." The authors then attempt to explain away this disturbing finding by alleging a lack of precision in definitions of this condition, but if this relationship was due to parental recall bias, it would have been seen in all the vaccine groups, including those who received any measles vaccine, but "the significant clustering is only seen in recipients of the MMR, indicating that this is likely to be a true effect."

- "In statistical terms," the AIA critics continue, "the data set is of limited size despite assurances that the findings are based on a large study. The absolute defence of the MMR vaccination in the discussion section of the paper is out of all proportion to the weak scientific evidence presented in the findings. Indeed the findings indicate the opposite of the defence given."

- The authors allege that the surge in autism incidence occurred just prior (after 1984) to the introduction of the MMR in 1988, which they assert implied no relationship between the MMR and autism. However, what they failed to note was that because the MMR was newly available, it was also given to older children, including those born prior to 1987. These children would have also had the measles jab at 12 months of age, thus "the claims of the authors to have provided evidence of non-linkage are unsustainable."[13]

- *The study lacks control groups* to compare against, like a group listing the rates of occurrence of autism in children unvaccinated with either the monovalent vaccines or the MMR or those just vaccinated with only the monovalent (just the measles) vaccine. Without these control groups, one cannot say that a higher or lower number of children who were given the MMR would have developed autism relative to those who did not receive it.

- "It is clear," the AIA analysts continue, "that the study was commissioned to dismiss the hypothesis that there may exist a relationship between the MMR vaccine and autism. In reality the study is fatally flawed and statistically inadequate."

- "Despite clear findings supporting the relationship hypothesis, the authors discard their own clearly unexpected statistical findings and manipulate the results to 'prove' their own pre-existing hypothesis."

- The AIA called for the resignation of all key members of the study group that performed this "skewed and feeble study" for attempting to deceive the public as to the safety of the MMR vaccine.

- This study, like so many others, also fails to address the population of children that Wakefield and his colleagues described in the 1998 Lancet 12 study—children who regressed after the MMR and who also had symptoms of chronic intestinal inflammation confirmed by direct visual examination of their gut wall and by biopsy.

Conclusion: Another fraudulent study widely and irresponsibly quoted as supporting the non-linkage hypothesis.

---

10   Ibid.
11   Ibid.
12   Ibid.
13   Paul Shattock, Ibid.

THE FIRST REFUGE OF SCOUNDRELS?

"I regard consensus science as an extremely pernicious development that ought to be stopped cold in its tracks.
Historically, the claim of consensus has been the first refuge of scoundrels.
It is a way to avoid debate by claiming that the matter is already settled."

— *Michael Crichton*

Negative Study 4: Farrington, C.P.; Miller, E.; Taylor, B. "MMR and Autism: Further Evidence Against a Causal Association." *Vaccine.* 2001; 19: 3632-3635.

In this self-matched case series study of the same population as in the previous fraudulent Taylor study, and by the same authors, the researchers compared the rates of regression, parental concern, or diagnosis of ASD in specified periods (24, 36, or 60 months) after vaccination to all other periods for that individual and found no increased likelihood of ASD, regression, or parental concern occurring after vaccination compared with prior to vaccination. The authors allege, as the title clearly states, that this provided further evidence against a causal association.

Comment: This study is simply an extended analysis of the last study and suffers from exactly the same concerns that were raised in regard to that study.

Whether or not a child regresses before or after the MMR is not relevant if one is attempting to rebut the Wakefield Lancet 12 study.

Wakefield never contended that the MMR was the only, or even the primary, cause of autism. He merely noted that children who had autistic regression following the MMR vaccine and who also had chronic intestinal complaints appeared to exhibit inflammatory bowel disease from which the measles virus found in the immunization could be frequently isolated from those children's GI tracts. No such comparison was made in this study.

It is certainly feasible, given what we have learned, that children regressing prior to their MMR may have regressed due to mercury overload or for other reasons (pollution, acetaminophen exposure, other toxins, etc.) and those regressing after the MMR could be doing so due to factors associated with the MMR. The fact that the rates of problems at various times before and after the MMR were similar, therefore, proves nothing.

Conclusion: Another deceptive study that misleads the public in regard to the safety of the MMR vaccination. The study did not evaluate any subset of children who were similar to those evaluated by Wakefield et al. in the Lancet 12 study, and so it is not capable of either refuting or confirming those findings.

"Falsehood flies and truth comes limping after; so that when men come to be undeceived it is too late; the jest is over and the tale has had its effect."

— *Jonathan Swift*

Negative Study 5 (The "First Finnish Study"): Patja, Peltola, et al. "Serious Adverse Events after Measles-Mumps-Rubella Vaccination during a Fourteen-Year Prospective Follow-Up." *Pediatr Infect Dis J*, 2000; 19:1127-3; http://www.nccn.net/~wwithin/MMR.pdf

This is exactly the same study as that reviewed above in "Negative Report 1." In this case, the study was published as a more complete peer-reviewed article in the *Pediatric Infectious Diseases Journal* almost five years after the study was completed and, undoubtedly, not coincidentally, just prior to the appearance of another Wakefield study that was to be published implicating the MMR vaccine in relation to certain chronic inflammatory bowel conditions.

The comments and criticisms of this study are identical to those already provided in our evaluation of the aforementioned Negative Report 1; however, it is important to note that Patja and Peltola also fail in their report to account for the dramatic rise in autism and inflammatory bowel disease in Finland during the years this study was in progress in contrast to what the study's conclusions suggest.

Peltola alleged that there had been no rise in the incidence of autism during the time of the campaign to immunize all children in Finland with the MMR vaccine. That wasn't true. A Finnish research team evaluated all children born in two Finnish provinces between the years 1979 and 1994 and found an almost three-fold rise in the incidence of autism in those years and over four times as much in the 5-7 year age group compared to earlier data.[14]

Between 1992 and 2001, the prevalence rate per thousand of Crohn's disease and ulcerative colitis also doubled (a 100 percent rise) while the population of Finland only increased by 3 percent.[15]

After reviewing this poorly done study, the British Medical Council diplomatically warned, "The findings need to be interpreted with some caution, as cases of autistic spectrum disorder or bowel disorders not considered at the time attributable to MMR would not necessarily have been reported." There's an understatement!

In other words, the study's findings are in serious doubt because the authors undoubtedly undercounted the autism and bowel disorder cases, and by so doing, made their claims as to the safety of the MMR vaccination invalid.

It is a shame and a tragedy that these faulty studies based on the same questionable data and inappropriate criteria have been so widely quoted as offering proof of the lack of association between the MMR vaccine and autism and inflammatory bowel disease. They, of course, do no such thing!

"Strange times are these in which we live when young and old are taught in 'Falsehoods School,' and the one man who dares to tell the truth is called at once a lunatic and a fool."

— Plato

Negative Study 6: Dales, L.; Hammer, S.J.; Smith, N.J. "Time Trends in Autism and in MMR Immunization Coverage in California." *JAMA* 2001; 285; 1183-85.

In this retrospective study, Dales and associates reviewed the MMR coverage rates for California children born in 1980-1994 and found no correlation between the observed steady increase in autism from 1980 (44 cases per 100,000 live births) to 1994 (208 cases per 100,000 live births) and the MMR coverage rates, which were "much smaller and of shorter duration." The first MMR was licensed in the U.S. in 1971.

The children assessed were 5-6 years of age at the time of the surveys (1980-94) when the awareness of autism was not as widespread as it is today.

They concluded: "These data do not suggest an association between MMR immunization among young children and an increase in autism occurrence."[16]

Comment: The authors provide six different reasons why *the data they studied is of insufficient quality* for the purposes of drawing any conclusions. They then, as doctor Yazbak rightfully points out, "go ahead and draw a conclusion anyway."[17]

The 1999 California Department of Developmental Services repeatedly emphasizes that its "data cannot be interpreted as measuring trends in the actual incidence of autism." But the authors of this study decided to use this data for just that purpose.

---

14   Kielinen, M.; Linna, S.L.; Moilanen, I. "Autism in Northern Finland." *European Child & Adolescent Psychiatry. 9:162-167 (2000.)*
15   Statistical Branch of the Social Insurance Institution of Finland.
16   Ibid.
17   www.whale.to/vaccine/aut1.html

Why is the data inaccurate for the purposes of determining autism incidence?

- "Because it wasn't known how many children with autism had not enrolled in the system."

- "Because the system had expanded and matured over time."

- "Because the proportion of children enrolling in the system who were born outside of California may have changed over time."[18]

In addition, the study suffered from other *critical flaws*. To whit:

- "A detailed investigation into the apparent increases in autism cases" in regard to their being real or artifactual was in progress, but the results were still unknown.

- Individual immunization records on the children were not examined, so it was not known how many children received the combined MMR versus "separate injection of the measles, mumps and/or rubella components."

Conclusion: A study that bases its results on data of questionable accuracy must thereby have its "improperly drawn conclusions" called into question. Lenny Schafer, editor of *FEAT Daily Newsletter*, asks, "What could be the real purpose of this misleading exercise, if not for propaganda?"[19]

Indeed!

In addition, this study did not evaluate that subset of children who autistically regressed after MMR and who also manifested symptoms of chronic intestinal problems, and cannot, therefore, be used to refute or confirm the Wakefield Lancet 12 study or any of the other similar studies previously reviewed.

> *"When you seek a new path to truth, you must expect to find it blocked by expert opinion."*
>
> *— Albert Guérard*

Negative Study 7: Kaye, J.A. et al. "MMR Vaccine and the Incidence of Autism Recorded by General Practitioners: A Time Trend Analysis." *BMJ*. Feb 24, 2001; 322: 460-463.

The researchers analyzed data from the UK general practice research database in order to "estimate changes in the risk to autism and assess the relation of autism to the…MMR vaccine." The subjects were autistic children aged 12 years or younger who were diagnosed between the years 1988-99 with further analysis of boys aged 2-5 born 1988-93.

What Kaye and colleagues found was that the incidence of newly diagnosed autism increased by seven times from 1988 to 1999 while during that time the prevalence of MMR remained steady at 95 percent.

They concluded that "the data provide evidence that no correlation exists between the prevalence of MMR vaccination and the rapid increase in the risk of autism over time."

Comment: Kaye and colleagues suggest that because the immunization schedule was constant for the MMR and the increase in autism gradual, there is no evidence of an association. Marc Baltzan, consultant physician, and Michael Edwardes, research fellow at Royal Victoria Hospital Division of Clinical Epidemiology, take issue with this conclusion.

They point out that increasing diagnostic awareness could explain some of the increased incidence of ASD and they wonder whether the noted trend toward earlier vaccination might have been a factor in the alleged rise in incidence.

---

18   Ibid.
19   Ibid.

Although not convinced by arguments in favor of a link between the MMR and autism, they state that, "we submit that the argument given by Kaye (et al.) is too simplistic to reassure us that there is no link between MMR and autism."[20]

Dr. F. Edward Yazbak also takes issue with the findings. He points out that the "cohort of the children chosen was born between the years 1988-1993. MMR was introduced in the United Kingdom in 1988, and an uptake of 90-95 percent is unlikely to have been achieved from the first year." In other words, the assumption *that the immunization schedule was constant is highly unlikely.*

Dr. Yazbak also notes that the authors "effectively excluded children born before 1988 who may have been vaccinated in or after 1988." *This would serve to skew the true incidence figures.*

Dr. Yazbak states that, "the study did not mention how many children received two MMR vaccinations," and that many of the 114 boys selected "could have succumbed after the second MMR vaccination (booster)."[21]

Yazbak further asserts that the MMR "was previously given alone at 15 months or later. Then the age was lowered to 12-14 months and other vaccines were administered concomitantly, increasing the immune antigenic insult at a younger, more susceptible age and effectively increasing the incidence of autism."

Yazbak is also disturbed by the exclusion in this study of girls with autism. He would have preferred a breakdown of the 290 children in the 1990-1999 birth cohorts by sex and year of birth. "A larger proportion of girls among the 176 cases excluded might have been relevant to the completeness of the autism figures," he maintains.

He also questions the accuracy of the diagnoses of autism as neither the DSM-IV nor the ICD-10 criteria were systematically used in the United Kingdom, which he felt "creates further doubts about the significance of the findings." This concern also troubled epidemiologist Liam Smeeth and others who noted that "only 81 percent of the cases were reported to have been referred by a specialist, raising questions about the validity of the diagnoses used by Kaye, et al." [22]

Dr. Yazbak points out that "before 1988 the incidence of autism was 1 in 10,000;" and "after 1988-the year MMR was introduced—it leapt to 8 in 10,000. By 1992 it was 29 in 10,000. Kaye et al cannot exonerate MMR without offering a reasonable explanation for the increase."

"Until safety studies on MMR are independent of drug companies and are large scale and comprehensive," Yazbak alleges, "and until researchers review with parents the documented adverse reactions of bowel disease and autism, the triple jab (MMR) remains suspect."

Kreesten Madsen, in the second paragraph of his 2002 *NEJM* paper, maintains that this study, along with six other epidemiological studies that we review,[23] "lack sufficient statistical power to detect an association (between MMR vaccination and autism), and none has a population-based cohort design."[24]

In addition, and *most importantly,* the Kaye study's conclusion is faulty in that it totally ignores the fact that other obvious risk factors like thimerosal-preserved vaccines, pesticide exposure, pollution, vaccine adjuvants, etc., could and likely did account for part of the rise in autism during the years of this study, which in no way excludes the MMR immunization as being part of that causality.

And the Kaye et al. study, as is true of all the others thus far discussed, did not investigate the select group of children with similar symptoms to those evaluated in the Wakefield Lancet 12 study, i.e. those with autistic regression and

---

20 www.ncbi.nlm.nih.gov/pmc/articles/PMC1120793

21 Ibid.

22 Ibid.

23 The other five studies that Madsen alleges lack sufficient statistical power to detect an association between MMR vaccine and autism are: The Taylor *Lancet* study of 1999; The Dales *JAMA* 2001 study; The Fombonne *Pediatrics* study of 2001; The Patja *J. of Ped Inf Diseases* 2000 study; The Taylor *BMJ* study of 2002.

24 Madsen, M.D., Anders, Hviid et al. *New England Journal of Medicine.* November 7, 2002.

intestinal inflammation symptoms following the MMR vaccine, and so cannot be used to refute that study and its conclusions.

Conflicts of Interest: The Kaye study was supported by the Boston Collaborative Drug Surveillance Program, which itself is supported by grants from at least 8 pharmaceutical companies, including those that manufacture immunizations.[25]

> *"It's difficult to get a man to understand something when his salary depends on him not understanding it."*
>
> — Upton Sinclair

Negative Study 8: Fombonne, Eric; Chakrabati, S. "No Evidence for a New Variant of Measles-Mumps-Rubella-Induced Autism." *Pediatrics*. 2001, Oct; 108(4).

A number of additional studies purport to show no link between the MMR vaccine and autism. One of the next to be published was an early study authored by Drs. Fombonne and Chakrabarti, which was *specifically designed to show this alleged lack of linkage.*

The authors maintained that if there were indeed a new kind of autism characterized by intestinal symptoms and regression, that a number of predictions based on that assumption would be supported by data, but they weren't.

They then concluded that, "No evidence was found to support a distinct syndrome of MMR-induced autism or of "autistic enterocolitis. These results add to the recent accumulation of large-scale epidemiologic studies that all failed to support an association between MMR and autism at population level...."

The critical flaw in this study is that those predictions were based on faulty assumptions and questionable data, to whit:

Prediction 1: "Childhood Disintegrative Disorder [their term for regressive autism] has become more frequent."

What was found: Fombonne & Chakrabati allege that the incidence of CDD at the time of the study was an incredibly low 1 in 16,666 children and had not changed.

Critique: They presented no valid evidence to substantiate their data or claim. Their estimate of the prevalence of CDD was *magnitudes lower* than other estimates at the time (like those of the CDC, for example). See Figure 2 in Chapter 1, which shows the dramatic increase in delayed onset autism relative to birth onset autism after the mid-1980s.

Conclusion: Fombonne's data and assertions are unsubstantiated and, in fact, incorrect. Prediction 1 is not disproven, as the authors allege, and is very likely true.

Prediction 2: "The mean age of first parental concern for autistic children who are exposed to MMR is closer to the mean immunization age than in children who are not exposed to MMR."

What was found: The authors did not find any statistically significant difference between the two groups. The mean age of the children who had been exposed to the MMR prior to the onset of their symptoms was 19.2-19.3 months and was 19.5 months in those who had the MMR after the onset of symptoms. Although the difference tends to support the prediction, the difference in ages was not statistically significant.

Critique: The two authors present no argument as to why their assertion is valid. Why does there have to be a difference between the two groups? The absence of a difference proves absolutely nothing.

---

25   www.whale.to/a/yaz12.html

Childhood Disintegration Disorder (equivalent to delayed onset autism) most likely has a number of causal factors. Children who became autistic prior to their getting the MMR could have had a monovalent measles vaccine precipitating their autism, or their autism could have been induced by synergistic exposures to thimerosal, pesticides, pollution, immunization excipients, antipyretics or any number of other factors, none of which were addressed in this study. No one has suggested that there is only one cause for autism. Indeed, the evidence overwhelmingly indicates otherwise.

Conclusion: The assumption underlying the prediction is invalid. The absence of a difference between the two groups proves nothing and does not discredit the hypothesized causative association between delayed onset autism following an MMR vaccine in a susceptible subset of children.

Prediction 3: "Regression in the development of children with autism has become more common in MMR-vaccinated children."

What the authors found: "They found that the rate of developmental regression reported in the post-MMR sample (15.6 percent) was not different from that in the pre-MMR sample (18.4 percent) and therefore there was no suggestion that regression in the development course of autism had increased in frequency since MMR was introduced. The study also found that…the subset of autistic children with regression had no other developmental or clinical characteristics, which would have argued for a specific etiologically distinct phenotype."[26]

Critique: There is no reason to assume that the likelihood of autistic regression due to MMR would be any different than regression caused by other factors (like thimerosal, pollution, etc.), which the authors made no attempt to account for, and they again erred in framing their hypothesis to suggest that the sole cause of regression in autism is the MMR vaccine. There is also no evidence presented that children with regressive autism differ from autistic children who don't regress, but fail to progress.

In addition, their sample sizes were too small to use reliably in a statistically-based study (a pre-MMR sample of 98 autistic children and a post-MMR sample of 68 autistics) since "a few cases either way would impact upon their conclusions.[27.] There is also no reason to presume that MMR-induced autism would result in a "distinct phenotype" (presentation) of autism, so not finding one is irrelevant.

Conclusion: Invalid assumption, invalid prediction, invalid conclusion.

Prediction 4: "The age of onset for autistic children with regression clusters around the MMR immunisation date and is different from that of autistic children."

What they found: There was no difference in the age at which parents of autistic children with or without regression detected the first autistic symptoms in their child, and the time interval between the MMR vaccination and the onset of observable symptoms was the same in both groups.

Critique: Again, the authors present no scientific argument as to why the two groups should differ. Some children who develop autism between the first and second years of life regress and others fail to progress. Some show evidence of both presentations. There appears to be a spectrum of severity in the presentation and progression of symptoms in autistics. Regression following the MMR may happen within days of getting the immunization or may present weeks or months later.

Conclusion: Invalid assumption, prediction, and conclusion.

Prediction 5: "Children with regressive autism have distinct symptoms and severity profiles."

What they found: No distinct symptoms and severity profiles were noted in children with regressive autism.

Critique: There is no justification for the assumption that distinct symptoms and severity profiles should be found.

---

26   http://www.safeminds.org/news/documents/Vaccines percent20and percent20Autism. percent20 Epidemiology percent20Rebuttal.pdf
27   Ibid.

If any autistic children in this study had presented with chronic gut issues, they should have received appropriate diagnostic workups that included examinations of their intestines (ileo-colonoscopies) and biopsies of inflamed areas to look for the presence or absence of measles vaccine associated virus. This was not done in this study. Autistic enterocolitis may not present with sufficient external manifestations that would allow such children to be characterized by particular symptoms and severity profiles.

Conclusion: Invalid assumption, prediction, and conclusion.

Prediction 6: "Regressive autism is associated with gastrointestinal symptoms and/or inflammatory bowel disorder."

What was found: "In the epidemiologic sample, gastrointestinal symptoms were reported in 18.8 percent of children. Constipation was the most common symptom (9.4 percent), and no inflammatory bowel disorder was reported. Furthermore, there was no association between developmental regression and gastrointestinal symptoms."

Critique: The children in the study did not have visual or laboratory assessments of their GI tract, and so no conclusions would be possible in this regard. In addition, there is *no justification* for the assumption that regressive autism is associated with GI symptoms.

Remember, what Wakefield's group found was that children who had *both* chronic severe intestinal symptoms *and* autistic regression following their MMR vaccination *also presented* with a distinct intestinal pathology: inflammation and lymphonodular hyperplasia. That in no way implies that all or even most regressive autism is associated with GI symptoms or inflamed intestines, although GI symptoms are certainly common in autistic children.

Conclusion: Invalid prediction, invalid assumptions, invalid conclusion.

Critique from the *independent* and widely acclaimed *Cochrane Review*:[28]

> This study was assessed as having a 'high likelihood' of bias. In fact, the number of biases and their likelihood to negatively impact the study 'was so high that interpretation of the results was impossible.'

> "The population description in this study raised doubts about the generalizability of the conclusions to other settings. This study failed to report complete vaccine identification information, including lot numbers, adjuvants, preservatives, strains, product and manufacturer. There was a lack of adequate description of exposure (vaccine content and schedules) in the study. This study failed to report any vaccine strains at all and failed to provide descriptions of all outcomes monitored.

> The Fombonne and Chakrabarti study is flawed in a variety of ways. The biggest weakness is in its misinterpretation of the actual hypothesis of an association between a specifically defined sub-group of children and the exposure (MMR) of interest. It is on this erroneous understanding that the authors' assumptions are based. The assumptions are not valid and any findings based on them are consequently of little interest.

> The inadequate study design [in terms of poor definitions of cases, controls, and exposures] also means that any other uses to which the data might be put are extremely limited.[29]

Overall Conclusion: Professor Fombonne fails yet again. This flawed and biased study was undoubtedly designed to exonerate the MMR link to autism. It fails completely in that regard because the study relies on disproving hypotheses that are invalid to begin with.

---

28   The Cochrane Collaboration is an "international network of more than 28,000 dedicated people from over 100 countries" who analyze and review research studies for accuracy and relevance. Their reviews are alleged to be "internationally recognised as the highest standard in evidence-based health care." http://www.cochrane.org/cochrane-reviews.
29   "Vaccines and Autism—What Do Epidemiological Studies Really Tell Us?" Coalition for Safeminds PDF.

"Where large sums of money are concerned, it is advisable to trust nobody."

— *Agatha Christie*

Negative Study 9: (The Second Finnish MMR Study): Annamari, Makela. "Neurologic Disorders after Measles-Mumps-Rubella Vaccination." *Pediatrics*. (November 2002); 110:957-963.

In this *retrospective* study, 535,544 Finnish children aged 1-7 who were vaccinated between November 1982 and June 1986 were evaluated to see whether any association could be found between MMR vaccination and encephalitis, aseptic meningitis, and autism. "Changes in the number of *hospitalizations* for autism throughout the study period were searched for." Children with autism were further evaluated to see whether they had been *hospitalized* for inflammatory bowel disease.

Dr. Makela found that of the children who had been vaccinated, 199 had been hospitalized for encephalitis, 352 for autistic disorders, and 161 for aseptic meningitis. She found no increased occurrence of meningitis or encephalitis during the study period (three months following the vaccination) nor any increase in hospitalizations for autism or inflammatory bowel diseases.

Dr. Makela concluded that she did not find any association between MMR vaccine and encephalitis, meningitis, and autism.

Critique: The following critiques by the independent *Cochrane Review*, The Institute of Medicine, Science-based-medicine.com, ageofautism.com, and Edward Yazbak, M.D. are quoted from: http://www.ageofautism.com/2011/05/vaccines-and-autism-what-do-epidemiological-studies-really-tell-us.html.

What the *Cochrane Review* said:

> This study was "weakened" by the loss of 14 percent of the original birth cohort and the effects of the rather long time frame of follow up. What the impact of either of these factors was in terms of confounders is open to debate.

> The long follow up for autism was due to the lack of a properly constructed causal hypothesis.

> The study failed to report complete vaccine identification information, including lot numbers, adjuvants, preservatives, strains, product and manufacturer.

> There was an inadequate description of exposure (vaccine content and schedules).

> The authors provided 'inadequate' explanations for missing information, even though there were clearly missing unintended-event data on as many as 20 percent of the participants.

> The study had discrepancies in reporting of denominators and was classified to be at moderate risk of bias.

What the Institute of Medicine (IOM) said:

> The study suffered from one primary limitation: its exclusive reliance on hospitalization records. This made it impossible to identify children with ASD who were not hospitalized, but rather seen in an outpatient setting.... While the authors stated that it is common in Finland for children with autism to be admitted to the hospital for observation and testing, a diagnosis of autism does not always involve hospitalization.

In other words, an unknown and likely large body of data from children diagnosed with autism outside a hospital setting (which is where *most children* in other countries around the world are diagnosed) makes the conclusions reached by the authors of this study highly questionable.

What sciencebasedmedicine.com said:

It agreed with the IOM: "Using 'hospitalizations' as criteria for finding children with autism (is) not a good way to find autism cases."

What ageofautism.com said:

> The study fails to make explicit the exact definition of 'caseness,' particularly with respect to autism. The criticisms leveled at the study are crucially important in this respect. First, there is a failure to differentiate between autism per se, and the sub-group who are proposed to be at increased risk (i.e. those with regressive onset).

> There is also a degree of circularity in the statement that those whose encephalitis was 'unrelated to vaccination' were excluded. To deselect particular cases before analysis, on the basis of a proposed non-relationship between exposure and outcome is poor epidemiological practice. Further, it implies that decisions about causality were made after the event, on the basis of criteria which were not made explicit to the reader.

> Subacute sclerosing panencephalitis is widely acknowledged to be a known, albeit rare (and invariably fatal), side effect of the measles vaccination and it can occur years after the immunization is given, so it is difficult to understand why an episode of encephalitis not occurring in temporal proximity to an MMR vaccination should be excluded from consideration.

> The most problematic factor, however, is in the assumption that children hospitalized 'for autism' somehow represent the very well defined group of children that are proposed to be at risk of an adverse event following vaccination. This assumption simply has no validity, and neither, therefore, do any conclusions based on data related to this group.[30]

What critic Edward Yazbak, M.D. said:

> The whole study is based on one comparison. If the children in the first group developed symptoms of encephalitis and meningitis within two weeks of vaccination and many did, then causation is implied (medically and medico-legally). In this case, a comparison with the control group is meaningless and the author's conclusion is unwarranted.

Conflict of Interest: "Dr Makela was partially supported by a grant from Merck & Co., a manufacturer of the MMR vaccine." [31]

Conclusion: This study suffers from a number of fundamental problems. The basis of the study, the assumption that encephalitis, meningitis, and autism would causally manifest only within a three-month window following the MMR is preposterous and scientifically unjustified.

As mentioned, measles encephalitis following an MMR, measles vaccine, or measles infection has been known to occur *years* after the inoculation.

Autism symptoms may (but need not) start to manifest within three months following the MMR, but the diagnosis is rarely made that quickly. As a result, many children in this study who should have been included weren't.

The Makela "team" also erred in disregarding the many autistic children diagnosed outside of a hospital setting.

For these reasons, as well as the many appropriate criticisms listed above, the study and its conclusions *must be regarded as invalid.*

---

30   Ibid.
31   Ibid.

"Statistics are like a bikini. What they reveal is suggestive, but what they conceal is vital."

— *Aaron Levenstein*

Negative Study 10 ("The" Danish MMR Study"): "A Population-Based Study of Measles, Mumps and Rubella Vaccination and Autism." Madsen, Kreesten Meldgaard; Hviid, Anders; Thorsen, Poul, et al., *New England Journal of Medicine*. November 7, 2002; http://content.nejm.org/cgi/content/full/347/19/1477.

In this retrospective study, the researchers allegedly reviewed the MMR and autism status of all the children born in Denmark between 1991 and 1999, a total of 537,303 in all, of which 440,655 (82 percent) had received the MMR vaccine.

The aim of the study was "to assess whether an association prevails between MMR vaccination and…autism." The researchers identified 422 children with other autism spectrum disorders and 316 with autism for a combined rate of about 1 child in 730.

What the researchers alleged to have discovered was that the MMR-exposed children had a 17 percent *lesser risk* of having an autism spectrum disorder than did the non-exposed group.

They concluded: "This study provides strong evidence against the hypothesis that MMR vaccination causes autism."

Conflicts of Interest: Financial Support for this study was provided by the Danish National Research Foundation, the National Vaccine Program Office and National Immunization Program, the CDC, and The National Alliance for Autism Research (NAAR). The NAAR had a member of the CDC on its board at the time of this study, and the NAAR has received funding from Merck, a manufacturer of the MMR vaccine.

Critique: This "research" purported to show an apparent *protective effect* from the MMR inoculation. That finding should immediately raise one's index of suspicion. What we have learned from some of the previously reviewed thimerosal studies is that when researchers find a protective effect for an agent known to be harmful, like thimerosal (or in this case the MMR vaccine), we must take a much closer look at that study. It should come as no surprise that big concerns were found in this study as well, to whit:

An insufficient number of children with autism in the study had their diagnosis and records verified, according to Walter Spitzer, Professor Emeritus of Epidemiology at McGill University (and his colleagues). Dr. Spitzer made these concerns clear in a letter to the *NEJM* in 2003, stating, "without a multidisciplinary review of original lifetime records as well as double verification in a large descriptive single cohort, important errors would have been unavoidable, both in classification and numbers for the numerators."[32]

Statistical Chicanery?

The manner in which the data were collected and analyzed *could readily lead to an erroneous conclusion*, Professor Spitzer alleged. For example, he maintained that, "if…one assumed a vulnerability to MMR-induced disease in 10 percent of the regressive ASD cases, with 95 percent of this group being vaccinated, and if 80 percent of the non-regressive ASD cases were also assumed to be vaccinated, then the odds ratio for MMR as a risk factor for regressive autism would be 4.17." That would mean that MMR would indeed be a risk factor for regressive autism by a factor of over 4.

However, Dr. Spitzer continued, if children with autism, *regardless of sub-types*, were *combined* and compared against non-affected controls, the odds ratio would plummet to just 0.97. "Thus a small non-statistically significant reduction in uptake of MMR in the 90 percent of non-regressive autistic children would mask a strong causal association in a small subgroup."[33]

---

32   http://www.safeminds.org/news/documents/Vaccines percent20and percent20Autism. percent20Epidemiology percent20Rebuttal.pdf
33   Ibid.

There was also a "substantial underrepresentation of autism diagnoses and vaccination status for children born in the later study years." Drs. Yazbak and Goldman expressed this concern in their letter to the *American Physicians and Surgeons Journal*. In other words, *children did not have time to acquire the autistic diagnosis as a result of MMR vaccination before being excluded from the study.*

In Denmark, children were being diagnosed as autistic at five years of age or over, so many of the children in the study would not have been diagnosed as being autistic during the study period, and many of the children born in the last two years of the study (1997-98) would not yet have even received an MMR vaccine.

This "substantial under-representation of autism diagnosis and vaccination status for children born in the later study years" would skew the study results to show no association between MMR and autism when such an association was actually likely.[34]

Why was the association likely? Well, it turns out that the prevalence of autism was actually *increasing* during the years of the study, and it rose from 8.4 children per 100,000 births in 1986 (before the licensure of the MMR vaccination in 1987) to 71.4 children per 100,000 in the year 2000 "making the adjusted prevalence rate-ratio 4.7 for the post-licensure period compared with the pre-licensure period. This suggested a temporal association between the introduction of MMR vaccination in Denmark and an almost five-fold increase in autism cases," and it would support the hypothesis that the MMR was a causative factor in promoting autism.[35]

Note that prior to the introduction of the MMR vaccine in Denmark in 1987, autism prevalence rates were actually declining slightly, but after the MMR was introduced, there was a steady increase in the prevalence of autism (almost 15 percent growth).

The cases of autism presumed to be caused by the MMR *would be masked* by autism brought on by other factors, like other vaccinations, and by autism present shortly after birth (congenital autism due to other causes).

"The effect of relevant data has been diluted by irrelevant data," according to Ulf Bränell, who analyzed the Madsen study. "If the intention is to compare the effects of vaccines on children," he continued, "it is appropriate to compare vaccinated with unvaccinated children only after vaccination."

"Mixing such data with data concerning children prior to vaccination," Bränell maintains, "only serves to obscure the issue and make any effects much harder to detect. At the same time the impression is given that the study is based on far more observations than is in fact the case.... In the final analysis, the conclusions drawn by the authors of the study are based on a mere 10 cases per year. Given the numerous sources of error and the unclear definitions of the concepts used, this is totally inadequate."[36]

Dr. Bränell goes on to say that, "The design of the study means that the older cohorts (1992-1995) contribute far more person-years to the study. This means that just as in the English studies, any increase in the risk of autism over time is practically impossible to detect." Hence, "The data presented in the study provides no basis whatsoever for the conclusions drawn by the authors," he alleges.[37]

"All the sources of error identified in the study distort it in the same direction: obscuring the role of the MMR vaccine and exonerating it from any suspicion that it may cause autism. This strongly indicates deliberate fraud," Bränell concludes.[38]

Drs. Goldman and Yazbak reanalyzed the data from this study, but this time they also included children *over the age of five* (who were excluded in the study by Madsen et al.). What they found was that *the Danish autism rate had risen eightfold* over the period since the introduction of the MMR vaccination.[39]

---

34   Ibid.
35   Ibid.
36   http://www.motgift.nu/Div/SIEM/ MMRE2E.html
37   Ibid.
38   Ibid.
39   *J of Amer Physicians and Surgeons.* 2004;9(3):70-75.

Another investigator, Dr. Samy Suissa of McGill University, also did his own analysis of the 2002 Madsen et al. data and contrary to the Madsen finding of no association between the MMR and the rise in autism, he found just the opposite. Within two years of the MMR vaccination, autism incidence rose to 27 cases per 100,000 children as opposed to just 1.45 cases per 100,000 children who had not received the MMR vaccination.[40]

According to John Gilmore, executive director and founder of the autism Action Network:

> [T]he Thorsen group didn't do the study using the straightforward, conventional way. The data showed a much higher number of autism cases in the MMR vaccinated group than in the unvaccinated group, and if they did it the usual way they would have had to conclude that the MMR may cause autism. So instead of comparing cases of autism, they compared "life-years" with autism, and "life years" without autism.
>
> In short that means if a child was 8 years old at the end of the study period and that child was diagnosed with autism, when he was 6, he would be counted as 2 "life years" with autism, but 6 "life years" without autism. If this sounds devious, irrational and confusing it is, by design. It was necessary to come up with a way to avoid showing that there was a greater rate of autism among the children who got the MMR. And this is the method they chose to do it.[41]

Conclusion: This widely quoted study was almost assuredly deliberately designed to show through epidemiologically unacceptable means and analysis that there is no connection between the MMR vaccine and autism. It exemplifies statistical chicanery at its best.

The study's conclusion is not valid because the study is not valid. In actuality, the dramatic *increase* in autism prevalence in Denmark *after* the introduction of the MMR vaccine lends support to the contention that the MMR inoculation is *causally linked* to the epidemic of autism now manifest worldwide, and competent independent reanalyses of this study's data bolster that contention.

> *"Be prepared to analyze statistics, which can be used to support or undercut almost any argument."*
>
> *— Marilyn vos Savant*

A Negative Review: Wilson, Kumanon et al. "Association of Autistic Spectrum Disorder and the Measles, Mumps and Rubella Vaccine—A Systematic Review of Current Epidemiological Evidence." *Archives of Pediatrics & Adolescent Medicine*. July 2003.

In this *review* of twelve medical studies that purported to examine the association between the MMR vaccination and autism spectrum disorders, the authors concluded that, "The current literature does not suggest an association between ASD and the MMR vaccine; however, limited epidemiological evidence exists to rule out a link between a rare variant form of ASD and the MMR vaccine."

Critique:

1. This was *not a medical study but rather a review* of previous epidemiological studies, and as we have seen (and will soon see) the literature that was reviewed is highly suspect, so conclusions drawn on the basis of those studies must be suspect as well.

2. *None* of the "positive" studies listed in Chapter 23 that found an association between the MMR and autism were reviewed in this study, which indicates a pernicious and scientifically unacceptable selection bias on the part of the reviewers.

---

40   Stott et al. *J of Amer Phys and Surg*. 2004; 9(3): 88-91.
41   http://www.ageofautism.com/2013/09/round-2-cdcs-poul-thorsen-lying-in-plainsight

3. Other potential biases: "This review was supported by a grant from the Canadian Institutes for Health Research, Ottawa, Ontario. Dr Wilson is a Canadian Institutes for Health Research New Investigator."[42] The CIHR is a government-funded entity, and its sponsored studies *often suffer from bias manifesting as incomplete reporting of data*, as is the case with this review.

An-Wen Chan and associates, "sought to determine whether outcome reporting bias would be present in a cohort of (CIHR) government-funded trials subjected to rigorous peer review," and they found that "a median of 31 percent… of outcomes measured to assess the efficacy of an intervention…and 59 percent…of those measured to assess the harm of an intervention…per trial were incompletely reported."

They concluded that, "selective reporting of outcomes frequently occurs in publications of (allegedly) high-quality government-funded trials."[43]

In other words, when the CIHR sponsors a study, be highly skeptical of its conclusions. That same rule would, of course, apply to any study in which the sponsors or researchers had a conflict of interest or bias.

> *"It's quite easy to take a positive result (showing harmful effects) and turn it falsely negative….*
> *Any competent epidemiologist can employ tricks of the trade when certain results are desired."*
>
> — *David Michaels, author of* Doubt Is Their Product:
> How Industry's Assault on Science Threatens Your Health

Negative Study 11: Smeeth, Liam; Fombonne, Eric et al. "MMR Vaccination and Pervasive Developmental Disorders: A Case-Control Study." *The Lancet.* September 11, 2004.

In this matched case control study, which utilized the UK General Practice Research Database, Smeeth and associates compared a group of 1,294 children diagnosed with pervasive developmental disorder (PDD) born in the year 1973 or later who were diagnosed as having PDD between the years 1987 and 2004 with 4,469 age and sex matched controls.

"1,010 cases (78.1 percent) had MMR vaccination recorded before diagnosis (of PDD), compared with 3671 controls (82.1 percent) before the age at which their matched case was diagnosed. After adjusting for age at joining the database, the odds ratio for association between MMR and pervasive developmental disorder was 0.86."[44]

In statistical terms, this meant there was no association between a child receiving the MMR and the likelihood of that child becoming autistic.

"Findings were similar," the authors continue, "when restricted to children with a diagnosis of autism, to those vaccinated with MMR before the third birthday, or to the period before media coverage of the hypothesis linking MMR with autism…. Our findings," they conclude, "suggest that MMR vaccination is not associated with an increased risk of pervasive developmental disorders."

Comment: Dr. Andrew Wakefield commented on this study in September 2004.[45] He pointed out several critical "failings" that make the study's conclusions scientifically unsound.

The study as designed is incapable of rebutting the "Wakefield hypothesis" as outlined in the infamous Lancet 12 study.

Wakefield's findings suggested, as we have repeatedly noted, that there exists a subset of children who both show

---

42   Ibid.

43   "Outcome reporting bias in randomized trials funded by the Canadian Institutes of Health Research." *CMAJ.* September 28, 2004. Vol. 171. No. 7 doi: 10.1503/cmaj.1041086.

44   Ibid. abstract.

45   www.informedchoice.info/MMR.html

developmental regression after the MMR vaccination and also demonstrate symptoms and signs of inflammatory bowel disease and evidence of long-term infection with measles virus.

As we have seen, a number of studies both by Wakefield and others have provided evidence that backs this hypothesis.

However, this study and all the others thus far reviewed (and to be reviewed) are incapable of addressing that hypothesis because they all declined to study the appropriate group, and as the authors of this study so state: "We were not able to separately identify the subgroup of cases with regressive symptoms to investigate the hypothesis that only some children are vulnerable to MMR induced disease and that this is always regressive."

Interestingly, Smeeth, Fombonne, and colleagues consulted with both Dr. Wakefield and epidemiologist Dr. Scott Montgomery when they were designing the current study. According to Wakefield, "We made it absolutely clear that they should specifically look at children with regressive autism. They ignored this specific advice."

The study *lacks statistical validity*. Epidemiologists in Sweden and Cambridge have confirmed that even if the study had included the correct group (children with regressive autism and GI symptoms following the MMR jab), "the study would need to have included at least 3,500-7,000 children with autism, 3-6 times the actual number examined, in order for the study to have any validity at all."[46]

In other words, this study's conclusions are statistically invalid, hence they are meaningless.

The validity of the autism diagnoses provided in this study are also suspect, because the more stringent criteria for validating the diagnosis of autism utilized by the authors in their 2001 study were not followed and thus significantly weakened in this study, to whit:

- "Children with a possible diagnosis of autism will be identified from their electronic health records." This was done in just 25 percent of cases.

- "All diagnoses will be validated by a detailed review of hospital letters…" This was not done.

- "All diagnoses will be validated by "using information derived from a parental questionnaire." This was not done either!

- "The second and third steps were not performed," according to Dr. Wakefield. Only 25 percent of cases had their records examined and no questionnaires were used. "There were other significant changes in the methodology which were also not explained in the present paper," Wakefield adds.

Therefore, he concludes, "This paper meets neither the criteria for testing the original question or those laid down by the authors themselves."[47]

There were no controls unexposed to MMR and inadequate explanations for missing information, according to the *Cochrane Review.*

Conflicts of interest: Eric Fombonne has been paid to testify on behalf of vaccine manufacturers supporting the hypothesis that immunizations don't promote autism. Co-author A.J. Hall was a member of the UK's Joint Committee on Vaccines and Immunizations and was also compensated by Merck for research done on a hepatitis B vaccine.

Conclusion: Another failed study that lacks statistical validity, that evaluated the wrong group of autistic children, that failed to utilize stringent criteria for the diagnosis of autism, that was instituted by researchers with significant conflicts of interest, and that reached scientifically unsound and, therefore, unwarranted conclusions.

---

46   Ibid.
47   Ibid.

CONSPIRACY:

*"surreptitious or covert schemes to accomplish some end,
most often an evil one."*[48]

Negative Study 12: "Age at first measles-mumps-rubella vaccination in children with autism and school-matched control subjects; a population based study in metropolitan Atlanta." DeStefano, Frank; Bhasin, T.K.; Thompson, W.W. et al. *Pediatrics*. February 2004.

Frank DeStefano, co-author of the highly manipulated "Verstraeten study," and his four colleagues conducted a case-control study of African-American children in Atlanta, Georgia. They compared ages at first immunization with the MMR between autistic and non-autistic children and found that "the overall distribution of ages at MMR vaccination among children with autism was similar to that of matched control children."

This suggested a lack of association between the MMR and the likelihood of a child becoming autistic.

Or did it?

Comment: The DeStefano Group found that more cases (of autism) than controls were vaccinated before 36 months. They calculated the overall odds ratio for this difference as being 1.49 (about one and a half times the risk). That's actually significant and implies a possible link between MMR and autism!

The odds ratio increased to 2.34 for children aged 3-5, and this figure is likely to have been underestimated as a significant number of the children analyzed were too young to have as yet been diagnosed with autism.

The odds ratio for children given the MMR vaccination by 36 months and becoming autistic with a normal IQ was even higher at 2.54.

What is more, "The odds ratios were increased to 3.55 in a subgroup analysis adjusted for birth weight, multiple gestation, maternal age and maternal education, thus strengthening the association between age at exposure to MMR and autism."[49]

The odds ratio is a measure of the association between an exposure (the MMR vaccine in this case) and an outcome (autism). It represents the odds that an outcome (autism) will occur given a particular exposure (the MMR vaccine), compared to the likelihood (odds) of the outcome (autism) occurring in the absence of that exposure (MMR).

The higher the odds ratio (above 1), the more likely the exposure and the outcome are related. An odds ratio of 3.55 in this study means that exposure to MMR increases the risk of autism by slightly over 3.5 times.

So this research paper, which purported to show no support for the link between the MMR inoculation and autism, actually did the opposite by bolstering the association between MMR and autism.

This association was noted by the independent *Cochrane Review*, which also found the study suffering from a "moderate" risk of bias (it was being kind) and having the highest rate of excluded cases of all the studies it reviewed. The study was also criticized for offering "inadequate explanations" for missing data.[50]

Brian Hooker, an associate professor at Simpson University, reanalyzed the data from this CDC study after being tipped off by a then unnamed CDC "whistleblower," and confirmed that, "The present study provides new epidemiologic evidence showing that African American males receiving the MMR vaccine prior to 24 months of age or 36 months of age are more likely to receive an autism diagnosis."[51]

---

48   Dictionary.reference.com/browse/conspiracy

49   Coalition for Safe Minds. *Vaccines and Autism: What Do Epidemiological Studies Really Tell Us?* p. 26.

50   Safe Minds Ibid.

51   Hooker, B. "Measles-mumps-rubella vaccination timing and autism among young African American boys: a reanalysis of CDC data." *Translational Neurodegeneration*. 2014, 3:16. http://www.translationalneurodegeneration.com/content/3/1/16

The Final Nail in the Coffin?

So how is it that the data from this study actually show a clear association between the MMR vaccine and autism, yet DeStefano and his CDC colleagues, allegedly analyzing the same data, were able to conclude that there was no such association?

Easy answer: *The DeStefano team intentionally omitted relevant data.* It did so by eliminating from the study (for no valid scientific reason) any child not having a Georgia birth certificate. This effectively reduced the sample size being studied by 41 percent and resulted in "eliminating the statistical power of the findings and negating the strong MMR-autism link in African American boys."[52]

How do we know this? One of the coauthors of this study, and the aforementioned secret "whistleblower," Dr. William Thompson, confessed, in a statement made in August 2014, that the DeStefano et al. study, of which he was a coauthor, *intentionally omitted relevant data.*

His statement included the following:

> My name is William Thompson. I am a Senior Scientist with the Centers for Disease Control and Prevention, where I have worked since 1998. I regret that my coauthors and I omitted statistically significant information in our 2004 article published in the journal *Pediatrics.* The omitted data suggested that African American males who received the MMR vaccine before age 36 months were at increased risk for autism. Decisions were made regarding which findings to report after the data were collected, and I believe that the final study protocol was not followed.[53]

Conflict of Interest: Dr. DeStefano and all the coauthors work for the CDC.

Conclusion: This CDC-sponsored study actually *supports* the MMR-autism link, and not, as the authors suggest, a lack of an association. It is clearly a fraudulent study and should be retracted. If you didn't hear anything about Dr. Thompson's confession on your TV or radio or read anything about it in your local newspaper, don't be surprised. Mainstream corporate media protects its sponsors by controlling what the public gets to know. A whistleblower's "whistle" is only effective if it is heard.

"A lie told often enough becomes the truth."

— *Vladimir Lenin*

Negative Study 13: Honda, Hideo; Rutter, Michael et al. "No effect of MMR withdrawal on the incidence of autism: a total population study." *Journal of Child Psychology and Psychiatry*. February 8, 2005.

The MMR vaccination was first introduced to Japan in April 1989. Prior to that time, Japanese children had received only the separate measles and rubella vaccines and no mumps vaccine. Several brands of MMR were available at that time, including the MMR containing the dangerous Urabe strain of mumps vaccine that caused meningitis in children.

So many reports of meningitis followed the MMR that public confidence in the MMR declined and the MMR program was officially terminated just four years later in April 1993. The immunization policy that followed the discontinuation of the combined MMR vaccine was the recommendation to *inoculate sequentially* Japanese toddlers with the monovalent (just one antigen) measles, mumps, and rubella immunization. These were injected one at a time *every four weeks* starting at 12 months of age.

In this study, researchers Hideo Honda and Michael Rutter analyzed the cumulative incidence of autistic spectrum disorders (ASD) up to age seven for children born from 1988 to 1998 in a ward of Yokohama, Japan, in order to compare the ASD incidence before and after the MMR inoculation program was discontinued.

---

52   http://www.greenmedinfo.com/blog/breaking-whistleblower-names-cdc-scientists-covering-vaccine-autism-link

53   http://www.naturalnews.com/046630_CDC_whistleblower_public_confession_Dr_William_Thompson.html#ixzz3C2NKOcAp

They allege to have found that, "The MMR vaccination rate in the city of Yokohama declined significantly in the birth cohorts of years 1988 through 1992, and not a single vaccination was administered in 1993 or thereafter. In contrast, cumulative incidence of ASD up to age seven increased significantly in the birth cohorts of years 1988 through 1996 and most notably rose dramatically beginning with the birth cohort of 1993."

They concluded that the "MMR vaccination is most unlikely to be a main cause of ASD, that it cannot explain the rise over time in the incidence of ASD, and that withdrawal of MMR in countries where it is still being used cannot be expected to lead to a reduction in the incidence of ASD."

Comments: What the authors suspiciously *failed to note* was that there was a dramatic rise in the annual incidence of ASD from 20 per 10,000 population before MMR (prior to 1988) to 86 (per 10,000)…for children born in 1990, shortly after the MMR was introduced. The ASD incidence more than quadrupled!

The incidence subsequently *fell 35 percent* to c. 56 (per 10,000) for children born in 1991 [when MMR usage was in decline].[54] These statistics would thus support a link between the MMR vaccine and the incidence of autism in Japan. This is just the *opposite* of what Drs. Honda and Rutter allege.

But how to account for the rise in incidence of ASD in 1994? A possible explanation is that during the years 1991-1994, the single entity vaccine policy, which had been used successfully prior to the introduction of the MMR vaccine, was gaining re-acceptance and the rise in ASD cases could be partly accounted for by the increasing usage of single dose measles, mumps, and rubella vaccines.

Since the single vaccines (the measles, mumps, and rubella) were given in close temporal proximity (just four weeks apart) after the MMR was discontinued (as opposed to one year apart as Dr. Wakefield had recommended), in biological terms, this amounted to "overlapping exposure."

In other words, as far as the children's bodies were concerned, they were still getting the biological equivalent of the MMR. This would account for the data showing a rise in autism incidence after the MMR was introduced, followed by a fall after it was discontinued, followed by another rise as the substitute single entity immunizations were again being widely utilized.

The alleged continued rise in ASD cases after 1994 could also be explained by inaccuracies in the incidence data for ASD. Redistricting occurred in the Yokohama ward under study at that time, and the ASD incidence data subsequently appeared not to be as accurate as reflected in significant increases in the "confidence intervals on the point estimates of ASD incidence (which) increase(d) in parallel with this demographic change."[55]

A confidence interval is a statistical term that predicts with a reasonable degree of certainty that a certain parameter, in this case the ASD incidence in Yokohama, will fall somewhere between the upper and lower limits of the listed range. The wider this range, the less certain the incidence data is.

Conclusion: The authors' conclusion regarding the alleged lack of linkage between the MMR and autism spectrum disorders is incorrect. In fact, this study's data actually supports the contention that the MMR vaccine is causally related to the autism epidemic because "ASD numbers increased and decreased in direct proportion to the total number of children vaccinated with the three live viruses," whether from the combined MMR or the sequentially administered measles, mumps, and rubella vaccines.[56]

This study, as is true of all others thus far reviewed, did not specifically address the issues and findings that characterized the subset of children that Dr. Wakefield and his colleagues examined in the Lancet 12 study, and so, it cannot be used to refute the findings in that study.

Conflicts of Interest: The authors claimed no conflicts; however, coauthor Dr. Michael Rutter clearly was highly con-

---

54   www.whale.to/a/wakefield55.html
55   Wakefield Ibid.
56   Coalition for Safe Minds. *Vaccines and Autism: What Do Epidemiological Studies Really Tell Us?* p.32..

flicted. He has been a paid expert witness for manufacturers of the MMR vaccine, and was at the time "a board member of the Wellcome Foundation, a front foundation for Glaxo SmithKline, a vaccine maker…[and] a key witness in the case against Dr. Andrew Wakefield…."

Dr. Rutter's failure to list his conflicts of interest didn't seem to upset the Fitness to Practice Panel that was prosecuting Dr. Wakefield, who had been unjustly criticized for his alleged failure to disclose his irrelevant involvement with the Dawbarn's law firm.

Negative Study 14: Fombonne, Eric. et al. "Pervasive Developmental Disorders in Montreal, Quebec, Canada: Prevalence and Links with Immunizations." *Pediatrics*. July 2006.

In this study, which we previously reviewed (see Chapter 16), Dr. Eric Fombonne and associates surveyed over 37,000 children over an eleven-year period (1987-98) in Montreal, and looked at their exposure to thimerosal by two years of age and also their MMR coverage.

These children were typically given the MMR at 12 months of age; however, children born after 1995 received a second MMR booster at 18 months of age. Fombonne alleged that "PDD rates significantly increased during the same period when MMR uptake rates significantly decreased," and the "PDD prevalence went up at the same rate before and after the second MMR was introduced in 1996…. These results ruled out an association between MMR and autism," he concluded.[57]

Comment: (We repeat part of our review of this study that pertains to the MMR vaccine). A "cumulative exposure" to a vaccine is supposed to be calculated by multiplying three independent variables: the dose per vaccination, shot frequency, and coverage rates (what percentage of the population received the vaccine). Dr. Fombonne and his research colleagues used one standard for defining cumulative exposure to thimerosal and another for evaluating the effects of the MMR vaccination. That's a "no-no."

For ethyl mercury exposure, Dr. Fombonne and his associates considered only the concentration of thimerosal in each vaccine and the vaccine frequency, but they *did not consider* the coverage rates.

The standard they used for MMR exposure ignored the dosage and frequency and included only the coverage rates. By so doing, they conveniently disregarded the fact that autism rates increased after the number of MMR shots was increased from one to two after 1996, although the coverage rates, as Fombonne et al. claim, *allegedly* went down minimally at that time. But the researchers are also incorrect in that allegation as well. (See Criticism 8 below.)

Contrary to Fombonne's assertion, *the doubling of the MMR vaccine shots actually did result in an increase in the cumulative exposure* (which Fombonne failed to calculate accurately) to the measles virus from the MMR vaccine, despite the alleged marginal decrease in the coverage rate. This failure to calculate the cumulative exposure correctly for both the thimerosal and the MMR analysis, and the use of different and incorrect criteria for defining the cumulative exposure to each is scientifically unsound and deceptive, and it totally invalidates the results and their interpretation.

According to Dr. Ayoub, Fombonne's group "ignored the potential impact of mass measles immunization campaigns in Quebec and Montreal that delivered a second dose of measles to a large number of infants and children throughout 1996. The subsequent rise in [pervasive developmental disorder] shortly after that campaign is clearly depicted in their figures and would lead us to believe this observation supports an association between PDD and MMR exposure."[58]

Competing for Fombonne's most egregious offense is his inappropriately associating the MMR vaccination rates in Quebec, 265 kilometers away from Montreal, with the alleged PDD incidence in Montreal.

Dr. Edward Yazbak, M.D. reviewed several published vaccine uptake surveys of *Montreal* MMR vaccine rates and

57   www.ageofautism.com.2011/vaccines-and-autism-what-do-epidemioloogical-studies-really-tell-us.html05/
58   Ayoub Ibid.

found that in children 24-30 months of age, those rates increased from 85.1 percent in 1983 (Baumgarten) to 88.8 percent in 1996-97 (Valiquette) and then jumped to 96 percent in 2003-04 (Health Department Survey), which suggests, as Dr. Yazbak confirmed, "that in Montreal pervasive developmental disorder prevalence and MMR vaccination rates were in fact increasing in tandem during the study period."

This, of course, is just the opposite of what Dr. Fombonne concluded: "Pervasive developmental disorder rates significantly increased when measles-mumps-rubella vaccination uptake rates significantly decreased."

How can we explain this discrepancy?

Fombonne analyzed the wrong data. As Dr. Yazbak put it in his letter to the journal *Pediatrics* (which declined to publish it): "The readers deserve to know why the authors compared developmental data from a specific group of children in Montreal with MMR vaccination data from the city of Quebec, some distance away."

Conflicts Statement from the Study: "In the United Kingdom, Dr. Fombonne has provided advice on the epidemiology and clinical aspects of autism to scientists advising parents, to vaccine manufacturers, and to several government committees between 1998 and 2001. Since June 2004, Dr. Fombonne has been an expert witness for vaccine manufacturers in US thimerosal litigation."

Conclusion: This study clearly illustrates why good peer review is critical. Dr. Ayoub took the time to reanalyze the study data and found many serious errors that render the study's conclusions meaningless. To whit:

- Dr. Fombonne and his colleagues did not sample a representative population of children from Montreal, although they could have.

- They also failed to recognize the different subgroups in that population that had differing immunization rates and different incidences of PDD. They, therefore, were unable to calculate accurately the incidence of PDD in the unrepresentative population that they did study.

- Their basic assumption about when thimerosal was no longer present in vaccines was incorrect. Their conclusions in this regard are, therefore, invalid.

- The researchers used different and incorrect standards in defining the cumulative dosage for the vaccines that contained thimerosal vs. the vaccine for measles, mumps, and rubella (MMR), and their definitions and calculations of cumulative dosage were, therefore, incorrect.

- They failed to account for the impact of giving twice as many MMR immunizations on the incidence of PDD in their study population, which, contrary to their assertions, *actually demonstrated a likely association between the MMR vaccine and pervasive developmental disorders.*

- And they analyzed the data from the wrong city (Quebec) in their erroneous determination that MMR vaccination uptake rates had decreased (which they may have in Quebec), but not in Montreal where they actually increased.

"The Republic's in trouble, we lie about everything. Lying has become the staple."

— *Seymour Hirsch*

Negative Study 15: D'Souza, Y.; Fombonne, E.; Ward, B.J. "No Evidence of Persisting Measles Virus in Peripheral Blood Mononuclear Cells from Children with Autism Spectrum Disorder." *Pediatrics*. 2006 Oct; 118(4):1164-75.

This study "sought to determine whether measles virus nucleic acids persist in children with autism spectrum disorder compared to control children." The researchers looked for the presence of several measles virus genes (for nucleoprotein, fusion, and hemaglutinin) in certain white blood cells (mononuclear cells) taken from the blood of 54 children with ASD as well as 34 developmentally-normal children.

The authors found that by using previously suggested techniques, a large number of positive reactions were seen in both the autism and control samples, but the researchers were able to discount these results by utilizing allegedly more rigorous techniques (evaluations of melting curves and amplicon band size).

When this was done, none of the samples in either group yielded evidence of the measles virus. There was also no difference in anti-measles antibody between the autism and control groups.

They concluded that, "There is no evidence of measles virus persistence in the peripheral blood mononuclear cells of children with autism spectrum disorder."

Critique: Once again researchers evaluated the wrong group.

D'Souza's group compared autistic children with non-autistic children, when it should have studied children who autistically regressed *after* the MMR and who also exhibited symptoms of chronic intestinal inflammation, the group that Dr. Wakefield and colleagues had evaluated in the 1998 Lancet 12 study.

Studying autistic children who do not meet these criteria does not and cannot negate the findings of Wakefield and his colleagues.

More importantly, whether or not the measles virus persists in mononuclear cells *has no bearing* on the supposition that the measles virus may induce autism in a subgroup of susceptible children.

And the finding of no difference between the autistic group and the control group in regard to anti-measles antibody levels runs counter to the findings of New Jersey Medical School researchers Dr. Oleske and Professor Zecca, who found that children with autism had increased antibodies to the measles virus as compared to non-autistic controls.[59]

This finding was confirmed by Dr. Vijendra Singh in two studies.[60]

The *Science Daily* (Oct 22, 2006) irresponsibly reported that this study, "provides conclusive evidence that the... MMR vaccine is not associated with the development of autism spectrum disorders (ASDs)." That statement is totally false. This study did not in any way prove that contention, nor was it designed to do so.

Co-author Brian Ward, Chief of Infectious Diseases at McGill University Health Center, stated, "We hope that our investigation of these earlier studies will finally clear the MMR vaccine of its link to autism and give parents confidence in their choice to accept vaccination of their children against this potentially fatal disease."[61]

Dr. Ward, whose conflicts of interest are listed in our critique of the next study, is not justified in that assertion or wish. The MMR link to autism still remains a highly likely possibility, and parental concerns regarding the safety of the MMR are certainly appropriate.

Negative Study 16: D'Souza, Yasmin; Ward, B.J. et al. "No Evidence of Persisting Measles Virus in the Intestinal Tissues of Patients with Inflammatory Bowel Disease." *Gut.* 2007 June; 56(6): 886-888.

In this study, the researchers attempted to detect the measles virus in intestinal biopsy samples from patients with inflammatory bowel disease and from control intestinal biopsy samples. They used the same techniques (Uhlmann and Kawashima primer) that had been used in previous studies that had found the measles virus in the gut tissue of patients with inflammatory bowel disease, and they noted that when using the Uhlmann primer, the measles virus was detected in all the samples, but they found these to be false positives when other allegedly more rigorous techniques were utilized.

Their results suggested that "non-specific amplification, contamination or both occurred in these studies." In other

---

59   Unpublished paper by Dr. Oleske and Professor Zecca, New Jersey Medical School, 1999.

60   Singh, V.K. et al. "Abnormal measles-mumps-rubella antibodies and CNS autoimmunity in children with autism." *J Biomed Sci.* 2002 Jul-Aug; 9(4):359-64. *and* Singh, V.K. et al. "Elevated levels of measles antibodies in children with autism." *Pediatr Neurol.* 2003 Apr; 28(4):292-4.

61   *ScienceDaily.* Oct 22, 2006.

words, the studies by Uhlmann, Kawashima, and others may have misidentified the measles virus in the biopsied gut tissue of patients with inflammatory bowel disease, due perhaps to their utilization of faulty laboratory techniques.

Conflicts of Interest: Dr. Brian Ward is heavily conflicted. He has appeared on a number of government advisory committees addressing the issues of vaccine safety, has testified for the U.S. and Quebec vaccine injury compensation programs, has conducted and participated in several government-sponsored studies of measles vaccine safety, and has conducted a number of industry-sponsored studies of non-licensed vaccines as well as a study of a licensed acellular pertussis vaccine.

Comment: D'Souza and colleagues are likely correct in their contention that Uhlman, Kawashima, and others may have misidentified the measles virus in gut biopsies. However, this study does not and cannot rule out the measles virus as a cause of inflammatory bowel disease or autism. The presence or lack thereof of the virus in gut tissue or elsewhere in no way exonerates the MMR or the measles virus as causative agents in these or other conditions.

For a parallel example, heart valve damage (secondary to rheumatic fever), a type of kidney disease called glomerulonephritis and a neurological condition abbreviated PANDAS, have all been shown to be caused by auto-antibodies to a particular type of streptococcus bacterium, which is generally long gone by the time these conditions are detected.

Likewise, the measles virus may indeed have elicited the pathology in those with inflammatory bowel disease and then "moved on." No one has suggested that the measles virus caused or was present in *all* children with inflammatory bowel disease.

Furthermore, this was not a study that examined the inflamed gut tissue of children with chronic bowel complaints who had regressed after the MMR, and only that kind of study is capable of legitimately challenging the findings of the Lancet 12 study.

> *"A lie gets half way around the world before truth has a chance to get its pants on."*
>
> — *Winston Churchill*

Negative Study 17: Hornig, Mady et al. "Lack of Association between Measles Virus Vaccine and Autism with Enteropathy: A Case-Control Study." *PLoS One*. September 2008.

In this case control study, the researchers were interested in determining whether 25 children with *both* gastrointestinal (GI) disturbances and autism were more likely than 13 non-autistic children with GI disturbances (the control group) to have measles virus present (and/or inflammation) in their gut tissue.

The researchers were also interested in determining whether there was a temporal relationship linking the MMR vaccination with the intestinal problems and the onset of autism.

In order to perform this study, all the children underwent ileo-colonoscopy (a procedure that utilized a special device that allows the operator to view the intestinal tract). Children had biopsies taken of areas of the gut that were inflamed, and the samples were sent to three separate labs in a blinded fashion for analysis for the presence of measles virus (RNA). *The findings from the three labs were consistent.* Measles virus was found in only one child in each group.

The investigators found no differences between case and control groups in regard to the presence of measles virus genetic material in the intestines of these children, and they stated that "GI symptoms and autism onset were unrelated to MMR timing."

Discussion: There are a number of serious problems with this study and its conclusions:

- The biggest one is that it was not designed to ask the correct question. The investigators didn't recruit for the subset of children with autism who regressed after MMR vaccination. This and the next concern render the study's conclusions almost meaningless.

- Not enough children were in the study to satisfy its statistical intent. The researchers found that 48 percent (over twice as many) of the autistic children developed intestinal problems after the MMR, compared to just 23 percent of controls.

The difference was not statistically significant, however, because the likelihood that the difference between the two groups was due to chance was calculated to be 2.6 out of 20 (p=0.13). To reach statistical significance, the likelihood of the difference being due to chance would have to have been equal to or less than 1 in 20 (p≤ 0.05). The data do certainly suggest that if the sample size had been larger, the results would likely have been significant.

- Similarly, the researchers report no significant differences in age of first MMR between the two groups, but the non-autistic group got the MMR later in life than did the autistic group. The time difference between the two groups again almost reached significance (p=0.15).

- There were also no true negative controls, like non-autistic children without GI disease or unvaccinated children.

- The researchers used unequal sample sizes. The control group had about half the number of children as the autistic group did.

- The analysts used *ordinal data* in regard to the time intervals between the MMR vaccination and the onset of symptoms rather than the more reliable *interval data*, which they could easily have utilized. Interval data allow statisticians to perform parametric tests, a type of analysis that leads to more reliable statistical results. The use of ordinal data would serve to weaken the statistical significance of the results.[62]

- *The two children in the study (one from each group) who had measles virus in their guts also had lympho-nodular hyperplasia.* Since inflammation of the gastrointestinal tract was commonly seen in both groups of children whose biopsies yielded no evidence of measles virus, one could surmise that had another inflamed area been biopsied, measles virus might have been found.

- It is also possible that measles virus could have initiated the GI concerns in both groups and then disappeared from the gut tissue. This is similar, as we have previously mentioned, to what happens in the case of rheumatic fever; the organism (beta strep) that initiates the disease is gone by the time the disease has manifested. As Dr. Wakefield puts it, "We need to consider that the MMR vaccine can cause autism as a hit-and-run injury, but not necessarily leave the measles virus behind."[63]

- According to a critique from the National Autism Association: "only a small subgroup of children was the correct phenotype to study." From page 7, "Only 5 of 25 subjects (20 percent) had received MMR before the onset of GI complaints and had also had onset of GI episodes before the onset of autism (P=0.03)." The other 20 autistic children in the study had GI problems, but the pathology developed *before* the MMR vaccine. Additionally, the controls all received the MMR vaccine and had gastrointestinal symptoms. The controls *should have been free of exposure to vaccine measles* in order to make a comparison relevant for purposes of causation. This is another example of "overmatching."

- The autism support group Safe Minds also critiqued the study design which "precluded assessment of a role for acute measles infection from MMR in a subset of children with autism and did not examine the role of other vaccines, vaccine components such as thimerosal, or other environmental exposures which can trigger gastrointestinal and immunological problems."

What some of the authors of this study had to say:[64]

Dr. Ian Lipkin: "This study confirms that kids with autism often have 'unrecognized and undertreated bowel complaints.'"

Dr. Mady Hornig: "These intestinal problems may well be linked to the developmental regression seen in about 25 percent of kids with autism."

---

62   http://vaxtruth.org/w ordpress/wp-content/uploads/2011/08/Only-5-of-251-final.pdf

63   http://www.ageofautism.com/2008/09/autis-rese arch.html?cid=129381262

64   www.whale.to/vaccines.flegg.html

Who supported this study? Well, what do you know? It was the American Academy of Pediatrics, thanks to a grant from the CDC. And both of these organizations "along with experts in virology and neurovirology, autism pathogenesis, and vaccine design and safety; representatives of the autism advocacy community; and study collaborators in an Oversight Committee…reviewed and agreed to all aspects of study design prior to data collection."

Comment: This was a study designed to fail and confuse. Dr. Wakefield had evaluated children who developed autistic regression and intestinal symptoms shortly after receiving the MMR. Only five children in this study met those criteria, an entirely inadequate number from which to derive any meaningful data.

It is important to understand that Dr. Wakefield never contended or implied that intestinal disease caused autism or that all intestinal disease is caused by the measles virus component of the MMR vaccine or that autism is always caused by the MMR vaccine.

In addition, the sample size for the autistic group was also *far too small* to yield meaningful results. The number of children in the control group was also inadequate, and the wrong control group was used. The use of ordinal data rather than interval data weakened the statistical relevance of the sought-after associations, and there was no discussion or evaluation of other potential confounding factors like what toxic exposures or immunizations the children were exposed to.

It is curious to note that only two children out of the 38 evaluated were found to have measles virus in their gut tissue. This finding conflicts with that of the Uhlmann et al. 1992 study, which found measles virus in the inflamed gut tissue of 82 percent of the autistic children,[65] and with the 2007 Steven Walker et al. study that found measles virus in 85 percent of the biopsy samples taken from 82 children with regressive autism,[66] and with the Bradstreet 2004 study that found measles virus in the biopsied intestinal tissue of all three autistic children evaluated.[67]

It is certainly possible, even likely, that the use of the Uhlmann and Kawasaki primers used in these studies to detect measles virus invalidates the study conclusions regarding the presence of measles virus in the samples collected, as these techniques have now been alleged to yield false positive results, but *in no way rules out measles as a causative agent in promoting the autistic state.*

The conflicts of interest in this study are also significant. The CDC, in conjunction with the American Academy of Pediatrics, engineered this study, and given the history of the CDC's involvement in the sponsorship of many previous suspect studies that purport to show no association between vaccines and autism, one must look upon their involvement with this study with a more than skeptical eye.

Negative Study 18: Baird, Gillian et al. "Measles Vaccination and Antibody Response in Autism Spectrum Disorders." *Archives of Disease in Childhood*. February 2008.

In this paper, the authors compared three groups of children born in the year 1990 in one area of southern England. Ninety-eight of the children had an autism spectrum disorder, some of whom had a history of regressive autism. Fifty-two children in one control group were classified as having "special needs." Ninety other control children were developmentally normal, and all had received at least one MMR vaccine.

The researchers drew blood on all the children to look for the presence of circulating measles virus so as to determine whether the children had persistent measles infection or abnormally-increased antibody levels to the virus.

No differences in measles virus presence or measles antibody levels were found in the three groups of children. Moreover, none of the autistic children evinced any bowel symptoms.

The authors concluded that their study, like other previous studies, demonstrated no linkage between the MMR vaccination and autism.

---

65   Uhlmann, V. et al. "Potential viral pathogenic mechanism for new variant inflammatory bowel disease." *Mol Pathol*. April, 2002; 55(2):84-90
66   Walker, S. et al. "Persistent Ileal Measles Virus in a Large Cohort of Regressive Autistic Children with Ileocolitis and Lymphonodular Hyperplasia: Revisitation of an Earlier Study." IMFAR May 2007.
67   Bradstreet, J.J. et al. "Detection of measles virus genomic RNA in cerebrospinal fluid of three children with regressive autism: a report of three cases." *Journal of American Physicians and Surgeons*. 2004; 9(2):38-45.

Critique: Once again, we see a deceptively-constructed study designed to obfuscate the MMR-autism linkage. We've made it clear that Wakefield and other investigators found the MMR-derived measles virus in the inflamed gut lining of many of the autistic children who had both regressed and developed bowel complaints shortly *after* the MMR jab.

No one, as we repeatedly emphasize, claimed that the measles virus persistently circulated in the blood in these children, so not finding the virus in the blood of the children that Baird's team investigated is *irrelevant* and does not negate Wakefield's findings.

In addition, only *some* of the children in this study had regressive autism, and *none* had any bowel disorder. That finding is highly suspect since chronic bowel complaints are very commonly reported in autistic children.[68]

Keep in mind that Wakefield never suggested that the MMR vaccination induced autism or caused intestinal disease in all or even in most children, and he did not suggest that all children with autism who had GI complaints had their symptoms induced by the measles virus or any other component of the MMR.

The inclusion in this study of children who did not have regressive autism, or who had regressed prior to their MMR shots, or who did not experience any bowel complaints was, therefore, not appropriate because Wakefield evaluated only those children who had regressed and had chronic bowel complaints *after* their MMR.

So the researchers in this poorly designed study did not evaluate the appropriate group of children, the children who exhibited the same clinical course and symptoms as those in the Wakefield studies, which means their conclusions as to the safety of the MMR are not warranted.

Elevated levels of measles antibody were indeed reported by Wakefield and others in many children who had both GI symptoms and autistic regression after their MMR shot. The presumed cause of this elevation of antibody levels may have been the chronic infection of the gut lining (or other tissue) by the measles virus.

So not finding elevated measles antibodies in the children in this study is not surprising or unexpected or relevant because *none of the autistic children studied had any intestinal symptoms at all.*

Conflicts of Interest: The sponsors of the study included the Department of Health and the Wellcome Trust. Researchers "MA and DB have given unpaid advice to lawyers in MMR and MR litigation. GB has acted as an occasional expert witness for the diagnosis of autism. AP receives royalties from SCQ and ADOS-G instruments. PBS has acted as an expert witness in the matter of MMR/MR vaccine litigation."[69]

> *"Truth is mighty and will prevail. There is nothing wrong with this, except that it ain't so."*
>
> — *Mark Twain*

Negative Studies 19 and 20: Mrozek-Budzyn, D. et al. "Lack of Association between MMR vaccination and Autism in Children: A Case-Control Study." *Przegl Epidemiol.* 2008; 62:597-604; *Pediatric Infect. Dis J.* 2010 May; 29(5):397-400. Doi: 10.1097/INF.0b013e3181c40a8a; PMID: 19952979; also published on Dec 1, 2009 online in *The Pediatric Infectious Disease Journal.*

Two essentially identical studies by researchers at Jagiellonian University in Krakow, Poland, purported to show that children who received either the MMR vaccine or single measles vaccine were actually at *lower risk* of developing autism. The studies were published in Polish in 2008 (in the Polish journal *Przegl Epidemiol.*) and then in English in the *Pediatric Infectious Disease Journal* in 2010.

Doctor Mrozek-Budzyn's team evaluated 96 children aged 2-15 with autism and compared them to 192 "healthy" controls matched to cases by year of birth, sex, and who their doctor was. The team also "considered the mother's age,

---

68   See previous study and Chapter 3.
69   Ibid.

medications used during pregnancy, generation time, perinatal injury and Apgar score in their analysis."[70]

The team found that, "Vaccinated children were at 72 percent reduced risk of autism compared to those who did not receive measles vaccine." They concluded that, "The study provides evidence against the association of autism with either MMR or single measles vaccine."

Critique:

- Once again, these studies did not evaluate children with intestinal issues who had developmentally regressed following the MMR, as was the case with the children evaluated in the Wakefield Lancet 12 study, so they cannot be used to refute the findings in that and subsequent studies of similarly affected children.

- The "control group" was exempted from the measles or MMR vaccine because of "developmental delays and disorders," making it an *inappropriate control group*.[71]

- In the Polish publication, it was revealed that only 34 of the 106 cases received the MMR at the "usual time" (before 18 months of age).[72]

- There were not enough children in this study to allow one to determine the role, if any, of the MMR vaccine as a cause of autism in children. It may be that all of the autistic children in this study were mercury poisoned, or had another etiology for their autism. The Polish immunization schedule requires babies to receive three Hepatitis B vaccinations and 3 DPT (not DTaP) vaccinations by 7 months of age, and *all of these contained 25 mcg of ethyl mercury as thimerosal.* [73]

- We don't know how many of the MMR-inoculated Polish children in these studies went on to develop intestinal inflammation and regressive autism. This issue was not addressed.

- Dr. Dorato Mrozek-Budzyn, the lead author, is a self-described, "Great supporter of vaccination." She is the director of a Polish government agency whose job is to track "parents who delay or refuse to vaccinate."[74]

- The finding of a seemingly protective effect from the MMR in regards to autism incidence makes the results of these flawed studies highly suspicious. The authors attempt to explain away this finding: "Our results would seem to provide a basis to believe that [M or MMR] vaccination is highly protective against autism, but the results cannot be interpreted in that way. This [supposed protective] effect is no doubt due to the fact that children with prior health conditions *were not vaccinated for measles*. In our study, autism was the earliest appearing (?) serious disease. Disorders and developmental delays caused by perinatal problems and problems in infancy may have exempted children from measles vaccination." [75]

Conclusion: These two virtually identical faulty studies do not and cannot absolve the MMR vaccine as a possible causative factor in promoting autism. The control group was totally inappropriate. Children with developmental delays and disorders may well be on the autism spectrum, and their dysfunctions could certainly be related to their prior immunizations. They would, therefore, likely have been at increased risk for autism, and the fact that children in the study with prior health conditions were not vaccinated with the measles or MMR makes the study's conclusions absurd.

"The fact that an opinion has been widely held is no evidence whatever that it is not utterly absurd; indeed in view of the silliness of the majority of mankind, a widespread belief is more likely to be foolish than sensible."

— *Bertrand Russell*

70   foodconsumer.org is.gd/5wN6f
71   http://www.ageofautism.com/2011/08/new-iom-report-on-vaccine-adverse-effects-shows-alarming-lack-of-good-science-safeminds-notes-parent.html
72   Ibid.
73   Ibid.
74   Ibid.
75   Ibid.

Negative Study 21: "Increasing Exposure to Antibody-Stimulating Proteins and Polysaccharides in Vaccines Is Not Associated with Risk of Autism." DeStefano, Frank; Price, Cristofer S.; Weintraub, Eric S. *Journal of Pediarics.* April 2013. http://jpeds.com/webfiles/images/journals/ympd /JPEDS DeStefano.pdf

In April 2013 the *Journal of Pediatrics* published a study by Frank DeStefano (Director of the CDC's Immunization Safety Office) and his associates in which 256 Autism Spectrum Disorder (ASD) children were matched to 752 comparable controls. The total number of antigens that each child received in any single day of vaccination and by two years of age was determined, and no difference between the two groups was found.

The researchers alleged that there is "no association between receiving 'too many vaccines too soon' and autism."[76]

The authors also point out "although the current vaccine schedule contains more vaccines than the schedule in the late 1990s, the maximum number of antigens that a child could be exposed to in 2013 is 315, compared with several thousand in the late 1990s." This is largely due to the substitution of the "old" pertussis vaccine, which induced the production of thousands of antibodies, with the newer acellular vaccine that stimulates the production of six or fewer antibodies.[77]

Comment: Although this was not designed to be a study that exonerates the MMR vaccine specifically as a cause of autism, we include it because its erroneous conclusions may suggest to some that vaccines, of which the MMR is one, are not causally linked to the current epidemic of autism and other related disorders.

Antigens are the chemical components in vaccines that stimulate the body to make specific antibodies that may provide immunity to the various diseases the immunizations are intended to protect us against. Antigens in vaccines are generally either proteins or chains of sugar molecules (polysaccharides).

Were the authors of this study justified in concluding that, "increasing exposure to antibody producing proteins and polysaccharides in vaccines during the first two years of life was not related to the risk of developing Autism Spectrum Disorder"?

Is that conclusion even relevant?

Not according to research scientist and study critic Brian Hooker, Ph.D. Dr. Hooker states, "Of all the papers I have reviewed over my 26-year career as a research scientist, this is perhaps the most flawed and disingenuous study I have encountered."[78]

"The basis for the study," according to Dr. Hooker, "is essentially a rehash of the data that was used to generate the fraudulent Price et al. 2010 *Pediatrics* study (Price et al. 2010. "Prenatal and Infant Exposure to Thimerosal from Vaccines and Immunoglobulins and Risk of Autism." *Pediatrics* 126:656)." (See Chapter 16 for a review of that study.)

The control children in this study were described as being "neurotypical" (i.e., developmentally and neurologically "normal"), but 25 percent of the supposedly "neurotypical" controls were not at all "neurotypical." They had autism symptoms like speech or language delays, learning disabilities, attention deficit hyperactivity disorder, tics, or had an individual education plan suggestive of a learning impairment.

Since many "autism cases were matched with 'cases' of other, similar neurodevelopmental maladies, you would expect to see no difference between the two groups," Dr. Hooker explains, so it's not surprising that no differences were seen. Children with tics, developmental and speech delays, or ADHD are not neurotypical and should not have been used as controls.

And like the flawed 2010 Price study and so many others previously referenced, this study also suffers from the same statistical malady known as "overmatching."

---

76   jpeds.com/content/JPEDSDeStefano
77   Ibid.
78   healthimpactnews.com/2013/can-we-trust-the-cdc-claim-that-there-is-no-link-between-vaccines-and-autism/

Overmatching, it may be recalled, occurs when cases and controls are too closely matched to each other. This clever statistical trick actually precludes finding a difference between cases and controls as "all differences (are) matched out case by case."[79]

Cases in this study "were matched with controls of the same age, sex, within the same HMO, same birth year and essentially the same vaccination schedule using the same vaccine manufacturers."[80] There was no difference in exposure to vaccines between cases and controls, so it is not surprising that no differences were found. That undoubtedly was Dr. DeStefano's intent.

A High Participant Refusal Rate

"Some epidemiologists consider a high study participation rate a hallmark of a 'good' epidemiologic study."[81]

However, in this study there was a high participant *refusal* rate. Over half (52 percent) of the contacted ASD cases declined to participate and 68 percent of the controls did as well. While low participation rates don't necessarily invalidate a study, they can result in unintended biases that weaken the statistical conclusions of the study.

The Real Fallacy...

However, the real fallacy is the premise of the study itself: that the number of antigens given a child is the only or primary relevant factor linking immunizations to the ASD epidemic.

It is feasible that certain common antigens present in both the earlier and current immunizations may be responsible for the increased incidence of autism and ADHD, which has nothing to do with the total number of antigens injected.

Likewise, it is possible and indeed likely that other constituents of the immunizations like aluminum, thimerosal, hydrolyzed gelatin, fetal cells, retroviral remnants, and formaldehyde may play a role in the causality of autism spectrum disorders.

Additionally, the nature, amount, and strength of each antigen present in an immunization is likely to be as (or more) pertinent in relation to autism causality than the number of antigens present.

"For example," Dr. Hooker explains, "'antigens' for the five antigen DTaP vaccines (e.g., Infanrix) include diphtheria toxoid, tetanus toxoid, pertussis toxoid, filamentous hemagglutinin and pertactin. The number '5' assigned in this category is merely the number of different antigens and doesn't account for each antigen's amount or relative strength.... Hence, the 'main independent' variable of 'number of antigens' within the DeStefano et al. study is meaningless," he concludes.

Missing the Point

"Finally," Dr. Hooker continues, "this type of study misses the point entirely that children with autism are physiologically different than neurotypical children. Numerous studies have shown genetic (e.g., James et al. 2006), morphological (e.g., Herbert et al. 2005) and biochemical differences (e.g., Waly et al. 2004) between these two populations. To perform a case-control study such as that presented in the DeStefano et al. 2013 paper assumes a genetically, morphologically, and physiologically homogeneous population, which is simply not the case.

"No one is claiming that children with autism or ASD got higher doses of vaccine antigens, thimerosal, MMR or whatever. What we know instead is that when our children received the same vaccines within the ACIP recommended schedule, they reacted differently."[82]

---

79   Ibid.
80   Ibid.
81   depts.washington.edu/epidem/Epi583/January20-08.pdf
82   Ibid.

As has been emphasized repeatedly, the CDC refuses to do a study that compares vaccinated and unvaccinated children. We know it is able to do that. The data are available in its VSD database. Indeed, Dr. DeStefano, it may be remembered, was the co-author of Dr. Verstraeten's nefariously manipulated study that initially showed significant adverse effects of thimerosal in vaccinated vs. unvaccinated babies in the first few months of life. (See Chapter 13.)

What Was Concealed...

Dr. Hooker alleges that, "the study authors hid data regarding the only valid part of the study" (i.e., prenatal thimerosal exposure) which showed that children exposed to just 16 micrograms of mercury in thimerosal *in utero were up to 8 times more likely* to receive a diagnosis of regressive autism.[83]

Conflicts of Interest: The CDC funded and designed this study and approved the protocol.

The CDC's own researchers, Eric Weintraub and Frank DeStefano, were key players in this study.

Cristofer Price, a coauthor of this study (and the manipulated Verstraeten study), was the lead author of the aforementioned fraudulent 2010 study that purported to exonerate thimerosal as a causative agent in promoting autism, and he is also an employee of Abt Associates, "a contract research organization whose largest clients include vaccine manufacturers and the CDC's National Immunization Program."[84]

Drs. Eric Weintraub and Frank DeStefano were also coauthors of the 2010 Price study.

Conclusion: The CDC strikes again with yet another deceptive bit of hocus-pocus cleverly disguised as a study, featuring inappropriate controls, extremely low participation of cases and controls, overmatching, and an unsound premise. Any conclusion that the study authors arrive at is, therefore, likely to be without merit.

Final Thoughts

We have analyzed twenty studies that purport to invalidate the link between the MMR vaccine and autism.

None of them do so.

And none of them specifically investigated children who regressed after the MMR vaccine and who also then had symptoms of intestinal inflammation, as did the children evaluated in the infamous Wakefield Lancet 12 study.

Do you wonder why none of these researchers attempted to replicate that study? It would have been easy to do. Did they fear that if they did so, they might prove Dr. Wakefield right?

Four of these "negative" studies, when properly analyzed, actually support the MMR-autism link.

Many of the studies appear to have been deliberately designed to distort the results so as to obfuscate the autism-MMR linkage. Some are out and out frauds.

There are thus no valid studies that exonerate vaccines as causative agents in promoting autism, and there are dozens of valid studies that confirm that linkage. The evidence is clear and compelling: *Vaccines do indeed cause autism!*

---

83   Price, C. et al. Thimerosal and Autism. Technical Report. Vol. I. Bethesda, MD: Abt Associates Inc. 2000. healthimpactnews.com/2013/can-we-trust-the-cdc-claim-that-there-is-no-link-between-vaccines-and-autism/
84   Safe Minds

"During my thirty-plus years as a research microbiologist in the Environmental Protection Agency's Office of Research and Development (ORD) and the University of Georgia, I experienced the far-reaching influence of corrupt special interests firsthand....

"My dealings with civil servants, corporate managers, elected officials, and other scientists expose the ease—and disturbing regularity—with which a small group, motivated by profit or personal advancement can completely hijack important areas of research science at even our most trusted institutions."

— John Stone[85]

In 2012 and 2013, outbreaks of measles occurred in large numbers of children and adults who had been vaccinated and who were living in areas of highly vaccinated populations in the North of England. The North of England outbreaks involved the same MMR vaccine in use in the USA, Merck's MMR II.[86]

---

85   http://www.ageofautism.com/2014/07/an-article-for-independence-day-the-american-revolution-and-health-tyranny.html?utm_source=feedburner&utm_medium=email&utm_campaign=Feed percent3A+ageofautism+ percent28AGE+OF+AUTISM percent29
86   https://childhealthsafety.wordpress.com/2015/02/08/officials-covered-up-massive-uk-measles-outbreak-in-highly-mmr-vaccinated-children-adults-officials-withheld-the-evidence-parents-not-warned-children-unprotected-bbc-directly-implica/

Chapter 26
The Aluminum Connection

"It is my opinion that most bureaucracies don't have a brain or a heart, but they do have a strong survival instinct."

— Boyd Haley, Prof. of Chemistry
in a letter to Congressman Dan Burton, 23 May 2001

WHY IS EXPOSURE *to Aluminum a Concern?*

Aluminum is the most abundant metal on the earth's crust. It has no nutritional function. In its metallic form, it is harmless; however, when humans are exposed to aluminum in its common ionic +3 form,[1] there are real dangers to consider because ionic aluminum is highly toxic to brain cells as well as to other tissues in the body.

How Are Humans Commonly Exposed to Aluminum?

Humans are exposed to aluminum constantly. The sources of aluminum exposure include:

- Aluminum cookware: Aluminum cookware is popular because it is light and inexpensive. When acidy foods like tomatoes are cooked in aluminum pots and pans, toxic aluminum ions are leached out from the pan's surface and enter the food.

- Aluminum cans: These are used as containers for soda and beer, which are both acidic. Aluminum does become ionized when exposed to these beverages and is ingested when the beverage is swallowed. "Even one beer or cola drink per day can lead to aluminum toxicity in susceptible individuals over time," according to Analytical Research Labs, Inc.[2]

- Antacids: Aluminum hydroxide is commonly found in a majority of over-the-counter antacids, like Maalox, Mylanta, and Rolaids.

- Anti-perspirants and cosmetics: Aluminum chlorhydrate is the usual ingredient in antiperspirants because it is readily absorbed through the skin and effectively inhibits the local sweat glands from producing perspiration. Aluminum is also used as a base in some cosmetics.

- Foods: Black tea, soy products, and many baking powders may contain aluminum in significant amounts. Processed cheese may contain the emulsifier sodium aluminum phosphate. An aluminum salt called potassium alum is used to bleach flour. Aluminum may be found as a drying agent in cocoa, salt, and other products. A 2012 survey in Taiwan by the Consumer's Foundation found that 66 percent of 24

---

1   +3 means each aluminum atom has lost three electrons.
2   www.arltma.com/Articles/AlumToxDoc.htm

randomly selected foods, like doughnuts, steamed buns, and seaweed, contained aluminum in *amounts that could pose a danger to children.*[3]

- Water Supplies: Aluminum may be found naturally in some water sources, and aluminum salts are also commonly added by local water authorities to remove solid wastes prior to further purification steps.

- Baby Formula: Researchers in Britain tested 30 (cow's milk) baby formulas for aluminum and found it present in all of them at elevated levels. Some formulas had 100 times more aluminum (4-65 ng/ml) than what is found in breast milk.[4] In the U.S., soy infant formulas were found to contain 600-1300 ng/ml of aluminum, according to research published in the journal *Pediatrics.* The aluminum's source was mineral salts used in the formula's production.[5]

- Hemodialysis: Individuals with renal failure must undergo dialysis in order to rid themselves of toxic substances, but aluminum is not efficiently removed by dialysis and may build up to toxic levels. The water that is used for dialysis can also present a real danger for the dialysis patient if it contains a significant amount of aluminum. "Dialysis dementia" is the name given to the condition of aluminum neurotoxicity that was once quite commonly seen in dialysis patients. Aluminum can also cause the bone disease osteomalacia and induce a type of anemia.

- Total Parenteral Nutrition (TPN) and IV dextrose (a sugar) and calcium gluconate solutions: TPN is the name given to the procedure for ensuring adequate nutrition in individuals who for various reasons are unable to eat, swallow, or digest foods normally. The TPN nutrients are often given intravenously directly into the bloodstream, and any aluminum in these nutrients or in the fluid injected can add to the toxic burden of this substance.[6] The FDA states that, "Studies show that aluminum may accumulate in the bone, urine and plasma of infants receiving TPN." They add "Aluminum toxicity is difficult to identify in infants…"[7]

- Glass jars and vials: It may surprise the reader to learn that glass containers, commonly assumed to be inert and safe storage vessels, contain significant amounts of aluminum (1.9 to 5.8 percent aluminum oxide) and this aluminum readily leaches from the glass container over time. "Storage containers contribute significantly to aluminum contamination of serum albumin products," for example.[8]

- Vaccines: Aluminum is used in some vaccines as an "adjuvant," a substance that increases the vaccine's effectiveness. In addition, "storing vaccines in glass containers can up the aluminum content by 200 times compared to storing vaccines in plastic containers," according to Chris Meletis, N.D.[9] Injected aluminum, as we shall see, is a major concern. So even if a vaccine does not contain aluminum, the element may enter the vaccine from the glass vial in which it is stored.

What Factors Influence How Aluminum Enters the Body and Affects the Body?

Dietary aluminum is usually not a serious concern for most healthy individuals, because most of the aluminum ingested is excreted in the stool. Normally, only 0.3 percent of the aluminum ingested is absorbed by the GI tract. The little that is absorbed is bound to various proteins in the bloodstream and eliminated by the kidneys. People with impaired renal function are, therefore, at greater risk for aluminum toxicity.

Absorption from the intestinal tract is enhanced by foods containing lactate (dairy products), citric acid (citrus fruits), or ascorbic acid (vitamin C), and by parathyroid hormone. A "leaky inflamed gut" is also likely to promote increased aluminum absorption.

---

3   www.taipeitimes,com/News/front/archive//2012/04/07 /2003529707
4   Chuchu, N. et al. "The aluminium content of infant formulas remains too high." *BMC Pediatrics.* 2013; 13:162f *and* Burrell, S.A.; Exley, C. "There is still too much aluminum in infant formulas." http://www.biomedcentral.com/1471-2431/10/63
5   *Pediatrics.* Vol. 101 No. 1 January 1, 1998. p. 148-153.
6   Poole, R.L. et al. *J Parent Enteral Nutr.* 2008; 32:242-246.
7   www.fda.gov/ohrms/dockets/98fr/oc0367.pdf
8   Bohrer, D. et al. *J. Trace Elem. Med. Biol.* 2003, 17:107-115.
9   http://www.wholehealthinsider.com/brain-health/alzheimers-and-autism-the-common-link/

Aluminum readily crosses the blood brain barrier. It can damage neurons by causing oxidative stress, which results in damage to essential cellular structures called neurofilaments.

Some experts believe that aluminum plays a role in the development of neuro-fibrillary tangles, commonly thought to be part of the pathological process that causes Alzheimer's disease.. "Exposure to aluminum in laboratory animals results in the development of neurofibrillary tangles and degeneration of cerebral neurons."[10]

Russell Blaylock and others theorize that the neurological dysfunction seen in autism is at least in part secondary to brain inflammation and overexcitation mediated by the neurotransmitter glutamate and also by inflammatory cytokines. Aluminum can exacerbate this cytotoxicity.

"High aluminum concentrations have been seen in post-mortem brain specimens of those with Parkinson's disease…."[11]

Autistic children have higher levels of aluminum than do non-autistic children.[12]

If the amount of aluminum entering the body exceeds the amount eliminated, then toxicity is likely, as the excess aluminum deposits in various organs and tissues. The elimination half-life of aluminum from the human brain is *seven years*! That means it can take seven years for just half of the aluminum in the brain to be eliminated, and that's assuming no more aluminum is entering the brain during that time![13]

How Much Aluminum Is allowed in Injectables by the FDA?

Certain intravenous (IV) solutions, like glucose (dextrose sugar) or mixtures of vitamins and minerals (TPN), often given to patients unable to eat or digest normally (like some premature infants and newborns), may contain aluminum in potentially toxic amounts.

The FDA warns that "aluminum may reach toxic levels with prolonged parenteral (IV) administration if kidney function is impaired. Premature neonates are particularly at risk because their kidneys are immature…."

"Research indicates that patients with impaired kidney function, including premature babies, who received parenteral (IV) levels of aluminum greater than 4-5 micrograms per kilogram (about 2.2 lbs) of body weight per day accumulate aluminum at levels associated with central nervous system and bone toxicity (for a tiny newborn this would be 10-20 micrograms and for an adult it would be about 350 micrograms."[14]

The hepatitis B vaccine, generally given on the first day of life and again at one month of age, contains *250 micrograms of aluminum*! However, the FDA insists that aluminum in vaccines is safe for infants.[15]

The studies they cite to support this contention allege that the "maximum amount of aluminum an infant could be exposed to over the first year of life would be 4.225 milligrams (same as 4,225 micrograms), based on the recommended schedule of vaccines. Federal regulations for biological products, including vaccines, limit the amount of aluminum…in individual doses to not more than 0.85-1.25 mg."[16]

The Mitkus et al. *FDA-sponsored study* that the FDA cites alleges that "the body burden of aluminum from vaccines and diet in the first year of life is significantly less than the corresponding safe body burden of aluminum…."[17]

But is that true in all babies, and should we feel comfortable with these FDA assurances?

10   Zheng, W. "Neurotoxicology of the Brain Barrier System: New Implications." *Clinical Toxicology*. 39 (7), 711-719, 2001.

11   Blaurock-Busch, E. et al. *Maedica (Buchar)*. Jan 2012; 7(1):38-48.

12   Blaurock-Busch, E. et al. *Maedica (Buchar)*. Jan 2012; 7(1):38-48.

13   Yellamma, K. *Toxicol Int*. 2010 Jul-Dec; 17(2): 106–112.

14   www.askdrsears.com/topics/vaccines/vaccine-faqs

15   www.fda.goc/BiologicsBloodvaccines/ScienceResearch/ucm284520.htm

16   Ibid.

17   Ibid. Keith, L.S. et al. "Aluminum toxicokinetics regarding infant diet and vaccinations." *Vaccine*; 2002:20 (Supplement 3): 513-17, *and* Mitkus, R. et al. "Updated aluminum pharmacokinetics following infant exposures through diet and vaccination." *Vaccine*. 29; 2011: 9536-43.

> *"Most dietary aluminum or mercury will be excreted.*
> *Injected aluminum is not easily removed...."*
>
> — *Dr. Chris Shaw*[18]

Should We Feel Comfortable with These FDA Assurances?

Not at all because it isn't just the total amount of aluminum injected or ingested over the first year of life that is a concern. It is *how much* aluminum a baby receives *each time* he or she gets vaccinated, how efficiently he or she excretes that aluminum, and how the toxicity of aluminum may be synergistically enhanced by the presence of other substances like the mercury in thimerosal,[19] and also by what route the aluminum enters the body.

The studies the FDA cites do not address these valid concerns, but we shall.

> *"There's not one single live human infant study that has ever been done to determine how much*
> *aluminum can safely be injected into a human infant. And I challenge anybody to show me just*
> *one such study, because I couldn't find it anywhere."*
>
> — *Dr. Bob Sears, Frontline Interview*

In addition, the Mitkus study did not compare babies who received aluminum in vaccines with those who had only received aluminum-free vaccines or had not been vaccinated at all to see whether there were any differences regarding the likelihood of their suffering any adverse consequences (like ADHD, developmental concerns, speech delays, or autism). It is only by so doing that one can determine whether aluminum in vaccines is a safety concern or not, but *this kind of study has never been done.*

How Did We Arrive at the Safety Limit for Aluminum (4-5 Mcg/Kg/Day)?

In 1997, a study was published that compared the fates of 100 preemies who had received a standard intravenous feeding solution containing aluminum (50 mcg/day equivalent to 25 mcg per kg body weight per day) with a matched set of another 100 preemies who had been given the same solution with much lower levels of aluminum (10 mcg per day or 5 mcg/kg/day). The babies given the high aluminum IV solutions showed *more impaired neurological and mental functioning* at 18 months of age compared to the low aluminum group.[20]

It appeared that up to 4-5 mcg of aluminum per kg could be given safely by IV to preemies each day with less adverse neurological consequences by 18 months of age. But would the low aluminum-exposed babies have shown any developmental deficits if followed for longer than 18 months? Would they later develop learning delays or hyperactivity? Would any have become autistic?

Babies in the 1990s received significantly less aluminum from vaccines (just DPT and HIB) than did those in the 2000s (when Hepatitis A and Pneumococcal vaccines were added). Would these additional sources of aluminum pose a greater risk?

These are important questions that still need answering.

---

18   www.ageof autism.com/2012/03/the-aluminum-threat-a-interview-with-chris-shaw.html
19   Babies are currently exposed to 25 mcg of mercury in thimerosal from the influenza vaccination given their mothers during the pregnancy and again when they are six months old and yearly thereafter as part of the recommended vaccination schedule. There are also "trace amounts" of thimerosal in many other vaccines that babies receive.
20   Bishop, N.J. et al. "Aluminum neurotoxicity in preterm infants receiving intravenous feeding solutions." *NEJM*. 1997, May 29; 336 (22): 1557-1561.

"I have taken a lot of histories of kids who are in trouble in school. The history is that developmental milestones were normal or advanced, and

They can't read at second grade,

They can't write at third grade,

They can't do math in the fourth grade,

And it has no relationship to the developmental milestones."

— Dr. William Weil, Pediatrician, Committee on Environmental Health, AAP
From minutes of the June 2000 CDC-sponsored Simpsonwood Conference, p. 216

What About Other Studies That Purport to Show Aluminum in Vaccines Is Safe to Use?

At a conference held in 2002, a group of doctors met to discuss the use of aluminum in vaccines. They concluded that aluminum was useful and likely not harmful, but they acknowledged that more research needed to be done regarding how aluminum is stored, transported, and excreted, and in particular in children.[21]

In 2004, the Cochrane Collaboration epidemiologists published a review of studies of one particular aluminum-containing DTP vaccine that had been compared to those with no aluminum. They found no side effect differences of significance, *except that the aluminum-containing DPT shot elicited more local reactions like pain, swelling, and redness.* They concluded that aluminum in vaccines is not a safety concern, and they unjustifiably suggested that no further studies needed to be done.[22]

As Doctor Robert Sears so aptly put it, "The Cochrane group closed the book on aluminum without even really opening it."[23]

The Global Advisory Committee on Vaccine Safety for the World Health Organization agreed with the Cochrane Group's conclusions and declared in 2008 that the use of aluminum adjuvants in vaccines posed no health risks.

Aluminum "Foiled" Again?

However, that conclusion was not justified because what has never been tested, and should have been, are the aluminum levels in babies after vaccination. What needs to be determined is: How much aluminum is stored in the brain and other tissues of those infants? What factors besides poor renal function (like genetic differences, for example) might place some babies at greater risk for aluminum toxicity? Are some children poor detoxifiers of aluminum? Does the presence of other vaccines containing aluminum or mercury induce additive or additional toxic effects?

"Fluoride, when combined with aluminum, forms a compound that can destroy numerous hippocampal (a brain structure) neurons at a concentration of 0.5 parts per million in drinking water. It seems that aluminum readily combines with fluoride to form this toxic compound.... Fluoraluminum compounds...can activate G-proteins."

— Russel Blaylock, M.D., c 2004
"The Truth behind the Vaccine Cover-up"

---

21   Eickhoff, T.C.; Myers, M. "Workshop Summary: Aluminum in Vaccines." *Vaccine*; 2002:20 (Supp): S1-S4.

22   Jefferson, T. et al. "Adverse events after aluminum-containing DTP vaccines: systematic review of the evidence." *The Lancet Infect. Dis.* 2004; 4: 84-90.

23   www.askdrsears.com/topics/vaccines/vaccine-faqs

How Much Aluminum Is in the Vaccines That Babies and Children Commonly Receive?

At 2, 4, and 6 months of age, babies injected with recommended vaccines receive 1250 mcg of aluminum at each of those visits.[24] The FDA limits the amount of aluminum per day to 50 mcg for adults and 20 mcg per day for children.

Table 26.1 lists the current recommended schedule for the common vaccines that contain aluminum. Table 26.2 provides data on the aluminum exposure from vaccines at various ages.

Table 26.1. Vaccine Schedule and Aluminum Content of Vaccines[25]

Vaccine	Aluminum content in micrograms/shot	Generally given at:
HIB (PedVaxHib brand only-All other single HIBs are Al-free)	225	2,4,6 & 18 months
Hepatitis B	250	Birth, 1 month & 6-18 months
DTaP (Diphtheria, Tetanus & acellular Pertussis)	170-625 (depending on manufacturer)	2,4,6 & 18 months & 5 yrs.
Pneumococcus	125	2,4,6 & 18 months
Hepatitis A	250	1st dose 12-23 months 2nd dose 6-18 months after 1st
Pentacel (DtaP, Hib, Polio combo)	330	2,4,6 & 18 months & 5 yrs.
Pediarix (DtaP, Hib, Polio combo)	850	2,4,6 & 18 months & 5 yrs.
HPV-Human Papilloma Virus	225	3 doses starting at 11-12 yrs. of age

Table 26.2. Aluminum Exposure from Vaccines at Various Ages[26]

Age at Vaccination	Minimum Aluminum Exposure (in mcg)	Maximum Aluminum Exposure (in mcg)
Birth	250 from hepatitis B vaccine	250 from hepatitis B vaccine
1 month	250 from hepatitis B vaccine	250 from hepatitis B vaccine
2 months	295 (if lowest Al. content vaccines are used)	1225 (if max aluminum brands + 3rd Hep B given)
4 months	295 (if lowest Al. content vaccines are used)	1225 (if max aluminum brands + 3rd Hep B given)
6 months	295 (if lowest Al. content vaccines are used)	1225 (if max aluminum brands + 3rd Hep B given)
12 months	250 (from 1st Hep A)	250 from 1st Hep A
18 months	295 (if lowest Al. content vaccines are used)	1225 (if max, aluminum brands + 2nd Hepatitis A given
2-5 years	170 (from lowest aluminum DTaP at 5 years)	625 (from highest aluminum -containing DTaP)

---

24   mcg=microgram
25   Table 26.1 data from: www.askdrsears.com/topics/vaccines/vaccine-faqs & www.cdc.gov/vaccine/schedules/hcp/imz/child-adolescent.html
26   Table 26.2 data from: www.askdrsears.com/topics/vaccines/vaccine-faqs

If we accept 5 mcg of aluminum per kilogram body weight per day as the upper limit of a safe dose then that would mean that a six-pound newborn should have no more than 14 mcg of aluminum per day injected.

The hepatitis B vaccine given on the day of birth contains 250 mcg of aluminum! That's 18 times higher than safety levels allow!

Are There Any Studies Comparing Aluminum Excretion in Term and Preterm Infants?

Yes. A group of French researchers did just that and published their results in the *Journal of Parenteral and Enteral Nutrition* in 1992. They studied two groups of premature infants, and compared the aluminum content of their serum and urine with that of a control group of full-term healthy newborns over a three-month period. Dozens of samples were obtained from each of these groups. The results are summarized in Table 26.3.

Table 26.3. 1992 Study of Premature Infants [27]

Measurement	Term Newborns	Preterm: 28-32 Wk Gestation	Preterm: 33-36 Wk Gestation	Significant Difference?
Daily Al Intake*	0.42	0.64	0.52	Yes (p=0.5)
Plasma Al Level**	0.29	0.49	0.39	Yes (p=0.007)
Urine Al Level***	0.80	0.77	0.78	No

The results indicate that the aluminum intake and plasma aluminum levels were greater for the preemies than for the full-term infants, but *the aluminum excretion levels were similar in all groups.*

The researchers concluded that, "Although the metabolic consequences of the high aluminum intakes and blood levels we have observed in very low birth weight infants need to be assessed, these results suggest that more attention should be paid to the aluminum status and intake of healthy premature babies."[28]

These authors focused on the oral and enteral (IV) intake of aluminum in premature and term infants. They did not include the additional aluminum exposure from vaccines in their calculations.

Further studies in this regard are essential.

"A foolish faith in authority is the worst enemy of truth."

— Albert Einstein

What Additional Evidence Links Aluminum to Autism?

Adjuvants (additional substances like aluminum and squalene), which are and have been added to certain vaccines, have neurotoxic potential and may act in a synergistic fashion with other known neurotoxins like mercury.

Aluminum is well-established as a neurotoxin, and its toxicity is magnified many times when mercury, another neurotoxin, is present. Of the 32 currently recommended vaccines for children, 18 contain aluminum!

---

27   Table 26.3 Al= Aluminum; *mμmol/kg/day; **mμmol/L; ***mμmol of aluminum/mmol of creatinine
28   Bougle, D. et al. "A Cross-sectional Study of Plasma and Urinary Aluminum Levels in Term and Pre-term Infants." *JPEN*. Mar-Apr 1992 16(2):157-9.

Individuals who suffer from the aluminum-linked neurological disorder known as macrophagic myofasciitis (MAC-row-FAY-jik MY-oh-FASH-ee-EYE-tis) have been known to "harbor aluminum at the site of injection for up to 8 to 10 years after vaccination."[29]

This implies that aluminum from vaccines may be released from the injection site over many years in certain individuals.

Pediatrician Bob Sears published his concerns about the potential dangers of aluminum in vaccines in an article he wrote in 2008 for *Mothering Magazine* titled, "Is Aluminum the New Thimerosal?" He noted that, as with thimerosal, no adequate safety tests had been done to establish that aluminum was safe to inject into babies and children.

And it appears that his concerns were justified.

Lucija Tomljenovitch and Chris Shaw published a study in the *Journal of Inorganic Biochemistry* in 2011, in which they "examined the current childhood vaccine schedules for several western industrialized nations and compared them with autism rates in children.

"What they found was chilling: a highly statistically significant relationship between aluminum exposure from vaccinations and the number of ASD diagnoses in children."[30]

The authors examined data on autistic youth (aged 6-21 during the years 1991-2008) obtained from the U.S. Dept. of Education Annual Reports, which they correlated with the children's aluminum exposure from vaccines up to age 6.

They did the same analysis on data they collected from the United Kingdom, Australia, Canada, and three Scandinavian countries. They were also careful to eliminate confounding factors, like vaccines that were added after the relevant ASD prevalence studies.

What Tomljenovitch and Shaw found was a highly significant correlation between the total aluminum exposure from vaccines and the prevalence of autism spectrum disorder diagnoses for each year studied in every country studied.

"Hill's Criteria" were created to establish the likelihood of a cause-effect linkage between two variables, in this case aluminum from vaccines and ASD prevalence. The authors point out that their findings satisfy 8 of the 9 Hill's Criteria (one of these was not relevant), *thus establishing the likelihood that aluminum exposure from vaccines is also a cause of autism and related disorders.*[31]

While it is true that ecological studies like this one don't prove that aluminum in vaccines causes autism, they provide strong evidence that this assumption is highly likely, especially when these results were confirmed by another research team analyzing an entirely different database.

That research team, headed by Stephanie Seneff of MIT's Computer Science and Artificial Intelligence Laboratory, analyzed information from the Vaccine Adverse Event Reporting System (VAERS) database and *found a strong link between autism and the aluminum in vaccines.*

Using standard statistical techniques, the team identified "several signs and symptoms that are significantly more prevalent in vaccine reports after 2000...which [were] significantly associated with aluminum containing vaccines."

The researchers theorized that "children with autism diagnosis are especially vulnerable to toxic metals such as aluminum or mercury due to insufficient serum sulfate and glutathione," which aid in the detoxification process.

29   www.gaia-health.com/gaia-blog/2011-12-92/aluminum-adjuvant-in-vaccines-a-smoking-gun-autism-link/
30   www.gaia-health.com/gaia-blog/2011-12-92/aluminum-adjuvant-in-vaccines-a-smoking-gun-autism-link/
31   Tomljenovitch, L.; Shaw, C.A. "Do Aluminum Vaccine Adjuvants Contribute to the Rising Prevalence of Autism?" *J Inorg. Biochem.* Nov 2011.

The researchers also found a strong correlation between autism and the MMR vaccine, which they surmised might be due to an increased sensitivity to acetaminophen, a commonly prescribed fever medication.[32]

And there's more….

A landmark study by Professor Gayle Delong, published in the *Journal of Toxicology and Environmental Health* (Part A) in 2011, gives further support to the hypothesis that aluminum in vaccines causes autism in susceptible children.

In this study, Professor Delong analyzed "the relationship between the proportion of children who received the recommended vaccines by two years of age and the presence of autism or speech or language impairment in *each* U.S. state from 2001 and 2007."

What she found was startling.

"The higher the proportion of children receiving the complete battery of vaccinations by two years of age the greater the prevalence of autism and disorders of speech and language," she discovered. And the results were statistically significant.[33]

For every 1 percent increase in the vaccination rate, there was a concomitant increase of 680 children with autism and speech and communication disorders!

In her analysis, Professor Delong controlled for family income and ethnicity. "Neither parental behavior nor access to care affected the results," she maintained, and "vaccination proportions were not significantly related (statistically) to any other disability or to the number of pediatricians in a U.S. state."[34]

She concluded that, "The results suggest that although mercury has been removed from many vaccines, other culprits may link vaccines to autism," and she recommended further study in this regard.[35]

One of those "culprits" may most certainly be aluminum!

Since the number of vaccinations containing mercury decreased after 2000, while at the same time the number of vaccines containing aluminum increased, and since aluminum is a confirmed neurotoxin that dramatically increases the neurotoxicity of mercury, it is logical to look closer at this substance in regard to the persistent autism epidemic that has continued into the current millennium.

In a previously reviewed study (see Chapter 15), 39 confirmed autistic children 3-9 years of age were given urine tests for toxic metals both before (baseline) and after a chelation challenge using DMSA as the chelating agent.[36]

The purpose of the study, it may be recalled, was to see whether chelating these children with a *once-a-month* DMSA dose for a period of 6 months would improve their neurological and social functioning and reduce their toxic metal burden, and indeed, DMSA was found to be effective in removing cadmium, mercury, and lead; in reducing abnormal behaviors; and in improving communication and socialization skills.

In addition, the researchers discovered "There was a significant positive correlation between baseline urine aluminum & body use, taste, smell, touch responses, and total Childhood Autism Rating Scale (CARS) scores."

In other words, the more aluminum found in the urine at baseline, the more severe the autism.

"This indicates that a higher aluminum exposure is associated with increased impairment in these body functions and higher total CARS (scores)," the researchers maintained.

---

32   Seneff, S. et al. "Empirical Data Confirm Autism Symptoms Related to Aluminum and Acetaminophen Exposure." *Entropy.* 2012; 14(11): 2227-53.
33   Ibid. abstract.
34   Ibid.
35   Delong, G.A. "Positive Association Found between Autism Prevalence and Childhood Vaccine Uptake across the U.S. Population." *J Tox Env Hlth.* 2011; 74(14):903-16. Doi: 10.1080/15287394/2011.573736.
36   Blaucok-Busch, Eleanor et al. "Efficacy of DMSA Therapy in a Sample of Arab Children with Autistic Spectrum Disorder." *Maedica: A Journal of Clinical Medicine.* Vol. 7. No.3, 2012.

"Since aluminum is a known neurotoxin, there is no safe level."
Seneff, S. et al. *"Empirical Data Confirm Autism Symptoms Related to Aluminum and Acetaminophen Exposure."*

Entropy 2012; 14(11): 2231.

How Does Aluminum Get from the Vaccine Site to the Brain?

A recent well-done study by Zakir Kahn and associates has added to our knowledge of how the aluminum adjuvant (alum) in vaccines moves from the injection site into the brain.

Using fluorescent tracers, the researchers discovered that aluminum in test mice follows a particular indirect path to the brain by way of the local lymph nodes initially, and then through the lymph system to the thoracic duct, which connects to the bloodstream.

From the bloodstream, the aluminum was found to go primarily to the spleen. From the spleen, the aluminum then re-enters the bloodstream, crosses the blood brain barrier, and enters the brain. The blood brain barrier is known to be *suboptimal* in newborns, making them *more susceptible* to neurological toxicity than older children or young adults.

This passage from the injection site to the brain takes time, but the process is sped up dramatically by a particular immune system stimulating substance (a cytokine) called CCL2.

CCL2 "recruits" a variety of immune cells (monocytes, dendritic cells, and others). Some people with certain genetic variants produce larger amounts of CCL2 than are optimal. These people are likely to be at greater risk for aluminum neuro-toxicity, and for them, "even small amounts of injected alum can be disastrous."

The study authors conclude that, "It is likely that good tolerance to alum may be challenged by a variety of factors including overimmunization, blood-brain-barrier immaturity, individual susceptibility factors, and aging that may be associated with both subtle blood-brain barrier alterations and a progressive increase of CCL2 production."[37]

Conclusion: We conclude that more than sufficient evidence exists to implicate the aluminum adjuvants used in many childhood vaccines as causative agents in promoting autism and related disorders in susceptible babies. We need to get aluminum, mercury, and all neurotoxins out of vaccines immediately.

ALUMINUM PROMOTES IRON AND COPPER MEDIATED OXIDATIVE STRESS

"It is known that aluminum displaces iron from its normal carrier proteins, transferrin and ferritin. This causes free iron to accumulate in the blood and brain, leading to high levels of oxidative stress.
"It has also been shown that aluminum worsens the oxidative stress caused by copper in the brain."[38]

— Blaylock

"I take a very low view of 'climates of opinion.'"

— C.S. Lewis

---

37   Khan, Zakir et al. "Slow CCL2-dependent translocation of biopersistent particles from muscle to brain." *Biomed Central Medicine.* doi: 10.1186/1741-7015-11-99.
38   Blaylock, Russell. *The Blaylock Wellness Report.* Nov 2010 Vol. 7, No. 11; and Becaria, A. et al. *J Alzheimer's Disease.* 2003; 5:31-38.

Chapter 27
Vaccines and the Vaccine Schedule

"Every dogma has its day."
— Anonymous

H ow Effective and *Safe Are the Vaccines Given to Babies and Children?*
The DPT and DTAP Vaccines

The DPT and DTaP vaccines given to babies at 2, 4, 6, and 18 months, and again at 4-5 years of age are designed to protect the child against three bacterial diseases: pertussis, diphtheria, and tetanus.

Pertussis (whooping cough) is a contagious, debilitating disease that manifests as a chronic cough, respiratory distress, and fever. Symptoms may take months to resolve. Pertussis can affect people of all ages and is especially devastating to young infants. The lung infection and unremitting cough interrupt sleep and can lead to difficulty in getting enough oxygen, which can cause convulsions and even death. The usual organism that causes pertussis is a bacterium called Bordatella pertussis, but a related bacterium known as Bordatella parapertussis may also cause whooping cough symptoms.

Tetanus (lockjaw) is a potentially fatal condition caused by a toxin released from the bacterium Clostridium tetani. Clostridial spores generally gain entry into the body via contaminated wounds. The Clostridial toxin causes painful muscle spasms (tetany) that can affect the jaw and muscle groups throughout the body.

Diphtheria is another bacterially-caused disease. The bacterium (Corynebacterium diphtheria) infects the throat and causes a pseudo-membrane to form with associated pain, fever, and swelling of the tonsils and local lymph nodes. The skin may also be affected, and 20 percent of diphtheria patients have heart involvement (myocarditis). One in ten gets a peripheral neuropathy (numbness, tingling, and pain in the extremities). Fatalities can occur.

The Pertussis Vaccine

The first vaccine for pertussis was developed at the beginning of the twentieth century; however, it was not widely used until the 1930s and '40s. This vaccine was made up of components of the entire organism ("whole cell"), and in 1946, it was combined with vaccines for tetanus and diphtheria to make the DPT shot (which contained thimerosal and aluminum). This immunization caused serious side effects in many, especially from the pertussis component. In 1981, Japan switched to an allegedly less troublesome *acellular* form of pertussis vaccine (DTaP) and the U.S. followed in 1996.

The DTaP vaccine administered at 2, 4, 6, and 18 months, and again at 4-5 years of age contains antigens from only one of the organisms (Bordatella pertussis) that cause whooping cough (pertussis). Also found in this triple vaccine are an inactivated toxin (a toxoid) from the organism (Corynebacterium diphtheria) that causes diphtheria plus inactivated cultures from the organism (Clostridia tetani) that causes tetanus.

Potentially troublesome components in this vaccine include *aluminum* (170 mcg), a "trace" of *thimerosal*, plus *gelatin*, and *formaldehyde*. GlaxoSmithKline makes a five in one shot (Pediarix*) that combines the DTaP with inactivated polio and hepatitis B viruses. The GSK vaccine has even more *aluminum* (850 mcg!) plus antibiotics *neomycin, polymyxin B, and the toxin formaldehyde.*

Does the DTaP Immunization Cause Fewer Side Effects than the DPT?

Safety: According to a 1987 study, the acellular DTaP vaccine decreased "mild" reactions like fever and pain by 60 percent as compared to the whole cell DPT shot, but *both promoted similar rates of severe reactions.*[1]

A later Swedish study confirmed the finding of less severe mild reactions with the DTaP; however, the scientists also noted that severe reactions like loss of muscle tone (hypotonia) and signs of brain inflammation (encephalitis) were noted in *1 out of every 106 DTaP vaccinated babies.*[2]

Table 27.1. lists studies that highlight these *serious* side effects, including neurological damage, seizures, ADHD, developmental delay, asthma, and sudden death.

Table 27.1. Pertussis, DT & DPT Vaccine Side Effects[3]

Journal	Year	Side Effects Found
NEUROLOGICAL-27 studies		
JAMA	1933	Neurological damage, convulsions, death
Pediatrics	1948	Coma, neurological damage, retardation, Cerebral palsy, death
Lancet	1950	After DT shot: mental retardation and paralysis in one child
J.of Pediatrcs	1955	Child with convulsions and death within hour of a DPT shot
J.of Pediatrics	1957	Myoclonic seizures and developmental delay after DPT shot
BMJ	1958	107 cases of neurological damage after pertussis vaccination
Arch. Dis. Ch.	1974	This study linked the DPT vaccine with mental retardation
DMW	1974	German study documented 59 cases of convulsions after pertussis vacc.
Lancet	1977	160 DPT reactions; 65 had ADHD, convulsions and mental defects
Devel.Biol Std	1979	Persistent screaming, shock, neurological damage, and death in 13.
BMJ	1981	DPT likely to have caused hospitalization of children with neurol. damage
Pediatrics	1981	DPT: more screaming, sleepiness & seizures than controls (DT injected)

---

1   Noble, G.R. et al. *JAMA*. 1987; 257:351-356.

2   Blennow, M. et al. *Pediatrics*. 1989; 84: 62-27.

3   *From Neil Z. Miller "Vaccine Safety Manual"; pp 91 ff and references page 319 ff.

Journal	Year	Side Effects Found
Lancet	1983	Greater risk of seizures after DPT
BMJ	1993	10 yrs. post DPT-children more likely to have neur. adverse effects
Misc.	1967-1993	At least 13 other studies link DPT vacc. with neurological side effects.
ASTHMA-5 studies		
JAMA	1994	Links DPT shot with 5 X higher risk of asthma
Epidemiology	1997	Links pertussis vaccine with asthma (1 in 5 children)
Thorax	1998	140 percent increased risk for asthma associated with pertussis vaccine
JMPT	2000	Increased risk for asthma in those given DPT or tetanus vaccine
JACI	2008	If vaccinated on schedule—2X risk to get asthma as those w. delayed DPT
DEATH-8 studies SIDS = Sudden Infant Death Syndrome		
J of Pediatrics	1982	DPT likely cause of sudden infant death in Tennessee Study
Neurology	1982	70 percent of babies who died of SIDS had pertussis vacc. within 21 days prior
J of Pediatrics	1983	DPT likely to cause sudden infant death in some children
JADC	1987	Death of twin babies shortly after they received the DPT shot
AJ of Pub Hlth	1987	Sudden infant death much higher within three days of DPT shot
JAMA	1987	37 cases of sudden death following pertussis vacc. in Japan (1970-74)
Pediatrics	1988	After Japan moved 1st DPT to 2 yrs of age, babies stopped dying of SIDS
Am J of Epidem	1992	8X greater risk of death within 3 days of DTaP shot

The Aborigine Cot Deaths (SIDS) Mystery

In the 1960s and '70s, Australian health officials began a mass vaccination program of the indigenous aborigine population. A good many of the babies so inoculated were somewhat malnourished, and as many as *1 in 2 died shortly after their immunizations* against pertussis and other diseases.[4]

The puzzling cause of these sudden infant deaths was discovered by local physician Archie Kalokerinos. He was able to prevent these "cot deaths" by giving the babies a small amount of vitamin C (100 mg/month of age) prior to their immunizations. Apparently, many of the aborigine babies were vitamin C deficient, and the combination of the immunization and the vitamin C deficiency was responsible for the "cot deaths."[5]

The implication of these findings is that it would be a good idea to supplement babies with vitamin C prior to their receiving a DPT or other immunization.

Efficacy: Death rates from whooping cough in the U.S. and Great Britain had declined dramatically in the years

---

4   Miller, N.Z. *Vaccine Safety Manual.* p. 93.
5   Ibid.

preceding the introduction of the pertussis vaccine, and they continued to decrease after its introduction in the late 1930s.[6]

It is not clear to what extent the decline in incidence of pertussis over the years may be ascribed to the effectiveness of the vaccine or to what extent immunity is maintained after either a DPT or a DTaP inoculation. It is clear, however, that both the efficacy and the endurance of these immunizations are far from optimal. See Table 27.2. for documentation of these assertions.

Local epidemics of pertussis are common *and occur almost yearly* in the U.S. (and worldwide), often in highly immunized populations. In the past decade, multiple outbreaks have occurred in Vermont, California, Ohio, Colorado, Pennsylvania, and Texas, for example.[7]

Pertussis continues to be a concern despite the high immunization rate among children and teens. In 2012, 42,000 whooping cough cases were recorded by the CDC, "a fifty-year high." Most of these were in young children followed by young teens.

One possible explanation for this resurgence of pertussis in highly immunized populations is that the acellular pertussis vaccine currently in use, while reducing or eliminating symptoms of whooping cough in many, does not prevent the colonization or spread of the organism. The original pertussis vaccine did prevent this spread, however.[8]

In other words, individuals who are immunized with the DTaP vaccine and infected with Bordatella pertussis bacteria may be asymptomatic, but they are still capable of spreading the infection to others.

Why Is the Acellular Pertussis Vaccine in the DTaP Relatively Ineffective?

The answer isn't clear. The now largely discarded whole cell (DPT) vaccine is likely more antigenic (more likely to induce immunity) because it contained particular antigens that induce immunity to pertussis that may not be present in the acellular (DTaP) vaccine. Unfortunately, these additional antigens also provoked more severe reactions.

Another possibility is that some of the whooping cough cases are the result of mutated pertussis organisms that lack a particular antigen (pertactin) found in the acellular pertussis vaccine. That was true in over 90 percent of the sampled organisms in a Philadelphia outbreak in 2011-2012 as reported in the *New England Journal of Medicine*.[9]

It may be that some cases of pertussis are caused by related organisms, like B. parapertussis, for example, which none of the pertussis vaccines are designed to protect against.

Whatever the reason, it is clear that the DTaP and DTP vaccines carry substantial risks, are not as effective or as enduring as would be desired, and need to be improved upon if whooping cough outbreaks are to be curtailed. Serious consideration needs to be given to excluding harmful substances from all vaccines and honestly weighing the benefits and risks of vaccination and making this information available to all so that intelligent informed consent can be obtained prior to inoculation.

The Diptheria Vaccine

As was the case with whooping cough, the death rate from diphtheria declined dramatically (by 88 percent) in the U.S. in the first three decades of the twentieth century, and this occurred *before* the introduction of the diphtheria vaccine.[10]

---

6   Cherry, J.D. *Curr Probl Pediatr.* Feb 1984; 14(2):1-78.

7   www.cdc.gov/pertussis/outbreaks/index.html

8   Wafgel, Jason et al. "Acellular pertussis vaccines protect against disease but fail to prevent infection and transmission in a nonhuman primate model." *PNAS.* 11-25-13. Published online.

9   http://www.clinicaladvisor.com/pertussis-mutations-may-explain-whooping-cough-epidemic/article/279440/

10   Dublin, J. et al. N.Y. Metropol. Life Ins. Co. *Twenty-Five years of Health Progress.* (1937): p. 56.

Table 27.2. Efficacy of DPT or DTaP Immunizations in Preventing Pertussis[11, 12]

YEAR	Journal	Claimed Efficacy
1988	Pediatrics	63-91 percent
1988	Lancet	54-64 percent (Evaluation of 2 different DtaP vaccines)-placebo controlled study
1989	J of Pediatrics	40-45 percent
1997	J of Ped Inf Dis	80 percent
		Actual Efficacy
1965	Pub. Hlth Rprt	5 percent in Michigan outbreak after complete series of DPT vaccinations (Lambert H)
1979	Pediatrics	5 percent just a few years after complete series of DPT vaccinations (Pichichero, et al.)
1985	USDHHS 20th C.	46 percent of all reported cases (to CDC) were adequately immunized to pertussis.
1986	Vacc. Bulletin	In Kansas outbreak of pertussis, 90 percent were adequately immunized.
1993	NEJM July7	In Ohio outbreak of pertussis, 82 percent of affected children were "highly immunized."
1993	J Clin Microbiol	62 percent of pertussis cases were adequately immunized in a Canadian outbreak.
1997	MMWR: 9-5-97	74 percent of children <4yo with pertussis in VT outbreak were up to date on their shots.
1997	MMWR: 9-5-97	68 percent of all children 7-18 yo in Vermont outbreak had 4-5 DTaP inoculations.
2000	Emer Inf Dis	Pertussis endemic in Netherlands in 1996 despite "high vaccine coverage."
2003	Euro Surveillance	Pertussis outbreak in Cyprus in 2003 despite 98 percent vaccination rate.
2006	Israel Med Ass J	16 fold increase in pertussis between 1998 & 2004 despite excellent coverage.
2006	Can Med Ass J	DTaP not as effective as DPT and may not protect young children (Vickers, D. et al.)
2007	Clin Inf Diseases	5 yrs after 5th DTaP booster shot—low or no antibody to pertussis toxin in teens.
2012	VT Dpt of Hlth	VT pertussis outbreak mainly in vaccinated children despite c. 90 percent vacc. rate
2012	NEJM (9-13)	In an analysis of the California 2010 pertussis outbreak it was found that "protection from disease after a fifth dose of DTaP among children who had received only DTaP vaccines was relatively short-lived and waned substantially each year."

Starting in 1896, an antitoxin to the diphtheria organism's secretions was available, but it was made from horse serum, and it could and did cause severe anaphylactic reactions in many recipients. Some individuals died within minutes of receiving the antitoxin.

11   Data from Miller, NZ *"Vaccine Safety Manual;* pp 108-109
12   Klein NP, et al *N Engl J Med* 2012; 367:1012-1019

In 1929, 90 percent of the doctors surveyed by the American Medical Association opposed the use of the antitoxin, not only on the grounds that the reactions to the substance were both too severe and too frequent, but also because the diphtheria antitoxin didn't even seem to work in preventing disease progression.[13]

A new (toxoid based) diphtheria vaccine was introduced to the U.S. in 1920, but it was not widely used until it was combined with the tetanus and pertussis vaccines in the 1940s (to make the DPT, DT, and later the DTaP immunizations).

In 1938, Dr. D.C. Okell admitted in *The Lancet*, "If we…told the whole truth (about the ineffectiveness of and the dangers of the diphtheria vaccination) it is doubtful whether the public would submit to inoculation."[14]

Diphtheria vaccine was compulsory in German-occupied France in the early 1940s, yet diphtheria prevalence actually increased after its introduction from 14,000 cases in 1941 to 47,000 just two years later. In contrast, Sweden did not immunize against diphtheria at all during that time period, yet the disease almost disappeared there.[15]

In diphtheria outbreaks in Chicago in 1969, over 50 percent of the cases had been partially or completely immunized prior to their contracting the disease. In still another outbreak, 61 percent had been adequately immunized.[16]

There were outbreaks of diphtheria in Eastern Europe and in some of the former Soviet states in the mid-1990s, and many of those contracting the disease were fully immunized.[17]

Both the Food and Drug Administration (FDA) in 1975 and 1999 and the *British Medical Journal* in 2000 criticized the effectiveness of the diphtheria vaccine and booster. The FDA said, "diphtheria may occur in vaccinated individuals (and that)…the permanence of immunity induced by the toxoid…is open to question." The *British Medical Journal* found the adult DT booster shot to be "insufficient to obtain adequate protection." In 1999, the FDA found the diphtheria vaccines given to children in 1998 were "too weak to protect against diphtheria."[18]

The prevalence of diphtheria in the U.S. since the 1990s has been negligible. Diphtheria can be spread by inhalation and by contact with the skin ("cutaneous"). After 1979, the definition of diphtheria came to mean only diphtheria spread by inhalation. This resulted in a dramatic (and factitious) 95 percent drop in cases the following year, and the number of cases has remained low since that time. During the 11 years between 1995 and 2005, only 14 cases of diphtheria were reported in the U.S. That's less than two cases per year in the entire country![19]

The Tetanus Vaccine

Tetanus is, thankfully, a very rare disease. The incidence has declined from about 200 cases per 100,000 wounds in the mid-1800s to 0.44 cases per 100,000 wounds in the 1940s. The decline is likely due to better wound hygiene. From 1995 to 2005, the U.S. was averaging 35 cases and four deaths per year, primarily in those over the age of 50.[20]

A vaccine made from tetanus toxoid was manufactured in 1933. It was combined in the 1940s with diphtheria toxoid and the pertussis vaccine to make the DPT vaccine. The DTaP vaccine has taken the place of the DPT now for children under five years of age.

Safety: Reactions to this vaccine are *common* and can be *severe*. The less severe side effects include local pain,

---

13   *JAMA*. March 16, 1929.

14   *Lancet*. Jan 1938.

15   Elben. "Vaccination Condemned." (LA Better Life Research). Data taken from government statistics in N.Y. and Mass, and *The Vaccination Inquirer* (Sept. 1947).

16   Mendelsohn, Robert S. *How to Raise a Healthy Child in Spite of Your Doctor*. New York, NY: Ballantine Books, 987. p 245.

17   Hardy, I.R. et al. *Lancet*. 1996; 347; 1739-44, *and* Prospero, E. et al. *Europ J Epidem* 1997; 13:527-534.

18   FDA Nov 20-21, 1975, *and* Vellinga, A. *BMJ*. 1-22-00; 320:217, *and* www.cnn.com CNN Interactive. Jan 29, 1999.

19   CDC; *MMWR* April 6, 2001 *and Pink Book* Sept 13, 2006.

20   Miller, N.Z. *Vaccine Safety Manual for Concerned Families and Health Practitioners*. 2nd ed. Santa Fe, NM: New Atlantean Press, 2011. p. 55.

swelling, fever, and chills. Serious documented side effects include *neurological and paralytic disorders, arthritis, anaphylactic shock, neuropathies, and death.* In one study, 8 out of every 10 subjects receiving the combined diphtheria-tetanus (DT) vaccine had local reactions and *a quarter of the subjects experienced systemic reactions.*[21]

Neurological disorders that follow the tetanus shot include *convulsions, neuropathies* (pain in peripheral nerves), *myelitis, brachial neuritis, and ascending paralysis.*

A 1981 study revealed that the tetanus booster vaccinations caused the ratio of two important immune cells, the T-helper and T-suppressor lymphocytes, to fall below normal in a manner that parallels the abnormal ratio seen in the disease AIDS.[22] *This suggests that the tetanus booster suppresses the body's ability to combat infection for a period of time.*

The injection of tetanus toxoid induces the formation of antibodies to that substance, and it was found in the 1980s that too frequent injections of tetanus toxoid could cause the levels of antibody to tetanus toxoid to skyrocket. This, in turn, could and did lead to allergic hypersensitivity reactions, autoimmune diseases (like lupus), and high fever (an "Arthus" reaction).[23]

The tetanus vaccine can cause *joint inflammation* and *rheumatoid arthritis* in some. This fact was brought out in a 1989 study in the *Journal of Rheumatic Disease.*[24]

Efficacy: After the initial series of five DPT shots (at 2, 4, 6, and 18 months, and at age 5 years), it is recommended to get a booster tetanus shot (usually combined with diphtheria toxoid) every ten years. It isn't clear that this recommendation is based on good science, however. Tetanus has occurred in fully vaccinated people, even in one case in a subject with tetanus antitoxin antibody levels twenty times higher than were thought necessary to provide protection against this organism.[25]

Elderly people do not respond to tetanus toxoid immunization as well as younger individuals do. Their response is less intense and of shorter duration. *Vitamin E* supplementation may help in this regard. Older subjects who received the tetanus immunization after ingesting 200 mg of vitamin E daily for more than six months produced more antibodies to tetanus toxin than did the control population.[26]

The Polio Vaccines

Polio is a disease caused by a virus that normally just infects the intestinal tract. Most (95 percent) infected individuals exhibit few or no symptoms. Others may have a fever, sore throat, joint pains, vomiting, and headache. In rare cases (1 out of 1000), the virus can infect the nervous system, causing weakness or paralysis. If the respiratory muscles are affected, the disease can be life-threatening. It is spread by fecally-contaminated hands via ingested foods, water, or even airborne droplets.[27]

Even in cases where paralysis occurs, there is usually a full recovery, although this may take months or even years. Symptoms, like muscle weakness and pain, sometimes return after years of being symptom-free. This condition is called "Post-Polio Syndrome," and occurs in up to 50 percent of those previously affected.

For some reason, susceptibility to polio increases if the individual has had an injection (in the muscle or under the skin) of a vaccine or even an antibiotic. This has been documented in a number of studies. In one of these studies, published in the *Journal of Infectious Diseases* in 1992, children who received the DPT shot were significantly more likely to contract poliomyelitis for 30 days following the injection than were the controls. This may be due to the tetanus vaccine's

---

21   *PDR.* 2001.

22   Eihl, M. et al. *NEJM* 11-22-81:1307-1313.

23   CDC. "Adverse Events Following Immunization." *MMWR.* 1985; 34: 43-47. *and* CDC. *MMWR.* 1985; 34: 405f, *and* CDC. *MMWR.* 1996; 45: 22f.

24   Jawad, A.S. et al. "Immunization Triggering Rheumatoid Arthritis." Vol. 48. p. 174.

25   Miller, N.Z. *Vaccine Safety Manual, and* Katz, K.C. et al. *CMAJ.* 2000 163(5); 571-573.

26   Burns, E.A. et al. *J of Geriatr Ontology.* 48(6); B231-B236 *and* Meydani, S.N. et al. *JAMA* 1997; 277(17): 1398-1399.

27   Miller, N.Z. *Vaccine Safety Manual.*

effects in diminishing the T-helper/T-suppressor ratio and, thereby, increasing susceptibility to viral infections.[28]

Nutrition also plays a key role in one's susceptibility to polio. Studies show that *a higher incidence of polio occurs in countries that consume the most sugar.* The phosphoric acid in soda has been shown to cause a loss of calcium from bones, and calcium deficiency is associated with increased risk for polio as well.[29]

People tend to drink more soft drinks and eat more sweets like ice cream in the summer months when the weather is hot, and that is when polio incidence appears to increase. Dr. Benjamin Sandler found a link between the consumption of sugars and starches and the risk for polio. In 1949, he warned the residents of North Carolina to decrease their consumption of sweets and starchy foods, and they did. Carolinians decreased their consumption of sugar by 90 percent and the prevalence of polio declined from 2,498 cases in 1948 to just 229 cases in 1949.[30]

Unfortunately, the Rockefeller Milk Trust joined forces with soft drink manufacturers to dismiss Dr. Sandler's findings as a fluke. By the next year, the sale of sugary foods was "back to normal" and the rate of polio climbed accordingly.[31]

A 1973 study supported the link between sugar and increased risk for infection by showing that sugar inhibited the ability of certain immune cells to ingest (phagocytize: FA-go-sit-eyes) bacteria. This inhibition lasts for many hours.[32]

Safety: The vaccine in use today is the killed-virus injection, a variant of the original Salk vaccine, which actually caused polio in many and had to be withdrawn.[33]

The oral, live (attenuated), and popular polio vaccine developed by Dr. Sabin has been replaced because of its ability to cause poliomyelitis in some immunized individuals. Ironically, the oral vaccine itself was the principal cause of all the polio seen in the U.S. since 1961.[34]

A *five-year* analysis of the VAERS (Vaccine Adverse Event Reporting System) database revealed "13,641 reports of adverse events following the use of the oral polio vaccine," including *6,364 emergency room visits, 540 deaths*, and an average of eight cases of polio per year.[35] Keep in mind that the VAERS database greatly under-reports adverse events.

African green monkey kidney cells were used to develop both the Salk and Sabin polio vaccines. Unbeknownst to both Salk and Sabin, those kidney cells were infected with a cancer-causing virus, later identified as simian virus 40 (SV-40), which was resistant to the formaldehyde that Salk had used to kill the polio virus in his vaccine.

So *both* the injectable and the oral vaccines were contaminated with this harmful live virus, and estimates are that up to 100 million Americans, as well as many others around the world, were exposed to SV-40, which has now been identified in certain bone cancers, brain cancers, lung cancers, and leukemias. And the incidence of these cancers appears to be higher in those exposed to this virus from their polio immunizations than in those not so exposed.[36]

Worse, it is likely that a mother who received an SV-40 contaminated polio vaccine could pass that virus on to her offspring. Indeed, "Children of mothers who received the Salk vaccine between 1959 and 1965 had brain tumors at a rate thirteen times greater than mothers who did not receive those polio shots."[37]

African green monkey kidney cells also harbor many other viruses, including the simian immunodeficiency virus, which is very similar to the AIDS virus and may be a variant. It is possible that one or more of the original polio vac-

---

28   Ibid. p. 47.
29   Ibid. p. 47-48.
30   Ibid. p. 48
31   Ibid.
32   "Role of Sugars in Human Neutrophilic Phagocytosis." *American Journal of Clinical Nutrition*, 26: November, 1973. p. 1880-84.
33   Miller, N.Z. *Vaccine Safety Manual*. p. 50.
34   Ibid.
35   Ibid.
36   Ibid. p. 56.
37   Ibid. p. 56.

cines may have even played a key role in the spread of the AIDS epidemic.[38]

According to microbiologist Dr. Howard Urnovitz, as many as *26 monkey viruses may have contaminated the original Salk vaccine.*[39] Another of these was the *respiratory syncytial virus*, which causes severe lung disease (bronchiolitis) in many infants.[40]

The current injectable (IPV) killed-virus immunization can cause an ascending paralysis (much like polio) called Guillain-Barrè syndrome, and infant death has been temporally associated with this immunization. Today's polio vaccines are still manufactured using either monkey kidney cells (U.S.) or human diploid cells (Canada) and contain formaldehyde as a preservative as well as two antibiotics (neomycin & streptomycin).

Efficacy: The live virus vaccine is still used in many parts of the world today because it is less expensive than the injectable, killed vaccine, and because it is contagious. It can spread attenuated polio virus from the immunized individual to others who are not immunized and thereby confer "herd immunity."

However, the three weakened viruses in the oral vaccine can mutate (recombine with each other) to form new and more dangerous versions of the virus that are now capable of causing paralytic polio. This appears to have been the cause of sporadic outbreaks in many countries around the world in recent years, even in children who have received as many as 10 vaccine doses.[41]

It is a commonly held belief that the polio immunizations are highly effective and are the reason why polio has been virtually eradicated in the U.S., and that appears to be the case. The hope is that by massively immunizing the world's population, we may be able to eradicate completely this menace to our health. That is indeed a noble goal. But if we are at the same time injecting other viruses found in the kidney cells (or diploid cells) used to grow these viruses for the vaccines, shouldn't we first identify these potential and real risks?

However, studies show that the polio *death rate* was decreasing (except during and shortly after WWII) prior to and after the introduction of the polio vaccines in both Great Britain and the U.S.

It isn't clear, therefore, that the vaccines contributed significantly to the continued decline after their introduction. It is likely, however, that a good diet, low in refined carbohydrates and sugars, plus good hygiene, might dramatically decrease our susceptibility to polio viruses.

WHO IS MINDING THE STORE?

"Who's minding the store when the FDA has allowed drug companies to produce vaccines grown on contaminated monkey kidneys?"

— *Barbara Lee Fisher*

"Half the people in this country are baby boomers and were born between the years 1941 and 1961 and are at high risk for having been exposed to polio vaccines contaminated with monkey viruses."

— *Dr. Howard B. Urnovitz, microbiologist*

Scientists in 1992 discovered how to synthesize the polio virus in a test tube, so eradication of this virus cannot be entirely certain and is likely impossible, because the polio genome is known.[42]

---

38   Kyle, W.S. "Simian Retroviruses, polio vaccine, and origin of AIDS." *Lancet.* 1992; 339:600-601.
39   Ibid. p.62.
40   Miller, N.Z. *Vaccine Safety Manual.* p. 61.
41   Ibid. 62-63.
42   "The test-tube synthesis of a chemical called poliovirus. The simple synthesis of a virus has far-reaching societal implications." *EMBO Rep.* 2006 Jul. 7 Spec No: S3-9. PMID: 16819446.

Influenza Vaccines

Influenza is the name given to a highly contagious respiratory illness caused by three families of constantly mutating viruses (A, B, and C). These viruses vary in their ability to spread, as well as in the severity of the disease they promote.

Most sufferers have congested noses, coughs, fevers, muscle aches, and other pains and decreased appetites. The illness may last anywhere from a few days to a week or more. In vulnerable populations, like the elderly, infants, or the infirm, complications, like bacterial pneumonia, may occur, which in some instances have resulted in death.

Natural immunity to influenza viruses is difficult to maintain as novel mutated strains appear from one year to the next, and immunity to one strain may not protect against another.

Currently, five licensed "flu" vaccines are available that are injected, and one (FluMist) that is sprayed into the nose. The problem with designing a flu vaccine is that it is not entirely possible to predict which varieties of flu viruses will be causing concerns the following year, and mistakes have been made in the past in this regard.

The manufacture of these influenza vaccines entails the inoculation of the chosen viruses into live chicken embryos (eggs), and then, after an appropriate incubation period, killing the viruses with formaldehyde. *Thimerosal* is the preservative, generally at *25 mcg mercury per dose*, in the multi-dose vials. Other potentially troublesome additives (like MSG and gelatin) are often also present.

Safety: The "flu shot" is famous for causing symptoms that mimic the disease itself. Pain at the injection site, body aches, chills, fever, and malaise are commonly reported side effects. These usually abate after several days, but not in everyone.

Safety and efficacy testing for these yearly immunizations has not been required by the FDA, which is a major concern. In 1976, the CDC told Americans to fear the "deadly swine flu epidemic" predicted for that year, and many were immunized. The epidemic never materialized, but hundreds of those immunized came down with a paralytic condition known as the Guillain-Barré syndrome, and many died or were left with permanent disabilities. Thousands of lawsuits were filed and billions were paid by the government in compensation.[43]

A 2005 *Lancet* review of relevant influenza vaccine studies in children revealed that not only were *no adequate safety studies done*, but there was good evidence that the vaccine manufacturers systematically "suppressed safety data" in this regard.[44]

"FluMist'" is a live, albeit attenuated, influenza virus vaccine that is given nasally, and in those with weakened immune systems may actually cause full blown influenza symptoms. It was shown in a large study that FluMist' was associated with 'a statistically significant increase in asthma or reactive airway disease' in children less than five years of age, and up to 9 percent of the babies who wheezed required hospitalization.[45]

In addition to paralysis and asthma, other serious side effects likely to have been caused by the "flu shot" include *brain swelling and damage (encephalitis), muscle and nerve damage, and death.*

Deaths from the influenza virus itself are uncommon, and when they occur, they are generally in the elderly.[46] It is not clear how many deaths and long-term side effects the vaccines themselves cause.

Efficacy: The CDC admits that flu "vaccine effectiveness varies from year to year, depending on the degree of similarity between" the vaccine strains and circulating strains of the virus. As has been mentioned, the CDC sometimes errs in its predictions and the expected flu strains don't materialize. This happened in the 1994/1995 1997/1998, 2003/2004 and 2014/2015 flu seasons.[47]

---

43   Miller, N.Z. *Vaccine Safety Manual*. p. 66.
44   Jefferson, T. et al. *Lancet* 2005; 365 (Feb 26): 773f.
45   Miller, N.Z. *Vaccine Safety Manual*. p. 67.
46   CDC Natl Vital Statistic Reports
47   Miller, N.Z. Ibid. p. 71-72 *and* CDC.

Effectiveness of Flu Vaccine in Children

Although the CDC and the American Academy of Pediatrics recommend influenza vaccine be given to children as young as 6 months of age, a large review of *all* the studies done up to 2004 revealed that there was *no evidence that the flu vaccine was effective in children under the age of two years.* Indeed, the efficacy was the same as that of a placebo! The flu vaccines did not reduce mortality, hospital admissions, serious complications, or community transmission of influenza.[48]

In a 2006 report, 51 studies involving 260,000 children were analyzed and the researchers found that in children older than 2 years of age, the flu vaccine was just 33-36 percent effective, similar to that expected from a placebo. The lead author stated that, "We just cannot understand how you can vaccinate millions of small children in the absence of convincing scientific evidence that the vaccines make any difference."[49]

Another children's study published in 2008 came to similar conclusions. In this study, the "flu" vaccines were not shown to reduce influenza-related doctor or hospital visits.[50]

Effectiveness of Influenza Vaccines in Healthy Adults

The Cochrane Collaboration researchers reviewed 25 vaccine efficacy studies in healthy adults under 65 years of age and concluded the *vaccines were ineffective.* They "did not affect hospital stay, time off from work, or death from influenza or its complications," and concluded that "universal immunization of healthy adults is not supported" by the data.[51]

Effectiveness of Influenza Vaccines in the Elderly

Those same researchers also analyzed 62 of the best studies on the efficacy of influenza vaccines in an elderly population and again concluded that the vaccines were of little or no help. *For those living in the community, the vaccines did not protect against influenza or prevent pneumonia.* For those living in a *group home*, the vaccines were minimally or not at all effective against the influenza virus and were only 46 percent effective in preventing pneumonia, even in years when the vaccine and circulating virus were identical.[52]

Effectiveness of Influenza Vaccines in Health Care Workers

In most of the country, health care workers who care for the aged population are required to be current on their yearly influenza immunizations. A thorough review of all the health staff vaccination program studies revealed that *immunizing health care workers to influenza is not beneficial.* Giving healthcare workers influenza immunizations does not reduce "the incidence of influenza or its complications in the elderly in institutions." In simple terms, these programs don't work![53]

Other Studies Also Show the Influenza Vaccine Program to Be Remarkably Ineffective

A 2005 study showed that over a twenty-year period, as immunization rates increased in the elderly, there was no corresponding decline in influenza or pneumonia-related deaths. The authors concluded that vaccination benefits were "overestimated."[54] A 2006 U.S. study found that influenza vaccination was ineffective "for preventing influenza cases, deaths or hospital admissions," and in that same year, a British study came to the same conclusion.[55]

In another investigation, researchers compared children in schools in which all students were vaccinated to influenza with children from control schools who weren't. While the *families* of the inoculated students did experience

48   Jefferson, T. et al. *Lancet.* 2005; 365 (Feb 26): 773f.
49   Alliance for Human Resource Protection www.ahrp.org.
50   Szilagyi, P.G. et al. "Influenza vaccine effectiveness among children 6 to 59 months of age during 2 influenza seasons." *Arch Ped & Adolescent Med.* 2008; 162(1): 943f.
51   Rivetti, D. et al. "Vaccines for preventing influenza in healthy adults." The Coch Collab (Cochrane Database of Systemic Reviews). 2004(3): # CD001269.
52   Rivetti, D. et al. "Vaccines for preventing influenza in the elderly." The Coch Collab (Cochrane Database of Systemic Reviews). 2006(3): #CD004876.
53   Thomas, R.E. et al. The Coch Collab (Cochrane Database of Systemic Reviews). 2006 (3); #CD005187.
54   Simonson, L. et al. *Arch Int Med.* 2005; 165: 265-272.
55   Geier, B.A. et al. *J Am Phys Surg.* 2006; 11(3):69f, *and* Jefferson, T. "Influenza Policy vs. Evidence." *BMJ.* 2006; 333:912f.

milder flu symptoms, both the *children who were vaccinated and their families had significantly higher hospitalization rates than did the control schools, and the children had significantly more symptoms of influenza post-vaccination*, including serious adverse events in four students.[56]

And it gets even worse. Children who get yearly "flu" shots appear to be *more susceptible in the future to dangerous varieties of the virus* than children who contract seasonal influenza infection itself, say researchers in a 2009 *Lancet* study.[57]

Similarly, mice vaccinated against seasonal flu strains died when exposed to alternate strains. Unvaccinated mice survived the exposure.[58]

Conclusion: The influenza vaccines appear to do more harm than good. They are ineffective in children under two and minimally or not at all effective in older children and adults, including the elderly living at home, and are only minimally beneficial in preventing pneumonia in elderly individuals who reside in group homes.

Influenza vaccines may increase the risk for asthma, neurological side effects, and even death. Repeated yearly influenza immunizations may increase the risk of getting Alzheimer's disease and more severe reactions to future virulent strains. These vaccines have not been tested for safety and efficacy, and the multidose vials contain neurotoxic mercury as thimerosal. They are also not cost-effective.[59]

If forced by law or circumstance to get an influenza immunization, it would be wise to request the single dose vial without thimerosal.

> *"Influenza vaccines are approved for use in older people despite any clinical trials demonstrating a reduction in serious outcomes."*
>
> — *Johns Hopkins scientist, Peter Doshi, Ph.D.*

Hepatitis A Vaccine

Hepatitis A is a contagious viral liver infection generally acquired by ingesting contaminated food or water; however, transmission from person to person is possible if careful hand washing is not practiced since the virus is shed in the stool. Its manifestations vary from person to person. Some get a fever, malaise, fatigue, and abdominal pains and may become jaundiced. Others, especially young children, are often asymptomatic, but may still be capable of spreading the disease. Deaths from liver failure are rare. Infection with hepatitis A virus generally provides lifetime immunity.

The CDC estimates there are about 20,000 cases per year in the U.S., most of which are unreported, and that there has been a 90 percent decline in incidence in the last twenty years. In 2005, only 208 cases of hepatitis A were reported in children less than five years of age and only fourteen of these were in children under the age of one year. Most of those infected recover completely with no after-effects, although recovery may take several months.[60]

Hepatitis A vaccine was introduced in 1995, and it is routinely given to all children over the age of one year and to adults at risk. For children, it is recommended to give two injections six months apart starting at one year of age. There are currently three vaccines available for hepatitis A: Vaqta®, Havrix®, and Twinrix®. The latter combines the hepatitis A vaccine with that for hepatitis B and is recommended for adults only. All the vaccines are made using aborted human fetal tissue (diploid fibroblasts) and *contain aluminum and formaldehyde as well as aborted fetal tissue and retrovirus remnants.*

---

56   King, Jr., J.C. et al. *NEJM*. 2006; 355:2523f.
57   Bodewes, R. et al. "Yearly Influenza Vaccinations: A Double-Edged Sword?" 9(12):784f.
58   Bodewes, R. et al. *PloSOne*. 2009; 4(5):e5538.
59   Bridges, C.B. *JAMA*. 10-4-2000; 285:1655f.
60   http://www.cdph.ca.gov/Health Info/discond/Documents/CDCHepAGeneralFactSheet.pdf

Safety: Several serious, albeit rare, conditions have been reported to occur after exposure to these vaccines. These include Guillain-Barrè paralysis, brain inflammation (encephalitis), low platelets (thrombocytopenia), cerebellar ataxia (muscle coordination difficulty), asthma, allergic reactions, and even *autism*. (See below). Common less severe side effects include fatigue, headache, pain at injection site, and loss of appetite.[61]

Efficacy: Hepatitis A was declining in the U.S. prior to the introduction of the vaccines in 1995. There were about 55,000 cases reported in the U.S. in the early 1970s and the number reported by the early 1990s declined to less than 25,000 cases per year. In 2005, only 4,488 cases were reported in the U.S.[62]

There were just 2,979 *reported* cases of hepatitis A infection in 2007 and only 1,398 in 2011, representing an *estimated* 2,800 *actual* acute cases, according to the CDC. It isn't clear to what extent the vaccine contributed to this decline, but the current rate of infection with this virus in the U.S. is currently about one case for every 100,000 individuals.[63]

Merck, the maker of Vaqta* hepatitis A vaccine, in its product handout reveals that after 6 years *children and teens who received two doses of this vaccine had suboptimal levels of protective antibody in their serum*. So we don't know how long protection from hepatitis A infection (if any) that might be attributable to this vaccine lasts, but it is obviously not for very long.

Hepatitis B Vaccine

The hepatitis B virus is another organism that infects the liver and may cause symptoms similar to those of hepatitis A. These include weakness, fever, nausea, vomiting, muscle aches, and jaundice (yellowing of the skin and the whites of the eyes) in 77 percent. And as with hepatitis A infections, there are individuals who are infected with hepatitis B who can spread the virus, but who exhibit no symptoms of the disease.

The disease runs its course over a matter of months and then abates in 95 percent of cases, and it confers *lifetime immunity*. In 5 percent of cases, the individual is unable to rid himself of the virus and the infection becomes chronic and may cause serious consequences, like liver damage in about 20 percent. Infants and young children are more prone to having a chronic infection than are older individuals, but the disease is rare in this age group. In 2005, only *four* children under four were reported to have hepatitis B! The disease is thought to cause some 4,500 deaths annually in adults.[64]

The virus in infected individuals is found in saliva, stools, semen, and blood, and it is spread through sexual contact, contaminated needle sticks, and in the case of newborns, by passage through the birth canal. According to the CDC, "The number of acute cases of hepatitis B decreased by 36 percent overall during 2007–2011, from 4,519 cases to 2,890 cases…." However, the number of reported cases vastly underestimates the actual number of cases in the U.S. About 55 percent of hepatitis B patients require hospitalization and 1.3 percent of reported cases die from the disease.[65]

The current hepatitis B vaccines were developed in the 1980s and were mandated for use in babies and children in 1991 by the Advisory Committee on Immunization Practices. They are manufactured from genetically-engineered (recombinant) yeasts, and many brands are available around the world. The two currently licensed in the U.S. are Merck's Recombivax HB*, which contains *formaldehyde* and *250-500 mcg of aluminum* and GlaxoSmithKline's Engerix-B*, which also contains aluminum plus "trace" amounts of *thimerosal*.

Safety: The initial clinical trials that established the safety of these vaccines were woefully inadequate. They evaluated only 147 healthy infants and children who were monitored *for just five days* after their inoculation. Adults who received the vaccine were also monitored for only five days after the injection, and 15 percent of them had side effects

---

61   *J Public Health & Epid.* 6(9): Sept. 2014; p. 271ff. *and* CDC.
62   CDC.
63   http://www.cdc.gov/hepatitis/Statistics/2011Surveillance/Commentary.htm#hepA
64   CDC.
65   http://www.cdc.gov/hepatitis/Statistics/2011Surveillance/Commentary.htm #hepA

during that short period of time, including pains in the back, head, neck, abdomen and joints.

Neil Z. Miller, author of *The Vaccine Safety Manual*, has compiled an impressive list of published studies that reveal the numerous documented side effects of the hepatitis B vaccines. Many of these are *autoimmune disorders.*

At least 17 studies document *vision and hearing impairments* that have occurred after hepatitis B immunization. These include *hearing loss* and *vision problems* like uveitis, optic neuritis, epitheliopathy, occlusion of the central retinal vein, bilateral white dot syndrome, and neuropapillitis. All of these conditions can and do impair vision.[66]

At least 15 studies link the hepatitis B vaccine with *serious blood disorders* like inflamed blood vessels (vasculitis), eosinophilia (an allergic blood disorder), low platelets, which can lead to easy bruising and bleeding, erythromelalgia, a rare disorder that causes burning sensations in the hands and feet, polyarteritis nodosa, another variety of vascular inflammation, and pancytopenia (the technical name for a marked diminution in the number of all the blood cells).[67]

At least 14 studies have found a variety of *skin disorders* occurring after the hepatitis B shot. These include erythema nodosum (tender red nodules usually on the legs), lichen planus (*LIKE-en PLANE-us*: an itchy skin eruption), erythema multiforme (*err-ith-THEME-uh MUL-TEE-for-mee*: an inflammatory rash, skin atrophy (loss of elasticity, increased wrinkling and thinning of the skin) and others.[68]

At least 14 studies link the hepatitis B vaccination with *arthritis*, including cases of polyarthritis (involving many joints), rheumatoid arthritis, Reiter's syndrome (inflammation of the joints, eyes, and urinary tract), and Sjogren's syndrome (dry eyes, dry mouth, fatigue, and joint pain).[69]

And at least 34 studies link the hepatitis B vaccination with a variety of serious *neurological and autoimmune conditions* like multiple sclerosis and other demyelinating conditions (myelin is the insulating sheath that surrounds nerve cells), neuropathies (nerve inflammation causing pain and numbness), lupus (a debilitating autoimmune disorder), and many others, including *diabetes.* See Table 27.3 for details on these studies and others.[70]

Table 27.3. Journal Articles Linking the Hepatitis B Vaccine Disorders:

Year	Journal	Article
Arthritis—14 Studies		
1990	BMJ.	"Hepatitis B vaccine associated with erythema nodosum and polyarthritis." v301: 345
1990	J of Rheum.	"Reactive arthritis after Hep B Vaccine." v17:1250-1251
1994	Brit. J Rheum.	"Acute seropositive rheumatoid arthritis after Hepatitis B vaccination." October; 33(10):991
1994	BMJ.	"Reiter's Syndrome & Reactive Arthritis after hep. B Vaccination." July 9; 309(6967):1513
1994	BMJ.	"Reiters Syndrome attributed to Hepatitis B Immunisation." Dec; 309(6967):1513
1994	BMJ.	"Hepatitls B Immunisation and Reactive Arthritis." Dec 304(6967): 1514
1995	Scand J Rheum.	"Arthritis after Hepatits B Vaccination: report of 3 cases." 24(1):50-52
1995	Scand J Rheum.	"Rheumatological Manifestation following Hepatitis B Vaccination…" 24:50-52
1995	Irish Med J.	"Psoriatic Arthropathy" March-April 88(2): 72. (Showed links between Hep B Vacc. & arthropathy)

66   Miller, N.Z. *Vaccine Safety Manual.* p. 182-187.
67   Ibid.
68   Ibid.
69   Ibid.
70   Ibid.

Year	Journal	Article
1997	Brit. J Rheum.	"Patients with Inflam. Polyarthritis after immunization…. IP." March; 36(3):366-369
1997	Brit. J Rheum.	"Polyarthritis associated with hepatitis B vaccination." February; 36(2):300-301
1998	J of Rheum.	"The development of rheumatoid arthritis after hepatitis B vaccination." Sept.; 25(9):1687-93
1999	Rheumatology	"Rheumatic disorders developed after hepatitis B vaccination." Oct.; 38(10):978-83
2000	Arthr & Rheum.	"Sjogren's syndrome occuring after hepatits B vaccination." Sept.; 43(9)
Autoimmune and Neurological Disorders—36 Studies		
1983	NEJM.	"Polyneuropathy assoc. with administration of hep B vaccine." Sept 8; 309(10):614-615
1988	Amer J Epidem.	"Postmarketing surveillance for neurol. adverse events after hep B vacc—first 3 yrs." Feb 37(s):337f
1988	Arch Int Med.	"Myasthenia Gravis after general anesthesia and hep B vaccination." December; 148(12): 2685
1991	Lancet.	"CNS demyelination after immunization with recombinant hep B vaccine." Nov 9;338(8776):1174f
1992	Nephron.	"Systemic lupus erythematosus and vaccination against hepatitis B." 62(2): 236
1992	Clin Inf Dis.	"Evan's Syndrome triggered by hepatitis B vaccine." 15: 1051 (Evan's synd is a rare blood disorder)
1992	Therapie (Fr.)	"Peripheral facial paralysis following vaccination against hep B." 47: 437
1992	Inf Disease News	"Other side of the coin." Ltr by BAWaisbren re CNS demyelination; 1992; 5:2
1993	J of Hepatology	"Transverse myelitis following hepatitis B vaccination." Sept. 93; 19(2):317-318
1993	La Nouv Pr Med.	"Acute myelitis after hepatitis vaccination." Dec: 22(40):1997f
1993	Clin Inf Dis.	"Multiple sclerosis and hepatitis B vaccination." Nov; 17(5): 928-9
1994	Arch Ped Adol Med.	"Lupus erythematosus disseminatus & vaccination against hep B virus." 1:307-309
1994	Acta Neur Scand.	"Acute cerebellar ataxia after immunization with recombinant hep B vaccine." 89(6):462f
1995	J Neur Nsur Psych.	"CNS demyelination after vaccination against hep. B & HLA haplotype." Jun; 58(6):758-9
1995	Amer J Neur Rad.	"MR imaging in a case of post-vaccination myelitis." 16(3): 581f
1996	Nephron	"Systemic lupus erythematosus following hepatitis B vaccine." 74(2):441
1996	Ann Derm Vener.	"Cutaneous Lupus erythematosus & buccal aphthosis after hep B vacc…" 123(10):657f
1996	J of Hepatology	"Leukoenncephalitis after recombinant hepatitis B vaccine." June; 24(6): 764f
1996	NEJM.	"Cryoglobulinemia after Hep B vaccine." Aug; 335(5):335
1996	J of Autoimmunity	"Vaccine-induced autoimmunity." Dec 9(6):699-703
1997	Indian J of Ped.	"Guillain-Barre Syndrome associated with hepatitis B vaccination." Sept-Oct; 64(5): 710f

Year	Journal	Article
1997	J Korean Med Sc.	"Acute myelitis after hepatitis B vaccination." June; 12(3) 249f
1997	Orl Surg…Orl Endo.	"Mental nerve neuropathy after hepatitis B vaccination." June; 83(6):663f
1997	JAMA.	"Hair loss after routine immunizations." Oct 8; 278(14):1176f
1998	Neph Dial Trnsplnt.	"Systemic Lupus Erythem. & Thrombocytopeinic purpura…after hep B vacc." 13(9):2420f
1999	Am J of Gastroenter.	"The bald truth." 94(4):1104 (describes hair loss after hepatitis B vaccination)
1999	Autoimmunity	"Lumbosacral acute demyelinating myeloneuropathy following hep. B vaccination." 30: 143f
1999	Neurology	"Encephalitis after hep. B vaccination…encephalitis or MS?" July 22; 53(2):396f
1999	Presse Med.	"Acute transverse cervical myelitis following hepatitis B vaccination…" Jul 3-10; 28(24):1290f
2000	Neurology	"Development of multiple sclerosis after hep. B vaccination." 54 (Supp 3):A164
2000	J Med Assoc Thai.	"Guillain-Barre syndrome following recomb. Hep. B vaccination…" 83(9):1124f
2001	Clin Inf Disease	"Two episodes of leukoencephalitis assoc with Hep B vacc. in single patient." Nov 15; 33: 1772f
2004	Neurology	"Recombinant Hep. B vaccine and the risk of MS: a prospective study." 63:838-42 (risk found!)
2006	Chinese Med J.	"Multiple sclerosis after hepatitis B vaccination in a 16 year-old patient." 119(1):77-79
2008	Neurology*	"Hep B vaccine and risk of CNS inflammatory demyelination in childlhood." Oct 8 (online)
2008	Neurology*	"Hepatitis vaccines and pediatric multiple sclerosis. Does timing or type matter?" Dec 17 (online)
Miscellaneous Disorders—6 Studies		
1994	Lancet.	"Liver dysfunction and DNA antibodies after hepatitis B vaccination." Nov; 344(8932);1292f
1995	Clinical Nephrology	"Nephrotic syndrome after recombinant hepatitis B vaccine." May 43(5) 349
1996	New Zealand Med J.	"Childhood immunization and diabetes mellitus." May 24; 195**
1996	New Zealand Med J	"The diabetes epidemic and the hepatitis B vaccine." May 24; 366**
1997	Intensive Care Med.	"Liver inflammation and & acute respiratory distress syndrome…" January; 23 (1):119f
2000	Pediatric Nephrology	"Nephrotic syndrome following hepatitis B vaccination." Jan; 4: 89-90

* Found statistically significant risk of multiple sclerosis in childhood more than 3 yrs after Hep B vaccination!

** "The incidence of (juvenile) diabetes rose 60 percent in NZ following a massive hepatitis B immunization program…. The CDC initiated a study to verify our findings. Their preliminary data…shows hepatitis B immunization, when given starting after 8 weeks of age, is associated with a 90 percent increase in the risk of diabetes…. Our data… shows that vaccine-induced diabetes may occur three or more years following immunization."[71]

71   J. Barthelow Classen, M.D.; Congressional Hearing; May 18, 1999. List of studies derived from *The Vaccine Safety Manual* by Neil Z. Miller

Adverse Reactions Outnumber Cases of the Disease

In 1996, *872 serious events* occurred in children under the age of 14 after their hepatitis B vaccination, including *hospitalizations, emergency room visits, permanent disabilities, and 48 deaths.* By contrast, only *279 cases of hepatitis B* reported in children less than 14 years of age that same year. "From 1992 through 2005 there were 36,788 hepatitis B vaccine-related events reported to the Vaccine Adverse Events Reporting System (VAERS) in all age groups, including 14,800 serious adverse events and 781 deaths (SIDS?)."[72]

When the number of serious or fatal reactions to a vaccine far outnumbers the cases of the disease it is alleged to protect against, it is certainly time to reevaluate the need for that vaccination.

Efficacy: Scientists often determine vaccine efficacy by discovering whether there has been a sufficient enough rise in antibody levels to the disease organism in question to provide protection from the infecting agent. This is generally measured after the final dose of the vaccination series has been given. *In the case of the hepatitis B vaccine, those protective antibody levels are found to be suboptimal or undetectable just 4-10 years after the series has been completed in 40 to 60 percent of those so vaccinated.* There are many studies documenting vaccine failure after immunization with these vaccines.[73]

One recent study may well be the final "nail in the coffin" regarding the need to inject infants with the hepatitis B vaccine. "The researchers followed 259 babies born to hepatitis-B-positive mothers for two years in order to determine whether vaccinating such babies prevents asymptomatic occult (asymptomatic) HBV (hepatitis B virus) infection.

Occult HBV infection is diagnosed when a person tests negative for hepatitis B surface antigen (HBsAg) while testing positive for HBV DNA. It's thought that the HBsAg mutates in occult HBV such that it can't be detected by conventional lab tests, making it often difficult to diagnose in addition to the fact that rarely are there clinical symptoms associated with occult infection.

The researchers found that while the vaccine may help prevent *overt* HBV transmission, *it was not effective in preventing occult HBV infection in up to 40 percent of the babies* born to hepatitis B-positive mothers. This was true whether or not the babies also received hepatitis B immune globulin (HBIG), which is used to prevent the development of hepatitis B. The babies were still infected with the virus, although it was not making them clinically ill. They could still suffer the dire consequences of chronic hepatitis and not be aware that they were infected.[74]

Conclusion: The current hepatitis B vaccines cause a variety of serious and sometimes fatal reactions in an unacceptably large number of individuals, especially children. Many of these appear to be autoimmune reactions. The number of babies who contract hepatitis B infections is small and their risk of acquiring the infection if their mother is not infected is close to zero. However, their risk of having potentially serious reactions, *including autism*, is ever present and far exceeds their risk of acquiring the disease.[75]

The waning protection afforded to babies from these immunizations over the years is likely to be suboptimal by the time they reach the age they are more likely to engage in those activities, like unprotected sexual encounters or injected illicit drug use with contaminated needles, which are the usual risk factors for acquiring this disease. And the vaccine does not even prevent many babies born to hepatitis B infected mothers from being infected with the virus.

It thus makes no sense routinely to immunize all babies to hepatitis B. The risks clearly outweigh any possible benefit. Mothers should be tested for the organism, and if hepatitis B is not present, there is no reason to immunize the child.

---

72   Ibid. p. 190 from NVIC data.

73   Ibid. p. 196.

74   Pande, C. et al. "Hepatitis B vaccination with or without hepatitis B immunoglobulin at birth to babies born of HBsAg-positive mothers prevents overt HBV transmission but may not prevent occult HBV infection in babies: a randomized controlled trial." *J Viral Hepat.* 2013 Nov; 20(11):801- doi: 10.1111/jvh.12102. Epub 2013 Apr 23.10.

75   *Annals of Epidemiology.* Sept 2009: 19(9); 659. This study was performed on babies who received the hepatitis B vaccines that contained thimerosal and aluminum.

> *"We estimate there are 10,000 cases of (hepatitis B) vaccine-induced diabetes in the U.S. each year. On average each case may cost $1 million in lost productivity and medical expense."*
>
> — J. Barthelow Classen, M.D., coauthor of:
> *"Childhood immunization and diabetes mellitus."* New Zealand Med J. *1996; May 24; 195*
> *"The diabetes epidemic and the hepatitis B vaccine."* New Zealand Med J. *1996; May 24; 366*

Measles Vaccine

Safety: The first measles vaccines were developed in the 1960s. An inactivated measles virus vaccine was developed in 1963, but it was ineffective and was discontinued in 1967. The attenuated live virus vaccine has been used since that time and has been associated with a variety of side effects, some of them serious. These include encephalitis, brain damage, seizures, sensory and immune system impairments, *autism*, blood disorders, allergic reactions, atypical measles, digestive and lymphatic disorders, and death. Serious side effects are more likely to occur in babies, teens, and older individuals.[76]

According to a 1995 study published in *Lancet*, people who received the measles vaccine were 2½ times more likely to come down with Crohn's disease and 3 times more likely to develop ulcerative colitis than were those unvaccinated to the measles virus.[77] A variety of other studies support this association.[78]

We've already reviewed the many studies that link the MMR vaccination with autism, and we have shown the studies that allege otherwise to be faulty.

Efficacy: (See also Chapter 20.) Measles used to be an extremely common childhood disease, but deaths from this infection were uncommon and declined by 98 percent in both the U.S. and Great Britain *prior* to the introduction of the measles vaccines.[79] Infection with the virus confers lifelong immunity in most individuals.

There are 20 known wild-type strains of measles, and the naturally acquired antibodies from measles infection confer immunity to 18 of these strains, whereas the measles vaccine in the MMR provides *short-lived* immunity and is unable to inactivate 10 of these strains in most vaccinated individuals.[80]

The MMR vaccination, nevertheless, does prevent measles in many, but protection doesn't last long, and outbreaks of the disease have occurred in populations where as many as 97 percent had received the vaccination. Many other examples of vaccine failures during measles outbreaks have been documented in a number of published studies.[81]

Within a year of receiving the MMR, a person's protective antibody levels dropped by 59 percent in one study, and booster shots didn't confer long-lived immunity either. Just one year after the measles (MMR) booster shot, antibody levels dropped back to about where they were prior to the booster dose. Currently, the MMR is administered at age 12-18 months and again at 5 years prior to the start of school attendance.[82]

The use of the MMR immunization has unfavorably changed the dynamics of who now gets infected with measles during outbreaks. Prior to the widespread use of the measles vaccine, 97 percent of cases occurred in children less than 15 years of age, an age when serious side effects are less common. Mothers, who had acquired natural immunity from childhood measles infection, were also able to pass their protective antibodies on to their babies, thereby shielding them from this infection for many months after birth.

---

76   Miller, N.Z. *Vaccine Safety Manual*. p. 114-118.
77   Thompson, N.P. *Lancet*. 1995; 345:1071f.
78   Miller, N.Z. *Vaccine Safety Manual*. p. 116-117.
79   See declining mortality graphs below.
80   Ibid. p. 123.
81   Ibid. p. 120-122.
82   Ibid. p. 120.

Since 1977, there has been a shift in the age of susceptibility to measles to the high-risk older age groups and to infants. "By 1999, the CDC confirmed that at least 50 percent of all measles cases were still occurring in high-risk age groups that had not been susceptible to measles during the pre-vaccine era." Adolescents and young adults are more prone to getting measles-related pneumonia and liver abnormalities than are younger children.[83] Infants less than one year of age are also now at greater risk for catching measles due to the decline in natural immunity in their mothers.

In an attempt to immunize babies to measles in impoverished communities in Africa, Haiti, Mexico, and Los Angeles, researchers tested two new *unproven high titer* vaccines to measles with *tragic consequences*. The vaccines, which were administered to the babies at just five months of age, dramatically *increased* their deaths from a variety of *other childhood diseases*. The immunizations appeared to have *lowered the babies' immunity*![84]

The new vaccines not only didn't save lives, but they actually *significantly increased the death rate* in these unfortunate poor children who were being used as "guinea pigs." *One out of six babies died in Senegal within three years of receiving the shot.* The CDC, which had lied on several points in the L.A. part of the study, ultimately confessed that "a mistake was made" and these vaccines were eventually discontinued.[85]

Conclusion: The measles vaccine component of the MMR raises significant safety concerns and does not confer immunity to measles for very long, even with booster dosing. Its use has resulted in a potentially-harmful shift of measles-associated side effects, like pneumonia, to more at risk populations (infants and young adults). *Its lack of efficacy and short duration of protection mean that it is unlikely to be able to eliminate measles in any given population, nor is it likely to be able to confer herd immunity even at very high vaccination levels due to its incomplete coverage of all wild measles virus strains and its short duration of protection against the strains it does protect against.*

Mumps Vaccine

Mumps, like measles, was once a common childhood infection that generally causes a fever, aches, malaise, and fatigue. The mumps virus usually infects the salivary glands beneath the ears, causing local pain and swelling. In teens or older men, the virus can invade the testes, usually only one, and this infection can result in decreased sperm production in that gland. Rarely, the virus can infect the brain, causing meningitis, from which full recovery is the norm. Patients generally feel better after 3-4 days of illness. The illness generally confers lifelong immunity to the disease.

Vaccine: The live virus mumps vaccine was invented in 1967 and put into general use in the 1970s. It is now combined with the measles and rubella vaccines to make the MMR immunization currently in use today.

Safety: (See also Chapter 20.) Different strains of the virus have been shown to produce different side-effect risks, as we have previously noted. Merck's "Jeryl Lynn strain" seemed to cause less meningitis than did Glaxo SmithKlein's "Urabe" strain. It may be recalled, however, that the Jeryl Lynn strain has also been associated in several studies with serious neurological events like aseptic meningitis. The risk for coming down with meningitis (17-34 days) after the MMR inoculation is about one child out of every 350-3500 children.[86]

As is true with the hepatitis B vaccine, the mumps vaccine has also been associated with an increased risk of the vaccine recipient becoming an insulin-dependent diabetic. This was confirmed in at least 8 studies published in peer-reviewed journals. The onset of this form of diabetes (Type I or "juvenile diabetes") has been seen in as little as 10 days following the vaccination, but it may take months before the symptoms manifest. In the 1960s, 92 percent of the patients with mumps were less than 14 years old, but because the immunization changed the susceptibility demographics, by 2004, 79 percent of all cases of mumps occurred in the higher-risk older population.[87]

---

83   Ibid. p. 123

84   Ibid. p. 124-128.

85   Ibid. p. 127 and Cimons, M. "CDC says it erred in measles study." *L.A. Times* June 17, 1996.

86   Miller, N.Z. *Vaccine Safety Manual.* p. 129-130.

87   Ibid. p. 130.

Efficacy: As we pointed out in an earlier chapter, serious questions have been raised regarding the effectiveness of the mumps component of the MMR vaccine. It may be recalled that two "whistle-blower" Merck scientists claimed that *Merck falsified data* regarding the efficacy of its mumps vaccine (Jeryl Lynn strain) by testing it against a weakened strain of mumps virus and by doctoring the vaccine with animal antibodies.

These dishonest manipulations artificially inflated the vaccine's efficacy and resulted in the U.S. government, a major purchaser of vaccines, paying hundreds of millions of dollars for a vaccine that does not provide adequate immunization.[88]

Evidence to support this alleged lack of efficacy comes from a number of studies. See Table 27.4.

Table 27.4. Mumps Vaccine Efficacy Studies

Year	Source	Findings
1981	MMWR	94 percent of mumps cases in a highschool outbreak had been immunized to mumps. *Vaccinated teens were 2X as likely to contract mumps as those unvaccinated.*
1987	Minn. Dept of Health	82 percent of 769 cases of mumps in schoolchildren with mumps were immunized.
1988	JAMA	119 stockbrokers caught mumps following a vaccination campaign.
1991	J of Infect. Disease	99 percent of mumps cases in Tennessee schoolchildren had been vaccinated to mumps.
1993	Lancet	Japan stopped MMR because it was causing contagious mumps in those vaccinated.
2006	JAMA	30 percent of >70,000 mumps cases in GB epidemic were immunized to mumps! And 82 percent of the population had had mumps vaccinations.
2006	CDC/MMWR	92 percent had one mumps vacc & 74 percent had 2 mumps vaccines in outbreaks in U.S. in 2006. The median age of persons who caught mumps was 21 years!

Conclusion: Mumps, a relatively benign infection, generally confers lifelong immunity to most individuals. Mumps vaccine does not! Protection is short-lived, and the mumps vaccine is associated with significant safety risks (*meningitis, diabetes, and orchitis* [testicle inflammation] in teen boys or older males, and other side effects). It also puts more susceptible populations (babies, teens, and adults) at greater risk for complications.

Rubella Vaccine

Rubella is a mild infection in most individuals, lasting only a few days and associated with minimal symptoms, like low grade fever, malaise, and aches and pains. Infection with the virus conveys lifelong immunity in most individuals. However, the *virus* is dangerous to the fetus *in the first trimester* of pregnancy and increases the risk for serious birth defects, *autism* (see Chapter 20), and *juvenile diabetes* in up to 25 percent of those afflicted (see above in this chapter.)

The first live virus vaccine for rubella was developed in 1969, and an improved vaccine was licensed in 1979. Merck manufactures Merovax II rubella vaccine and combines it with measles and the Jeryl Lynn mumps vaccine to make the MMR vaccine it calls "M-M-R II." An identical vaccine that also includes the chickenpox (varicella) virus is branded as "ProQuad."

Safety: The rubella vaccine has been associated since its inception with serious side effects including arthritis, joint

---

88   http://www.court housenews.com/2012/06/27/47851.htm & www.beyondconformity.org.nz/hilarys-desk/mercks-illegal-mmr-smokescreen-continues

and muscle pains, encephalitis, Guillain-Barre paralysis, nerve inflammation (neuritis, neuropathy, and optic neuritis), anaphylaxis, diabetes, blood disorders, chronic fatigue syndrome, low platelets (thrombocytopenia), and death.[89] Tables 27.5 and 27.6 list the studies that associate this vaccine with a number of serious complications.

Efficacy: Infection during childhood with the rubella virus confers lifetime immunity to the disease in 85 percent of those infected.[90] The vaccine, on the other hand, does not. In a 1971 outbreak in Wyoming, 73 percent of cases of rubella were in vaccinated individuals.[91]

A 1973 study in Australia reported that 80 percent of army recruits vaccinated to rubella just four months earlier came down with the disease. In 1980, *Pediatrics* revealed that 15 percent of children vaccinated against this disease came down with the infection, and three studies published in 1980, 1985, and 1987 confirmed that antibodies against rubella virus were not at protective levels in 15 percent of the adult population, including women of childbearing age. This is the same percentage that was susceptible before vaccinations against rubella began![92]

Antibody levels against the rubella virus were shown to fall by 50 percent after four years in one study, and 50 percent of all rubella cases were in vaccinated populations in another study. And two studies showed that high levels of antibodies were not necessarily protective against rubella infection.[93]

Nevertheless, following vaccine licensure in 1969, rubella incidence declined rapidly. Each year from 1992 through 2000, fewer than 500 cases were reported; each year since 2001, fewer than 100 cases have been reported—a 99 percent decline compared with the pre-vaccine era…. From 1995 to 2000, an average of five cases of congenital rubella syndrome were reported annually; since 2001, an average of one congenital rubella syndrome case has been reported annually."[94]

Conclusion: The rubella vaccine program, which was initiated to prevent congenital rubella syndrome (CRS), has been very effective in reducing the number of cases of rubella and congenital rubella syndrome.

However, the vaccine has many undesirable side effects and does not promote lasting immunity in all. One must weigh the documented serious risks of this vaccination against its proven ability to prevent rubella infection and congenital rubella syndrome in making one's decision as to whether or not to immunize against this condition.

Haemophilus Influenzae Type B (Hib) Vaccine[95]

The Hib organism is a dangerous bacterium that children under three years of age are especially susceptible to. Hib bacteria can cause a range of serious and occasionally fatal infections, including meningitis, cellulitis, epiglottitis (throat infection), and pneumonia, but not influenza (the "flu"). Influenza is a viral disease. Many people carry the Hib organism asymptomatically, but they may infect others.

There was a dramatic 400 percent rise in Hib infection rates between 1946 and 1986, coincident with the increasing use of the DPT vaccine in babies. This may not be a coincidence.[96]

It may be recalled that the tetanus booster was shown to inhibit immune function (see "The Tetanus Vaccine" above in this chapter) for a month or so after the inoculation. Several studies have shown that immunizations and the DPT, in particular, can make a child more susceptible to other infections, including paralytic polio.[97]

In 1975, Japan postponed immunizing babies to pertussis until age two years, and the haemophilus meningitis rate in the under two year-olds declined significantly, while meningitis in the 2-3-year old population "skyrocketed."[98]

89   VAERS Reports
90   *Canad Med Assoc J.* July 15, 1983
91   Miller, N.K. *Vaccine Safety Manual.* p. 138.
92   Ibid.
93   Ibid. p. 138-9.
94   http://measles.emedtv.com/rubella/rubella-statistics.html.
95   Pronounced "hem-OPH- i-lus In-floo-EN-zee"
96   *Pediatrics.* 1972; 50(5):723f
97   *J Inf Dis* 1975; 1313(6):749f *and J Inf Dis*1992; 165:444f.
98   *Lancet* (4016088): 881f *and* Scheibener, V. *Vaccination: 100 Years of Orthodox Research.* 1993. p. 133

Table 27.5. Twenty-Two Rubella Vaccine Studies: Joint Pains and Arthritis are Common Side Effects

Year	Source	Finding
1969	NE J of Med	Arthritis is a frequent side effect of inoculating women with rubella vaccine
1969	A J of Diseases Child.	Transient arthritis is common in children after rubella inoculation
1971	AJDC	10 percent of children inoculated with rubella vaccine developed joint problems
1971	Am J of Epidemiology	25 percent to 50 percent of women in their 20s and older had joint pains after rubella vaccination
1972	JAMA	46 percent of women >25 yo developed arthritis following rubella vaccination
1972	Am J of Epidemiology	Joint reactions common in children following rubella vaccination
1972	Journal of Pediatrics	Documented joint problems in babies 2-7 weeks after rubella vaccination
1972	Amer J of Public Health	Joint symptoms common after an area-wide rubella immunization campaign
1973	A J of Diseases in Child	Reported on several children with recurrent arthritis following rubella inoculation
1977	J of Arthritis & Rheum	Documented chronic arthropathy (joint pain) following rubella vaccination
1980	Merck Labs: 2 studies	1 out of 4 women at greater risk for joint pains & arthritis post-rubella vaccination
1982	Am J of Epidem Lancet	Joint reactions and rubella associated arthritis common after rubella vaccination
1984	Lancet	Chronic arthritis lasting at least 7 years reported in women after rubella vaccination
1985	J of Infect Diseases	Documented arthritis in women after rubella vacc lasting at least 20 years in one lady
1986	Annal Rheum. Disease	55 percent of women developed arthritis & joint pain within 4 wks of rubella vaccination
1991	US Vacc Safety Comm	Verified that rubella vaccine induces long-term and short-term arthritis
1992	Clinical Infect Diseases	Documented cases of chronic arthritis following rubella vaccination
1996	J of Arthr & Rheum	Chronic arthropathy and musculoskeletal symptoms are associated with rubella vaccine
1997	JAMA	Chronic arthropathy and musculoskeletal symptoms are associated with rubella vaccine
1998	J of Infectious Diseases	Rubella Vaccine induces "joint manifestations"
2002	Clin & Exper Rheumat	Statistically signif. risk of chronic arthritis 10-11 days post rubella & Hep B vaccinations

Table 27.6. Seventeen More Rubella Vaccine Studies: Other Complications

Year	Source	Neurological & Blood Disorders
1970	JAMA	Reported Paralysis following rubella vaccination
1972	J of Pediatrics	Loss of Sensation & Difficulty Walking
1972	NY St J of Med	Thrombocytopenia (low platelet syndrome)
1974	Am J Dis Child	Neuroligical Disorders (POLYNEUROPATHY lasting for yrs in 1 out of 500)
1977	Brit Med J	Diffuse Myelitis
1982	Arch of Neurol	Neuritis & Myelitis
1991	NE J of Med	Hearing loss after measles and rubella vaccination
1994	Europ J of Ped	Guillain-Barre ascending paralysis
Diabetes After Rubella Vaccination?		
1978 2005	Lancet 1-14-78 NIH Pub 06-3893; 2005	Juvenile diabetes rates have skyrocketed (1 out of 500 children & teens today) since the start of the mumps (1967) and rubella (1969) mass vaccination programs. (*Lancet.* Jan 14, 1978 and NIH Pub 06-3892 2005.)
1982	Infect. Immunit.	Rubella vaccine-specific complexes that attack the insulin producing cells found in 2/3 of vaccinees
1986	Diabetes	Rubella virus induced diabetes in hamsters
1989	Am J Clin Path	Rubella infected human pancreatic islet cells have diminished capacity to produce insulin.
1997 Apr. 16	Congressional Testimony	Dr. Coulter analyzed the above studies & concluded: "Diabetes after rubella vaccination probably represents a combined effect: the virus attacks the islet cells of the pancreas in an organism which has already been weakened by an autoimmune reaction to the same virus."
Chronic Fatigue Syndrome (CFS)?		
1986	J of Immunol	Rubella virus suspected as cause of CFS
1988	Medical Hypoth	IgG antibody levels to rubella virus correlate with intensity of CFS symptoms
1991	Clinical Ecology	Study confirms vaccine strain of rubella virus is one cause of CFS

So the rise in Hib infections in the forty years prior to 1986 may indeed be related to the increased rate of DPT inoculation in babies.

Vaccines: Today three Hib vaccines are available for babies as young as 6 weeks of age. Hib vaccines were optional in 1988 (given initially at 15 months of age) and mandated in 1990 (to start at 2 months of age) in the U.S., and include Hib TITER, ActHIB, & PedVacHIB.

There are also three Hib vaccines that are combined with other immunizations: TrHIBit (with DTaP), Comvax (with hepatitis B), and Pentacel (with DTaP, hepatitis B, and IPV [polio]).

Pentacel, TriHIBit, Comvax, and PedvaxHib all contain aluminum (170-333 mcg per dose). In the 1990s, most of the Hib vaccines also contained *thimerosal*, and "trace amounts" remain in some of the current vaccines.

Safety: The Hib vaccine has been associated with a number of adverse events and illnesses, including Guillain-Barré ascending paralysis, paralysis of the spinal cord (transverse myelitis), aseptic meningitis, *sudden infant death*, and (as is true with hepatitis B and rubella vaccines) *diabetes*.[99]

---

99   Inst. of Medicine. "Adverse events assoc with childhood vaccines…" Wash DC 1994; *Europ J of Peds* 1993; 152:613f; *J of Peds* 1989; 115:743f; *Pediatrics* 1993; 92:272f; *NEJM* 1990323(2)1393f; *Pediatrics* 1987; 80:270f; *J Clin Invest* 1984; 74:1708f *and* VAERS.

Thanks to an excellent ten-year Finnish study of over 200,000 children, we now know that *Hib vaccines increase the risk of diabetes*. One group of children received no Hib vaccine, a second group received only one dose of Hib, and the third group received all four doses. The risk of diabetes was determined at ages 7 and 10 years, and the results were startling. There was a *linear* and *significant* increase in the risk of diabetes as the number of Hib inoculations increased, and the risk at 10 years was greater than the risk at 7 years.[100]

Table 27.7. Hib Vaccine Diabetes Risk Per 100,000 Children[101]

AGE	No Doses of Hib	One Dose of Hib	4 Doses of Hib
7 years	207	237	261
10 years	340	376	398

"Based on an annual birth rate of 4 million children, in the United States alone this [increased risk of diabetes] translates into 2300 additional (and avoidable) cases of diabetes every year. Each case of insulin dependent diabetes is estimated to cost more than $1 million in medical costs and lost productivity."—Neil Z. Miller, *Vaccine Safety Manual*, p. 202

As is true with both the tetanus and pertussis vaccines, the *Hib vaccine appears to hamper immunity for at least a week following vaccination*, making the child more susceptible to infection, including from the Hib bacteria itself.[102]

Adults may also be at increased risk for other types of invasive Haemophilus infections (other than type b) as a result of the Hib vaccination campaign in children. These non-type b infections have increased in adults and so have non-Hib bacterial infections.

Efficacy: The Hib vaccines are effective and have significantly reduced the number of children who contract the disease. Cases of Hib meningitis have declined dramatically. However, this may have come at a cost because now other types of bacterial meningitis, like those caused by Streptococcus pneumoniae and Neisseria meningitides, have dramatically increased.[103]

And the vaccine is far from 100 percent effective. According to the CDC, from 1998 to 2000, 32 percent of all children aged 6 months to 5 years with confirmed Hib disease had been given three or more inoculations of the Hib vaccine.[104]

In the January 15, 1987 edition of *Pediatric Notes*, Gellis reported that of all the children who contracted HIB at least 3 weeks after their shot, more than 70 percent developed meningitis.[105]

When the Hib vaccine is combined with other vaccines (like the DTaP), the vaccine becomes *less effective* and antibody levels are *significantly* (5-10 times) lower.[106]

The Hib vaccines only protect against the typable (encapsulated) forms of the haemophilus organism. Most forms of haemophilus are not encapsulated and not typable.

Conclusion: The Hib vaccines have significantly reduced the incidence of Hib infections in children, but they appear to make recipients more susceptible to other infections and to increase the risk for childhood (Type I) diabetes and SIDS.

---

100   *BMJ*. 1999; 318:1169f.
101   Table 27.7 from England and Wales depicting childhood mortality rates and many other similar mortality graphs may be seen at: http://www.whale.to / vaccines/decline1.html.
102   Package inserts for Wyeth, Sanofi, & Merck Hib Vaccines.
103   *Clin Inf Dis*. 2007; 44:810f.
104   CDC. Jan 8 2007.
105   *Pediatric Notes*; 11: 2.
106   *The Lancet Interactive*. Dec 11, 1999.

Pneumococcal Vaccine for Children

The pneumococcus ("new-muh-COCK-us") bacteria (now known as Streptococcus pneumoniae) causes a variety of quite serious illnesses, including pneumonia, meningitis, ear infections (otitis media), sinus infections, and sepsis (blood infections). The incidence of pneumococcal disease has increased significantly since the introduction of the Hib vaccines in the late 1980s, and currently, there are about 10-30 cases per 100,000 individuals resulting in approximately 200 deaths annually. Infants, the elderly, and those with compromised immune systems are particularly susceptible to infections by these organisms.

Currently, only one vaccine (Prevnar 13˚ by Wyeth) has been approved (2010) for use in children. It is designed to protect against just 13 of the 90 or so strains of pneumococcal bacteria that cause disease in man. It replaced the Prevnar 7 vaccine which was licensed in 2000. Babies generally receive the Prevnar 13 vaccine at 2, 4, 6, and 12-15 months of age.

Safety: The vaccine contains a *diphtheria toxin* (CRM) and an *aluminum* adjuvant (125 mcg of aluminum per shot) to bolster the immune response. The neurotoxic aluminum content of each Prevnar injection exceeds the FDA recommended maximum of 4-5 mcg/kg/day for all babies who weigh less than 25 kg (55 lbs), which is virtually all babies less than 18 months of age, the very ones for whom the shot is intended!

Acute adverse reactions to the vaccine are common and include pain at the injection site, irritability, loss of appetite (20 percent), diarrhea, and vomiting (13 percent). Even more serious adverse reactions to the vaccine occurred in 8.2 percent of babies who received Prevnar 13, according to the product insert, and include cessation of breathing (apnea), seizures, wheezing, autoimmune conditions, and sudden infant death, among others.

A Diabetes Connection?

Dr. Barthelow Classen, who published a study linking the Hib vaccines to an increase in juvenile diabetes, is concerned that the Prevnar 13 vaccine, like the Hib vaccines, might also promote diabetes in children. Both the Hib and pneumococcal vaccines are *conjugate* vaccines. Both use the diphtheria toxin as an immune stimulator.

An Autism Connection?

Concern also exists that conjugate vaccines, like the HIB and pneumococcal vaccines, might promote autism. Both of these organisms are encapsulated, and their capsules contain certain carbohydrate antigens (polysaccharide sugars) that engender an effective immune response *only in adults and older children, but not in infants.*

Babies do not produce antibodies when injected with the polysaccharide antigens from these encapsulated organisms, and they don't even produce antibodies when infected with the disease organism itself.[107]

In order to promote an effective immune response in babies to Haemophilus type b and pneumococcal bacteria, scientists attached (conjugated) a reactive protein molecule (modified diphtheria toxin) to the polysaccharide antigens, and they added an *aluminum* adjuvant. The resultant vaccines were then able to provide effective immune protection from the diseases caused by these bacteria, but this benefit may have come at a cost.

This inability of infants to react to carbohydrate antigens coincides with a period of "intense myelination" of the brain neurons. It is theorized that this period of hypo-responsiveness to these bacterial polysaccharide antigens protects the infant brain from autoimmune attacks directed at the myelin sheath and other neurological structures.

According to B.J. Richmand, "[C]onjugate vaccines may have disrupted evolutionary forces that favored early brain development over the need to protect infants and young children from capsular bacteria." He hypothesized that, "[T]he introduction of the Hib conjugate vaccine in the U.S. in 1988 and its subsequent introduction in Denmark and Israel could explain a substantial portion of the initial increases in Autism Spectrum Disorders in those countries. The continuation of the trend toward increased rates of ASDs could be further explained by increased usage of the vaccine."[108]

---

107   www.ccrc.uge.edu/~rcarlson/Vaccines.pdf
108   Richmand, B.J. "Hypothesis: conjugate vaccines may predispose children to autism spectrum disorders." *Med Hypotheses*. 2011 Dec; 77(6):940-7.

Efficacy: It is difficult to say how effective this vaccine is as doctors rarely subtype an organism in their workup for treating a bacterial infection, so it is difficult to know to what extent this vaccine has helped in reducing pneumococcal infections. The vaccine is designed to protect against only the 13 included strains of Pneumococcal bacteria, and it isn't beneficial in the prevention of infection from other serotypes of this organism.

To complicate matters further, it is known that the organisms' capsular type can change (mutate) by recombination. This can result in making the vaccine recipient more susceptible to other strains of the bacteria not included in the vaccine.[109]

As Neil Miller points out in his book *The Vaccine Safety Manual*, "During 2000, the year in which Prevnar (then Prevnar 7) was licensed, 65 percent of all pneumococcal cases were caused by strains in the vaccine. By 2004, just 27 percent of all pneumococcal cases were caused by vaccine strains...furthermore, the non-vaccine strains isolated from patients' respiratory tracts were more resistant to antibiotics and multi drug treatments."[110]

In 2007, researchers published data again showing that pneumococcal infection by non-Prevnar strains of the organism were replacing those targeted by the vaccine. "The incidence of non-PCV 7 serotype disease more than doubled among Alaskan native children" in the few years since the vaccine was first introduced, and *the new strains were more dangerous*; more children needed to be hospitalized for pneumococcal diseases like pneumonia and empyema (pus in the lung) than had been the case previously.[111]

Efficacy for otitis media (middle ear infection): Wyeth, the manufacturer of the Prevnar 13 vaccine, states in its product insert that "children who received Prevnar appear to be at increased risk of otitis media (middle ear infection) due to pneumococcal serotypes not represented in the vaccine." The brochure goes on to say that, "because otitis media is caused by many organisms other than serotypes of streptococcus pneumonia represented in the vaccine, protection against all causes of otitis media is expected to be low."

Nevertheless, the results of a Kaiser Permanente Efficacy trial indicated that Prevnar significantly reduced the risk of otitis media, especially for those children who had frequent ear infections and ear tube placement.[112]

Efficacy for pneumonia prevention: Another Kaiser study of young children showed a dramatic reduction in the incidence of pneumococcal disease after the licensing of the Prevnar 7 vaccine in February 2000.

However, *the decline began a year prior to the licensure of the vaccine*, so it is isn't at all clear that the vaccine was responsible for the continued decline in incidence.[113]

Varicella (Chickenpox) Vaccine

Chickenpox is a relatively benign, albeit highly contagious, childhood disease caused by the Varicella-Zoster virus. It is spread by direct contact with a patient or by inhaling airborne viruses from a sneeze or cough. The illness manifests with cough, fever, malaise, and a skin eruption consisting of itchy, raised, fluid-filled vesicles, which gradually crust over and which appear mainly on the trunk and face. These lesions, which last about a week or so, heal without scarring in most cases. After the illness abates, the virus remains in a dormant state in the nerve tissues. The illness usually confers life-long immunity.

A late complication of chickenpox is *shingles*, an often painful eruption that represents a reactivation of the once dormant virus, and which can occur years or even decades after the initial childhood infection has resolved.

Like most childhood viral infections, the disease tends to be more severe in adults, especially men, and in the immune-compromised. Chickenpox is rarely fatal. However, women who are infected with the varicella virus early in a pregnancy may pass the virus to their baby, which can result in a variety of serious birth defects and malformations.

109   Coffey, T. et al. *J Mol Microbiol*; 1/98; 27(1):73f *and* Lipsitch, M. et al. *Emer Infect Dis*. May/June 99; 5(3):336f *and* Lipsitch, M. *PNAS*; 6/97; 94(12)657f.
110   p. 209 *and* Farrell, D.J. et al. *Ped Inf Dis J*. 2007; 26(2):123f.
111   Singleton, R.J. et al. *JAMA*. 4/25/7; 297: 1784f.
112   www.fda.gov/ohrms/dockets/ac/02/slides/3854S1_03.ppt
113   http://www.medscape .org/view article/445087_1

Vaccine: A vaccine to prevent chickenpox was invented in 1974 to be given primarily to children with leukemia or impaired immune systems. Merck's Varivax® vaccine for chickenpox was licensed in 1995, and shortly thereafter, it became part of the mandated childhood vaccine schedule for children older than one year of age.

Safety: Varivax is an attenuated live virus vaccine and causes adverse reactions in 67 out of every 100,000 recipients, according to a CDC/FDA study of the VAERS database. Of these reactions, 4 percent were deemed serious or life-threatening and included bleeding disorders, seizures, anaphylaxis, and death. The younger the child, the greater was the risk of having a serious adverse reaction.[114]

Fever, injection site pain, and a chickenpox-like rash are also commonly reported side effects of the vaccine. Individuals who have been vaccinated with Varivax can transmit the virus to others. This is of special concern for pregnant women and the immune-compromised. There are also numerous reports of vaccine recipients coming down with shingles.

As is the case with the other vaccines that offer protection from what used to be common childhood illnesses (rubella, measles, chickenpox and mumps), the new immunization schedule is likely to shift chickenpox disease to older age groups (teens and adults) who have higher complication rates. "Before the vaccine was introduced most cases of chickenpox occurred in children between 3 and 6 years of age. By 2004, only 30 percent of chickenpox cases were in children under the age of 6 years…. Adults are 10 times more likely to require hospitalization and 25 times more likely to die from chickenpox than children."[115]

Efficacy: Varivax probably does not induce lifelong immunity, and two injections are recommended. It is not 100 percent effective. There have been a number of reports indicating that adequately immunized children and adults still came down with chickenpox. Nearly 10 percent of all cases of chickenpox reported were in those previously immunized with Varivax.[116]

Varivax and Autism: Does the Varivax vaccine promote autism? It appears that it might. Research by Theresa Deisher et al. revealed that *both Varicella and Hepatitis A* immunization coverage was significantly and linearly correlated to autistic disorder cases: the greater the coverage, the higher the prevalence of autism. The suspected reason for this, as has been previously discussed, is the presence of aborted fetal DNA and cell fragments as well as retrovirus remnants in these immunizations. (See Figure 27.7.)[117]

Rotavirus Vaccine

Rotaviruses, which exist in many subtypes, are common intestinal pathogens that can cause fever, diarrhea, and vomiting in children, especially in the winter months. Babies are especially vulnerable to this infection and are very prone to dehydration, which can lead to death in some if appropriate interventions (IV or oral fluids) are not taken. Rotavirus-infected babies in poor countries are often unable to get proper medical attention and are, therefore, more likely to die as a result. In the U.S., about 20 deaths and many hospitalizations occur each year as a consequence of this disease.[118]

Vaccine: The FDA (Food and Drug Administration) prematurely approved the Wyeth-Lederle "RotaShield" vaccine in 1998 without first doing adequate long-term follow-up studies. This was a mistake. The FDA and the CDC were both aware of potentially serious concerns regarding the vaccine prior to its approval, and those concerns proved to be justified. The vaccine was pulled off the market just one year later when it was found that RotaShield was associated with numerous cases of intussusception, a potentially lethal form of intestinal obstruction, and indeed, many babies died after receiving the vaccination, and many more were hospitalized.[119]

114   Wise, R.P. et al. *JAMA*. Sept 13, 2000; 1271 f.
115   Miller, N. *Vaccine Safety Manual*. p. 221 and 225.
116   Chavez, S.A. et al. "Loss of vaccine induced immunity to varicella over time." *NEJM*. March 15, 2007; 356:1121f/
117   *J Public Health & Epid*. 6(9): Sept 2014; p.271ff
118   CDC.
119   *MMWR Weekly*. Nov 5 1999; 48(43) 1007.

Conflicts of Interest?

This tragedy should have been prevented. Were conflicts of interest at play in the decision making of the FDA and CDC members who approved this vaccine?

- 60 percent of FDA committee members who voted "yes" on licensing the RotaShield vaccine had financial ties to either its manufacturer, Wyeth-Lederle, or to Merck or Smith Kline Beecham, companies that were developing their own rotavirus vaccines.

- 50 percent of the CDC's advisory committee members also had similar ties to industry.

On June 15, 2000, a concerned Congress held a hearing to investigate the process by which vaccines are approved. It was chaired by Congressman Dan Burton who was appalled by what the committee discovered. "No individual who stands to gain financially from the decisions regarding vaccines that may be mandated for use should be participating in the discussion or policymaking for vaccines," he stated.[120]

But the FDA had no desire to change its procedures in this regard. "Both the law and policies allow us to use people who have financial ties," countered Linda Suydam, the FDA's senior associate commissioner at that time, and to this day, the decision-making process regarding the approval of vaccines remains largely unchanged.[121]

Consider, for example, the FDA's approval of Merck's new rotavirus vaccine RotaTeq®, which was licensed in 2006 in large part based on a positive study of this vaccine published in January of that year in the New England Journal of Medicine. Two of the authors of that study were Paul Offit and H. Fred Clark, co-owners of the patent on RotaTeq, who clearly stood to gain financially by its approval. Other members of the study team had financial ties to Merck or to GlaxoSmithKline (another maker of a rotavirus vaccine, RotaRix®, approved by the FDA in 2008).[122]

RotaTeq Safety: The four living strains of rotavirus (G1-G4) in the RotaTeq vaccine are grown in Vero cells from the kidneys of African green monkeys. The vaccine, which is administered at 2, 4, and 6 months of age, *more than triples the risk of having intestinal bleeding (including from intussusception)* as compared to babies who received a placebo (according to the 2006 *New England Journal of Medicine* study previously alluded to), and over twice as many babies had seizures within seven days after receiving the vaccine than did babies in the placebo control group.[123]

Other side effects seen more frequently in RotaTeq vaccine recipients than in controls include skin inflammation (dermatitis), vomiting, and diarrhea. The vaccine has not been studied in relation to the other 8 vaccines given to babies between 2 and 6 months of age (polio, diphtheria, tetanus, pertussis, hepatitis B, pneumococcus, Haemophilus, and Influenza). No one knows whether there is a cumulative or synergistic toxicity from this large combination of antigens because there are no studies.

RotaRix Safety: This vaccine *significantly increases the risk of death from pneumonia*, diarrhea, convulsions, bronchitis, and Kawasaki disease (a serious illness that can adversely affect the heart) in children who receive it, compared to children who receive a placebo inoculation.[124]

The risk of death in the placebo group was 29 babies for every 20,000 individuals, but the death rate in the RotaRix group was higher at 37 babies per 20,000 population. As Neil Z. Miller points out, "For every one million babies who receive this vaccine, we can expect 1,850 to die. However, if we leave them unvaccinated, just 1,450 will die—400 babies per every million would be saved by not vaccinating them! As of April 2008, more than 25 million doses had been distributed worldwide. In addition twice as many babies died from diarrhea when compared to the non-vaccinated babies."[125]

---

120   Gov't Reform Committee Hearing; June 15, 2000 *and* Reuters Medical News; Aug 24, 2000.
121   Ibid.
122   Vesikari, T. et al. *NEJM.* 1-5-06; 354:23f.
123   Vesikari Ibid. and Merck product insert.
124   Product Insert *and* Ruiz-Palacios, G.M. et al. *NEJM.* Jan 5, 2006; 354: 11f *and* Linker, A. "Study: GSK vaccine may increase risk of convulsion, death." *Triangle Business J.* Feb 15, 2008.
125   *Vaccine Safety Manual.* p. 221.

Efficacy: Both vaccines are over 95 percent effective at preventing severe rotavirus infections after the series of three immunizations has been completed, and both reduce the hospitalization rate for infections caused by the rotavirus strains included in the vaccine. However, the efficacy of the RotaTeq vaccine declines to only 63 percent just one year after the last inoculation, according to the Merck product insert.

> *"An Italian court recently awarded damages to a boy who developed autism as an injury from the GlaxoSmithKline's Infanrix Hexa vaccine, a combined vaccine for polio, diphtheria, tetanus, hepatitis B, pertussis and Haemophilus influenza type B…. Internal GlaxoSmithKline documents revealed five acknowledged cases of autism resulting from Infanrix Hexa among the children enrolled in the trials for the shot," as well as at least 65 cases of sudden infant death likely to have been caused by the vaccine (they occurred within 10 days of vaccination).[126]*

Review

In this chapter, we have briefly summarized the safety, efficacy, and risk data of all the vaccines that children under the age of five are mandated to receive in 2014 in the U.S. We have noted that some, like the influenza, mumps, rubella, rotavirus, and hepatitis B vaccines appear to cause far more harm than good, and this may be true for many of the others as well.

If a vaccine postpones an illness, like chickenpox, mumps, or measles, from a less vulnerable younger population to a more vulnerable older population, are we really benefitting society in the long run? If a vaccine protects against certain germ varieties, which then results in other equally dangerous competitors rising to the fore, are we better off?

It is clear that many vaccines promote autism, ADHD, neurological harm, developmental and speech disorders, autoimmune diseases like arthritis, childhood diabetes, multiple sclerosis, and asthma as well as sudden infant death, among other concerns. Are these reasonable tradeoffs for the temporary benefits that vaccines are alleged to provide?

Table 27.7 summarizes some of these concerns.

HPV Vaccines: "a Giant Deadly Scam?"

> *"Dr. Diane Harper was a leading expert responsible for the Phase II and Phase III safety and effectiveness studies which secured the approval of the human papilloma virus (HPV) vaccines, Gardasil™ and Cervarix™. Dr. Harper also authored many of the published, scholarly papers about the vaccines. She is now the latest in a long string of experts who are pressing the red alert button on the devastating consequences and irrelevancy of these vaccines. Dr. Harper made her surprising confession at the 4th International Conference on Vaccination which took place in Reston, Virginia.*

> *"Her speech, which was originally intended to promote the benefits of the vaccines, took a 180-degree turn when she chose instead to clean her conscience about the deadly vaccines so she 'could sleep at night.' HPV vaccines, she points out, are unlikely to have any effect on the rate of cervical cancer and the vaccines are known to have serious side effects like paralysis, seizures, blood clots and death. 98 percent of HPV-infections resolve, usually in less than 2 years, and there is no evidence that the vaccines actually reduce the risk of getting cervical cancer. Each vaccine only works on 4 of the 40 HPV strains that cause cervical cancer, 'so the chance of it actually helping an individual,' says Dr. Harper, 'is the same as the chance of being struck by a meteorite.' Over 15,000 girls have reported adverse side effects from just the Gardasil vaccine. 'Dr. Harper has been the victim of a relentless campaign attempting to discredit the validity of her claims.'"[127]*

---

126   https://us-mg205.mail.yahoo.com/neo/launch?.partner=sbc&.rand=508ir3ben1u3l#malhttps//mg205 .mail.yahoo .com/neo/launch?.partner=sbc&.=50 8ir3ben1u3l#mail

127   http://www.healthfreedoms.org/lead-developer-of-hpv-vaccines-comes-clean-warns-parents-young-girls-its-all-a-giant-deadly-scam/

Table 27.7. Summary of Vaccines, Their Efficacy, and Potential Harm[128]

VACCINE	Efficacy	Autism ADHD	Neurolog. Harm	Death	Diabetes Type I	Arthritis & Auto-immune	Other
Diphtheria	See DPT	YES if Hg Present	YES if Hg is in vaccine	YES			Hg=Mercury
Pertussis	See DPT	YES if Hg In vaccine	YES if Hg is in vaccine	YES			Asthma-5 studies
Tetanus	5 years??	YES if Hg in vaccine	YES if Hg is in vaccine	YES		YES	↓ Immunity for wks
DPT	5-80% Wanes over time (5-10y)	YES if Hg in vaccine	YES-27 Studies	YES-8 studies SIDS			Decreased immunity for weeks
Measles	1-2 years ?	See MMR	See MMR	YES			
Mumps	1-2 yrs?	See MMR	Meningitis		YES		
Rubella	< 4 years?	See MMR	Encephalitis	YES	YES -5 studies	YES-21 studies	Autism if fetal cells used
MMR	1-2 years?	YES	YES	YES	YES	YES	
Hepatitis A	Up to 6 years	YES	YES				Asthma
Hepatitis B	4-10 year protection in 50% of vaccinees	YES	YES-36 studies	YES	YES	YES- 40+ studies	Vision & hearing impairment; Blood & skin disorders. Many studies
Haemophilus	Effective for 1-2 yrs	YES if Hg Present		YES SIDS	YES		
Pneumococcus	Uncertain	?			?		
Rotavirus	1 year or so			YES			Intussusception
Polio oral	Excellent but duration unknown	? if grown on fetal cells	YES	YES			May cause polio-myelitis (& autism?)
Polio-killed	Same as oral	? "—"	YES				
Influenza	Minimal or none for <2y or elderly. Slight for others.	Likely if Hg present in vaccine	YES- Guillain-Barre paralysis	YES			Influenza-like illness. ↑ risk for hospitalization.
Varicella (Varivax)	90%?; Duration unknown	YES if fetal cells used	YES	YES			Shingles?

---

128   Data from Neil Z. Miller; Vaccine Safety Manual and other sources previously alluded to.

What About the Vaccine Schedule Itself? Does Any Evidence Show That Giving a Lot of Vaccinations Increases the Risk of Autism and Other Neurological Disorders?

Yes. A Generation Rescue special report published in 2009 reviewed the vaccine schedules, autism incidence, and the under 5 year-old mortality rates in 34 countries around the world and found that, "The United States has the highest number of mandated vaccines for children under 5 in the world (36, which is double the Western world average of 18), the highest autism rate in the world (1 in 150 children),[129] 10 times or more than the rate of some other Western countries, but only places 34th in the world for its children-under-5 mortality rate."

The U.S. not only has the highest infant mortality rate of the 34 countries evaluated, but also has the highest autism prevalence relative to the countries that immunize substantially less. Table 27.8 compares the vaccine schedules (2006), published autism rates, and under-five mortality for select countries. The column labeled "U.S. Autism Rate Multiplier" lists a number that represents how many times higher the U.S. autism rate is compared to each country listed.[130]

Table 27.8. Vaccine Schedules, Autism Rates, and Under Five Mortality for Select Countries131

Country	No. of Mandatory vaccines to age 5y	Autism Rate	U.S. Autism Rate Multiplier	Mortality Rate per 1000 children < 5yo	Mortality Rate Worldwide Rank
U.S.A.	36	1 in 150*		7.8	34
Iceland	11	1 in 1,100	7.3x	3.9	1
Sweden	11	1 in 862	5.7x	4.0	2
Japan	11	1 in 475	3.2x	4.2	4
Norway	13	1 in 2,000	13.3x	4.4	5
Finland	12	1 in 719	4.8x	4.7	6
France	17	1 in 613	4.1x	5.2	11
Israel	11	1 in 1,000	6.7x	5.7	17
Denmark	12	1 in 2,200	14.6	5.8	18

Generation Rescue concluded that, "The analysis lends credibility to the relationship between vaccines and autism and challenges the public view of both the Centers for Disease Control and American Academy of Pediatrics that more vaccines are always positive for public health."[132]

Another analysis published in 2011 of the international infant mortality rates statistically regressed against the number of routine vaccine doses given to babies supported the Generation Rescue study findings. The authors of this study found a "statistically significant correlation between increasing number of vaccine doses and infant mortality rates… (p=0.0009)." They suggest that, "a closer inspection of correlations between vaccine doses, biochemical or synergistic toxicity, and infant mortality rates is essential."[133]

---

129   Now 1 in 50-58 children (2015)
130   http://www.rescuepost.com/files/gr-autism_and_vaccines_world_special_ report1.pdf
131   Adapted from Generation Rescue Special Report April 2009; p. 3
132   Generation Rescue, April 2009. http://www.rescuepost.com/files/grautism_and_vaccines_world_special_ report1.pdf
133   Miller, N.Z.; Goldman, G.S. *Hum Exp Toxic.* Sept 2011; 30(9):1420f.

Is There Other Evidence That Excessive Immunizations Can Cause Harm?

Yes. Japanese researchers found that "Repeated immunization with antigen causes systemic autoimmunity in mice...."

In this underpublicized study, the scientists repeatedly injected mice especially bred *not* to be prone to auto-immune disease with a bacterial antigen. No significant immune abnormalities were detected after seven im-munizations, but *after the eighth injection, all the mice developed autoimmune disease.* Every mouse showed an undesirable transformation of an important immune cell (the CD4 T cell) into a cell that could and did induce autoimmune disease.

This suggested to the "surprised" researchers that "overstimulation of (the) immune system beyond its self-organized criticality inevitably leads to systemic autoimmunity." In other words, over-stimulating the immune system with too many immunizations is likely to promote autoimmunity.[134]

The implications of this study and their likely relevance to the development of autism are clear. The American Acad-emy of Pediatrics has been recommending more and more immunizations for children in the U.S. for over two de-cades. American children, as has been noted, already get many more immunizations than do children in most other countries, and they have the highest prevalence of autism.

Babies in the U.S. get immunized in utero (flu shot to mother), on the day of birth (Hep B) and again at one month (Hep B), two months (DTaP, HIB, IPV, PCV, RV), four months (DTaP, HIB, IPV, PCV. RV), six months: (DTaP, HIB, IPV, PCV. RV, Flu), twelve to fifteen months (HEP B, HIB, PCV, MMR, Varicella), and again at 18 months (DTaP, Hep A, Flu), 30 months (Hep A, Flu), 42 months (Flu), and at 4-6 years (DTaP, IPV, Flu, MMR, Varicella).[135] That's 36 shots for 14 different diseases, with more on the way.

Autoimmune disease targeted against brain and nervous system substances (like myelin basic protein and brain tis-sue), as we have pointed out (Chapter 3), is a common finding in autistic children, as is brain inflammation. Could the aggressive U.S. immunization program be the reason why so many American children regress into autism in the second year of life? Could this be a consequence of the induction of autoantibodies from the excessive number of immunizations (26) they are receiving in the first year of life?

Doesn't this possibility deserve to be studied before the program is expanded even further?

Is There Any Evidence That Children Who Have Not Been Vaccinated Are Healthier Than Those Who Have Been?

Yes, if the results of a recent ongoing survey are valid.

A comprehensive evaluation of vaccinated vs. unvaccinated children's health was initiated in 2010 by two websites www.impfshaden.info and by www.vaccineinjury.info. The respondents were primarily from the U.S., the UK, Can-ada, and Australia. As of October 2013, over 7,500 surveys have been reviewed.

What has been discovered thus far is:

- Less than 10 percent of unvaccinated children suffer from allergies of any kind. This compares with 40 percent of children in the U.S. ages 3-17 reporting an allergy to at least one allergen and 22.9 percent with an allergic disease.

- 0.2 percent of *unvaccinated* children suffer from asthma. This compares with 14-15 percent of vacci-nated children with asthma in Australia, 4.7 percent in Germany, and 6 percent in the USA.

- 1.5 percent of unvaccinated children suffer from hay fever. This compares with 10.7 percent in Germany.

134   Tsumiyama, K.; Miyazaki, Y.; Shiozawa, S. "Self-Organized Criticality Theory of Autoimmunity." *PLoS ONE.* Dec 31, 2009; 4(12): e8382. doi:10.1371/journal.pone.0008382; http://www.plosone.org/article/info:doi/10.1371 /journal. pone.0008382

135   DTaP=Diphtheria, Tetanus, acellular Pertussis (whooping cough); HIB=Haemophilus Influenza B; IPV=Inactivated Polio Vaccine; PCV=Pneumococcal Vaccine; RV=Rotavirus Vaccine; MMR=Measles, Mumps, Rubella (German measles); Flu=Influenza Virus; HEP=hepatitis (A or B)

- 2 percent of unvaccinated children had neurodermatitis. This auto-immune disorder affects over 13 percent of children in Germany.

- ADHD was present in only 1-2 percent of the unvaccinated children. This compares with nearly 8 percent of children in Germany with ADHD and another 5.9 percent borderline cases. [The incidence in the U.S. is 8 percent or more.]

- Middle ear infections are very rare in unvaccinated children (less than 0.5 percent). In Germany, 11 percent of children suffer from this problem. Less than 1 percent of unvaccinated children had experienced sinusitis. This compares with over 32 percent of children in Germany.

- Only 4 unvaccinated children out of the 7,600+ total surveys reported severe autism. In all 4 cases, however, the mother tested very high for mercury.[136]

So, unvaccinated children appear to have fewer allergies, less asthma, less neuro-dermatitis, less sinusitis, fewer ear infections, *less ADHD, and less autism* than their vaccinated counterparts.

Has Anyone Tried a Less Aggressive Vaccination Schedule?

Yes, indeed. Dr. Elizabeth Mumper, a pediatrician and Medical Director of the Autism Research Institute, has done just that. Her modified vaccine and well-baby visit schedule is shown in the following table, and includes all the immunizations that a child will need in order to enter kindergarten.[137]

Note that the hepatitis B shot and the MMR are not given until at least 2 years of age. Varicella vaccine is discussed at age 1 year and may not be given until age 5. No "flu" shots or rotavirus vaccines are given. "Prevnar" (a brand of Pneumococcus [Streptococcus pneumoniae] vaccine) is given at the usual times, as are the DTaP, HIB, and IPV vaccines. Mothers in her practice do not get the flu vaccine during pregnancy.

Dr. Mumper followed 294 children in her practice who were born in or after 2005 for up to 8 years (to at least 26 months of age). All were given immunizations according to the table schedule. None of these children had autism. The CDC estimate of autism prevalence for that cohort of 8-year-old children is 1 in every 50 children. On that basis, it would be expected that at least 5 of the children in her practice would be autistic. Her results were *significant* at a probability of 0.014 (that means there were 14 chances out of a thousand that the difference was due to chance). Her study was published in the *North American Journal of Medicine and Science* in July 2013.[138]

Twelve of the children (6 boys and 6 girls) included in the study had an older sibling with autism. That would statistically make it even more likely that a child in her practice would be autistic (the risk for a boy becoming autistic if an older sib is, is 26 percent and for a girl 9 percent), but none of these high risk children came down with autism.

Dr. Mumper is cognizant that this is a small study so it is difficult to ascribe her good results to just the change in the immunization schedule alone. She does not use acetaminophen in her practice and is cautious about prescribing antibiotics. She encourages mothers to breast feed, puts her children on probiotics, and has them on pesticide-free diets.

On the basis of what we now know about vaccine risks, it is certainly more than appropriate to rethink and reassess the entire vaccination program. If Dr. Mumper's findings continue to be supported by good research, her modified immunization schedule and modest practice suggestion changes might well be a good compromise solution for the pro- and anti-vaccine factions and could serve as a foundation for a revised vaccine schedule.

Dr. Robert Sears offers yet another alternative vaccine schedule (see Table 27.9). If utilizing this schedule, it would be wise to avoid thimerosal-containing influenza immunizations. It is not known whether this schedule reduces vaccine risks (like autism & ADHD).

---

136   http://www.getholistichealth.com/37851/survey-results-are-unvaccinated-children-healthier/
137   http://www.ageofautism.com/2013/08/weekly-wrap-another-medical-practice-with-a-sane-vaccine-schedule-and-no-autism-.html
138   Vol. 6; No.3; p134 ff

Table 27.9. Dr. Mumper's Modified Vaccine & Well Child Visit Schedule

Age	Visit	Vaccine
2 months	Well child visit	HIB, Polio (IPV)
3 months		DTaP, Prevnar
4 months	Well child visit	HIB, IPV
5 months		DTaP, Prevnar
6 months	Well child visit	HIB, IPV
7 months		DTaP, Prevnar
15 months	Well child visit	HIB
18 months	Well child visit	DTaP, Prevnar
2 years	Well child visit	MMR
4-5 years	Well child visits	DTaP, IPV, MMR, varicella (max of 2 /visit)

Well child visits with no vaccines at 1, 8, 9, and 12 months and at 3 & 4 years of age. Varicella vaccine discussed at 12-month visit & Hep B at the 2-year well baby check.[139]

Table 27.10. Dr. Robert Sear's Alternative Vaccine Schedule to Age 6

Age	Vaccine
2 months	Rotavirus & DTaP
3 months	PCV& Hib
4 months	Rotavirus (second dose) & DTaP (second dose)
5 months	PCV (second dose) & Hib (second dose)
6 months	Rotavirus (third dose) & DTaP (third dose)
7 months	PCV (third dose) & Hib (third dose)
9 months	Polio & Influenza (and given every year until at least 19 years old)
12 months	Polio (second dose) & Mumps (separated from MMR)
15 months	PCV (fourth dose) & Hib (fourth dose)
18 months	DTaP (fourth dose) & Varicella
2 years	Rubella (separated from MMR) & Polio (third dose)
2 ½ years	Hep B & Hep A
3 ½ years	Hep B (second dose) & Measles (separated from MMR)
4 years	DTaP (fifth dose) & Polio (fourth dose)
5 years	MMR (second dose of each vaccine)
6 years	Varicella (second dose)

A study by Theresa Dreisher and colleagues, illustrates the *linear* link between the Chickenpox (Varivax) and Hepatitis A vaccines and autism prevalence. This supports the supposition that these vaccines cause autism. This study was previously discussed in Chapter 24. It may be recalled that these vaccines may contain fragments from aborted fetal cells as well as a retrovirus.[140]

139   *North American Journal of Medicine and Science.* July 2013. Vol. 6; No.3; p. 134f.
140   Dreisher, Theresa et al. *J Public Health & Epid*; 6(9); Sept. 2014; p. 282-3.

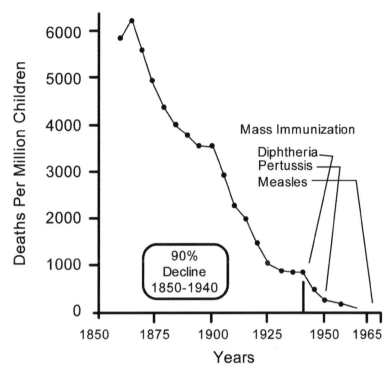

Figure 27.1. England and Wales: Deaths of Chidren Under 15 Years Attributed to Scarlet Fever, Diptheria, Whooping Cough, and Measles[141]

Mortality rates from many infectious diseases declined dramatically in the U.S. England, Wales, Australia, and the Dominican Republic prior to the introduction of antibiotics and immunizations.

For example, there was a 90 percent decline in child mortality in England and Wales from measles, scarlet fever, diphtheria, and whooping cough in the period from 1850 to 1940. Similar declines were seen in the U.S. as depicted in Figure 27.1.

Also note that mortality from diseases for which there were no immunizations, like scarlet fever, also declined significantly long before antibiotics were discovered.

> *"The decline in infectious diseases in developed countries had nothing to do with vaccinations, but with the decline in poverty and hunger."*
>
> — *Dr. Buchwald, M.D.*

---

141   http://www.whale.to/a/graphs.html

Chapter 28
Toxins and Other Substances Implicated in Causing Autism, ADHD, and Related Disorders

"History is apt to judge harshly those who sacrifice tomorrow for today."

— *Harold MacMillan*

WHAT OTHER SUBSTANCES *Besides Mercury and Aluminum Are Implicated in Causing Autism?*
Toxins from Waste Sites and Polluted Air

As we discussed (Chapter 18), there is good statistical support for the association between autism prevalence and proximity to toxic waste sites.

In Minnesota, it may be remembered, investigators found a significant increase in autism in children who lived close to superfund waste sites compared to those who did not. The researchers found that the autism rate among school-children living within a 20-mile radius of toxic waste sites was nearly *twice* that of children living farther away from such sites.[1]

Similarly, a study of San Francisco Bay area children showed a significantly increased risk of becoming autistic in direct relationship to their exposure to hazardous airborne pollutants, particularly to diesel exhaust particles, metals (mercury, cadmium, and nickel), and chlorinated solvents.[2]

The dangers of living too close to a freeway were confirmed in a 2012 study by Heather Volk and colleagues at the Children's Hospital of Los Angeles and the University of Southern California. Volk's team found that children who lived within 300 meters (c. 1,000 feet) of a freeway had double the autism risk compared to those who lived at distances greater than 1,400 meters from the freeway. Proximity to smaller roadways did not show associations with autism.[3]

And in 2013, the same team found that children with autism were *three times* as likely to have lived in close proximity to a freeway during their first year of life as compared to children whose development was normal. Exposure to traffic pollution during pregnancy also increased the child's risk of becoming autistic.[4]

---

1   DeSoto, M.C. "Ockam's Razor and Autism: The case for developmental neurotoxins contributing to a disease of neurodevelopment." *Neurotoxicology.* 2009. doi:10.1016/j.neuro.2009.03.003

2   Windham, G.C. et al. "Autism spectrum disorders in relation to distribution of hazardous air pollutants in the San Francisco bay area." *Environ Health Perspect.* 2006. 114(9):1438–4.

3   Volk, H. et al. "Residential proximity to freeways and autism in the CHARGE study." *Env Health Perspect.* 2011 June; 119(6): 873-877.

4   Volk, H. et al. "Traffic-Related Air Pollution, Particulate Matter, and Autism." *Journal of the American Medical Association Psychiatry.* January 2013.

Other researchers looked at hazardous air pollutant exposure from around the time of birth and found, "Perinatal exposures to the highest versus lowest quintile (fifth) of diesel, lead, manganese, mercury, methylene chloride, and an overall measure of metals were *significantly* associated with ASD, with odds ratios ranging from 1.5 (for overall metals measure) to 2.0 (for diesel and mercury). In addition, linear trends were positive and *statistically significant* for these exposures (P < .05 for each)."

In other words, the greater the pollution exposure, the greater the risk of autism. "For most pollutants," the authors state, "associations were stronger for boys (279 cases) than girls (46 cases) and significantly different according to sex…. Perinatal exposure to air pollutants may increase risk for ASD," they conclude.[5]

It has been found that toxic substances found in small particles from traffic-polluted air are capable of reaching the brain directly, and that adverse brain changes in adults are seen after just *one hour* of exposure to diesel exhaust.

In an Australian study, serum levels of brain-derived neurotrophic factor did not increase as they should after twenty minutes of cycling near a major road, but they did increase when the exercise was repeated in a clean air environment. Brain-derived neurotrophic factor is an important substance linked to proper brain development, learning, and memory.[6]

And a very important study by Ming Xue and associates examined the relationship between population proximity to toxic landfills in New Jersey and the incidence of autism and found a significant correlation. The research team also looked at the relationship between the number of "Superfund" toxic waste sites and autism in the lower 48 states and found that (with the exception of Oregon) a statistically significant correlation (p = 0.015) existed between the *number* of these sites and the rate of autism in each and every one of the other 47 states.[7]

Pesticides: Research Links Organophosphate (OP) Pesticides with ADHD in Children

Organophosphate insecticides damage human brain cells by blocking an important enzyme (acetylcholinesterase). "The half-life of organophosphate pesticides is 6 hours in normal adults, but an astonishing 36 hours in infants."[8]

Children are exposed to OP pesticides mostly from eating foods that have been sprayed with these neurotoxic chemicals. Seventy percent of insecticides currently in use are classified as being organophosphates. The most common organophosphate contaminated foods eaten by children are peaches, apples, grapes, green beans, and pears.[9]

One such OP pesticide called Malathion® was found in 28 percent of frozen blueberry samples, 25 percent of strawberry samples, and 19 percent of celery samples in a 2008 U.S. study. Crops commonly sprayed with these noxious chemicals include wheat, corn, and cotton, and they are also used to kill fleas on cats and dogs and to eradicate mosquitoes and termites.

In a government-sponsored survey between the years 2000 and 2004, 1,139 U.S. children aged 8-16 took part. Of those children, 150 (13 percent) had symptoms of ADHD according to their parents. Urine samples were obtained from all the children, and these samples were analyzed for the presence of six common agricultural *organo-phosphate* pesticides. Their presence was detected in 94 percent of the children!

One out of five of the children (20 percent) with *above average* amounts of pesticide in their urine had ADHD, but in the children who had no detectable amounts of pesticide in their urine, the incidence of ADHD was half that amount (one in ten).[10]

"Each 10-fold increase in urinary concentration of organophosphate metabolites was associated with a 55 percent to

5   Roberts, A.L. et al. "Perinatal Air Pollutant Exposures and Autism Spectrum Disorder in the Children of Nurses' Health Study II Participants." *Environ Health Perspect.* DOI:10.1289/ehp.1206187

6   Knibbs, Luke and Morawska, Lidia. *Environmental International.* 2012 Nov 15; 49:110-4.

7   Ming, Xue et al. "Autism Spectrum Disorders and Identified Toxic Land Fills: Co-Occurrence Across States." *Environmental Health Insights.* 2008:2.

8   Philip Landrigan, MD, Dean of Global Health, Mount Sinai Hospital, at the 2015 Integrative Healthcare Symposium.

9   FoodNews.org

10   Bouchard, Maryse et al. *Pediatrics.* June 2009.

72 percent increase in the odds of (having) ADHD," said lead study author Maryse F. Bouchard of Harvard University. "This is the first study to link exposure to pesticides at levels common in the general population with adverse health effects," she added.

Pesticides may enter the body via ingested produce and less commonly from breathing air near farm-sprayed fields or from contaminated water or surfaces. This study didn't specify the origin of the pesticides found in the children's urine, but since these weren't farm-raised children or children of agricultural workers, the likely origin of their pesticide exposure would have been from the pesticide-sprayed foods they were eating.

The EPA regulates how much pesticide may remain in food, but the results of this study suggest that either the foods being eaten by many of the children had excessive amounts of pesticide residue in violation of EPA standards, or alternatively, that the amount of pesticide allowed in foods now considered safe really isn't. In other words, even tiny, allowable amounts of pesticide may adversely affect brain chemistry.

Additional Studies Showing Harm to Children from Organo-Phosphate (OP) Pesticides

A number of studies published in the journal *Environmental Health Perspectives* clearly demonstrate that children born to mothers who were exposed to these dangerous chemicals showed evidence of serious neurological dysfunction.

In a Columbia University study, seven-year-old children born to mothers who were exposed to the now banned organophosphate pesticide chlorpyrifos were found to have significantly lower IQs and working memory.[11]

These findings were confirmed in a Mt. Sinai study that found prenatal exposure to OP pesticides resulted in having children with impaired perceptual reasoning.[12]

U.C. Berkeley scientists found that female farm workers with high organo-phosphate pesticide exposures gave birth to children who had dramatically lower IQ scores at seven years of age.[13]

EPA researcher Devon Payne-Sturges estimated in a 2009 study that 4 out of 10 children (40 percent) tested by the CDC from 1999 to 2002 had unsafe levels of organo-phosphate pesticides in their bodies.[14]

> *"The primary federal law that governs chemical management in the United States, the Toxic Substances Control Act (TSCA) of 1976, is not protective of the health of children and pregnant women and has not undergone any meaningful revision since its passage.... Since then, of the tens of thousands of chemicals that are in commerce, the TSCA has been used to regulate only FIVE chemicals or chemical classes...."*
>
> *— American Academy of Pediatrics*

"Studies by Furlong and Holland in a California agricultural region have shown that infants are more at risk for organophosphate toxicity than older children and adults because their systems are less able to detoxify these chemicals.[15] The most sensitive newborn was found to be 65 to 130 times more affected than the least sensitive adult."[16]

A study of children of mothers who live in close proximity to farm areas sprayed with pesticides showed a 6.1 times increased risk of a child becoming autistic in the mothers with the highest pesticide exposure as compared to those with the lowest exposure.[17]

---

11 Rauh 2011
12 Engel 2011.
13 Bouchard 2011.
14 *Environmental Health Perspectives* 2009.
15 Ibid.
16 http://west town.monthlymeeting.net/friendly-households/food/news-and-events/organic-food-101-keeping-pesticides-out-of-your-food.
17 Roberts, Eric et al. "Maternal residence near agricultural pesticide applications and autisms spectrum disorder among children in the California Central Valley." *Env Health Perspectives.* 115(10) October 2007.

In a 2006 published study, 23 children aged 3-11 had their urinary pesticide levels measured while on a "conventional" diet and then again after five days on an organic diet. Metabolites of the pesticides Malathion and Chlorpyrifos were readily detectable in the urines of the children eating conventionally-sprayed produce, and they dropped to undetectable levels when the children were given the organic diet, only to return to detectable levels again when the children resumed the conventional diet.[18]

These study findings suggest that we all should eat only organically-grown produce, and getting farmers to grow all their crops organically ought to be the goal of agricultural policy worldwide. It's also important never to use organophosphate pesticide-containing flea collars for household pets or use these toxins in and around the home.

A good website in this regard is globalstewards.org, "an online resource of environmental tips for sustainable living and information about exciting environmental solutions that are speeding the shift toward a sustainable way of life."

Acetaminophen (Paracetamol)

Acetaminophen (Tylenol™ brand and others) is a widely used non-prescription pain relieving substance that is also commonly utilized to reduce fevers. It is recommended for use in babies and children to prevent and treat fever and pain associated with certain immunizations like the MMR. However, there is now evidence that acetaminophen may be a cause of autism in some children.

Acetaminophen has also been shown to directly damage brain cells, specifically the Purkinje (per-KIN-jee) cells, which results in excessive branching of neuronal extensions called dendrites.[19]

Purkinje cell loss is noted commonly in autistic children, especially in the vermis of the cerebellum, which functions to normalize bodily posture and locomotion. This results in *increased brain volume* due to replacement of those cells with white matter. Autistic children have been shown to have increased brain volume.[20]

The reason why immunizations are given is to stimulate an antibody response to the disease entity being immunized against. Acetaminophen has been shown to *inhibit* the production of antibodies after immunization, thus defeating the purpose of getting an immunization.[21]

Acetaminophen is detoxified in the liver via four chemical pathways. Many autistic children don't break down (detoxify) acetaminophen well due to impaired functioning of one of the major detoxification pathways called "transsulfuration."

This impairment results in the overproduction of another breakdown product of acetaminophen abbreviated NAPQI, which is quite toxic to the liver. Normally, NAPQI itself is metabolized to a safer substance (a mercaptide), but that process requires adequate amounts of glutathione, which is often deficient in autistic children, and NAPQI excess promotes a deficiency of glutathione, which sets up a vicious cycle.

Since glutathione is necessary for detoxification of many substances, including mercury, deficiencies set the stage for increased toxicity in autistic individuals

Levels of NAPQI have been shown to increase even in individuals taking just the *recommended amount* of acetaminophen. NAPQI has also been shown to damage mitochondria, and mitochondrial impairment is commonly seen in autistic children, as we have noted.

Sonic hedgehog sounds like the name of a character in a children's videogame, but it is actually the name of a substance necessary for the normal development of the brain and immune system. Its production is stimulated by cholesterol, which, as we have noted, is often decreased in autistic children. NAPQI also inhibits the production of

---

18   Chensheng, Lu et al. "Organic diets significantly lower children's exposure to organophosphate pesticides." *Env Health Perspectives*. 2006; 114; 260-263.

19   *J Toxic and Envir. Health*. Mar-Dec 2006; 9(6) 485f. *J Toxic and Envir. Health*. Mar-Dec 2006; 9(6) 485f.

20   "Acetaminophen induces apoptosis in posterior cortical brain neurons." *Basic Clinical Pharmacology and Toxic*. 2011 July 20, 1742f.

21   *Lancet* 2004; *Alt Med Review*. Vol 14. No. 4; 2009; Yamoura. *Biolog. Pharm Bull*; 2002 25(2); Torres, B. "Is fever suppression involved in autism?" *Pediatrics*. Sept 2, 2003; 319f;

sonic hedgehog, which might thereby contribute to some of the neurological and immune dysfunctions commonly observed in autistic individuals.

Trans-sulfuration reactions, which involve the transfer of a sulfur atom from one molecule to another, can be impaired by a substance (HPHPA) secreted by a variety of toxin-producing bacteria in the gut called Clostridia. Acetaminophen detoxification via this trans-sulfuration pathway is thus impaired in the presence of HPHPA, which also increases the production of toxic NAPQI.

Clostridia are commonly found in autistic individuals, and their metabolites are known to interfere with the actions of a particular brain enzyme (dopamine beta hydroxylase) that metabolizes the neurotransmitter dopamine. The end result of this interference is an excess of dopamine and a decrease in the production of another neurotransmitter called norepinephrine (see Chapter 7).

Excesses of dopamine can manifest clinically as obsessive-compulsive, stereotypic behaviors that are commonly seen in those with autism.

Individuals with norepinephrine deficiency often show reduced exploratory behavior and diminished learning in novel environments. These characteristics are also commonly observed in autistics.

Increases in dopamine production may be diagnosed by measuring the levels of a dopamine metabolite (homovanillic acid) in the urine. Likewise, a surrogate marker for norepinephrine sufficiency or insufficiency called VMA (vanilyl mandelic acid) may also be measured in urine.

We have already reviewed the Schultz et al. study that confirmed that the use of acetaminophen (but not ibuprofen) in conjunction with the MMR vaccine dramatically increased the odds (4-8 times) of a child becoming autistic (see Study 19, Chapter 23).[22]

There is also a more recent study (2013) by Bauer and Kriebel that correlated the prenatal use of acetaminophen with autism and autism spectrum disorders. The authors also found that when acetaminophen became commonly used to diminish "circumcision pain after 1995, there was a strong correlation between country-level autism/ASD prevalence in males and a country's circumcision rate" in the 9 countries analyzed. "A very similar pattern was seen among U.S. states."[23]

Further support for the acetaminophen-autism linkage comes from the island of Cuba. On January 13, 2012, Dr. William Shaw, Ph.D. biochemist and director/owner of the Great Plains Laboratory, presented a webinar on the acetaminophen connection to autism.

He learned that Cuba has an *alleged* very low incidence of autism (1 case for every 59,259 people—or almost 300 times less than the incidence in the U.S.) even though it has an "aggressive" immunization campaign. (That unusually low rate of autism is certainly suspect, however.) By the age of 6, Cuban children have received 34 vaccines, and the compliance rate is about 99 percent.

How to explain the alleged low incidence of autism in Cuba?

One possible explanation for this finding is the increased exposure of Cuba's inhabitants to sunlight, which increases the production of protective vitamin D, but Dr. Shaw suggests another possibility.

Cuban children aren't given acetaminophen for fever; instead, they receive another medication called *metamizole*. Dr. Shaw theorizes that since the immunization schedules of the U.S. and Cuba are similar, the low incidence of autism in Cuba might well be due to Cuban parents not using acetaminophen for their children's fevers.

22   Schultz, Stephen T. et al. "Acetaminophen (paracetamol) use, measles-mumps-rubella vaccination, and autistic disorder." *Autism.* 2008; Vol. 12, No. 3, 293-307.

23   Bauer, A.Z., Kriebel, D. "Prenatal and perinatal analgesic exposure and autism: an ecological link." *Environ Health.* 2013; 12:41. doi: 10.1186/1476-069X-12-41 *and* quoted from Shaw, William. "Increased Acetaminophen use Major Cause Autism, Attention Deficit with Hyperactivity, and Asthma." *Journal of Restorative Medicine.* Vol. 2, No. 1, Oct 2013, p. 14-29(16).

He notes that the increased use in the U.S. of acetaminophen for fever reduction paralleled the rise in autism incidence and prevalence, and that during the two "Tylenol scares" (when the Tylenol brand of acetaminophen was briefly taken off the market), the prevalence of autism in the U.S. fell slightly.

Dr. Shaw published his findings in the *Journal of Restorative Medicine* in the October 2013 issue.[24]

The purported ASD/acetaminophen link has been further backed up by two 2014 studies. In one, a group of New Zealand scientists evaluated 871 children with behavioral concerns suggesting ADHD and found a correlation between acetaminophen use by women during their pregnancy and increased risk of ADHD in their children.[25]

In the second smaller study, researchers evaluated a group of 64 children and their mothers and confirmed that acetaminophen use during pregnancy is associated with an increased risk for developing hyperkinetic disorders (ADHD).[26]

It is important to note that the dosage of acetaminophen listed on the package container may not always have been accurate and that overdosaging was, therefore, likely at times. Johnson and Johnson, the maker of Tylenol, has been found guilty of poor manufacturing practices on several occasions (recent Tylenol recalls occurred in March of 2010 and 2011). Some of their recalled batches were mislabeled in terms of content amount and contained potentially liver-damaging quantities of acetaminophen.

The obvious message here is do not use acetaminophen for children's pain or fever, and do not use acetaminophen during pregnancy either.

Antibiotics

Antibiotics are the proverbial "double-edged sword." They are vital for treating certain infections, but that benefit comes at a cost. Antibiotics often destroy beneficial gut bacteria, while allowing the overgrowth of more dangerous organisms. Their use can promote the development of resistant organisms, and they have a variety of other side effects depending on the antibiotic, some of them dangerous.

Children are often exposed to antibiotics in their first few years of life, commonly as treatment for middle ear infections (otitis media). Children with autism have more ear infections during their first three years than do neuro-typical kids. Almost 20 percent also experienced a severe vaccine reaction.[27]

A frequently used antibiotic for otitis media is amoxicillin, either given alone or in combination with clavulanate (Augmentin®, for example).

Preliminary studies by Professor Boyd Haley found that amoxicillin and tetracycline increase thimerosal-induced neuronal death. In other words, it takes less mercury to damage the brain when these antibiotics are present. Tetracycline is not used in children anymore, as it causes tooth staining, but amoxicillin is still widely prescribed.

A study examining the relationship between otitis media occurrence and autism *severity* among school-aged children with autism spectrum disorders between the ages of 7-9 was presented at the International Society for Autism Research in May 2011. The researchers found that "children with at least one occurrence of otitis media during their development had significantly higher autism severity scores compared to those without an occurrence."

It isn't clear from this study whether it was the infection itself and possible consequent diminishment in hearing acuity that was related to the worsening of the child's autism score or the use of antibiotics given to the child for the ear infection or both.

24   Shaw, William. "Increased Acetaminophen Use Major Cause Autism, Attention Deficit with Hyperactivity, and Asthma." *Journal of Restorative Medicine.* Vol. 2, No. 1, October 2013, p. 14-29(16).

25   Thompson, J. et al. "Associations between acetaminophen use during pregnancy and ASDHD symptoms measured at ages 7 and 11 years." *PLoS One.* Sept 24, 2014.

26   Liew, Z. et al. "Acetaminophen use during pregnancy, behavioral problems and hyperkinetic disorders." *Jama Pediatrics.* 2014; 168(4): 313ff.

27   Konstantareas, M.M.; Homatidis, S. "Ear infections in autistic and normal children." *J Autism Dev Disord.* Dec 1987; 17(4):585-94.

The study authors concluded that "The occurrence of otitis media during development could play an important role in autism severity and symptom expression among children in a critical age range for skill development. Importantly, the present effects observed coincide with other language, processing, and behavioral deficits in ASD populations specific to this particular age group."[28]

Researcher Joan Fallon found in her study of 206 autistic children that they averaged about *ten* episodes of middle ear infection by three years of age, and Augmentin was commonly prescribed for these infections. She suggested a mechanism by which the clavulanate in Augmentin might promote autism by inducing neuronal death via the production of urea and neurotoxic ammonia.[29]

So both of the antibiotics in Augmentin (amoxicillin and clavulanate) may promote autism and magnify its severity. Further research in this regard needs to be carried out to confirm or refute these associations.

Terbutaline (ter-BYOOT-uh-leen)

Terbutaline is a drug licensed for the treatment of asthma. It acts on certain receptors (Beta-2 Adrenergic Receptors/ B2Ars) in the smooth muscle cells lining the respiratory tract (bronchi) and relaxes those muscles, thereby opening up the airway to make breathing easier. Terbutaline also acts on the muscles lining the uterus and can inhibit contractions that occur during labor. It is not approved for this use, but physicians desiring to inhibit premature labor commonly use this drug (intravenously via a pump) off-label (not approved by the FDA) for just this reason.

In 1997, the FDA warned doctors that terbutaline was not effective at prolonging pregnancy long-term and had a number of undesirable side effects, including heart failure in the mother, but obstetricians appear to have ignored this warning. Of the over 300,000 prescriptions for terbutaline written in 2002, 63 percent were for pregnant women.[30]

A study was done comparing fraternal twins born to mothers who had received terbutaline during the pregnancy with twins whose mother hadn't been given the drug. What the scientists found was that the likelihood of both twins having autism was significantly greater for those whose mothers had been prescribed terbutaline. This finding may just be coincidental, or it may be that the mothers who needed the terbutaline bore twins who were for other reasons at greater risk for becoming autistic, or the terbutaline itself may have played a role in this regard.[31]

A possible mechanism linking terbutaline with autism was suggested by the authors of the aforementioned study. The B2AR receptor that terbutaline acts on is a cell membrane protein that is necessary for normal brain development. Animal studies indicate that terbutaline over-stimulates this receptor, causing it to produce excess cell-to-cell signals, which very well might result in abnormal brain development in certain susceptible children perhaps in association with exposure to various environmental insults. This would put some children at greater risk of becoming autistic.[32]

Evidence from animal studies supports this hypothesis. Rats exposed to terbutaline during the late pregnancy period experienced neuronal injury and scarring in the brain. They manifested certain structural abnormalities in the hippocampus (important for memory) and the cerebellum (important for coordinating muscle movements) that are similar to those seen in individuals with autism. The rats also had decreased numbers of Purkinje cells, and were also *significantly more susceptible* to the neurotoxic pesticide *chlorpyrifos* later in life. As we have previously noted, a decreased ability to detoxify is characteristic of many on the autism spectrum.[33]

---

28 "Examining the Relationship between Otitis Media Occurrence and Autism Severity among School Aged Children with Autism Spectrum Disorders between the Ages of 7-9." INSAR Conference; May 13, 2011.
29 "Could one of the most widely prescribed antibiotics amoxicillin/clavulanate 'augmentin' be a risk factor for autism?" *Med Hypotheses.* 2005; 64(2):312-5.
30 http://usautism.org/content/interview_terbutaline_2005.htm
31 Witter, F.R. et al. *Amer J Obst Gyn.* Dec 2009; 201(6):553f.
32 Ibid.
33 Rhodes, M.C. *J Pharm Exp Ther.* Feb 2004; 308(2): 529f.

Conclusion: The jury is still out on the role that terbutaline may play as a possible cause of autism and related disorders, but it is clear from a more recent (2011) FDA warning that terbutaline should not be administered to a pregnant mother, except under very extraordinary circumstances, as the risks appear to far outweigh any possible benefits.[34]

Fluoride

"Fluoride" is a chemical substance (the anion of the toxic gas fluorine) that is added to many brands of toothpaste and also the water supply in a good part of the U.S., ostensibly to prevent tooth decay, but in reality, fluoride is actually a harmful substance and is *ineffective* as a cavity preventer *when ingested*. It only prevents dental decay when applied topically.[35]

Fluorosis: This term describes a permanent mottling of the teeth caused by fluoride ingestion during the formative years when the teeth are developing and haven't as yet erupted.

Studies have shown that the incidence of fluorosis increases as the fluoride content in drinking water increases. However, increased amounts of fluoride in the water do not show any benefit in reducing tooth decay. Fluorosis may be disfiguring, but in itself, it is not the major concern with fluoridation.

Bone density decrease in young girls: A 2006 study provides some evidence that fluoride ingestion hampers bone mineralization in girls.[36]

Adverse effects on IQ in Children: The most damaging aspect of fluoride exposure is its adverse effect on the brain. Thirty-nine studies conclude that *fluoride (like lead) lowers the intelligence of children as measured by IQ tests*. In 32 of these studies, the source of the fluoride was from the water.[37]

In a recent Chinese study, for example, neonatal exposure to fluoride from the local water was found to cause a 7-point drop in IQ scores as compared to the control group with significantly lower exposure to fluoride.[38]

For a list of all the studies that associate fluoride exposure with lower IQ, see http://fluoridealert.org/studies/brain01/.

Seven studies found no such association, but all these "negative" studies are suspect. In one of these studies, for example, the control group was supplemented with fluoride in amounts equivalent to the active group, so it is not surprising that no differences were found.[39]

In another, the Li 2010 study, the researchers compared two groups of children, both of whom had equal fluoride exposure; however, one group had fluorosis and the other did not. Again, it is not surprising that no differences in IQ scores were found.[40]

What Levels of Fluoride in Water Cause IQ Reductions?

According to FluorideAlert, "IQ reductions have been significantly associated with fluoride levels of just 0.88 mg/L among children with iodine deficiency (Lin 1991). Other studies have found IQ reductions at 1.4 ppm[41] (Zhang 2012); 1.8 ppm (Xu 1994); 1.9 ppm (Xiang 2003a,b); 0.3-3.0 ppm (Ding 2011); 2.0 ppm (Yao 1996, 1997); 2.1-3.2 ppm (An 1992); 2.3 ppm (Trivedi 2012); 2.38 ppm (Poureslami 2011); 2.45 ppm (Eswar 2011); 2.5 ppm (Seraj 2006); 2.85 ppm (Hong 2001); 2.97 ppm (Wang 2001, Yang 1994); 3.1 ppm (Seraj 2012); 3.15 ppm (Lu 2000); 3.94 ppm (Karimzade 2014); and 4.12 ppm (Zhao 1996)."[42]

34   http://www.Fda.gov/drugs/drugsafety/ucm243539.htm
35   http://fluoridealert.org/issues/studies/
36   Levy, S.M. et al. "Associations of fluoride intake with children's bone measures at age 11." *Community Dentistry and Oral Epidemiology*. 2009; 37(5):416-
26.   Heller, K.E., et al. "Dental caries and dental fluorosis at varying water fluoride concentrations." J of Public Health Dentistry. 1997; 57: 136-143.
37   http://fluoridealert.org/studies/brain07/
38   Choi, A.L. et al. "Developmental fluoride neurotoxicity: a systematic review and meta-analysis." *Environ Health Perspect* 2012; 120: 1362-1368.
39   Broadbent. 2014. http://fluoridealert.org/studies/brain07/
40   Ibid.; http://fluoridealert.org/studies/brain07/
41   ppm=parts per million
42   http://fluoridealert.org/studies/brain01/

Does Fluoride Exposure Promote Autism and ADD/ADHD?

There are no hard data, but there is a good likelihood that fluoride has a role in promoting these conditions at it is known to poison virtually all enzyme systems even at doses as low as 1 part per million, the amount allowed in the water that we drink.[43]

Fluoride Accumulates in the Body, So Levels Increase Over Time

According to Professor Emeritus Jonathan Forman: It is now known that such vital organs as the kidneys, thyroid, aorta (main heart artery), liver, lungs and others can be the sites of an unusually high fluoride build-up. No matter how small the amount of fluoride in the diet, a part of it tends to accumulate in the body.

When the water supply is fluoridated, the intake of the individual is considerably increased and the accumulation in the body increases accordingly. There is no clear-cut pattern as to the degree of retention among individuals. Further, it accumulates in certain organs in an unpredictable way. Some individuals may store up to 100 times more fluoride in certain tissue than others. This has given rise to concern over fluoride's possible role in chronic disease.

Fluoride is an enzyme poison and medical authorities recognize that disturbances of the enzyme system are a cause of disease."[44]

Fluoride Contaminated With Arsenic

The fluoride added to our water supply and toothpaste comes from a toxic byproduct of the phosphate fertilizer industry, and *it often contains arsenic as a contaminant.* "In 2000 the National Sanitation Foundation (NSF) released the results of its tests that showed fluoridation chemicals can add as much as 1.66 ppb (parts per billion) arsenic to the finished water (which exceeds the EPA allowed maximum of 1 ppb arsenic). NSF found that about 40 percent of the fluoridation chemicals it tested were contaminated with detectable levels of arsenic."[45]

Fluoridated Water Causes Lead to Leach Out of Older Pipes

A number of studies, including a recent one done under very controlled conditions, has shown that the form of fluoride added to water (fluorosilicic acid) causes lead to leach out of pipes in homes built before 1946, when lead solder was commonly used to join copper pipes. Children living in these homes have been shown to have higher lead levels. Lead, like fluoride, is highly neurotoxic and causes a diminishment of IQ.[46]

Are There Other Sources of Fluoride Besides Water and Toothpaste?

Yes. There are two fluoride-containing pesticides that are of concern: *cryolite and sulfuryl fluoride.* Cryolite is commonly sprayed on grapes, especially white grapes, so non-organic grape products may contain unacceptable levels of fluoride. "According to data from the USDA (2005), the average fluoride levels in grape products are:

- White grape juice = 2.13 ppm (also used as a base for other juices)

- White wine = 2.02 ppm

- Red wine = 1.05 ppm

- Raisins = 2.34 ppm[47]

---

43   "Fluorine and fluorides act as direct cellular poisons by interfering with calcium metabolism and enzyme mechanisms. *Handbook of Poisoning: Prevention, Diagnosis and Treatment*, 11th Edition, 1983. "Fluoride is an enzyme poison, in the same class as cyanide, oxalate, or azide...it is capable of a very wide variety of harmful effects, even at low doses." (James B. Patrick, Ph.D., antibiotics research scientist.)

44   (Dr. Jonathan Forman, M.D., world-renowned specialist in allergy, Professor-Emeritus of Ohio State University, former editor of the *Ohio State Medical Journal*, editor of *Clinical Physiology*, in a statement on behalf of Medical-Dental Committee on Evaluation of Fluoridation.

45   http://fluoridealert.org/issues/water/fluoridation-chemicals/

46   http://fluoridealert.org/issues/water/fluoridation-chemicals/

47   http://fluoridealert.org/issues/sources/f-pesticides

Cryolite may also be found in a wide variety of fruits and vegetables: "Apricot, broccoli, Brussels sprouts, cabbage, cauliflower, citrus fruit, collards, eggplant, kale, kiwifruit, kohlrabi, lettuce, melon, nectarine, peach, pepper, plum, pumpkin, squash (summer & winter), tomato, and a number of berries (blackberry, blueberry, boysenberry, cranberry, camu camu, loganberry, raspberry, strawberry, youngberry)."[48]

Sulfuryl fluoride is commonly used as a fumigant and *virtually all cocoa powder, dried beans and walnuts and 69 percent of dried fruits are contaminated with this pesticide.* (See http://fluoridealert.org/issues/sources/f-pesticides/ for more details.)

Conclusion: Fluoride is a neuro-toxin that causes a loss in IQ in children, as well as fluorosis and bone mineralization issues. It is a potent enzyme poison, and it accumulates in the body over time. Fluoride added to the water supply does not significantly prevent dental caries. It, therefore, makes no sense to be adding it to our water supply.[49]

Phthalates

Phthalates (THAL-ates) are a ubiquitous class of chemicals commonly found in cash register receipts, plastic tubing and containers, vinyl flooring, shampoos, fragrances, cosmetics, pesticides, nail polish, children's toys, and wall coverings. They may enter the human body by direct contact with the skin, via ingestion and through inhalation. They have been shown to exert harmful effects on the thyroid gland and can cause "testicular-based androgen insufficiency" in both animals and humans.

A recent study published in the journal *Environmental Health Perspectives* examined the long-term effects of *prenatal* exposure to phthalates. To accomplish this, researchers measured phthalate metabolites in the urines of pregnant women in the third trimester of pregnancy and then evaluated the children's behavior and executive functioning at ages four to nine years.

What they found was alarming. Increased concentrations of maternal phthalate metabolites were associated with a greater incidence of conduct and attention problems as well as depression and low scores on global executive functioning and emotional control. The scientists concluded that "behavioral domains adversely associated with prenatal exposure to…phthalates…are commonly found to be affected in children clinically diagnosed with conduct or attention deficit hyperactivity disorders."[50]

In another study reported in the journal *PLOS One*, researchers found that mothers with increased phthalate exposure during pregnancy gave birth to children whose IQ scores by age seven were 6 points lower than children with lesser exposures.[51]

Two other studies of Korean children's urinary phthalate metabolites support these findings. Researchers in both studies found an association between children's urine phthalate metabolite concentrations and poor attentional performances for ADHD, and in the more recent study, "a genetic influence of this association" as well.[52]

Conclusion: Pre- and post-natal exposures to phthalates may be a cause of attentional deficits, lower IQ, and conduct disorders in children, and there are likely genetic predispositions that can magnify the adverse effects of these pervasive toxins.

Bisphenol A

Bisphenol A is a known endocrine disruptor found in certain plastic (polycarbonate) food and drink containers, including baby bottles, that can leach into foods stored in those containers and cause harm. Bisphenol A has been found in breast milk.

---

48   Ibid.
49   http://www.thelancet.com/journals/laneur/article/PIIS1474-4422 percent2813 percent2970278-Neurobehavioural effects of developmental toxicity; Philippe-Grandjean, M.; Landrigan, Philip J. *The Lancet Neurology*. March 2014; Vol. 13, Issue 3, p. 330–338.
50   Engel, S.M. et al. "Prenatal Phthalate exposure is associated with childhood behavior and executive functioning." *EHP*; Apr 2010; 118(4): 565f.
51   *PLOS One*; December 10, 2014. [Epub ahead of print]
52   Kim, B.N. et al. "Phthalates exposure and ADHD in school-age children." *Biol Psych*. Nov 15 2009; 66(10): 958f. *and* Park, S. et al. "Association between urine phthalate levels and poor attentional performance in children with ADHD." *Intl J Environ Res Public Health*; July 2014; 11(7) 6743f.

According to an article published in the *Federation of American Societies for Experimental Biology Journal* (FASEB), "Epoxy resins containing BPA are also used as lacquers to coat metal in items, such as food cans, bottle tops, and water supply pipes."[53]

In the November 2014 issue of the *FASEB* journal, researchers report on their study in which they found that exposure to Bisphenol A at a dose *significantly below* the current FDA Tolerable Daily Intake predisposes rodent offspring to *food intolerances* in adulthood. In this placebo-controlled study, the researchers exposed one group of pregnant rats to low doses of Bisphenol A and then fed the pups of those pregnancies egg albumin when they had reached adulthood. The bisphenol A exposed rats, but not the controls, showed evidence of intestinal inflammation and activation of a variety of inflammatory immune cells.[54]

The researchers concluded that "the naïve immune system of the neonate is vulnerable to low doses of BPA that trigger food intolerances later in life."[55]

Bisphenol A is also well-known as an endocrine-disrupting substance. Bisphenol A free products may contain bisphenols S or F, which, unfortunately, also appear to be potent endocrine-disrupting chemicals.[56]

Ways to Attenuate the Adverse Effects of the Bisphenol Chemicals

There are research studies that show that genistein (from soy, coffee, and clover), alpha lipoic acid, certain probiotics (Bifidobacterium breve and Lactobacillus casei), folic acid, black tea, royal jelly, and the bacteria found in kimchee may be able to lessen the adverse effects of the bisphenols.[57]

Conclusion: The bisphenols found in plastics are pervasive and undesirable additions to our environment. Products labeled as "bisphenol A free" may still contain other harmful bisphenol chemicals. It would be wise to exercise an abundance of caution and limit human exposure to Bisphenols A, S, and F, especially in pregnant women, babies, and children.

"If you don't read the newspaper, you're uninformed.
If you read the newspaper, you're mis-informed."

— *Mark Twain*

In the US 1,500 newspapers, 1,100 magazines, 9,000 radio stations, 1,500 TV stations, 2,400
publishers are all owned by only SIX corporations!

— *www.Storyleak.com#sthash.razN5M1t.dpuf*

---

53   Menard, S. et al. "Food intolerance at adulthood after perinatal exposure to the endocrine disruptor bisphenol A." *FASEB J.* November 2014; 28:4893-4900.

54   Ibid.

55   Ibid.

56   Eladek, S. et al. "A new chapter in the bisphenol A story: bisphenol S and bisphenol F are not safe alternatives to this compound." *Fertility and Sterility*, Published online Dec 1, 2014. http://www.fertstert.org/article/S0015-0282 percent2814 percent2902351-6/abstract

57   http://www.greenmedinfo.com/blog/research-bisphenol-bpa-causes-100x-more-harm-previously-imagined?page=2

Chapter 29
Genetically Modified Foods

"Money talks. Many listen!"

— *Anonymous*

WHAT ARE GENETICALLY-MODIFIED *Foods?*

The traditional genetic manipulation of plants (and animals) through the tried and true, albeit time-consuming, process of selecting and cross-breeding those with desirable characteristics has benefitted mankind for centuries. As a result, we have bred edible plants that are richer in nutrients, more resistant to pests and diseases, and hardier and more adaptable to harsher climates and poor soils.

However, the 1970s marked the beginning of a novel way of creating new plants (and animals) that has scary implications for mankind's future. In that decade, it became possible to transfer genes from one species to another by utilizing a particular plant parasite or by forcefully "shooting" certain desired DNA fragments carried by a plant virus into plant or animal cells where these genes had never existed before. Those cells could then be made to grow into mature plants or animals that carried the new genetic trait.

Scientists were now able to insert a spider gene into goat DNA so goat milk would contain spiderweb protein. Pig skin could now resemble cowhide after the insertion of the appropriate cow gene, and in 1982, the first transgenic plant, an antibiotic-resistant tobacco plant was created.

Scientists use an antibiotic resistance gene coupled to the "alien" target gene in order to determine whether or not the desired gene transplant was successful. Unfortunately, *this antibiotic resistance can be transferred to gut bacteria when that genetically-modified food is eaten.* That can be a serious problem if the now antibiotic-resistant intestinal organisms cause infection at some later point in time.

When the alien genetic material is introduced into the DNA of a plant, it must be accompanied by an *activator* that turns the gene switch to "ON." Unfortunately, *there is no accompanying OFF switch,* so the newly inserted gene directs the cell to pump out the foreign protein continuously, and this happens in every cell in the plant.

The activator is usually the cauliflower mosaic virus without its protective outer coat. This virus winds up in every cell of the plant and is consumed when that plant is eaten.

The creation of transgenic tobacco was followed by genetically-engineered cotton in 1990, and other genetically-engineered plants soon followed. Companies, like Monsanto, that had invested millions of dollars in this new technology began making huge profits as growers in ever-increasing numbers became enamored with these new man-made "miracle" plants and animals. Assurances were made of higher yields and reduced costs. Those proved to be false promises.

It was now possible, we were told, to turn farm "fields into factories (that produce) anything from life-saving drugs to insect-resistant plants." But those insect and pesticide resistant plants are now proving to be a major concern! By 2004, over 8 million farmers in 17 countries were growing these genetically-modified crops, especially soy, corn, cotton, and canola (rape seed). And what is more, we were reassured, this technology was safe. These new transgenic creations were alleged to be just like their natural predecessors, only better.

FDA Ignores Its Own Scientists' Warnings Regarding GM Foods' Possible Dangers

In 1992, the Food and Drug Administration (FDA) of the United States, the regulatory agency tasked with assuring the safety of the foods that we eat, declared, "The agency is not aware of any information showing that foods derived by these new methods differ from other foods in any meaningful or uniform way," so, incredibly, *no independent safety studies* were required to be carried out. None! It would be up to the obviously conflicted food producers themselves to assure the safety of their products.

However, this declaration of safety ran counter to the reasoned advice given by the FDA's own scientists who, rightly fearing potentially serious side effects from this new technology, urged their politically-appointed superiors to require long-term safety studies of these new genetically-modified foods to be undertaken *before* these "pseudo-foods" were allowed to be used for human or animal consumption.

Their sage warnings were ignored, however, and their serious concerns were kept secret until 1999 when a lawsuit forced the FDA to open its records to public scrutiny, and it was then learned that it was the White House that had pressured the FDA to promote genetically-modified crops.

One of those political appointees at the FDA was Michael Taylor, who was placed in charge of *policy development* at the agency. Mr. Taylor was highly conflicted, however. He was not a scientist, but rather, an attorney who had worked for Monsanto, a leader in developing genetically-modified foods, and would later become its vice president. He succeeded in quashing the FDA scientists' admonitions and recommendations.

As a result, millions of humans and animals around the world have now eaten and continue to consume these never adequately safety-tested abnormally genetically-modified foods. "The Grocery Manufacturers of America estimated in 2003 that 70–75 percent of all processed foods in the U.S. contained a genetically-modified ingredient."[1]

Genetically-modified plants have proven to be a cash cow for the industry leaders like Monsanto. "The global value of biotech seed alone was US $13.2 *billion* in 2011, with the end product of commercial grain from biotech maize, soybean grain and cotton valued at approximately US $160 billion or more per year."[2]

So how did the biotech food producers demonstrate the safety of their genetically-modified crops? They performed their own animal feeding safety studies, and by 2007, there were twenty such peer-reviewed studies and, not surprisingly, none showed that the genetically-modified foods posed any harm to the animals.

But these biased studies were uniformly substandard in that they failed to look for organ dysfunctions in the animals studied, and the researchers used a variety of statistical tricks and investigational chicanery to mask any potential risks. Sound familiar?

These "creative ways to avoid finding problems," according to Jeffrey M. Smith, author of *Genetic Roulette*, included testing the feed on just older animals instead of the more sensitive young ones, using inadequate sample sizes and the wrong controls, mixing the GMO feed with non-genetically-modified feed, limiting the duration of the feeding trials, using inadequate detection methods, ignoring animal deaths and sickness, and others. As Smith points out, "They've got 'bad science' down to a science."[3]

1   https://en.wikipedia.org/wiki/Genetically_modified_crops
2   Ibid.
3   Smith, Jeffrey M. *Genetic Roulette: The Documented Health Risks of Genetically Engineered Foods*. Fairfield, Iowa: Yes! Books, 2013. p. 3.

All Is Not Well in "Monsanto-Land"

But there is also *good science* that points to the very real dangers posed by these unwarranted experiments on human and animal health. Inserting genes through bioengineering processes can have undesired and unexpected consequences. The following findings demonstrating that assertion are adapted from *Genetic Roulette*.[4]

- Scientists developed the genetically-modified "Flavr Savr" tomato, but it proved toxic to rats. They developed stomach lesions and 7 of the 40 tested died within 2 weeks. Nevertheless, it was approved, but fortunately for us, never marketed.

- Scientist Arpad Pusztai developed a genetically-modified potato with a gene for a *non-toxic* lectin from the snowdrop plant that made the potato resistant to insect attack, but the genetically-modified potato now caused abnormal intestinal growths and other undesirable side effects in animals and was notably deficient in many nutrients.

- A bacterium ("germ") known as Bacillus thuringiensis (Bt for short) makes a toxin that kills the corn rootworm and other insects. Monsanto scientists allege that the Bt-toxin is safe for humans and animals, despite the findings from their own study that showed otherwise.

- Monsanto scientists had inserted the gene for the Bt-toxin into corn plants and then fed the corn to rats over a 90-day period. Studies show that *the Bt-toxin in crops is thousands of times more concentrated and is continuously produced in every plant cell. The rats developed liver and kidney lesions, had abnormal white and red blood cell counts, and increases in their blood sugar levels.* The corn was nevertheless approved for human consumption. When humans eat plants containing the Bt-toxin gene, they are also ingesting this potentially harmful toxin. It cannot be washed off as it can when organic corn is sprayed with the toxin.

- Similarly, rats fed potatoes containing the gene for the Bt toxin were found to have abnormal intestinal growths, and sheep, cattle, water buffalo, and other ruminants died after grazing in Bt cotton fields.

- Farmers reported that pigs fed genetically-modified corn had low conception rates, false pregnancies, and increases in sterility.

- 12 cows in Germany died after being fed a variety of Bt corn.

- "Roundup'" is Monsanto's brand of its big money-making herbicide *glyphosate*. The company wanted to use it as an agricultural herbicide, but couldn't, as it would also have killed the farm crop in addition to the weeds. They found out how to insert a gene into corn, soy, cotton, and other plants that renders them resistant to glyphosate. These plants are referred to as "Roundup Ready."

- Mice fed Roundup Ready soy had liver and testicular cell problems, showed decreases in key digestive enzymes, and had abnormal pancreas cell nuclei. Most of their offspring died within weeks of birth. Glyphosate causes birth defects in animals at levels even lower than those used in agricultural spraying.[5]

- When humans eat Roundup Ready corn or soy, they are also eating glyphosate. It's in the seed! "The only human feeding trial ever published confirmed that genetic material from Roundup Ready soy transferred into the gut bacteria of three of seven human volunteers." These bacteria produced the glyphosate-tolerant protein.[6]

- Nature adapts to stresses, and weeds have adapted to glyphosate. Farmers are now seeing new glyphosate-resistant "super-weeds" invade their fields, which necessitates spraying with much larger quantities of Roundup (glyphosate) weed-killer, which then incorporates in greater amounts into the crop plants that we consume.

- Roundup-resistant corn, soy, and beet plants have lower levels of copper, iron, and zinc, and their cel-

4   Ibid.
5   http://earthopensource.org/files/pdfs/Roundup-and-birth-defects/RoundupandBirthDefectsv5.pdf
6   *Genetic Roulette*. p.130.

lular manganese metabolism is significantly reduced compared to non-genetically-modified plants.[7]

- Likewise, Roundup-resistant soybeans require 50 percent more water than their non-GMO counterparts.[8]

- Rabbits fed Roundup Ready soy had significant enzyme level changes in their livers, hearts, and kidneys.

- Glyphosate and aluminum are synergistically toxic![9]

- The foreign genes inserted into the genetically-modified plants may elicit an unwanted immune response. Soy allergies "skyrocketed in the UK after genetically-modified soy was introduced."

- Given a choice, animals invariably avoid genetically-modified foods. This behavior has been observed in cows, pigs, geese, squirrels, elk, deer, raccoons, mice, and rats. In the photo below, GMO and organic corn were left outside, and as can be seen, the animals that ate the corn preferred the organic and left most of the GMO corn untouched.

- One widely used process for inserting foreign genes into cells actually involves blasting micropellets of tungsten, gold, or silver coated with the desired gene into a culture of plant cells and hoping that the gene will find its way into the cellular DNA.

The process is literally hit or miss, and most attempts at gene transfer are unsuccessful, and the implanted gene, if it does find a "home" in the foreign DNA, may not wind up in the optimal spot in the chromosome. *This unnatural genetic engineering process is most assuredly not the same as traditional plant or animal breeding* and carries grave risks that are just now beginning to be realized.

When foreign genes are randomly inserted in this manner, they can and do disrupt the function of the natural genes and, thereby, "mess up" the genetic code near the insertion site. Some parts of the DNA are invariably scrambled and others are simply deleted. Many of the host genes have been found to change their levels of expression after a single gene was inserted. These unpredictable mutations and changes in gene expression may manifest as undesired and even dangerous changes in the plant's chemical makeup. *Hundreds of thousands of further mutations may occur* as the genetically-modified stem cells are multiplied in tissue cultures and then differentiated into seedlings.

According to Arden Anderson, Ph.D. "Inflammation is the universal response to consuming GMO Foods."[10]

"Every study, including those by the industry itself, shows adverse reactions by animals that eat GMO crops. These adverse reactions include inflammatory bowel, indigestion, cramping and diarrhea, reflux, stomachaches, behavioral changes, nondescript inflammatory responses that include skin irritations, achy joints, aching muscles, soreness, headaches, runny nose, cough and potentially more serious consequences to include endocrine disruption, liver and kidney decline."[11]

One potentially devastating problem seen both in animals and humans is the trend of *declining fertility* that has paralleled the rising use of genetically-engineered foods. Pregnant rats and hamsters fed genetically-modified foods *were sterile by the third generation*. Will the same thing happen to us? No one knows. There are no studies![12]

The genetic engineering of plants and animals creates many other potentially serious problems and concerns. The reader is encouraged to review two books by Jeffrey M. Smith, *Seeds of Deception* and the aforementioned *Genetic Roulette*, for more information and studies in this regard. Both books are highly referenced.

---

7   Zobiole, L.H.S. et al. *Plant Soil.* 2009; 328:57-69.

8   http://www.gmwatch.org/latest-listing/51-2012/14164-glyphosate-and-gmos-impact-on-crops-soils-animals-and-man-dr-don-huber.

9   Seneff, S. et al. "Aluminum and Glyphosate Can Synergistically Induce Pineal Gland Pathology: Connection to gut Dysbiosis and Neurological Disease." *Agr Sci* 6(1) 2015.

10   Anderson, Arden. "The Dangers of GMOs." http://www.cpmedical.net/articles/the-dangers-of-gmos?utm_content=the-dangers-of-gmos&utm_source=nl20130801m&utm_campaign=nl&utm_term=ctype-M&utm_medium=email

11   Ibid.

12   Ermakova, I. EcosInfo. 2006; 1:4-10.

Uh oh!

A study reveals that 30 percent of Pediasure samples being fed to children in hospitals were contaminated with glyphosate which "effects heart tissue and facilitates serious heart rhythm problems," says cardiologist Joel Kahn, M.D.

"Ye gads," he exclaims, "glyphosate in Pediasure is frightening."[13]

How Do Genetically-Modified Foods Affect Autistic Individuals?

The answer: It isn't clear. We just don't have enough information, but there are animal lab experiments and relevant observations that suggest that genetically-modified foods cause abnormal behaviors and reactions in animals that parallel those seen in autistic children.

Autistic children often show signs of anxiety and frequently prefer to stay by themselves.

- Lab rats fed GM corn and soy became very agitated and preferred to stay by themselves.[14]
- Lab mice showed similar reactions.[15]
- So did pigs.[16]

A disproportionate number of autistic children have digestive ailments.

- A number of studies point to intestinal problems occurring commonly in autistic individuals. These include bloating, diarrhea, gassiness, abdominal pain, inflammation, intestinal permeability, and imbalances in intestinal bacteria.[17]
- Intestinal problems also seem to plague animals fed genetically-modified corn and soy. Emeritus Professor Don Huber notes, "When you look at the intestine on those pigs fed the GM feed, the lining is deteriorated and the critical microbial balance is drastically changed."[18]
- "The small intestines in GM-fed livestock are typically thin and can tear easily as they're removed from the carcass. The same organ from a non-GMO fed animal…is much stronger."[19]
- Pigs fed GM diets had inflammation and ulcerations in their stomach linings. Pigs fed conventional non-GM feed did not.[20]
- When Danish farmer Borup Pedersen fed his pigs GM food, many experienced bloating, diarrhea, and loss of appetite. Some pigs died. After he switched them to non-GM foods, the pigs' vitality returned, their intestinal symptoms vanished, and their milk production and conception rate increased.[21]
- After only ten days of being fed genetically-modified potatoes, lab rats showed significant changes in the lining of their stomachs and intestines.[22]

13   http://www.naturalhealth365.com/herbicide-brain-damage-leaky-gut-1281.html

14   Ermakova, I.V. "Diet with the Soya Modified by Gene EPSPS CP4 Leads to Anxiety and Aggression in Rats." 14th European Congress of Psychiatry. Nice, France, March 4-8, 2006; and Ermakova, I.V. "Genetically modified soy leads to the decrease of weight and high mortality of rat pups of the first generation." Preliminary studies. Ecosinform. 2006; 1:4–9.

15   Hogendoorn, H. "Genetically Modified Corn (Zea mays) and Soya (Glycine soja) or Their Natural Varieties – Do Mice Have a Preference?"

16   http://www.responsibletechnology.org/autism

17   Buie, T. et al. "Evaluation, diagnosis, and treatment of gastrointestinal disorders in individuals with ASDs: a consensus report." *Pediatrics.* Jan 2010; 125 Suppl 1:S1-18; Buie, T. et al. Preliminary findings in gastrointestinal investigation of autistic patients. 2002. Summary: Harvard University and Mass General Hospital; Valicenti-McDermott, M. et al. "Frequency of gastrointestinal symptoms in children with autism spectrum disorders and association with family history of autoimmune disease." *J Dev Behav Pediatr.* 2006 Apr; 27(2 Suppl):S128-36; Wasilewska, J. et al. [Gastrointestinal abnormalities in children with autism] [Article in Polish]. *Pol Merkur Lekarski.* 2009 Jul; 27(157):40-3. de Magistris, L. et al. "Alterations of the Intestinal Barrier in Patients with Autism Spectrum Disorders and in Their First-degree Relatives." *J Pediatr Gastroenterol Nutr.* 2010 Oct; 51(4):418-24; http://www.autismbiomed.com/gut-diet.html

18   http://www.responsibletechnology.org/autism

19   Ibid.

20   Ibid.

21   Ibid.

22   Ewen, S.W.; Pusztai, A. "Effects of diets containing genetically-modified potatoes expressing Galanthus nivalis lectin on rat small intestine." *Lancet.* 1999; 354:1353-1354.

- "According to US hospital discharges and ambulatory admissions records data, inflammatory bowel disease in the US population skyrocketed by 40 percent since the introduction of GMOs."[23] This, of course, doesn't prove that genetically-modified foods are the cause of these conditions, but they certainly must be considered as a possible contributor to this dramatic increase in the incidence of intestinal inflammation (which is a common finding in autism).

- The Bt-toxin found in many GM crops, including corn, kills insects by damaging cells lining their digestive tracts as well as their gut bacteria. *In high concentrations* that same toxin damages human intestinal cell membranes in less than 24 hours.[24]

- Most of the corn now sold in the U.S. is genetically-modified and contains the Bt-toxin. It is possible for the gene, which codes for the Bt-Toxin, to transfer to intestinal bacteria, which would then be able to produce this toxin in amounts sufficient to damage the gut lining and promote food allergies, inflammation, and a host of other maladies. Food allergies and intestinal inflammation are common in autistic individuals.

- "The bacteria living inside us play an important role in digestion, immunity, detoxification, and even the production of nutrients." There is a great deal of anecdotal evidence that animals fed genetically-modified corn and soy exhibit dramatic changes in the balance of their intestinal flora, often manifesting as a "horrible stench" emanating from their intestinal tracts.[25]

- Glyphosate, found in most corn and soy products, is patented as a microbiocidal agent. It will kill intestinal microorganisms. The rise in autism prevalence in the 1990s parallels the use of glyphosate (Roundup) on corn and soy. Is this just coincidence? While associations don't prove causation, the fit is compelling.[26]

- "A 2011 Canadian study conducted at Sherbrooke Hospital discovered that 93 percent of the pregnant women (and 67 percent of non-pregnant women) they tested had Bt-toxin from Monsanto's corn in their blood. And so did 80 percent of their unborn fetuses."

- Why did so many women have the toxin in their bloodstreams? Were these Canadian mothers eating corn products every day? Or was there another explanation? Was their intestinal tract now infested with Bt-toxin producing bacteria? If the gene for the glyphosate resistance protein can and does transfer to gut bacteria, why couldn't the gene for Bt-toxin? Have we been turning our guts into pesticide factories by consuming GM corn? It is obvious that more studies to evaluate this concern need to be done, and quickly.[27]

- Both *glyphosate*, an herbicide and microbicide, and *Bt-toxin*, a pesticide, can kill beneficial intestinal bacteria and promote the growth of unfriendly bacteria like Clostridia. This is believed to be the cause of the increase in botulism noted in German dairy farms. The ramifications of this dysbiosis will be discussed in Chapter 32."[28]

- Clostridia produce a variety of toxins and causes diseases like gangrene, botulism, and tetanus. Autistic children have been found to harbor this bacterium species in greater number and variety than non-autistic controls. (The ramifications of this dysbiosis will be discussed in Chapter 32.)

Could genetically-engineered foods containing these two toxins (glyphosate and Bt-toxin) be contributing to this problem? Wouldn't it have been good to have studied this concern before releasing these potentially harmful foods for public consumption?[29]

23   http://www.responsibletechnology.org/autism

24   Mesnage, R. et al. "Cytotoxicity on human cells of Cry1Ab and Cry1Ac Bt insecticidal toxins alone or with a glyphosate-based herbicide." *J. Appl. Toxicol.* 2012; doi: 10.1002/jat.2712

25   http://www.responsibletechnology.org/autism.

26   Sustainablepulse.com; http://articles.mercola.com/sites/articles/archive/2013/12/05/adhd-glyphosate.aspx?e_cid=20131130Z1A_DNL_artTest_B4&utm_source=dnl&utm_medium=email&utm_content=artTest_B4&utm_campaign=20131130Z1A&et_cid=DM34178&et_rid=353606974

27   Aris, A.; Leblanc, S. "Maternal and fetal exposure to pesticides associated to genetically-modified foods in Eastern Townships of Quebec, Canada." *Reprod Toxicol.* 2011 May; 31(4):528-33. Epub 2011 Feb 18.

28   Krüger, M., Shehata. A.A, Schrodl, W., Rodloff, A. "Glyphosate suppresses the antagonistic effect of Enterococcus spp. on Clostridium botulinum." Anaerobe..

29   Yuli, Song et al. "Real-time; PCR quantitation of Clostridia in feces of autistic children." *Appl. Environ. Microbiol.* Nov 2004. Vol. 70. No. 116459-6465.

It is uncertain to what degree these genetically-modified "foods" contribute to the autistic condition. What is clear is that genetically-modified plants are not the same as conventionally-hybridized plants. Genetically-modified foods pose such grave dangers for human and animal-kind that they all should be immediately taken off the market, and no consideration of reintroducing them for human or animal consumption should be entertained until sufficient *independent* safety trials show them to be truly safe.

We should demand FDA leadership that is ethical, unbiased, and respects science! At the very least, consumers have a right to know what they are eating. Genetically-modified produce needs to be labeled as such. If not grown organically, a great likelihood exists that any canola, corn, and soy you are eating is genetically-modified and likely contains glyphosate, and now even *non-GMO wheat is often sprayed with glyphosate prior to harvest, so only organic wheat products are safe to eat!*

How Can We Identify GM Foods?

The best way is to *eat only organic produce*, preferably locally grown. Organic implies non-GMO. A lot of produce these days can be identified by the PLU code often found on a sticker on the fruit or vegetable. The PLU codes on produce allow the laser scanners in grocery stores to identify what is being purchased, but they also provide useful information concerning the ingredients in products.

If the five digit PLU number starts with:

- An 8, the food was genetically-modified or engineered.
- A 9, the food was organically grown.
- A four-digit number PLU code means the item was neither organic nor genetically-modified, i.e., it was conventionally grown (using pesticides and herbicides perhaps).

"I refute the claims of the biotechnology companies that their engineered crops yield more, that they require less pesticide applications, that they have no impact on the environment and of course that they are safe to eat....
The scientific literature is full of studies showing that engineered corn and soya contain toxic or allergenic proteins."

— Thierry Vrain, former pro-GMO scientist

Roundup (glyphosate) herbicide is found in 75 percent of Mississippi air and rain samples according to a U.S. Geological Survey.[30]

"Glyphosate residues cannot be removed by washing and they are not broken down by cooking. (They) can remain stable in foods for a year or more, even if the foods are frozen, dried or processed."[31]

On March 19, 2015, glyphosate was declared a probable carcinogen by the International Agency for Research on Cancer. The announcement was published in the prestigious medical journal Lancet Oncology.

doi:10.1128/AEM.70.11. 6459-6465.2004 and Finegold, S. et al. "Gastrointestinal microflora studies in late-onset autism." *Clin. Infect. Dis.* 2002; 35(Suppl. 1):S6-S16.

30   Majewski. *Environ Toxicol and Chem.* Feb 19, 2014.

31   Kruger, M. et al. *J Env Anal Toxic.* 4(2).

And Yet Another Story That Might Sound Familiar

In 2012, French scientist Gilles-Eric Sèralini published a study in the journal *Food and Chemical Toxicology*, which revealed that laboratory rats fed a particular genetically-modified corn (Monsanto's NK603) and *followed for two years* developed *cancerous tumors* that were larger and occurred earlier than in controls.

The females died 2-3 times faster than controls and more rapidly. The GM-fed rats caused disruptions in sex hormone balance. The *pituitary, liver, and kidneys were all affected adversely* by the GM feed in both male and female rats.[32]

The authors found that, "lower levels of…glyphosate, at concentrations well below officially set safety limits, induce severe hormone-dependent mammary, hepatic and kidney disturbances." They went on to recommend long-term safety studies on GM edible plants and pesticides.[33]

This study rocked the manufacturers of GM foods. There was no fraud or manipulation of the data, and no conflict of interest.

Monsanto tried to attack the study by saying Sèralini used the wrong rat breed (Sprague-Dawley) and didn't evaluate enough of them (10 rats in each group), but the same journal had published a similar study (2004) using the same breed of rat, the same number of rats (10), and the same GM corn, but *in that study, sponsored by Monsanto, the rats were only followed for 3 months*, an inadequate amount of time to look for the long-term effects of genetically-modified "Roundup Ready" corn.

Not surprisingly, the industry-sponsored 90-day study found no adverse effects from the GM rat food.

What was Monsanto to do in order to quash this troublesome new study?

That was easy.

It influenced the *Food and Chemical Toxicology (FCT)* journal to hire a former Monsanto scientist, Richard E. Goodman, to the new post of associate editor. He then asked Professor Sèralini to retract his study. Sèralini refused, stating that the study was peer-reviewed and no fault was found with the methodology. The *FCT* journal retracted the study anyway in November 2013.

Does anyone smell a rat?

In 2009, the American Academy of Environmental Medicine called for a moratorium on genetically-modified foods, and said that long-term independent studies must be conducted, stating: "Several animal studies indicate serious health risks associated with GM food, including infertility, immune problems, accelerated aging, insulin regulation, and changes in major organs and the gastrointestinal system…. There is more than a casual association between GM foods and adverse health effects. There is causation…."[34]

---

32   "Long term toxicity of a Roundup herbicide and a Roundup-tolerant genetically-modified maize." Food and Chemical Toxicology. Nov 2012; Vol. 50, Issue 11. p. 4221–4231.
33   Ibid.
34   http://articles.mercola.com/sites/articles/archive/2014/03/11/retracted-gmo-studies.aspx

Chapter 30
Toxic Peptides: The Opioid Excess Theory of Autism

"The chains of habit are generally too small to be felt until they are too strong to be broken."

— *William Shakespeare*

WHAT ARE OPIOID *Peptides, and How Did This Theory Originate?*

An early clue that foods might affect behavior came from patients suffering from celiac disease. Celiac disease is a condition in which individuals show a marked sensitivity to the protein gluten and its constituent gliadin. Gluten is found in certain grains like wheat, kamut, spelt, triticale, barley, and rye, and sometimes, in oats. Approximately one person out of every 100-130 individuals has this condition, and the vast majority of those affected have never been diagnosed and are unaware that they must avoid glutinous grains.

Individuals with gluten sensitivity who eat gluten-containing foods may lose significant digestive function secondary to a loss (atrophy) of the villi, the microscopic small intestinal "fingers" that produce digestive enzymes and absorb nutrients from the intestinal tract.

This "villous atrophy," which is not seen in all celiac sufferers, can result in nutritional deficiencies and intestinal complaints, and may surprisingly also manifest as psychiatric symptoms.

Kaser, in 1961, described celiac children as being "conspicuously quiet, turned inward, often weepy, often discontented or surly and apparently lack(ing) all joy in living. They can," he asserted, "take on negativistic and schizoid characteristics and may execute ceaseless stereotyped movements." These are, of course, symptoms noted commonly in autism.

At about that time (1960s-1970s), Dr. F.C. Dohan observed that gluten- and dairy-foods worsened the behaviors of many individuals with schizophrenia and children with behavioral disorders.[1]

In 1979, researcher Jaak Panksepp was struck by the similarity between autistic symptoms and the effects of naturally-occurring substances called *endorphins* that are produced by the brain and mimic the effects of narcotic substances like opiate drugs.[2]

Inspired by Dr. Panksepp's observations, Norwegian scientist Karl Reichelt began his research into food-derived urinary peptides that are able to attach to opioid receptors in the brain, immune system, and intestinal tract. These exogenous (coming from outside the body) endorphin-like molecules are now commonly referred to as "exorphins."

---

1   Dohan, F.C. in *The Biological Basis of Schizophrenia.* Hemmings, ed. London, Gr. Brit.: MTP Press, 1980.
2   Panksepp, Jaak. *A Neurochemical Theory of Autism.* 1979.

Dr. Reichelt found very elevated levels of these abnormal exorphin peptides in autistic children and also in schizophrenics. These peptides (small proteins) are generally just 3-7 amino acids long and contain sequences that match those of the opioid peptides from casein (casomorphin) and from gliadin and gluten (gliadorphin). Thus far he has identified at least 8 different unusual opioid peptides in the urine of autistic children.[3]

Subsequent research by Paul Shattock and Robert Cade has confirmed Reichelt's work and led to the theory of opioid excess as a cause of some of the symptoms seen in autism (as well as in schizophrenia).[4]

The opioid excess theory suggests that certain breakdown products of particular proteins from gluten, casein, and possibly soy, called opioid-like peptides, are prevented from being further digested due to abnormalities or deficiencies in the enzymes that break down these small protein fragments. A key enzyme that functions in this regard is DPP IV (Dipeptidyl Peptidase IV [four]), which is a metallothionein-dependent enzyme.[5]

It may be recalled (see Chapter 6) that metallothionein deficiencies and abnormalities (mutations) are common in autistic individuals. It is, therefore, understandable that inadequate amounts of DPP IV may be present in individuals with autism, which would then lead to inadequate breakdown of these morphine-like peptides, which might then leak through the gut wall, enter the bloodstream, and affix to opioid receptors in the brain, in the gut, and on certain immune cells.

In the brain, these narcotic-like peptides may promote a dull affect, a decreased ability to focus and pay attention, and a diminished response to painful stimuli. All of these manifestations are commonly observed in many autistic individuals.

And like narcotics, they may also be somewhat addictive. Many autistic children crave these exorphin-producing foods, especially wheat and dairy products, and may experience mild to moderate withdrawal reactions when these foods are eliminated from their diets.

In the GI tract, morphine and other narcotic agents tend to slow the movement of food. This can result in constipation. Children with high levels of these opioid peptides are also often constipated.

These morphine-like peptides eventually are excreted into the urine where they can be measured. Dr. Reichelt has been able to show that when the levels of these peptides in the urine are high, the child's autistic symptoms worsen, and conversely, when the levels decline, the symptoms improve.

He also showed that *they break down quickly at room temperature*, which is why some researchers have been unable to find them in the urine of autistic children. Reichelt and his colleagues assert that urine collected for this purpose *must be fast frozen or treated with acetic acid.*[6]

The morphine-like peptides include *casomorphin* from casein found in dairy products, *gliadorphin* (also called gluteomorphin), which comes from gliadin or gluten in gluten-containing grains, and *desmorphin*, whose etiology is unclear, but which is identical to a paralyzing toxin produced by a certain South American tree frog (the "poison dart frog"). Desmorphin has been found solely in the urines of some autistic children, but never in non-autistics.

Several studies have shown that a significant number of children who eliminate the dairy and grain foods that pro-

---

3   Reichelt, K.L. et al. "Can the pathophysiology of autism be explained by the nature of the discovered urine peptides?" *Nutr Neuroscience.* Feb 2003; 6(1) 19-28.

4   Cade, R. et al. "Autism and schizophrenia: intestinal disorder." *Nutritional Neuroscience* 3: Feb 2000, *and* Sun, Z.; Cade, R. "A peptide found in schizophrenia causes behavioral changes in rats." *Autism* 3: 85-96, 1999, and Sun, Z. et al. "Beta-casomorphin induces Fos-like reactivity in discrete brain regions relevant to schizophrenia and autism." *Autism* 3: 67-84, 1999. Cade, R. et al. "Autism and schizophrenia: intestinal disorder." *Nutritional Neuroscience* 3: Feb 2000, *and* Sun, Z.; Cade, R. "A peptide found in schizophrenia causes behavioral changes in rats." *Autism* 3: 85-96, 1999, and Sun, Z. et al. "Beta-casomorphin induces Fos-like reactivity in discrete brain regions relevant to schizophrenia and autism." *Autism* 3: 67-84, 1999.

5   Whitely, P.; Shattock, P. "Biochemical aspects in autism spectrum disorders: updating the opioid excess theory and presenting new opportunities for biochemical intervention." *Expert Opinion Ther. Targets.* Apr 2002; 6(2): 175ff.

6   Finvold, A.; Reichelt, K.L. "Peptides and Exorphins in the Autism Spectrum." 2012; Awares Internet Conference; Cymru, Wales; (Ed. A. Feinstein) p. 1-10.

mote the production of these peptides will manifest a dramatic improvement in their functioning. These studies confirm what the Autism Research Institute found in its 2008 survey of 27,000 families with autistic children.[7]

The peptides that derive from gliadin may also induce the production of antibodies against gliadin and certain brain cells (Purkinje cells in the cerebellum). This may account for some of the neurological symptoms seen in autistics.[8]

Gliadin peptide *has also been shown to induce autoantibodies* against certain digestive enzymes (aminopeptidases) that help break down peptides. Dr. Vojdani speculates that "dysfunctional membrane peptidases and autoantibody production may result in neuroimmune dysregulation and autoimmunity," which are common findings in autistics.[9]

Dr. Vojdani, in an earlier study, showed that autistic children, as compared to controls, produced significantly higher levels of antibodies (IgA, IgG, and IgM) against nine different neuron-specific antigens and three cross-reactive peptides (one from milk protein and the others from certain bacteria).

These findings suggest that a dysfunctional blood-brain barrier allowed these peptides to enter the brain where they promoted the production of antibodies that also cross-reacted with specific brain proteins.

This scenario could well set up a vicious cycle of inflammation promoting a "leaky" blood brain barrier, which would then allow more food substances to enter the brain and continue the cycle. "These results," says Dr. Vojdani, "suggest a mechanism by which bacterial infections and milk antigens may modulate autoimmune responses in autism."[10]

A 2005 study published in *Pediatrics* found that autistic children *with chronic intestinal complaints* produced more inflammatory substances (TNF-alpha & IL-12) when fed cow's milk protein and gliadin then did controls. This suggested that cow's milk protein and gluten grains may also play a causative role in the gastro-intestinal symptoms observed in children with autism spectrum disorders.[11]

The Structure of Casomorphin and Gliadorphin
tyr=tyrosine; pro=proline; phe=phenylalanine; ile=isoleucine; gln=glutamine; gly=glycine[12]

	1	2	3	4	5	6	7
Casomorphin:	tyr-	pro-	phe-	pro-	gly-	pro-	ile
Gliadorphin:	tyr-	pro-	gln-	pro-	gin-	pro-	phe

"Every time I talk to a mother of an (autistic) child or see a news story about autism on TV, I hear about or observe them eating foods rich in dairy or wheat.... They are addicted to the (foods) that are making them sick, just like a drug addict or alcoholic."

— John. B. Symes, DVM

7   www.alternativemedicine.com/autism/going-gluten-free-kids *and* Millward, C. et al. "Gluten- and casein-free diets for autistic spectrum disorder." *Cochrane Database Syst. review.* 2004; (2) CD003498; *and* Knivsberg, A.M., Reichelt, K.L. et al. "A randomized controlled study of dietary intervention in autistic syndromes." *Nutr Neuroscience.* Sept 2002; 5(4): 251ff, *and* Knivsberg, A.M.; Reichelt, K.L. et al. "Reports on dietary intervention in autism disorders." *Nutr Neuroscience.* 2001; 4(1) 25-37.
8   Vojdani, A. et al. "Immune response to dietary proteins, gliadin and cerebellar peptides in children with autism." *Nutr Neuroscience.* June 2004; 7(3): 15-ff.
9   Vojdani, A. et al. "Heat shock protein and gliadin peptide promote development of peptidase antibodies in children with autism and patients with autoimmune disease." *Clinic Diagn Lab Immunol;* 2004, May; 11(3):515ff.
10   Vojdani, A. et al. "Antibodies to neuron-specific antigens in children with autism: possible cross reactions with encephalitogenic proteins from milk... and streptococcus group A." *J Neuroimmunol.* Aug 2002; 129 (1-2): 168ff.
11   Jyonouchi, H. et al. "Evaluation of an association between GI symptoms and cytokine production against common dietary proteins in children with autism spectrum disorders." *J. Pediatrics.* May 2005; 146(5): 605ff.
12   http://www.biologicaltreatments.com/book/ch6.asp

Is There a Link Between Celiac Disease and Autism Spectrum Disorders?

There may be. A 2013 study in the *JAMA Psychiatry* journal found that while there was "no association between celiac disease or inflammation and *earlier* autism spectrum disorders, there was a markedly increased risk (3 times the risk) of autism spectrum disorders in individuals with normal mucosa but a positive celiac disease serologic test result." The latter include IgA/IgG antibodies to gliadin, endomysium, or tissue transglutaminase.[13]

Conclusion: The morphine-like opiates from gluten and casein (and possibly soy) produce foggy thinking, inattentiveness, irritability, addiction to the food, and constipation—all symptoms of morphine use/addiction. These food-derived opiate-like molecules may also have adverse effects on immune function and induce auto-immune disease. Evidence exists that IgA and IgG antibodies to gliadin, endomysium, and tissue transglutaminase may increase the risk of an individual becoming autistic.

Studies show that eliminating gluten and casein from the diet will improve symptoms in *many* (but not all) autistic individuals. It is, thus, appropriate to consider evaluating a diet free of dairy and gluten in individuals on the autistic spectrum.

---

13   Ludvigsson, J.F. et al. "A Nationwide Study of the Association between Celiac Disease and the Risk of Autism Spectrum Disorders." *JAMA Psychiatry.* Nov 2013, 70(11).

Chapter 31
Food Allergies, Intolerances, Additives, and Dietary Deficiencies

"One man's meat is another man's poison."

— Lucretius, 1ˢᵗ century BC

WHAT ARE SOME *Other Ways That Foods Cause Toxic Reactions in People?*
It surprises some people to learn that common, everyday foods like milk, wheat, soy, eggs, nuts, and beans can be harmful to many individuals. We have already seen that the genetic modification of our food supply can do harm, as can the incompletely digested products of gluten and casein (opioid peptides).

But allegedly beneficial foods can damage us in other ways and by other mechanisms. These include allergic reactions, hypersensitivity reactions, lectin incompatibilities, food intolerances due to other mechanisms, toxins in foods, and nutritionally-depleted "foods."

Food intolerances and allergies appear to be increasing worldwide. "According to a study released in 2013 by the Centers for Disease Control and Prevention, food allergies among children increased approximately 50 percent between 1997 and 2011." Why this is occurring isn't clear, but causes could include the effect of neonatal or childhood exposure to toxins like Bisphenol A (see Chapter 28), the increased presence of genetically-modified foods, and certain immunizations.[1]

Children with autism have been shown to have more allergies, particularly to foods, than their non-autistic peers, and these food allergies and intolerances do adversely influence autistic behaviors.[2]

What Are Allergies?

Allergies are abnormal immune reactions that cause the body to be inappropriately sensitive to substances that normally would not be expected to bother most people. Common allergens include pollen, dust, mold, animal danders, foods, insects, mites, many chemicals, and microorganisms.

---

1   http://www.foodallergy.org/facts-and-stats
2   Gurney, J.G. et al. "Parental report of health conditions and health care use among children with and without autism: national survey of children's health." *Archive of Pediatric Adolescent Medicine.* 2006; 160(8):825-830.

There are four types of allergic reactions:

Type I: These reactions can manifest as hives, swelling, difficulty breathing, sneezing, congestion, and anaphylaxis. They are initiated when allergens react with Immuno globulin E (IgE) antibodies on the surface of basophils (in blood) and mast cells (in mucous membranes). These immune cells release histamine and other reactive substances when stimulated by an allergic exposure. Histamine causes itchiness, hives, and swelling of tissues.

Some people refer to Type I allergies as the only "true" allergy and refer to Types II through IV below as "sensitivity reactions." In the end, the name we give to these reactions is of little importance.

Type II: This type of allergy manifests when other antibodies (IgG or IgM) bind to sticky molecules called lectins on red or white blood cell membranes. Complement (a mix of small immune-stimulating proteins) and K-Cells, a type of immune cell, can attach, agglutinating (clumping) the affected cells.

Type III: Caused when IgG antibodies form large antigen-antibody complexes. Complement proteins and neutrophils (bacteria-killing white cells) can attach to these complexes, which can deposit in tissues causing damage. These reactions are often delayed.

Type IV: Caused when large immune cells called macrophages interact with other immune cells (T-lymphocytes), which then migrate to the affected area, initiating the release of inflammatory chemicals called cytokines. This migration can take time, and these reactions may also be delayed by hours or even a day or so. The "poison ivy" (Rhus dermatitis) rash is an example of a Type IV allergy/sensitivity.

What Are Food Allergies?

Food allergies are adverse immune reactions to substances in the foods that we eat that can manifest in many ways. There are two major kinds of food allergies. These are immediate sensitivity reactions, mediated by immunoglobin E antibodies (IgE), and delayed sensitivity reactions mediated by immunoglobins A (IgA) and G (IgG), and in particular, by IgG4-a subtype of IgG. The latter are more properly referred to as "Type III hypersensitivity reactions," while the term "allergy," as previously noted, is now often reserved for just the Type I hypersensitivity reactions.

What Are Immediate (Type I) Allergies?

Immediate sensitivity reactions, also called Type I allergic reactions, can cause symptoms like wheezing, difficulty breathing, asthma, itchy, runny nose and eyes, hives, eczema, and intestinal distress.

The most serious reaction mediated by immunoglobulin E antibodies (IgE) is anaphylaxis, a potentially fatal condition characterized by severe swelling of the trachea and bronchi to such a degree that breathing is impaired. This is generally accompanied by hives, edema (abnormal fluid accumulation) of various body tissues, and intestinal symptoms. Individuals on the autistic spectrum are as susceptible to these allergies as are those who are not.

Approximately 6-8 percent of children and 3-4 percent of adults have IgE-mediated food allergies.[3]

Childhood peanut/tree nut allergies tripled between 1997 and 2008 from 0.6 percent to 2.1 percent. There has been a 265 percent rise in food allergy hospitalization among children. It isn't clear what is causing this epidemic of food allergies, but it isn't better diagnosing.[4]

Immediate sensitivity reactions generally start within minutes of exposure to the offending allergenic substance or food (antigens). The initial reaction is thought to be mediated by the release of histamine and other substances (leukotrienes and prostaglandins) from the aforementioned immune cells called mast cells and basophils.

---

3   Sicherer, S.H.; Sampson, H.A. "Food allergy." *J Allergy Clin Immune.* 2006; 117(suppl): S470-5; *and* Zeiger, R.S. "Food allergen avoidance in the prevention of food allergy in infants and children." *Pediatrics.* 2003; 111(6): 1662-1671.

4   CDC; *and* Sicherer et al. "US prevalence of self-reported peanut, tree nut and sesame allergy: 11-year follow-up." *JACI.* Vol. 125. No. 6. June 2010: 1322-1326 *and* Fraser, H. *The Peanut Allergy Epidemic.* New York, NY: Skyhorse, 2011. p. 124-126.

The allergenic substances that initiate these allergic responses include pollens, dust, mold spores, animal danders, dust mites, foods, bacteria, yeasts, various chemicals, and insect antigens.

A late (delayed) phase of the Immunoglobulin E-mediated allergic reaction often occurs 2-4 hours after exposure to the allergen and is thought to be mediated by substances called cytokines, which are released by particular immune cells.

Most individuals with Type I allergic reactions to foods are aware of which foods cause these reactions since the symptoms are generally obvious and discomfiting and begin shortly after the foods are ingested. The most common food allergens are from dairy foods, wheat, eggs, tree nuts, peanuts, and sea foods, but virtually any food can elicit IgE-mediated reactions.

Testing to confirm the presence of the antibodies to foods and other allergens can be done by any allergist via a variety of skin-testing techniques (prick, scratch, or intradermal) or with a blood test (RAST test). The latter is not as sensitive a test as are the skin tests, and may yield more false negative results (i.e., the RAST test may miss some allergens of importance). *None of these tests is 100 percent reliable* and both false positive and false negative results are not uncommon.

This type of food allergy does certainly manifest in autistic children and may affect behavior. There is some evidence that ADHD symptoms may worsen during the inhalant allergy season.[5]

In contrast, delayed (Type III) toxic immune complex-mediated hypersensitivity reactions are a major concern to autistic individuals and those with ADHD.

What Are Type III ("Delayed") Hypersensitivity Reactions?

According to Meridian Valley Lab: Type III reactions are mediated by a mixed group of antibodies, though IgG antibodies are the most common immunoglobulins that trigger these immune complex forming reactions.

Immune complexes are circulating antibodies coupled to antigens that activate, complement and trigger the release of inflammatory substances (cytokines). The resulting inflammatory cascade contributes to many undesirable health symptoms, including attention deficits, ear infections, joint pain, headaches, fatigue, eczema, and psoriasis, many of which are associated with food allergy.

Type III reactions are considered to be "delayed" because of the time required to form the immune complexes.[6]

Delayed sensitivity reactions to food allergens and other antigenic substances may occur shortly after exposure to the offending substance, but generally don't manifest until hours or even days after the exposure.

Delayed hypersensitivity reactions are often not obvious as the symptoms can vary greatly and may not occur in close proximity to exposure to the offending agent. The prevalence of this type of food sensitivity is not clear. Some estimates are that 45-60 percent of the population may have symptoms related to IgG food sensitivities.[7]

Children with autism are no exception. They were found to have higher levels of antibodies to dairy, wheat, and eggs than did their non-autistic peers in a 1995 study.[8]

ImmunoLabs in Florida has found that 95 percent of people tested for these sensitivities have significant reactions to one or more of the food allergens tested and note relief when the offending food is eliminated from the diet.[9]

This lab, and a number of others, tests for IgG-mediated food sensitivity reactions via an ELISA test (Enzyme Linked

5   Study presentations, American Academy of Allergy, Asthma and Immunology, Annual meeting, Denver. March 7-12, 2003.
6   http://meridianvalleylab.com/igg-allergy-testing
7   Shamberger, R. "Types of food allergy testing." *The Townsend Letter.* Jan 2008; 294: 71-72; *and* Breneman, J.C. *Basics of Food Allergy.* Springfield, IL: C.C. Thomas, 1978. p.8.
8   Lucarelli et al. "Food allergy and infantile autism." *Panminerva Medica.* Sept 1995.
9   Immunolabs.com.

Immuno-Sorbent Assay), which requires a blood specimen to be collected, centrifuged, and the serum separated and sent to the lab for analysis.

Conventional wisdom rejects these tests as unreliable, and indeed, many labs don't yield results that are reliable (reproducible/consistent) or have good predictive value (a positive reaction to a food correlates with symptoms).[10]

In this regard, it can be said that ImmunoLabs in Florida may be one exception to the rule. They have been doing IgG food allergy testing for decades, have performed millions of tests, have excellent reproducibility (send them a split sample with different names and get the same results), and have excellent predictability (eliminate the allergenic food and the symptoms abate).

This lab is so certain that its results will be of benefit to patients that it guarantees satisfaction or it will refund the cost of the test.

It has been my experience (over many years and hundreds of tests),[11] as well as the experience of many other clinicians, that the ImmunoLabs IgG food sensitivity test results do correlate with patient symptoms, and that the test is of immense value in that regard. As with IgE allergy testing, this test can also yield false positive and false negative results.

Do Any Studies Support the Use of IgG testing?

Yes, a number of research studies have demonstrated that IgG food sensitivity testing results correlate with symptoms, particularly intestinal symptoms (and migraine headaches).

Researchers in the Department of Gastroenterology at the Henan University of Science and Technology found great value in eliminating foods according to food-specific IgG antibodies in patients with irritable bowel syndrome and diarrhea.

"Specific immunoglobulin G (IgG) antibodies against 14 common food antigens in the serum were measured in 77 patients with (diarrhea and irritable bowel syndrome) and 26 healthy controls."[12] The researchers found food-specific IgG antibodies in about half (35) the symptomatic patients and just 15 percent (4 patients) in the control group.

"For 12 weeks following the serological testing, 35 patients with (diarrhea and irritable bowel) and food intolerance consumed diets that excluded the identified food…. After 4 weeks' dietary therapy, most symptoms of (diarrhea and irritable bowel) had improved. By 12 weeks, all symptom scores had decreased significantly compared with the baseline scores."

The authors concluded that, "The 12-week specific-food exclusion diets resulted in significant improvements in abdominal pain (bloating level and frequency), stool frequency, abdominal distension, stool shape, general feelings of distress and total symptom score compared with baseline in patients with (diarrhea and irritable bowel syndrome)."[13]

Another similar double-blind, placebo-controlled study by British researchers at St. George's Hospital Medical School in London was published in 2005 and arrived at the same conclusion. In this study, the authors evaluated immunoglobulin G4 (IgG$_4$)[14] antibody titers to 16 food allergens (milk, eggs, cheese, wheat, rice, potatoes, chicken, beef, pork, lamb, soya bean, fish, shrimps, yeast, tomatoes, and peanuts) in 25 patients with irritable bowel syndrome. Reactive foods were excluded for 6 months.

---

10   Miller, Sheryl B. "IgG Food Allergy Testing by ELISA/EIA What Do They Really Tell Us?" http://www.tldp.com/issue/174/IgG percent20Food percent20Allergy.html
11   The author has no financial or other connection to this lab or any other and has had no experience with other labs that may be equally reliable.
12   Abstract; Guo, et al.
13   Guo, H. et al. "The value of eliminating foods according to food-specific immunoglobulin G antibodies in irritable bowel syndrome with diarrhea." *J Int Med Res*. 2012; 40(1):204-10.
14   IgG4-is a relevant subtype of IgG antibody.

The authors noted that, "Symptom severity was assessed with a previously validated questionnaire at baseline, at 3 months and at 6 months. Rectal compliance and sensitivity were measured in 12 patients at baseline and at 6 months."[15]

What was found was that, "IgG$_4$ antibodies to milk, eggs, wheat, beef, pork and lamb were commonly elevated. Significant improvement was reported in pain severity ($p < 0.001$), pain frequency ($p = 0.034$), bloating severity ($p = 0.001$), satisfaction with bowel habits ($p = 0.004$) and effect of Irritable Bowel Syndrome on life in general ($p = 0.008$) at 3 months. Symptom improvement was maintained at 6 months. Rectal compliance was significantly increased ($p = 0.011$) at 6 months...."[16]

They concluded that, "Food-specific IgG$_4$ antibody-guided exclusion diet improves symptoms in (Irritable Bowel Syndrome) and is associated with an improvement in rectal compliance."[17]

A similar study by Dr. Zar and colleagues published that same year compared antibody titers (levels) of food specific IgG4 and also IgE (Immunoglobulin E) antibodies to 16 common food antigens in 108 irritable bowel syndrome patients divided into a diarrhea predominant group (52), a constipation predominant group (32), and a group with alternating constipation and diarrhea (24). A 43-person control group was also evaluated.

What the researchers found was that all three irritable bowel subgroups had significantly higher IgG antibody titers to 4 of the foods (wheat, beef, pork, and lamb) than did controls. There were no significant difference between the symptomatic and control groups in regard to antibody IgG4 antibody titers to the other foods and *no difference in IgE titers either.*

They concluded that, "Serum IgG4 antibodies to common foods like wheat, beef, pork, and lamb are elevated in Irritable Bowel Syndrome patients. In keeping with the observation in other atopic conditions, this finding suggests the possibility of a similar pathophysiological role for IgG4 antibodies in Irritable Bowel Syndrome."[18]

An elimination diet evaluation of the symptomatic patients was, unfortunately, not a part of this study, but it was an important part of the next one.

In a double-blind, placebo-controlled study published in the journal *Gut* in 2004, researchers investigated 131 individuals with chronic irritable bowel syndrome and measured their IgG food-specific antibodies to 29 different foods. Most of the participants reacted to 6-7 foods and had been ill for 10 years or so.

Patients were then given a true or a sham elimination diet and their symptoms were assessed at the end of 12 weeks, at which time those on the true elimination diet showed a 10 percent decrease in symptoms scores overall with a 26 percent improvement in those with the highest levels of IgG antibodies. However, only a minimal (placebo effect?) benefit was reported in those on the sham diet. The results were statistically significant.

In the second part of the study, the offending foods were reintroduced into the diet and symptom severity increased significantly by 83 percent in those on the true diet and by just 31 percent in the sham group, suggesting a placebo effect in those on the sham diet.

The investigators concluded that, "Food elimination based on IgG antibodies may be effective in reducing Irritable Bowel Syndrome symptoms and is worthy of further biomedical research."[19]

In another study published in 2008, Chinese researchers evaluated IgG levels in 82 children with chronic diarrhea and found that *milk* was the antigenic food that elicited the highest level of IgG response with pork being the least antigenic. The children were placed on a hypoallergenic diet eliminating the reactive foods. Symptom improvement was noted in 65 (79 percent) of the children in as little as one week after starting the elimination diet, and *by three months, all of the children had improved.*

---

15   Abstract.

16   Abstract (see below).

17   Zar, S. et al. "Food-specific IgG4 antibody-guided exclusion diet improves symptoms and rectal compliance in irritable bowel syndrome." *Scand J Gastroenterol.* Jul 2005; 40(7):800-7.

18   Zar, S. et al. "Food-specific serum IgG4 and IgE titers to common food antigens in irritable bowel syndrome." *Am J Gastroenterol.* Jul 2005; 100(7):1550-7.

19   Atkinson, W. et al. "Food elimination based on IgG antibodies in irritable bowel syndrome: a randomized controlled trial." *Gut.* Oct 2004.

The researchers concluded that "IgG mediated food allergy played a major causative role in the children's diarrhea and felt that food-specific IgG assessment should be part of the work-up of children with this condition."[20]

What we can see from these studies is that there is value in IgG food allergy testing when utilizing a reliable lab and that IgG and *not* IgE reactivity correlates better with symptoms of intestinal distress in patients with irritable bowel syndrome and children with diarrhea.

As we have previously noted, many of the symptom of irritable bowel are also seen commonly in autistic individuals, so IgG food allergy testing is recommended in these individuals as part of an appropriate biomedical workup. (See Appendix IA for many relevant references regarding autism and intestinal complaints.)

What Causes Food Allergies?

The digestive tract is designed to break down foods into their constituent parts so they can be readily absorbed and assimilated. This requires a complex "symphony" of biochemical events to be appropriately "orchestrated" by the stomach and intestines so that optimal digestion is achieved. Disruptions in this process can lead to an incomplete breakdown of food substances, which in turn can give rise to a variety of undesirable symptoms, like diarrhea, bloating, constipation, and pain, as well as the development of food allergies and sensitivities.

The intestinal tract is tasked with a difficult challenge. It must absorb food nutrients, while at the same time barring the entry of toxins, bacteria, viruses, parasites, and fungi. Intestinal immune cells must also evaluate which substances are safe and which are not, which ones to launch an immune assault against, and which ones to leave alone. It is for this reason that most of our immune system is situated in and near the digestive tract.

One of the ways the gut manages to bar unwanted substances from entering the bloodstream is by maintaining tight junctions between the cells that line the GI tract. Tight junctions prevent food substances and microorganisms from leaking between the cells that line the intestinal tract [from the lumen (inside) of the intestinal tract to the extracellular fluid (ECF)].

This means that the preferred way for nutrients to enter the circulation is by going *through* the intestinal cells and not *around* them. For example, this barrier action prevents large antigenic substances from incompletely digested foods from entering the bloodstream.

If tight junctions become "loose," then partially digested foods are able to pass through to the bloodstream where they may be misidentified as "foreign agents" and thereby elicit an immune response, including the production of antibodies to that food protein. The result is an "allergy" or "sensitivity" to that food.

What Causes a Loosening of Tight Junctions?

Intestinal bacteria, food allergies and sensitivities, toxins, radiation, intestinal infections, and malnutrition can disrupt tight junctions. This can lead to food allergies and intolerances, immune system abnormalities, and autoimmunity.

The increase in intestinal permeability caused by a loosening of the tight junctions between intestinal cells is commonly called "leaky gut."

What Are Lectins?

Lectins are "sticky" proteins, found protruding from the surface membranes of cells. They may cause cells to attach to one another (agglutinate), and are found in most plants, and in particular in grains (including wheat, rye, oats, corn, and barley) and in potatoes (and other "nightshades" like tomatoes and eggplant), as well as in dairy foods, beans, and peanuts. "The term 'lectin' was introduced in 1954 by Boyd and Shapleigh to indicate substances of non-immune origin which have the ability to agglutinate blood."[21]

20   Ou-Yang, W.X. et al. "Application of food allergens specific IgG antibody detection in chronic diarrhea in children." *Zhonggua Dang Dai Er Ke ZA Zhi.* 2008; Feb 10 (1): 21-4.
21   http://www.dadamo.com/science_nytech.htm

Lectin molecules bind to "glyco-proteins" (proteins with a sugar molecule at one end) on the surface of cells, and by so doing, may cause harm. Interestingly, virtually all foods contain these carbohydrate-binding lectins, to which certain people are intolerant.

Lectins are "thought to play a role in immune function, cell growth, cell death, and body fat regulation."[22]

Many lectins are relatively resistant to heating, stomach acids, and digestive enzymes. In some individuals, they may damage the gut lining, which in turn can lead to "leaky gut" and associated problems like food allergies and auto-immune diseases (like Type I diabetes [dairy lectins] and IgA nephropathy [wheat lectins]).[23]

Lectins, when consumed in excess, "can cause severe intestinal damage, disrupting digestion, causing protein loss and growth retardation, blocking glucose uptake and insulin receptors, contributing to Celiac Disease, and promoting the growth of harmful bacteria."[24]

Lectins can leak through a damaged "leaky" gut and bind to internal tissues and organs and in the process cause harm.[25]

"They can provoke numerous immune responses, including IgG and IgM sometimes IgE, and lymphocyte *mitogenesis.*[26][27]

Finally, they can agglutinate (clot) erythrocytes (red blood cells) leading to anemia, *sometimes with ABO specificity* (certain blood types may be more susceptible). In general, lectins can cause immune system exhaustion and failure to thrive."[28]

While allergy and IgG sensitivity testing will not reveal lectin intolerances, an elimination diet is a good way to discover whether certain lectins in foods are causing problems. This is achieved by eliminating all but a small select group of foods to which there does not appear to be any intolerance and then adding suspect foods back into the diet, one food at a time, looking for possible adverse reactions.

Lectins in foods can be reduced in amount by *soaking* (prolonged soak, rinse, drain and repeat several times), *sprouting, fermenting, or cooking the food*, but invariably some of the lectin molecules will remain, and their ability to do harm should not be underestimated. Red kidney beans, for example, contain a toxic lectin called *phytohaemagglutinin* (FIE-toh HEEM-uh-glue-tin-in) in such high amounts that as little as four soaked beans eaten *raw* can elicit symptoms. *Cooking* these beans inactivates over 90 percent of this harmful lectin.

Lectins may also be somewhat *neutralized* by ingesting the *sugar* at the end of the glyo-protein to which the lectin binds. This blocks the lectin attachment site and prevents the lectin from doing harm. A product called "Lectin Lock" (Vitamin Research Products) contains these lectin-binding sugars. This process may be helpful, but it does not inactivate all the lectins of concern.

It is also likely that adequate amounts of a gut-derived protective antibody called *secretory Immunoglobulin A (sIgA)* may offer protection to the gut lining from ingested lectins. *Mucin*, a substance found in the mucous layer that lines the GI tract, also protects the gut against the harmful effects of dietary lectins.

The production of both secretory IgA and mucin may be increased when the intestinal beneficial flora (microbes like Lactobacilli) are optimized.

---

22   http://www.precisionnutrition.com/all-about-lectins
23   Pierini, C. *Vitamin Research News.* Jan 2007. 21(1): 1-4.
24   http://www.biotype.net/diets/Lectin.pdf *and* Pusztai et al. "Local and Systemic Responses to Dietary Lectins." In: Liener, Sharon, & Goldstein (see below): p. 271-272 *and* Freed. "Dietary Lectins and the Anti-Nutritive Effects of Gut Allergy." In Hemmings, W.A. ed. *Protein Transmission through Living Membranes.* Elsevier/North Holland Biomedical Press, 1979. p. 411-422. *and* Liener, Irvin E.; Sharon, Nathan; Goldstein, Irwin J. eds. *The Lectins.* Orlando, FL: Academic Press, 1986. p. 529-552.
25   http://www.sciencedaily.com/releases/2007/08/070801091240.htm.
26   Refers to the replication of lymphocytes, an immune cell.
27   http://www.biotype.net/diets/Lectin.pdf *and* Goldstein & Etzler. *Chemical Taxonomy, Molecular Biology, and Function of Plant Lectins.* New York, Alan Liss, 1983. p. 1-29, 271-272; *and* Gell & Coombs. *Clinical Aspects of Immunology.* Philadelphia, PA: Lippincott, 1975, p. 763-779. *and* Breneman, James C. *Basics of Food Allergy.* Springfield, IL: Thomas, 1984. p. 10-229.
28   http://www.biotype.net/diets/Lectin.pdf *and* Gell & Coombs. *Clinical Aspects of Immunology.* Philadelphia, PA: Lippincott, 1975. p. 763.

Interestingly, the foods with the highest allergenicity also contain a high concentration of lectins. These are dairy, eggs, wheat, soy, peanuts, tree nuts, fish, and shellfish. This is probably not a coincidence, as lectins are believed to promote allergenicity. Oils from beans (soy) and other seeds (canola, corn, etc.) may also contain significant amounts of lectin molecules.

"Nachbar and Oppenheim (1980) found 30 percent of fresh and processed foods contained active lectins. Lectins from green salads, fruits, spices, seeds, dry cereals, and nuts (even after roasting) showed activity of potentially toxic lectins. Some of these lectins interact with serum or salivary components and bacteria from the oral cavity (Gibbons & Dankers, 1981)."[29]

There is a lot that we don't yet know about how food lectins interact with our physiology. What is known, as outlined by clinical nutritionist Krispin Sullivan, is that:

- Proteins institute most allergic and antigenic responses.

- Lectins are proteins found in large amounts in (certain) foods.

- Lectins are not easily removed from foods or rendered harmless to animals and humans.

- Lectins from soy, peanut and other beans, wheat germ and wheat, milk, peanut oil (and perhaps other seed oils including soy oil) and nightshades (potatoes, tomatoes, eggplant, pepper), in a variety of clinical studies have been shown to damage the gut lining, joints, kidney, pancreas and brain (and are even able to cross the blood-brain barrier).

- Lectins found in peanut oil have been implicated in atherosclerosis. Leaving open the possibility that other seed oils contain damaging lectins and that polyunsaturation and free radicals may not be the full picture on the dangers of polyunsaturated fats.

- A person may be more susceptible to lectin toxicity due to genetics, intensity of exposure, failure of immune factors to protect, viral infection, bacterial infection or gut permeability induced by medication or infection.

- Lectin toxicity (antigen-antibody response) can be "sub-clinical," i.e., not showing obvious symptoms for many years.[30]

It isn't clear how widespread lectin intolerance may be. Nachbar and others suggest that is probably very common.[31]

No evidence exists at this time that autistic individuals are more likely to suffer from lectin pathology than other persons. That being said, if intestinal or other symptoms have not been adequately addressed by other means, it would be wise to investigate the role lectins may play as causative agents of a variety of autistic manifestations, including chronic intestinal distress, and learning and behavioral issues.

What Other Substances in Foods Can Cause Harm?

There are, unfortunately, many substances commonly found in foods, especially processed foods, that are known to cause harm to the body. These include excitotoxins, artificial colors, preservatives, nitrites, endocrine-disrupting chemicals, and many others.

Excitotoxins

Excitotoxins are substances found in or added to foods and beverages that stimulate brain neurons. When in excess, they can over-stimulate and kill neurons. Common excitotoxins found in foods and beverages include monosodium glutamate, aspartame (NutraSweet®), cysteine (an amino acid), hydrolyzed protein, and aspartic acid.

---

29   http://www.krispin.com/lectin.html
30   http://www.krispin.com/lectin.html
31   http://www.naturaltherapypages.com.au/article/Lectins#ixzz2iafYPMkP

Monosodium Glutamate (Msg): MSG is the sodium salt of glutamic acid, an essential amino acid. We have taste receptors on our tongues for this flavor-enhancing substance, and like most things that are good for us in *optimal* amounts, too much glutamate can be harmful.

MSG is found naturally in the Japanese sea vegetable called Kombu, but most of those exposed to MSG get it by eating foods it has been added to as a flavor enhancer. Millions of pounds of MSG are used by the food industry every year.

According to the American Nutrition Association, "MSG is added to most soups, chips, fast foods, frozen foods, ready-made dinners, and canned goods. And it has been heaven sent for the diet food industry, since so many of the low-fat foods are practically tasteless.... Often MSG and related toxins are added to foods in disguised forms. For example, among the food manufacturers favorite disguises are 'hydrolyzed vegetable protein,' 'vegetable protein,' 'natural flavorings,' and 'spices.' Each of these may contain from 12 per cent to 40 per cent MSG."[32]

Brain neurons have receptors for glutamate. Glutamate is the main excitatory neurotransmitter and is essential for learning, attention, focus, and memory. Interestingly, it is also the precursor of a calming neuro-transmitter called GABA.

GABA is a neurotransmitter that engenders a feeling of peaceful satisfaction. It is also important in the acquisition of speech because it helps us to distinguish between the onset of a sound and background noise. An inability to filter background noise can lead to sensory overload, a common finding in autistic individuals. Low GABA levels also make seizure activity more likely.

The enzyme that converts glutamate to GABA (glutamic acid decarboxylase) also requires vitamin B6 (in its active form: "P5P") as a cofactor for its activity. Vitamin B6 plays a role in many chemical reactions pertinent to reversing autism and is one of the nutrients that has shown great success in this regard.

Autistic children often fail to convert glutamate to GABA in sufficient amounts. This leads to an imbalance that results in too much neuronal excitation (which can manifest as "stimming" behaviors) and too little GABA calming (which can promote speech impairment).

Glutamate opens calcium channels that allow the influx of calcium ions, which in turn activate the cell, a good thing, but the cell must then pump out the calcium in order to function again. This takes a lot of energy. Should excess glutamate enter neurons, the cells may be overstimulated, which can lead to their demise. Excess glutamate can also cause a breakdown of cell membranes, which causes the release of a particular fatty acid (arachidonic acid) that promotes inflammation.

Fevers, low blood sugar, nutritional deficiencies (magnesium in particular), and exercise can all magnify the harm done by excitotoxins. Magnesium, on the other hand, can close calcium channels and thereby reduce the adverse effects of excess glutamate. Zinc, GABA, glycine, and theanine are all natural calming agents that can also help attenuate the excitatory effects of excess glutamate.[33]

Dr. Russell Blaylock, author of *Excitotoxins: The Taste That Kills*, published an article in *Alternative Therapies in Health and Medicine* in 2009 in which he suggests that excitotoxins, like glutamate, may play an important role in promoting the neuro-degeneration and abnormal connectivity found in autistic individuals, and additionally, they may multiply the harmful effects of other neurotoxins.

He suggests that, "The interaction between excitotoxins, free radicals, lipid peroxidation products, inflammatory cytokines, and disruption of neuronal calcium homeostasis (balance) can result in brain changes suggestive of the pathological findings in cases of autism spectrum disorders."[34]

---

32   http://americannutritionassociation.org/newsletter/review-excitotoxins-taste-kills
33   Ibid.
34   *Altern Ther Health Med.* Mar-Apr 2009; 15(2):56-60.

Where MSG May Be Hiding

Additives that always contain MSG: Monosodium Glutamate, Hydrolyzed Vegetable Protein, Hydrolyzed Protein, Hydrolyzed Plant Protein, Plant Protein Extract, Sodium Caseinate, Calcium Caseinate, Yeast Extract, Textured Protein, Autolyzed Yeast, Hydrolyzed Oat Flour.

Additives that frequently contain MSG: Malt extract, Malt Flavoring, Bouillion Broth, Stock Flavoring, Natural Flavoring, Natural Beef or Chicken Flavoring, Seasoning, Spices.

Additives that may contain MSG and/or other excitotoxins: Carrageeenan Enzymes (Protease enzymes from various sources can release excitotoxin amino acids from food proteins.), Soy Protein Concentrate, Soy Protein Isolate, Whey Protein Concentrate.

Aspartic Acid & Nutrasweet® (Aspartame): Aspartic acid, found in aspartame, is another excitotoxin that should be minimized in the diet. It may also be added to processed foods, and the FDA does not require labeling of this potentially troublesome amino acid.

NutraSweet (aspartame) is an artificial sweetener that contains two amino acids: phenylalanine and aspartic acid. Studies show that aspartame can cause headaches ("Chinese Restaurant Syndrome"), cancer, neurological damage, and a host of other maladies. A list of 68 studies that point to the serious harm this product can engender may be found online at: http://aspartame.mercola.com/sites/aspartame/studies.aspx. Aspartame also releases toxic methanol, which in humans is metabolized to poisonous formaldehyde.[35]

Given the enormous body of evidence of harm that aspartic acid and aspartame may promote, it is wise to avoid using this artificial sweetener.

Cysteine ("SIS-tee-een"): This important amino acid is also an excitotoxin. It is commonly added as a dough conditioner, and as is true with aspartate (aspartic acid), there are no requirements that foods containing added cysteine be labeled. Interestingly, both cysteine and glutamate are found in the protective peptide glutathione, which is paradoxically not an excitotoxin.

Are They Really Safe?

"There are...double-blind studies suggesting that (cysteine, MSG and aspartate) are safe. A review of studies relevant to the safety and toxicity of glutamic acid (MSG), however, suggest that many of them are flawed."[36]

"For example, "in the case of MSG toxicology studies, the placebo used to test the excitotoxin glutamate is NutraSweet®, which contains the excitotoxin aspartate.

"It has been clearly shown in a multitude of studies that aspartate produces the identical destructive reactions on the nervous system as MSG. It would seem obvious even to the layman that you would not use a control substance to compare to a known toxin if the control contained the same class of chemical toxin.
But that is exactly what is being done."[37]

35   http://mercola.fileburst.com/PDF/ExpertInterviewTranscripts/Interview-DrMonte.pdf

36   Samuels, Adrienne. "Excitatory Amino Acids in Neurologic Disorders." *The New England Journal of Medicine*. 331(4): 274-5, July 28, 1994.

37   Blaylock, Russel L. Excitoxins: *The Taste That Kills*. Santa Fe, NM: Health Press, 1994. p. 200. From: http://americannutritionassociation.org/newsletter/review-excitotoxins-taste-kills

Is There a Connection Between Mercury Toxicity and Glutamate?

Yes, there is.

Researchers have recently discovered that *methyl mercury won't damage neurons unless glutamate is also present!*[38]

It is, therefore, likely that other forms of mercury, like the ethyl mercury from thimerosal, would have the same effect. *This suggests that excess glutamate will potentiate the toxicity of even low levels of mercury and vice versa.*

The bottom line for all of us is to minimize monosodium glutamate and other excitotoxins in our diets (and not inject mercury into our bodies). The many references included in Dr. Blaylock's revealing book, *Excitotoxins: The Taste That Kills,* will provide necessary scientific support for those attempting to influence authorities to ban or limit these potentially harmful ingredients.

Artificial Colors and Sodium Benzoate Preservative

It is common for many processed foods, particularly sweets (sodas, candy, cakes, desserts, cereals, etc.) to be *artificially* colored in order to enhance their eye appeal. Unlike the nutritionally beneficial *natural* colors from fruits and vegetables, chemically-manufactured artificial colors from chemical dyes and other sources offer no health benefits and have actually been shown to cause harm.[39]

In the early 1970s, a San Francisco allergist named Benjamin Feingold alerted the nation to the detrimental effects of food dyes and certain other harmful substances found in foods (like sugar, artificial flavors, natural salicylates, and certain preservatives).[40]

He suggested that these components could trigger hyperactivity and learning impairments in both children and adults, and he recommended an elimination diet to help determine which foods needed to be removed from the diet. He observed that by eliminating the offending foods, the symptoms in most affected individuals would improve dramatically.

Feingold's pronouncements were met with a lot of skepticism by the scientific community. Some studies, mostly industry-sponsored, failed to support his observations, while numerous others did.

Many of Feingold's assertions were affirmed in a 2004 meta-analysis by Schaband Trinh of a number of the aforementioned studies that found a link between food dyes and hyperactivity.

The authors concluded that dyes "promote hyperactivity in hyperactive children, as measured on behavioral rating scales" and that "society should engage in a broader discussion about whether the aesthetic and commercial rationale for the use of [artificial food colorings] is justified."[41]

"Two recent studies sponsored by the British government on cross-sections of British children found that mixtures of four dyes (and a food preservative, sodium benzoate) impaired the behavior of even *non-hyperactive* children.[42]

As a result, the British government told the food and restaurant industries to eliminate the dyes tested by the end of 2009, and the European Parliament passed a law that will require a warning notice on all foods that contain one or more of the dyes tested after July 20, 2010. The notice states that the dyed food "may have an adverse effect on behavior and attention in children" (Parliament accessed February 20, 2010).[43]

---

38   Aschner et al. "Methyl Mercury Alters Glutamate Transport in Astrocytes." *NeuroChem Intl.* 2000; 37:199.
39   Center for Science in the Public Interest. *Food Dyes: A Rainbow of Risks.*
40   Feingold, B.F. "Behavioral disturbances linked to the ingestion of food additives." *Del Med J.* Feb 1977; 49(2):89-94.
41   Schab, D.W.; Trinh, N.H. "Do artificial food colors promote hyperactivity in children with hyperactive syndromes? A meta-analysis of double-blind placebo-controlled trials." *J Dev Behav Pediatr.* Dec 2004; 25(6):423-34. PMID: 15613992
42   Bateman, Warner et al. (2004). "The effect of a double blind, placebo controlled, artificial food colourings and benzoate preservative challenge on hyperactivity in a general population sample of preschool children." *Archives of Disease in Childhood* 89: 506-511; & McCann, Barrett et al. (2007). "Food additives and hyperactive behaviour in 3-year old and 8/9-year old children in the community: a randomised, double-blinded, placebo-controlled trial." *Lancet* 370: 1560-1567.
43   Center for Science in the Public Interest. *Food Dyes: A Rainbow of Risks.*

Food Quality and Sufficiency

Is There Any Evidence That Improving the Diet or Supplementing with Nutrients Improves Behavior and Learning?

Yes! Professor Steven Schoenthaler and his associates did a number of studies that confirmed that diet plays a crucial role in improving all aspects of behavior and cognition in children and adults. It has been observed for some time that an impaired diet is associated with poor school performance, and the converse is also true: academic performance often improves when the diet improves.

Twelve early placebo-controlled studies support these findings; however, the studies were not without their limitations, so Dr. Schoenthaler and his colleagues then did another more rigorous double-blind, placebo-controlled investigation. The researchers wanted "to determine if schoolchildren who consume low-dose vitamin-mineral tablets (containing just half of the daily requirement for vitamins and minerals) (would) have a significantly larger increase in nonverbal intelligence than children who consume placebos in a study that overcomes the primary criticisms directed at the previous 12 controlled trials."

"Two 'working class,' primarily Hispanic, elementary schools in Phoenix, Arizona, participated in the study. Slightly more than half the teachers in each school distributed the tablets daily to 245 schoolchildren aged 6 to 12 years."

After three months the non-verbal IQs of the children were remeasured and compared to those taken at the study's onset. What was found was that many, but not all, of the children in the vitamin group had significantly higher IQ scores than did those in the placebo group.

The researchers concluded:

[V]itamin-mineral supplementation modestly raised the nonverbal intelligence of some groups of Western schoolchildren by 2 to 3 points but not that of most Western schoolchildren, presumably because the majority were already adequately nourished…. A significantly higher proportion of children in the active group gained 15 or more IQ points when compared to the placebo group ($p < 0.01$)….

> This study also confirms that vitamin-mineral supplementation markedly raises the non-verbal intelligence of a minority of Western schoolchildren, presumably because they were too poorly nourished before supplementation for optimal brain function. Because nonverbal intelligence is closely associated with academic performance, it follows that schools with children who consume substandard diets should find it difficult to produce academic performance equal to those schools with children who consume diets that come closer to providing the nutrients suggested in the U.S. RDA.
>
> The parents of school-children whose academic performance is substandard would be well advised to seek a nutritionally oriented physician for assessment of their children's nutritional status as a possible etiology.[44]
>
> In a related study in the same journal, Dr. Schoenthaler and an associate measured the effect of the same vitamin supplement on a group of previously disciplined, antisocial schoolchildren at the same schools and found that the vitamin supplemented group had a 47 percent reduction in antisocial behavior (threats, fighting, vandalism, being disrespectful, disorderly conduct, defiance, obscenities, refusal to work or serve, endangering others, etc.) compared to the control group.[45]

This finding was in agreement with numerous other studies, including two placebo-controlled trials, of institutionalized offenders aged 13-17 and 18-26 years whose antisocial behavior and acts of violence improved from

---

44   Schoenthaler, S.J. et al. "The effect of vitamin-mineral supplementation on the intelligence of American schoolchildren: a randomized, double-blind placebo-controlled trial." *J Altern Complement Med.* 2000 Feb; 6(1):19-29.
45   Schoenthaler, S.J. et al. "The effect of vitamin-mineral supplementation on juvenile delinquency among American schoolchildren: a randomized, double-blind placebo-controlled trial." *J Altern Complement Med.* 2000 Feb; 6(1):7-17.

approximately 26-40 percent on a nutrient-supplemented diet.[46]

Dr. Schoenthaler went even further. In a remarkable, landmark seven-year study, he investigated the effect of changing the diet of the over one million school children in 803 public schools in New York City, who in the 1978-79 school year ranked at the 39th percentile on standardized achievement tests given across the nation (California Achievement Test/CAT).[47]

The prior school year, the rankings were at the 43rd percentile. What had changed? For just the 1977-78 school year, the Board of Education had ordered a reduction in fat in the school food and the achievement test score rankings had improved, but for some reason, they abandoned that effort the next year and the scores dropped to the 39th percentile by the end of the 1979 season. That same year, the city's Board of Education, guided by Dr. Feingold's recommendations, now decided again to alter their school breakfast and lunch programs, but this time, the board ordered a reduction in sugar intake and it banned two of the many artificial food colorings. By the end of the next year (1980), the school system CAT score rankings had climbed dramatically from the 39th to the 47th percentile.

Bolstered by this success, the Board of Education then ordered the elimination of the other artificial colors, and as a result, the achievement test scores climbed still higher to the 51st percentile by the end of the 1979-1981 school year. No further dietary alterations were made in the 1981-1982 school season, and the children's test scores by the end of the 1982 season remained constant at the 51st percentile.[48]

Then the diet was changed again. The preservatives BHA (Butylated Hydroxy-Anisole) and BHT (Butylated Hydroxy-Toluene) were eliminated, and the achievement test scores rose even higher to the 55th percentile. New York City school children's achievement scores had climbed from the 39th to the 55th percentile by just improving their diet! Before these changes were made, the more meals the children ate at the school, the lower their test scores. The meals were actually causing harm.[49]

Further analysis of the data collected showed that the improvements were not uniform. *The children with the lowest achievement test rankings initially were the ones who improved the most.* "Before implementing the dietary changes, 12.4 percent of the one million students in New York City schools were performing two or more grades below the proper level. These were the "learning disabled" and "repeat failure" children.

By the end of 1983, only 4.9 percent of children were in that category. In other words, 7.5 percent of a million children—75,000 children—were no longer "learning disabled" low-achievers, but had become able to perform at the level normal for their age. These were the children whom no other efforts had helped. No other hypothesis fits: All changes were related to the dietary changes."[50]

So, What Have We Learned?

Science has confirmed what common sense has always suggested: A proper diet is vital for good mental and physical health, and conversely, that a bad or inadequate diet can have profound adverse effects on learning, behavior, and overall well-being. Influencing factors include food allergies, food intolerances, lectin sensitivities, toxic peptides from milk, wheat, and other foods, pesticide and herbicide residues on and in food, artificial colors, certain preservatives, excitotoxins, and genetically-modified foods.

Therefore, any given dietary regimen will not be appropriate for everyone because of individual tolerances, nutri-

46   Ibid. *and* Schoenthaler, S.J. et al. "The effect of randomized vitamin-mineral supplementation on violent and non-violent antisocial behavior among incarcerated juveniles." *Journal of Nutritional and Environmental Medicine.* Vol. 7. 1997, p. 343-352. *and* Gesch, C. Bernard et al. "Influence of supplementary vitamins, minerals and essential fatty acids on the antisocial behavior of young adult prisoners: randomized, placebo-controlled trial." *British Journal of Psychiatry.* Vol. 181. July 2002.

47   Schoenthaler, S.J.; Doraz, W.E.; Wakefield, J.A. "The Impact of a Low Food Additive and Sucrose Diet on Academic Performance in 803 New York City Public Schools." *International Journal of Biosocial Research.* 1986. Vol. 8(2): 185-195; *and* Schoenthaler, S.J.; Doraz, W.E.; Wakefield, J.A. "The Testing of Various Hypotheses as Explanations for the Gains in National Standardized Academic Test Scores in the 1978-1983 New York City Nutrition Policy Modification Project." *International Journal of Biosocial Research*, 1986. Vol. 8(2): 196-203.

48   ASUSAMD/Documents/NYC Schools Feingold changes improved CAT scores Schoenthaler.pdf

49   Ibid.

50   http://www.feingold.org/Research/BLUE/Page-11-Nyschools.pdf

tional requirements, digestive disabilities, and food sensitivities. That is to say, what is healthful for one person may harm another, but there are some overall common sense approaches to diet that would virtually apply to everyone.

These include eating wholesome organic produce as much as possible, thereby avoiding pesticide and herbicide residues and genetically-modified foods. It is also important to eliminate artificial ingredients (synthetic food dyes, preservatives, hydrogenated oils, excitotoxins, fluoridated water, etc.) and minimize processed foods, refined carbohydrates, and sugar in the diet. It is likewise a good idea to determine each individual's optimal diet based on his or her tolerances, allergies, and unique nutritional requirements.

Chapter 32
Microorganisms and Autism

"We feel justified in recognizing the existence of cases of mental disorders which
have as a basic etiological factor a toxic condition arising
from the gastrointestinal tract."

— *Armando Ferraro (neuropathologist) & Joseph Kilman (psychiatrist) 1933*

WHAT IS THE *Connection Between Microorganisms and Autism Spectrum Disorders?*
We Are Only About One-Tenth Human

Our intestinal tract, mouth, nose, sinuses, vaginal tract and skin are home to an estimated 100 trillion microorganisms (gut organisms are often referred to as "intestinal flora"). Hundreds of varieties of organisms inhabit these various surfaces. These include primarily bacteria and yeasts, but we may also be hosts to protozoans, viruses, and parasitic worms. Since there are about ten trillion "human" cells in our bodies, *the microorganisms that live in and on us outnumber our human cells by about ten to one.*[1]

The "Alien Organ"

When the number and kind of organisms that inhabit the human domain are in balance, all goes well, but when there is an imbalance in the number or type of these microflora, then disease may result. *Dysbiosis* is the term used to describe an imbalance in gut and surface bacteria and yeasts that cause harm. This vast array of non-human inhabitants has a profound effect on our own physiology and may be considered an organ in its own right—an alien organ if you will.

Probiotics, the Beneficial Germs

Certain gut organisms, called "probiotics," support optimal health. Some, for example, ferment fiber to make short chain fatty acids that are the food for the large intestinal cells (colonocytes). Others detoxify harmful substances, or make vitamins like vitamin K, or protect against the overgrowth of more harmful bacteria. Intestinal microbes influence the development of the intestinal immune system and its protective mucous layer, and they may even affect brain development and behavior.[2]

---

1   Sears, Cynthia L. "A dynamic partnership: Celebrating our gut flora." *Anaerobe.* 2005; 11 (5): 247–51.
2   O'Hara, A.M.; Shanahan, F. "The gut flora as a forgotten organ." *EMBO Rep.* 2006; 7: 688–693 and Macpherson, A.J.; Harris, N.L. "Interactions between commensal intestinal bacteria and the immune system." *Nat Rev Immunol.* 2004; 4: 478–485. and Heijtz, R.D. et al. "Normal gut microbiota modulates brain development and behavior." *Proc Natl Acad Sci USA.* 2011; 108: 3047–3052.

The beneficial bacteria include *Lactobacilli*, which mainly protect the small intestine, and *Bifidobacteria*, which protect the large intestine. A beneficial yeast, *Saccharomyces boulardii* (SACK-er-oh-MICE-eez boo-LARD-ee-eye), has been found to lessen the toxic effects of certain harmful bacteria known as Clostridia and to benefit those with diarrhea. Certain environmental factors, like antibiotics and certain diets, can disrupt the optimal microbiome of the gut.

Toxic Substances from Gut Organisms: Yeasts

Some intestinal micro-organisms may be harmful. Certain yeast species produce a variety of possibly toxic substances, like *arabinose*, a potentially troublesome sugar and a marker for the presence of harmful yeasts or their overgrowth, and *tartaric acid*, a toxic by-product of yeast fermentation.

Arabinose is known to inhibit the breakdown of table sugar (sucrose), which can lead to fermentation of that sugar in the gut by a variety of gut organisms. (Arabinose inhibits sucrase, the enzyme that "digests" sucrose).[3]

Dr. Shaw, of the Great Plains Lab, has studied two brothers with autism and profound muscle weakness whose autistic symptoms improved and whose *tartaric acid* levels declined when they were treated with an anti-fungal/anti-yeast remedy called *Nystatin*.[4]

Shaw also relates a similar case of a two-year-old boy who was developing normally until he was given an antibiotic for an ear infection at the age of 18 months, and subsequently developed *thrush*, a yeast (Candida) infection of the mouth and throat. The child regressed into autism shortly thereafter. He lost his speech, became very hyperactive, did not make eye contact, and was awake a good part of the night.

Dr. Shaw measured the boy's levels of urine organic acids (substances that give us biochemical clues regarding an individual's physiological functioning). Shaw found that the youngster had very elevated levels of many organic acids, including tartaric acid. The child's functioning improved dramatically and his abnormal levels of tartaric and other organic acids normalized after treatment with the yeast remedy Nystatin over a period of two months.[5]

Bacteria and Autism

Gut bacteria may also produce toxic substances. *Clostridia* are a family of bacteria that can cause diseases like tetanus, gangrene, and botulism. They are commonly found to overgrow in the intestines of autistic children and are capable of producing toxins (like p-cresol) that can adversely affect the brain. Another of these substances is abbreviated *HPHPA*. Both HPHPA and arabinose, as well as other marker substances, may be measured by getting a *urine organic acid test*. The Great Plains Lab is allegedly the only lab in the country currently able to measure levels of HPHPA and arabinose accurately.

Pediatric gastroenterologist Dr. Sophie Rosseneu has been studying undesirable gut organisms called *aerobic gram-negative* (these bacteria don't absorb the gram stain) *bacilli* (bah-SILL-eye). These include bacteria with names like Klebsiella, Proteus, Pseudomonas, Citrobacter, Acinetobacter, Serratia, and Enterobacter. While these are commonly present in small numbers in many people, they can cause harm if they are overabundant. Biologically speaking, overabundance is considered any amount over 100,000 organisms per milliliter of saliva or feces. The mechanism by which they cause harm is via the creation of toxic substances called *endotoxins*.

Almost all gut bacteria produce endotoxins, but the *aerobic gram-negative bacilli produce ten times more than do other common bacteria like E. coli.* The usual defense against these "bad guy" bacteria is the vast number of beneficial *anaerobic* flora that normally inhabit the intestinal tract. *Aerobic* refers to an organism that prefers (or can tolerate) living in air (oxygen) and *anaerobic* refers to organisms that die when exposed to air.

---

3   Osaki, S. *J Nutr.* Mar 2001; 131(3):796-9.
4   http://www.greatplainslaboratory.com/home/eng/candida.asp. and Shaw, W.; Kassen, E.; Chaves, E. "Increased urinary excretion of analogs of Krebs cycle metabolites and arabinose in two brothers with autistic features." *Clin Chem.* Aug 1995; 41(8 Pt 1):1094-104. Pubmed: 7628083.
5   Ibid. GPL.com

Dr. Rosseneu wondered whether children with autism harbored more of these harmful gut microbes than did non-autistic children. She did an as yet unpublished study of 80 autistic children who were experiencing constipation, abdominal pain, and overflow diarrhea and discovered that 61 percent had abnormal aerobic gram negative bacterial overgrowth and 95 percent had E. coli overgrowth. Candida was not found in excess.

She also found abnormalities in the intestinal lining layer in the autistic children that could explain some of their symptoms. She was able to show that by eradicating the abnormal gut flora with a three-month antibiotic (vancomycin) regimen, the autistic behavioral symptoms, as well as the GI abnormalities, both improved dramatically. Unfortunately, the improvements in symptoms did not persist after the antibiotic regimen was discontinued. The reoccurrence of the intestinal symptoms was most likely due to a recolonization of the children's intestinal tracts with the endotoxin-producing organisms.

A similar study was done by Sandler and colleagues who theorized that antibiotic use in autistic children "might promote colonization by one or more neurotoxin-producing bacteria, contributing, at least in part, to their autistic symptomatology." To test their hypothesis, they treated 11 children with regressive autism (who had diarrhea after exposure to a previously prescribed broad spectrum oral antibiotic) with vancomycin, a minimally-absorbed oral antibiotic that is usually effective in eradicating Clostridia species. The children's behavior was observed and graded prior to and after the vancomycin regimen in a blinded fashion. Eight of the ten who were evaluated showed significant improvement, albeit only while on the antibiotic and for just a short time after discontinuation.[6]

In a more recent study, researchers found elevated circulating levels of bacterial endotoxin and immune-inflammatory markers (IL-1 beta, IL-6, and IL-10) in 22 adult patients with severe autism as compared to 28 age-matched controls. These findings support the hypothesized role of intestinal bacterial endotoxins in promoting autism symptomatology.[7]

In another relevant study, biopsies of intestinal tissue in autistic children with gastrointestinal disease as compared to those of non-autistic children with gastrointestinal disease revealed that the autistic children commonly had impaired carbohydrate digestion and assimilation. In particular, the autistic children appeared to be deficient in the enzymes (disaccharidases) that break down double sugars (like sucrose—"table sugar"), and they also had an impaired ability to transport certain (6 carbon) sugars across cell membranes. *These findings were associated with dysbiosis.* This enzymatic defect can be overcome by avoiding foods with these sugars (The Specific Carbohydrate Diet).

These researchers also found that, "Deficient expression of these enzymes and transporters was associated with expression of the intestinal transcription factor, CDX-2." This suggested to the scientists that there is "a relationship between human intestinal gene expression and bacterial community structure."[8]

Other researchers have found that autistic children on average are colonized by significantly *fewer* varieties of bacteria, and the bacteria they are host to *differ in variety and amount* as compared to non-autistic children.[9]

6   Sandler, R.H. et al. "Short-term benefit from oral vancomycin treatment of regressive-onset autism." *J Chil Neurol.* Jul 2000; 15(7) 429f.

7   Emanuele, E. et al. "Low-grade endotoxemia in patients with severe autism." *Neurosci Letters.* Mar 8 2010; 471 (3) 162f. E pub Jan 25, 2010.

8   Williams, B.L. et al. "Impaired Carbohydrate Digestion and Transport and Mucosal Dysbiosis in the Intestines of Children with Autism and Gastrointestinal Disturbances." *PloS One.* Sept 16, 2011; 002458.

9   Kang, Dae-Wook et al. "Reduced Incidence of Prevotella and Other Fermenters in Intestinal Microflora of Autistic Children." July 3, 2013. DOI: 10.1371/journal.pone.0068322.

Table 32.1. Gi Micro-Organisms in Autistic Individuals as Compared to Healthy Controls

ORGANISM	AUTISM	COMMENTS
Number of Types of GI organisms	Decreased[1]	A decrease in the number of different species of bacteria may make autistic children more susceptible to the overgrowth of bacterial pathogens.
Prevotella copri	Decreased[1]	This is a beneficial carbohydrate fermenting bacterium. P. copri was significantly low in autistic children.
Coprococcus	Decreased[1]	A beneficial carbohydrate-fermenting bacterium
Veillonellaceae	Decreased[1]	A beneficial carbohydrate-fermenting bacterium
Sutterella	Increased[2] Found in c. 50 percent of autistics studied	This bacterium has been associated with intestinal disease. It was not found in non-autistic children with GI problems.
Bacteroides fragilis	Decreased[3]	"B. fragilis is able to ameliorate leaky gut by directly targeting tight junction expression, cytokine production, and/or microbiome composition." Other Bacteroides species were increased.
Faecalibacteria	Decreased[4]	Increased in well children.
Ruminococcus	Decreased[4]	Increased in well children
Caloromator	Increased[4]	Found in hot springs—heat-tolerant bacteria.
Sarcina	Increased[4]	Increased in those with delayed gastric emptying.
Clostridia	Increased[4]	Clostridia produce a variety of toxins.
Eubacterium	Decreased[4]	These are the "true" bacteria.
Bifidobacteria[4]	Decreased[4]	This is a beneficial bacterial genus.

1. Kang, Dae-Wook et al. "Reduced Incidence of Prevotella and Other Fermenters in Intestinal Microflora of Autistic Children." July 3, 2013. DOI: 10.1371/journal.pone.0068322

2. Williams, B.L.; Hornig, M. et al. "Application of Novel PCR-Based Methods for Detection, Quantitation, and Phylogenetic Characterization of Sutterella Species in Intestinal Biopsy Samples from Children with Autism and Gastrointestinal Disturbances." *mBio*. Jan 10, 2012; Vol. 3. No. 1. e00261-11. doi: 10.1128/mBio.00261-11.

3. Hsiao, E.Y. et al. "Microbiota Modulate Behavioral and Physiological Abnormalities Associated with Neurodevelopmental Disorders." http://dx.doi.org/10.1016/j.cell.2013.11.024

4. De Angelis, Maria et al. "Fecal Microbiota and Metabolome of Children with Autism and Pervasive Developmental Disorder Not Otherwise Specified." Published: Oct 9, 2013; DOI: 10.1371/journal.pone.0076993; PloS 1http://www.plosone.org/article/info percent3Adoi percent2F10.1371 percent2Fjournal.pone.0076993

In addition to endotoxin, arabinose, and HPHPA, certain intestinal bacteria (like Clostridia, Desufovibrio, and Propionibacteria) may produce *propionic acid*, which is a short chain fatty acid that is used as "fuel" for the cells lining the colon, but which in excess has been shown to cause neurological harm, at least in rats. Propionic acid is also sometimes used as a food preservative.

Rats treated with propionic acid had evidence of increased inflammation in their brains, reduced glutathione, increased oxidative stress, and mitochondrial dysfunction. *Infusions of propionic acid in test animals induced repetitive behaviors, hyperactivity, turning, object fixation, and seizures.* These findings, researcher Dr. Derrick McFabe points out, "are consistent with those found in ASD patients."

Butyric acid (found in butter) is another short chain fatty acid that in excess may produce similar reactions in lab rats. "We propose," McFabe adds, "that some types of ASD may be partial forms of genetically inherited or acquired disorders of altered short chain fatty acid metabolism, resulting in increased exposure to these enteric (refers to the intestine) metabolites at critical times during the life cycle."[10]

One probiotic, *Bacteroides fragilis* (BACK-ter-OID-eez fra-JILL-iss), was found in a 2013 study to be "selectively depleted in ASD children compared to matched controls, and most dramatically in those subjects with more severe GI issues." This organism "is able to ameliorate leaky gut by directly targeting tight junction expression, cytokine production, and/or microbiome composition." In a mouse model of autism, scientists were able to show that restoring depleted levels of B. fragilis *corrects* "gut permeability, alters microbial composition, and ameliorates defects in communicative, stereotypic, anxiety-like and sensorimotor behaviors." The mice that had the autistic behaviors also were found to have higher levels of a bacterial metabolite (4EPS).[11] When 4EPS was injected into normal mice, they too began to exhibit the same autism symptoms. A similar chemical, 4-methylphenol, has been found in high levels in the urine of some autistic children.[12]

So it appears that many autistic children are in a dysbiotic state wherein the number and variety of their intestinal bacteria differ from their non-autistic peers; consequently, they have an increase in troublesome organisms and a decrease in beneficial organisms. "A potential mechanism behind ASD symptoms could be neuro-active metabolites mediated by or produced by the microbiota, which could disseminate systemically and penetrate the blood-brain barrier."[13]

In a mouse model of autism, scientists were able to show that restoring depleted levels of B. fragilis corrects gut permeability, alters microbial composition, and ameliorates defects in communicative, stereotypic, anxiety-like, and sensorimotor behaviors. Hopefully, this same benefit will be realized in autistic individuals after supplementation with B. fragilis. Further research in this regard is needed. Unfortunately, most probiotic supplements on the market today do not contain this beneficial organism.[14]

The Streptococcal Connection to Autism

Streptococci (STREP-toe-COCKS-eye or "strep") are a family of bacteria that may be found in the human nose, throat, skin, and intestinal tract. Some members of this large family of organisms, beta-hemolytic strep for example, can cause diseases in humans, like "strep throat," which manifests as a sore throat, swollen neck lymph nodes, and often fever. The bacterium, which produces a toxin, is easily treated with a variety of antibiotics, but it can also be the source of several autoimmune conditions that cause heart disease (rheumatic fever), kidney disease (glomerulonephritis), and brain disease (PANDAS).

The acronym "PANDAS" stands for *Pediatric Autoimmune Neurological Disease Associated with Streptococcus.* The

---

10   http://www.psychology.uwo.ca/autism/researchinter-ests.htm. Patchell-Evans, Kilee. Autism Research Group. "Using Multidisciplinary Methods to Study Environmental Triggers in Autism Spectrum Disorder."

11   4-ethylphenylsulfate

12   Hsiao, E.Y. et al. "Microbiota Modulate Behavioral and Physiological Abnormalities Associated with Neurodevelopmental Disorders." *Cell.* Dec 19, 2013; Vol. 155. Issue 7. p.1451–1463.

13   Ibid.

14   Hsiao. 2013 Ibid. Illustration from http://www.cell.com/abstract/S0092-8674 (13)01473-6.

autoimmune reaction that results in PANDAS is directed at the basal ganglia, which results in a variety of brain disorders that may manifest as tics, unusual body movements (chorea), and obsessive-compulsive behaviors (OCD). Tics and OCD are often noted in autistic individuals. About 25 percent of people who have tics, OCD, and chorea have PANDAS, which can be difficult to treat.[15]

Dr. Vojdani (formerly the head of Immuno Sciences Lab) has found antibodies to the strep M protein as well as autoantibodies against neuronal tissue in samples taken from autistic children. Strep infection can promote the production of certain inflammatory substances like tumor necrosis factor (TNF) and nuclear factor kappa *B* (NFK-*B*). High levels of TNF are seen in those with tic disorders and in those with OCD.

Therapies for PANDAS-associated tic disorders and OCD include short courses on antibiotics, low dose Naltrexone, intravenous immunoglobulins, and plasmapheresis, and they have helped many with these disorders, but may be ineffective in some.

Dr. Kurt Woeller, an experienced autism clinician, has noted that autistic children who have OCD behaviors and/or tics may not do well on probiotics that contain a bacterium called streptococcus thermophilus.[16]

Protozoa and Autism

Protozoa are one-celled organisms that have the ability to move and may be parasitic. They include such organisms as the amoebae that cause dysentery, a disease characterized by diarrhea and dehydration, and Blastocystis hominis and Giardia lamblia, two protozoans that also cause intestinal symptoms.

Metametrix Lab did a study of protozoa in the intestinal tracts of 2-18-year-old children and adolescents on the autistic spectrum vs. non-autistic controls and found that about 2 out of 3 (69 percent) of the autistic children harbored these organisms as compared to only 30 percent of the control children. A majority of the protozoa were unclassified.[17]

It is not clear whether the increased protozoan presence in autistic children represents a cause of autism symptoms or is a result of this disorder. It is clear that certain protozoan parasites can cause gas, bloating, abdominal pain, and diarrhea, which are common symptoms in autism. A number of anecdotal reports testify to children with autism improving dramatically after their intestinal parasites had been successfully eliminated.[18]

Viruses and Autism

It is accepted science that a maternal rubella infection during pregnancy is a known cause of autism. We have shown that there is compelling research pointing to the link between autism and the live virus MMR vaccine administered to infants. It may be remembered that Dr. Yazbak also found that immunizing the mother-to-be with the MMR vaccine just before conception and during the pregnancy significantly increased the risk of autism in the baby (see Yazbak studies Chapter 23).

Researchers reporting in the *Journal of Child Neurology* document the case of a young child with encephalitis caused by an intestinal virus (enterovirus) who manifested developmental regression with autistic features as a result of the infection.[19]

In an animal experiment, scientists at the UC Davis Mind Institute found that activating the mother's immune system during her pregnancy damages the fetus's ability to make neuronal synapses, the essential connections between one nerve cell and another, and thereby provides a mechanism by which maternal viral infections or immunizations might increase the risk of having a child with autism spectrum disorder or schizophrenia.[20]

15   http://www.recoveryfromautism.com/index.php/articles/pediatric-autoimmune-neuropsychiatric-disorders-associated-with-streptococcal-infections-pan das-and-autism.html
16   http://www.recoveryfromautism.com/index.php/articles/autism-treatment-pandas-probiotic-problems-and-autism.html
17   http://pptu.lefora.com/topic/3752578/PPTU-AUTISM-ASD-high-incidence-PPTU-protozoa-auti#.VelOhBaxX-2
18   http://curezone.com/forums/fm.asp?i=1395519
19   Marques, F. et al. "Autism Spectrum Disorder secondary to enterovirus encephalitis." *J Child Neurol.* May 2014; 29(5):708-14.
20   Elmer, B.M. et al. "MHCI Requires MEF2 Transcription Factors to Negatively Regulate Synapse Density during Development and in Disease." *Journal of Neuroscience.* 2013; 33 (34).

In Chapter 24, we discussed several other mechanisms that could help explain the viral connection to autism. One study found that inherited or acquired defects in an enzyme (RNase L) that degrades viral RNA in a cell might be present in some autism-prone individuals and, therefore, could provide a link between viral infections and live virus vaccines, like the MMR, and autism.

Another study, authored by Theresa Deisher, found that the introduction of new vaccines containing aborted human tissue and *retroviral transcripts* (documented to be present in certain immune cells of autistic individuals) correlated directly with a dramatic rise in autism incidence on at least four occasions in the U.S., the United Kingdom, Denmark, and in Western Australia.

An important finding in the Deisher study was the discovery that "Varicella and Hepatitis A immunization coverage was significantly related to autistic disorder cases."

The viral inhibition of the enzyme abbreviated GAD (glutamic acid decarboxylase), which converts the excitatory neurotransmitter glutamate to the calming substance GABA (gamma amino butyric acid), provides another mechanism by which viruses (like the rubella virus) might promote autism. It has been shown that the GAD enzyme is often significantly decreased in autistic individuals, and that the rubella virus can further inhibit this enzyme.

Autistic individuals often suffer from non-specific inflammatory bowel disease, as Dr. Andrew Wakefield and others have shown. A Washington University School of Medicine study has found an association between inflammatory bowel disease and an increase in the *variety* of viruses in the digestive system. A large part of this increase in viral diversity was in the form of viruses that infect bacteria (bacteriophages). We do not as yet know whether a link exists between intestinal bacteria infected with phage viruses and inflammatory bowel disease. Further research is necessary to clarify this relationship.[21]

Stealth Viruses?

It appears that certain viruses escape immune detection and don't generate any immune response or inflammation. Dr. John Martin labels these as "stealth adapted viruses." Dr. Martin, who in 1995 was chief of the Immunology/Molecular Pathology Unit at the L.A. County Medical Center and a Professor of Pathology at USC, discovered that the polio vaccine had been contaminated with the simian cytomegalovirus, just such a "stealth" virus.

His research showed that the simian cytomegalovirus was capable of spreading from vaccinated individuals to others and that it caused neurological problems, and because it wasn't activating the immune response, its presence was being missed by medical staff. He presented his findings to the Institute of Medicine in November 1995.

Dr. Martin wanted to know whether other lots of polio vaccine were also contaminated with this "stealth adapted virus." He sent proposals to the CDC and FDA for grant money to finance such testing and (surprise, surprise) in short order found that his laboratory at USC was to be closed and his research funding was to be confiscated. Despite these obstacles, Dr. Martin (with alternative funding) continued his research into these stealth adapted viruses.[22]

Dr. Martin's further investigations revealed that "patient-derived stealth-adapted viruses caused severe neurological disease when inoculated into animals, without any accompanying inflammatory reaction."[23]

He found direct evidence for a stealth-adapted virus infection in patients with chronic fatigue syndrome *as well as a majority of patients with autism*, and that this infection damaged the mitochondria, rendering the individual "susceptible to environmental challenges."[24]

---

21   Norman, J.M. et al. "Disease-specific alterations in the enteric virome in inflammatory bowel disease." *Cell.* Jan 29, 2015.

22   http://www.ageofaut ism .com/2008/09/stealth-viruses.html

23   Ibid.

24   "Stealth virus isolated from an autistic child." *J Autism Dev Disorder.* 1995. 25:223-4. and http://www.ccid.org/stealth/faq.htm and Martin, W. John. *Stealth Adapted Viruses; Alternative Cellular Energy (ACE) & KELEA Activated Water: A New Paradigm of Healthcare.* Bloomington, IN: AuthorHouse, 2014.

Doctor Martin concluded that, "an autistic or severely learning disabled child should be considered as being stealth virus infected unless a negative culture shows otherwise." Fortuitously, he discovered an alternative cellular energy (ACE) pathway that is able to suppress the stealth viruses that are capable of evading the expected innate and acquired immune system detection and response.

Dr. Martin founded the Center for Complex Infectious Disease (CCID) where he continues his research. Many (but not all) autistic children have shown significant improvement in function after being treated with therapies that stimulate the ACE pathway. These improvements include, "markedly improved social interactions with far better eye contact, verbal speech, reading ability, attention span, and in one patient, the control of previously uncontrollable seizures, allowing for the discontinuation of seizure medication."[25]

Further information regarding this approach to stealth virus therapy may be had at www.iminhere.ca and www.s3support.com.

A Beneficial Stealth Virus?

Can stealth viruses sometimes be beneficial? The answer appears to be yes, at least for mice. Researchers found that a mouse intestinal virus called *murine nora virus* "can replace the beneficial function of commensal bacteria in the intestine." The virus was able to restore "intestinal morphology and lymphocytic function without inducing overt inflammation and disease."

This extraordinary virus was able to "offset the deleterious effects of treatment with antibiotics…. The new findings are the first strong evidence that viruses in the gastrointestinal tract can help maintain health and heal a damaged gut," the authors conclude. It is not known whether this virus or similar viruses play a role in human intestinal health.[26]

A Lyme Disease Connection to Autism?

Lyme disease is a serious infection caused by a bacterium called Borrelia burgdorfori, which is spread by tics. If treated early and appropriately with antibiotics, the infection can be eliminated; unfortunately, many people exposed to the bite of infected tics are not treated in the early stages of the disease when symptoms are minimal, so they go on to have chronic infections that are more difficult to eradicate. Infected mothers can pass the disease to their babies gestationally.

In a small unpublished study, 19 autistic children and 5 controls from 8 different states had blood drawn for the presence of the Lyme disease organism (using IFA and Western Blot IgG analysis). What the researchers found was that *26 percent of the autistic children tested positive for Lyme specific bands and none of the controls did.*[27]

In another study by Aristo Vojdani, presented at the 2007 Lyme-Autism Connection Conference, autism samples from different clinics in four states on the U.S. East and West Coasts showed positive results in 17-26 percent of those tested, supporting the findings in the aforementioned study.

In a case study of 102 children with gestational Lyme disease born to mothers with either treated or partially treated Lyme disease, it was found that their children, who weren't diagnosed until they were at least 1-5 years of age, actually had symptoms of Lyme disease present during infancy that were overlooked. These symptoms included ADHD (56 percent), irritability and mood swings (54 percent), light sensitivity (43 percent), sensory sensitivity (23-36 percent), anger or rage (23 percent), cognitive delay (27 percent), speech delay (21 percent), problems with reading and writing (19 percent), and a host of other detrimental symptoms and diagnoses, including autism (9 percent)![28]

---

25   http://www.ageofautism.com/2008/09/stealth-viruses.html
26   Kernbauer, E. et al. "An enteric virus can replace the beneficial function of commensal bacteria." *Nature 2014.* http://www.nature.com/nature/journal/vaop/ncurrent/full/nature13960.html.
27   www.liafoundation.org
28   Ibid. PDF slides from aforementioned 2007 Conference.

The findings in these preliminary studies warrant further research into the possible link between Lyme disease and autism and related disorders, and suggest that testing autistic children and those with ADHD for the presence of Lyme disease bacteria is appropriate.

Stealth Bacteria?

Dr. Dwayne Smith, Ph.D. believes that tiny, cell wall-deficient bacteria can commonly be found attached to Complex I in the mitochondria of many people with conditions ranging from cancer and Lyme disease to Parkinson's disease, COPD (Chronic Obstructive Pulmonary Disease), and even autism.

As is true with stealth viruses, these pleomorphic (many shapes and forms) bacteria don't appear to stimulate the immune system, and they impair energy production in the mitochondria by blocking electron flow, which is necessary for the production of ATP energy molecules.

Dr. Smith has developed a remarkable protocol for treating all these conditions (www.bxprotocol.com). The BX protocol was originally developed for treating cancers, but it appears to be beneficial for a host of various other health conditions in which mitochondrial dysfunction plays a key role. The downside of this protocol is the expense (roughly $17,000 for the first year). This will be discussed at greater length in the follow-up to this book titled *Reversing Autism* (pending completion).

Chapter 33
The Amy Yasko Hypothesis

"Those who have the privilege to know have the duty to act."
— *Albert Einstein*

AMY YASKO, N.D., *has a BS in chemistry and a Ph.D. in Microbiology, Immunology, and Infectious Diseases. She is also the co-founder of a successful biotech company involved in RNA and DNA research, diagnostics, and therapeutics.*

Dr. Yasko became interested in the problem of autism a number of years ago and has written two books, *Genetic Bypass* and *The Puzzle of Autism: Putting It All Together* (co-authored by Garry Gordon), explaining her approach to evaluating and treating autistic individuals.

Dr. Yasko hypothesizes, as do so many others, that autism is caused by certain genetic predispositions aggravated by particular environmental insults. In her research, she has traced the various complicated biochemical pathways leading to the autistic state.

Dr. Yasko agrees with Dr. Blaylock that excitotoxins like *glutamate* and *aspartate* represent one important cause of the dysfunctions seen in autism. Gluten from wheat and other grains and casein from milk and hydrolyzed yeast, as has been discussed, are some other sources of concentrated glutamate. Dr. Yasko integrates a great deal of what we know about the etiology of autism in her biomedical approach to treating autistic children and adults.

The Glutamate Connection

Glutamate, it may be recalled (see Chapter 31), is the main excitatory neurotransmitter and is essential for learning, attention, focus, and memory. As has been mentioned, it is also the precursor of the calming neurotransmitter abbreviated as GABA (gamma amino butyric acid).

GABA is a neurotransmitter that engenders a feeling of peaceful satisfaction. It is also important in the acquisition of speech because it helps us to distinguish between the onset of a sound and background noise. An inability to filter background noise can lead to sensory overload. Low GABA levels also make seizure activity more likely.

The enzyme that converts glutamate to GABA (glutamic acid decarboxylase) also requires vitamin B6 as a cofactor for its activity. Vitamin B6 plays a role in many chemical reactions pertinent to reversing autism, and it is one of the nutrients that has shown great success in this regard.

In autistic children, as we have noted, there is often a failure to convert glutamate to GABA in sufficient amounts. This results in an imbalance that results in too much neuronal excitation (which can lead to "stimming" behaviors) and too little GABA calming (which can lead to speech impairment).

One of the frequent findings in autistic children, Yasko points out, is the presence of a chronic viral infection (like measles). Viral infections (particularly rubella) are known to inhibit the conversion of glutamate to GABA. Excess copper, a common finding in 85 percent or more of autistic individuals, also inhibits GABA.

Excess glutamate, as has been mentioned, can damage and even kill neurons by allowing too much calcium to enter the cell, and it depletes glutathione and potentiates the toxicity of even low levels of mercury.[1]

One of the six receptors that glutamate attaches to is known as the NMDA receptor. When glutamate or other excitatory compounds (like aspartate) land on this receptor, they open a channel that allows calcium into the cell. It's the calcium that causes excitation in the cell. However, an excessive influx of calcium damages the neuron. *This reaction can be blocked with magnesium and zinc*, and both of these elements have been used successfully as supplements for autism.

As we have shown, autistic children exhibit elevated levels of these excitatory neurotransmitters. There is also some evidence indicating that autistic children also possess increased numbers of glutamate receptors. This isn't all bad, however; research has shown a link between increased numbers of glutamate receptors in mice and a superior ability to learn and memorize.[2]

Impaired Detoxification (Sulfation) in the Liver

The liver detoxifies huge numbers of chemical compounds by the processes of oxidation and by attaching other molecules like sulfate (a sulfur atom attached to several oxygen atoms) to them. The detoxified substances are then sent to the GI tract via the gall bladder. One of the enzymes in the liver that transfers sulfate groups to toxic substances is PST (phenol-sulfo-transferase).

Rosemary Waring found this enzyme to be low in almost all autistic children tested and, as a result, their ability to detoxify to be impaired. PST is necessary to detoxify salicilates (which have themselves been shown to suppress PST activity), food dyes, and other phenolic compounds. *This may help explain why children with autism or ADHD are especially sensitive to artificial colors.*[3]

The PST enzyme transfers a sulfate molecule from one substance to another. A deficiency of sulfate is found in a majority of children with autism, and this contributes to their poor ability to detoxify many substances. A lack of sulfur-containing foods in the diet of many autistic individuals is a likely contributing factor in this regard, as is a deficiency of vitamin B6, in particular in its active state as P5P (pyridoxine 5-phosphate). P5P is necessary in the conversion of cystathionine to *cysteine*, an important sulfur-containing amino acid found in glutathione and the metallothionein enzymes.

PST is also needed to add sulfate groups to connective tissue molecules called "GAGs" (glucosaminoglycans). If these are not sufficiently sulfated, the basement lining of the gut mucosa thickens, and this may contribute to the "leaky gut" so often noted in autistics. A lack of sulfated GAGs in the kidney promotes a loss of sulfate in the urine. The retention of sulfate by the kidney requires the activity of a sulfate transporter whose activity has been found to be blocked by *mercury*.[4]

---

1   Aschner et al. "Methyl Mercury Alters Glutamate Transport in Astrocytes." *NeuroChem Intl.* 2000; 37:199

2   Joe Tsien of Princeton in *Nature*. Sept 2, 1999.

3   Waring, R.H.; Klovrza, L.V. "Sulphur Metabolism in Autism." *Journal of Nutritional and Environmental Medicine*. 2000; 10: 25–32.

4   http://newtreatments.org/ga.php?linkid=252

Gastro-Intestinal Abnormalities

Autistic children often have impaired digestive and absorptive ability. This is due to decreased output of stomach acid, insufficient production of digestive enzymes and bile, and insufficient production of *secretin* (a gut enzyme that stimulates the pancreas to neutralize the stomach acid and to secrete digestive enzymes) and a deficiency of other hormones like *CCK* (cholicystokinin: which stimulates the gall bladder to release bile) and *Gastric Inhibitory Peptide*, which slows the release of acid into the digestive tract.

These digestive deficiencies promote the overgrowth of yeasts and other potentially harmful microorganisms in the gut. The normal, protective, and beneficial microflora (like Lactobacilli and Bifidobacteria) are often found in insufficient numbers. This often manifests as a drop in the levels of vitamin K, a fat-soluble vitamin produced in the intestinal tract by the action of beneficial bacteria on leafy green foods.

Vitamin K is well-known as a factor important in the clotting system. Less well-known are its roles in building bone *and in controlling hypoglycemic-related panic attacks*. Children with autism seem to be particularly susceptible to side effects from sugar ingestion; they are frequently dysbiotic (showing imbalanced gut organisms), and they often don't eat green-leafy vegetables.

The Streptococcal Connection

"Strep" germs produce a number of troubling substances, Dr. Yasko emphasizes. These include streptokinase, which can increase TNF (tumour necrosis factor); IL6 (inter-leukin 6), another inflammatory mediator; and NADase, an enzyme that depletes NAD, a vitamin B3 derivative, which is necessary for recycling glutathione.

TNF and IL6 are known to decrease methylation, which would serve to aggravate the 85 percent of autistic children who are undermethylated to begin with, and methylation reactions are necessary for the proper myelination of nerves and the "pruning" of excessive brain neurons. Autistic children show myelination delays in the outer area of white matter of the brain consistent with this hypothesis.

The Toxic Metals Connection

We live in a highly toxic world. Many of us harbor elevated levels of lead, mercury cadmium, arsenic, and other poisonous metals. Autistic children, as has been shown, have impaired detoxification systems (low glutathione, cysteine, lipoic acid, and metallothioneins) and can't excrete these dangerous substances well.

Dr. Bradstreet, it may be remembered, found the mercury burden in autistic children to be 8 times higher than in non-autistics. The main source of this mercury was the inclusion of thimerosal (which is almost 50 percent ethyl mercury) as the preservative in the immunizations given to babies and children.

Many practitioners serving the autistic community today believe in removing these harmful metals from the body by processes known as chelation or clathration. There are many chelating substances available today, like DMSA, EDTA, and DMPS.

Dr. Yasko prefers EDTA plus a unique, RNA-based process that she believes gets out the "bound" metals that the other agents miss. She claims that her chelating agents remove toxic metals "even with patients who have undergone extensive parenterally administered DMPS to the point that others have been convinced that mercury was no longer an issue."

Dr. Yasko points out that the thimerosal molecule may harm the body in three ways: 1) by poisoning the body with mercury, 2) by mimicking the nucleic acids (which it resembles structurally), and 3) by interfering with the actions of a number of enzymes (like the sulfate transporter in the kidney).

She hypothesizes that the thimerosal gets bound to the DNA molecule and thereby "hides" from the chelating agents. She further suggests that viral infections induce a particular form of metallothionein that effectively binds mercury and other toxic metals, but which gets trapped in cells. When these toxic metals are sequestered in cells, they may compromise immune function, which sets the stage for a chronic infection with viruses or other organisms.

She maintains that one must eliminate the chronic viral infection in order to eliminate the heavy metal burden. The best way to do this, she suggests, is with chelating agents like EDTA, DMPS, and DMSA, all of which also possess anti-viral properties. She and Dr. Garry Gordon have designed an oral RNA-based liquid product that they believe will effectively remove these toxic substances from the body.

Genetic Bypass

In her book, *Genetic Bypass*, Amy Yasko discusses a variety of undesirable genetic mutations that are commonly found in autistic individuals and suggests how to bypass certain of these genetic defects by supplementing with appropriate nutrients. The interested reader is encouraged to read her books in this regard; however, they are somewhat technical, not well-edited, and may be a bit difficult for the lay reader to understand.

Although there are no studies regarding the effectiveness of the Yasko approach to reversing autism, an abundance of anecdotal reports attest to the effectiveness of her therapies for many autistic individuals. A number of autism practitioners use her protocols with alleged great success.

Concerns regarding her therapies include the cost of the many supplements that she prescribes, the difficulty in getting autistic children to ingest all these supplements, and the conflict of interest regarding her recommending many of her own proprietary products. Figure 32.1 is an illustration of chemical pathways relevant to the Yasko hypothesis.

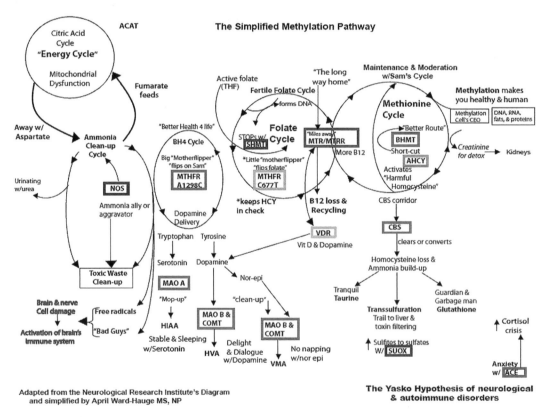

Figure 32.1. The Yasko Hypothesis of Neurological and Autoimmune Disorders

"American children are over vaccinated and over medicated, over fed, undernourished and have record levels of chronic illness and developmental delay....
"Our leading medical institutions have done more than merely fail us, their conduct lies at the root of the problem. Their agents have censored important science, manipulated data, intimidated honest scientists, and deceived the public.
"Worst of all, they have cloaked themselves in the mantle of science and 'evidence-based medicine' as they have circled the wagons to defend their policies, profits and programs. In the meantime, their conduct and behavior is perpetuating one of the most egregious and systematic episodes of scientific denial in human history."

— *The Canary Party Position Paper*[5]

---

5   http://canaryparty.net/index.php?option=com_content&view=article&id=46:the-canary-party-position-paper&catid=1:latest-news&Itemid=50

Chapter 34
The Perfect Storm

"It has become appallingly obvious that our technology
has exceeded our humanity."

— *Albert Einstein*

I N 1997, SEBASTIAN *Junger wrote a popular non-fiction book about the crew of the Andrea Gail, a fishing boat that got caught in a ferocious storm in 1991 in the north Atlantic and eventually capsized with the loss of almost all on board.*

Both the book and the movie based on it were entitled *The Perfect Storm* because the Andrea Gail met its tragic fate as a result of the highly unlikely and unfortunate confluence of two powerful weather fronts that collided with a third, a hurricane.

So, too, our children have been victims in recent years of a "perfect storm" of toxic encounters and dietary inadequacies that have resulted in 1 out of 6 having a neuro-developmental disorder and 1 in 68 having autism or a related autism spectrum disorder.[1]

In recent decades, we have exposed vulnerable babies and children to damaging levels of mercury and aluminum from their immunizations, many of which also contain other potentially harmful ingredients and even viruses. Pregnant women have been given mercury-containing injections on the irresponsible advice of the CDC, and additionally, they have often been prescribed autism-promoting acetaminophen for fever and pain, as have their offspring. Exposures to antibiotics, mercury, genetically-modified foods, and other toxics promote dysbiosis, allergies, inflammation, leaky gut, and neurological impairments.

Mercury from coal-fired plants, cement factories, fish, dental amalgams, and other sources has entered our food chain and augments the brain-damaging mercury contained in the recommended annual "flu" shot and in other immunizations as well. Pollution from cars, trucks, and toxic waste dumps also plays a key role in the noxious milieu to which many of us are exposed. Many of these environmental poisons are synergistically toxic.

The dramatic rise in cell phone use in recent years by pregnant women and children has been linked to a significant increased risk of behavior problems in those children so exposed. Many plant foods, like corn, soy, and canola, have been unnaturally genetically modified in a way that damages the plant's genetic code, increases undesirable mutations, decreases the plant's nutritional value (when sprayed with glyphosate), and promotes intestinal inflammation and possibly cancer and autism.

---

1   A 2014 parent survey suggests that the actual rate is 1 in 45 children aged 3-17. See http://www.cdc.gov/nchs/nhis.htm

And because glyphosate and BT toxin cannot be washed off of genetically-modified corn, soy, canola, and other sprayed crops, our population has been ingesting potentially harmful glyphosate herbicide/microbicide and BT insecticide in alarming amounts. Other brain-damaging organo-phosphate pesticides are additionally often found at significant levels in many non-organic vegetables.

Fluoride in our water and toothpastes has been shown to lower the IQ of children. And the typical American diet, replete with sugary drinks, artificial colors, preservatives, hydrogenated oils, artificial sweeteners, excitotoxins, and highly refined processed foods lacking in fiber and essential nutrients, undoubtedly plays a major role in promoting the neuro-developmental problems and learning disorders that are now epidemic in America and throughout the world.

Our babies and children have also been the recipients of ever-increasing numbers of immunizations with a resultant and likely relevant increase in conditions like allergies, arthritis, asthma, diabetes, sudden infant death, and a variety of serious neurological disorders including autism, hyperactivity, and attention deficit disorder.

The information presented in this book clearly illustrates the complexity of autism and its etiology. We should not be misled by those who claim we don't know what causes autism. We do. We now have a very good idea about the many damaging environmental influences, like immunizations, and exposures to mercury and aluminum, that promote autism in genetically-vulnerable children and by what mechanisms they do so. As we have shown, the evidence linking immunizations to autism is not just strong. It's overwhelming. Immunizations are indeed a major cause of autism, albeit not the only cause.

Tragically, the institutions and individuals supposed to protect the populace from this "perfect storm" of biological insults: the Centers for Disease Control and Prevention, the Food and Drug Administration, the World Health Organization, the American Academy of Pediatrics, and so many others, appear to be under the complicit, corrupting, pernicious influence of certain politicians, individuals, and corporations.

These conflicted entities have promoted the publication of deceptive and spurious studies that support their own questionable agenda, and they have played a key role in the censorship and suppression of contrary views, information, and studies. These once revered organizations have also unconscionably demonized non-conformist scientists and whistle-blowers whose valid research and views threaten the self-serving, biased pseudo-science that these institutions so often promote.

Our planet is in big trouble. The world population is increasing, as are demands for food and natural resources like oil, coal, minerals, and fresh water. Climate change predictions suggest that sea levels are rising and will continue to rise as glaciers melt. The rising waters are likely to swamp many coastal lands, cities, and islands.

As carbon dioxide levels soar, seas become increasingly acidic, which places the viability of the entire ocean ecosystem in jeopardy. Impactful weather events like droughts, floods, typhoons, and hurricanes are anticipated to become more severe and more frequent, and yet our oblivious industries continue to release huge amounts of potentially harmful chemicals and climate-damaging carbon dioxide into our air, water, and soil.

This "perfect storm" of horrendous events and exposures is growing in strength, and the results are likely to be devastating. "At today's rate, by 2025, one in two children will be autistic," warns MIT research scientist Stephanie Seneff.[2]

Have we gone mad? What kind of a world are we bequeathing to our children? Will our species even survive? We need to start now to take appropriate steps to calm this malevolent "storm," or it may sweep us all away.

"In the final analysis what are we doing?"

— Annette Piccirillo

---

2   http://althealthworks.com/2494 /mit-researchers-new-warning-at-todays-rate-1-in-2-children-will-be-autistic-by-2025/#sthash.Ics4zZqa.dpuf

Part IV
Some Appropriate Steps

Chapter 35
Preventing Autism Spectrum Disorders

"An ounce of prevention is worth a pound of cure."

— Ben Franklin

CAN WE DO *Anything to Decrease the Likelihood of a Child Having an Autism Spectrum Disorder?*
Yes. A number of steps can be taken to reduce the risk of a child becoming autistic. The following preventive measures are based on minimizing the known risks and causes of autism that we have discussed in this book. While we can't change a child's genetic predispositions to autism spectrum disorders, we can attempt to diminish the environmental factors that increase the risk of a child developing these maladies.

Suggestions for the Mother-To-Be

Ideally, the mother-to-be should be in optimal health. That entails eating an appropriate diet and minimizing toxic exposures. Suggestions in this regard include:

- Avoid immunizations just before, during, and post-conception if possible, and avoid immunizations that contain aluminum and mercury at any time. Forego the influenza immunization in particular.

- Drink non-fluoridated water and avoid fluoride toothpastes.

- Avoid mercury amalgams. Minimize aluminum exposure: avoid aluminum antiperspirants, aluminum cookware, etc.

- Minimize exposures to toxic pesticides and other harmful chemicals like lead, bisphenol A, and phthalates. Certain pesticides like Mirex and beta-hexachlorocyclohexane aren't broken down and are stored in animal fat. Reducing the intake of non-organic red meats may reduce such exposures.

- Reside in homes not located close to major roadways, cement plants, coal burning power plants, toxic waste dumps, or pesticide-sprayed farm fields.

- Eat wholesome foods, preferably organic. Wheat products should also be organic since wheat is often sprayed with glyphosate prior to harvest.

- Maintain optimal weight. Obesity increases autism risk.

- Ensure that levels of nutrients in the diet and especially selenium, zinc, vitamins C and D, and folic acid are optimal. A good quality prenatal vitamin and mineral supplement is suggested in this regard.

- Avoid/minimize refined carbohydrates, artificial colors, genetically-modified foods, hydrogenated vegetable oils, artificial sweeteners, excitotoxins, and fish that are high in mercury (tuna, swordfish, etc.)

- Ideally, allow several years between pregnancies.

- Avoid, if possible, the use of pitocin and terbutaline.

- Control blood sugar during pregnancy to help prevent diabetes, obesity, and hypertension.

- Avoid the use of cell phones during pregnancy.

- If possible, avoid all drugs during the pregnancy and acetaminophen in particular.

- Take appropriate steps to prevent or control preeclampsia.

Suggestions for the Baby and Young Child

- *Avoid all immunizations until the child is at least 3-4 years of age.* Or if immunizations are desired or required, *try a modified immunizations schedule* as per Dr. Mumper (see Chapter 27). Do not use any immunization that contains aluminum or mercury. Do not give any that have previously caused an adverse reaction (high fever, screaming, behavior change, regression, etc.). Give only one at a time and never if the child is ill.

- *Breast feed, if possible, for as long as possible.* Breast milk is considered the ideal food for babies. However, due to the release of megatons of largely untested and likely toxic chemicals into our environment every year, most women now produce breast milk that contains a variety of toxic substances. That being said, researchers Eric Dewailly and Joseph Jacobson showed that "contaminant exposure in maternal blood caused the same or far greater damage to the fetus than 10 fold higher exposure from breast milk. This damage, measured as impaired neurodevelopmental function, was present for years after (and possibly for life.)" The most important breast feeding is the first when immune-protective colostrum is produced.[1]

- Supplement with appropriate probiotics after birth.

- *Avoid soy.* If not breast feeding, it would be wise to avoid soy formulas like Isomil, Prosobee, and Nursoy. Soy formulas contain high levels of phytoestrogens and also very high levels of manganese, as much as 200 times the levels found in breast milk. Manganese is an essential nutrient, but in excess, it is neurotoxic. High levels of manganese in ground water have been shown to be associated with a significant IQ diminishment in children so exposed as well as "altered behaviors in adolescents." Fluoride in water increases the absorbability of manganese. Manganese excess can damage the dopamine-producing cells in the brain and has been linked to ADHD and criminal behavior.[2]

- *Feed organic foods whenever possible.* Avoid highly-processed foods, fluoridated water and toothpaste, conventionally-sprayed produce, genetically-modified foods, artificial colors, preservatives, hydrogenated oils, excitotoxins (MSG, etc.), artificial sweeteners, honey (a source of botulism bacteria), and fish that tend to have high levels of mercury. Identify food allergies and intolerances and remove those foods from the child's diet. Similac, Enfamil, and Gerber Good Start all contain genetically-modified ingredients.

- *Avoid acetaminophen.* It appears to be a risk factor for autism.

- *Minimize exposures to toxins.* This includes home and garden insecticide sprays and many household chemicals used for cleaning, stain removal, and painting or staining. Minimize exposure to aluminum by not cooking in aluminum pots and pans.

- *Minimize exposures to polluted air.* If you live near a major roadway, cement plant, power plant, conventionally-sprayed farm field, or toxic waste dump, make sure the baby's exposure to outside air is limited and that household air is filtered, or better yet, move.

- Don't let a child use a cell phone.

---

1   http://www.infactcanada.ca/breast milk_ contamination_is_not.htm
2   http://www.sciencedaily .com/releases/2010/09/1009 20074013.htm

Suggestions for the Rest of Us

- *Get educated and spread the word.* Countering the mountain of misinformation about autism spectrum disorders and the safety of vaccines is a formidable task.

As Dr. Suzanne Humphries says in her book *Dissolving Illusions: Disease, Vaccines and the Forgotten History,* "We have a highly profitable, lucrative religion that involves the government, industry, and academia. That religion is vaccination. People believe in vaccines. They'll tell you, they believe in vaccines. But you ask them what they know about vaccines and it will be almost nothing. In fact the people who argue the loudest usually know the least when it comes to trying to convince you to take the vaccine."

So we must educate ourselves in order to educate others about the truth regarding the myriad causes of autism spectrum disorders and, in particular, the harm that our current vaccination program appears to be causing.

In that regard, Dr. Humphries' aforementioned book, Neil Z. Miller's *The Vaccine Safety Manual,* and Kent Heckenlively and Judy Mikovitz's *Plague,* and those listed below are well worth reading.

Skyhorse Publishing is committed to publishing excellent books about autism and has a number of these on the subject of vaccinations. They include: *The Vaccine Court* by Wayne Rohde, *Callous Disregard* by Andrew Wakefield, Robert F. Kennedy Junior's book *Thimerosal: Let the Science Speak,* Anne Dachel's *The Big Autism Coverup,* Louis Conte and Tony Lyons' *Vaccine Injuries,* Louise Habakus and Mary Holland's *Vaccine Epidemic,* and Mark Blaxill and Dan Olmstead's *Vaccines 2.0.*

Support organizations, online sites and blogs that educate and promote the truth about autism and its myriad causes. These include:

Autism Research Institute (www.autism.com): This wonderful organization, founded by the late Dr. Bernard Rimland, pioneered the concept that autism is a reversible condition that can be therapeutically addressed by utilizing a scientifically-sound biomedical approach combined with appropriate therapies. ARI sponsors autism research and conferences, and the website provides a rich source of autism information on appropriate lab testing, how to locate a clinician, parent ratings of various treatments, drugs and supplements, and it provides in-depth information on various dietary, medical, nutritional, and behavioral treatments and therapies.

National Vaccine Information Center (www.nvicadvocacy.org): This site provides access to contact information for state legislators and provides free online training sessions for vaccine education and choice advocacy.

Age of Autism (www.ageofautism.com): This great online blog and information site, founded by Dan Olmsted and Mark Blaxill, provides frequent updates on autism-related issues, with pertinent comments from Anne Dachel and other contributors.

Dr. Mercola's website (www.drmercola.com): This free website provides a wealth of health information and interviews with leaders and researchers in the field of functional medicine.

Schafer Autism Report (www.sarnet.org/): This is a subscription-based email newsletter that provides the latest autism information compiled from news stories, websites, and research data.

Generation Rescue (www.generationrescue.org/): This organization, founded by Jenny McCarthy, advocates the view that autism and related disorders are primarily caused by environmental factors like vaccines and provides guidance and support in that regard.

Safe Minds (www.safeminds.org/): This organization is dedicated to eliminating toxic substances like mercury from vaccines and the environment. The site focuses on prevention and funds "research to find treatments that will lead to recovery for those living with autism."

National Autism Association (www.nationalautismassociation.org/): This organization supports the notion that toxic substances like mercury promote autism and provides support and information for parents of autistically-impaired children. They believe that autism is a biologically-based, treatable disorder.

The Canary Party (www.canaryparty.org): The Canary Party, according to its website, "is a movement created to stand up for the victims of medical injury, environmental toxins and industrial foods by restoring balance to our free and civil society and empowering consumers to make health and nutrition decisions that promote wellness." Its position paper is well worth reading, and it needs our support.

VOR (www.vor.net): VOR is an advocacy organization for people with developmental disabilities.

The Autism File: Publishes an excellent online free autism magazine. (4208 Love Bird Lane; Austin, TX 78730)

Be an activist and support legislation that encourages research into the environmental causes of autism, protects vaccine informed-consent rights and exemptions, supports GMO labeling laws, increases pollution controls, and promotes organic farming.

Write letters to the editor of local papers. Comment on autism site blogs. Get to know your local and state legislators and provide them with documentation supporting your views on appropriate legislation. Don't buy foods that contain GMOs. Contact companies that support the labeling of GMOs and thank them. Contact companies that have hampered the efforts to label GMOs and let them know how you feel. Vote for candidates that support all these efforts. Unite with like-thinking individuals and create local organizations that support the spread of accurate information regarding the causes of autism spectrum disorders and propose solutions for these problems.

Whistleblowers need to be protected and not prosecuted, especially those who have worked for the CDC (like William Thompson), the American Academy of Pediatrics, companies like Monsanto that manufacture genetically-modified plants, companies that manufacture vaccines, and the World Health Organization. Support them!

Chapter 36
Evaluating Individuals on the Autism Spectrum

"You get in trouble; you have to evaluate…"

— Robert Iler

THE WORKUP OF *any child on the autism spectrum starts with a proper evaluation by a knowledgeable health care provider who understands the complexity of the condition and its many genetic and environmental influences.*

A proper evaluation entails a thorough history and physical examination plus appropriate laboratory and other testing as indicated.

Do Appropriate Testing

Not all children require all the tests that are available. A qualified, *biomedically-trained* practitioner (usually an M.D. or N.D.) must guide the parent in selecting which tests to run.

A complete physical examination and history should be performed by the child's primary care clinician to ascertain the physical and developmental status of the child.

A specific evaluation for signs and symptoms of autism or ADHD should be part of the workup of children with developmental delays.

A detailed history is a necessary part of these evaluations. Specific questions should be directed at evaluating risk factors for these conditions like diet, exposure to medicines, immunizations, toxic substance, and antibiotics.

The clinician should investigate the mother's health during the pregnancy; establish when and if the child regressed and what factors improve or worsen the child's condition. Also, it is necessary to ascertain whether there is any history of hearing impairment, speech disability, socialization and developmental delay, OCD symptoms, ear infections, seizures, tics or major illnesses. Detail the child's abilities and disabilities and all parental concerns.

Some Basic Tests Generally Helpful for Most Autistic Children

1. A Comprehensive Digestive Stool Analysis.

2. An IgG food allergy test and/or an elimination diet.

3. A urine panel for organic acids, amino acids, toxic peptides, kryptopyrroles, succinyl purine, and also useful are urine sulfate & uric acid evaluations.

4. A complete blood count, liver panel and serum copper and plasma zinc are desirable.

5. A DMSA or DMPS-provoked urine for toxic metals test. Beware that these can yield false negatives. The reference ranges for this test are for *unprovoked* urine testing. Since there is really no safe level for lead and mercury, elevated excretion of lead, mercury, and other toxics on a provoked urine challenge test is likely to be meaningful, even though there is no reference range for provoked testing. It has been shown that asymptomatic volunteers have demonstrated elevated excretion of a variety of toxic metals on a provoked urine challenge. *This information is not relevant, however,* because individuals differ, as we have noted, in their ability to tolerate toxins, and many toxins exert their harmful effects over a period of many years. The presence of toxic metals on a provoked urine challenge test indicates that the toxin is still present and needs to be cleared.

6. Some practitioners also suggest doing thyroid function screens, antibody tests to myelin basic protein, and other neuronal antigens, metallothionein function evaluations, ceruloplasmin, a copper binding protein, serum evaluation of nutritional adequacy (vitamins D, B6, B12, folic acid, molybedenum, etc.)

7. Immune function testing may be indicated in those who are showing signs of immune dysfunction.

8. If indicated, evaluate testosterone and cholesterol levels, and look for the fragile X mutation.

9. A new test on the horizon is called the MELISA (Memory Lymphocyte Immuno-Stimulation Assay) test, and it may be used to measure the reactivity or sensitization of an individual to metals. This is not the same as direct toxicity from metals and may offer an additional area of investigation for autistic individuals. The test has been used to screen for the allergenic parts of a substance (a drug for example) that antibodies bind to and can be used to assay an individual's response to a given metal, like the amalgams used by dentists, for example.

10. Genomic testing (looking for enzyme mutations), including the DNA methylation pathway profile.

11. Porphyrin profile.

12. Strep antibody profile.

13. Hearing evaluation, if indicated.

14. Many other tests may be useful, (an EEG for seizure disorders, for example), but an informed practitioner can help in making the decision as to which tests should be performed and in what order.

Costs

A major concern in regard to these evaluations is cost. Lab studies are very expensive and may need to be repeated if abnormalities are found. Costs can range from hundreds to thousands of dollars, depending on which lab studies are required. A comprehensive autism panel at the Great Plains Lab, for example, costs $1,895, and one for ADHD or Tourette's costs $2,070 (January 2015 pricing). These evaluations are not always covered by health insurance programs, and the financial burden may fall on the parents of the affected individual.

Some Laboratories Commonly Used for These Evaluations

The listed labs were found to pass the *Autism Research Institute's reproducibility criteria.*[1]

- **Great Plains Laboratory** 11813 W. 77th St., Lenexa, KS 66214 USA Phone: 913-341-8949 Fax: 913-341-6207 (See: http://www.greatplainslaboratory.com/home/eng/pricing.asp for costs and a list of tests it performs.)

- **Metametrix Laboratory & Genova Diagnostics** are now one laboratory under the name **Genova Diagnostics**. (See: https://www.gdx.net/tests/alphabetical for a list of tests it performs.)

    Metametrix: 800 221-4640. http://www.metametrix.com & inquiries@metametrix.com

    Genova Diagnostics: 800 522-4762; http://wwwgdx.net Contact: info@gdx.net

---

1   http://www.autism.com/pdf/providers/Lab percent20Reliability percent201_10.pdf

- **Doctor's Data Laboratory**: 630 377-8139; See http://www.chelationmedicalcenter. com/lab_tests.html for a list of tests it performs.

- **ImmunoLabs**: www.immunolabs.com/ 800 231-9197. This lab specializes in allergy testing (IgG ELISA testing and IgE RAST testing).

- **Health Diagnostics and Research Institute** (formerly **Vitamin Diagnostics**): This lab performs a variety of tests, including functional nutrient status, allergy tests, toxic load, gut flora sufficiency, and others. Tel: 732 721-1234; http://www.europeanlaboratory.nl/

There are undoubtedly many other highly qualified laboratories. An informed health practitioner should be the one to determine which is best, and how to interpret the lab results.

> *"Research is showing that getting the (flu) shot one year might make the next year's vaccine less effective…. For more than a decade scientific papers have reported unexpected findings of lower effectiveness with repeated (influenza) vaccination—a strange negative effect of prior year vaccination on current year, but flu experts can't quite explain this curious effect of repeated vaccination."*
>
> *— Reported by the Canadian Press in January 2015[2]*
> *(but never mentioned in the American Press)*

Some Final Thoughts

This book has been a long journey for me, as author, and perhaps for you the reader as well.

We have discovered the many environmental contributors to the devastating epidemic of autism, ADHD, sudden infant death syndrome, autoimmune diseases like arthritis and childhood (Type I) diabetes, and a host of other maladies.

We now know that the current and proposed immunization program's many serious side effects have been largely suppressed, and the program needs immediate re-evaluation by non-conflicted scientists. Studies need to be done of vaccinated vs. non-vaccinated populations, and long-term evaluations of the current immunization program need to be carried out as well!

We have been appalled to learn that we have been betrayed by the very institutions, individuals, and companies that should be protecting us. Their conflicts of interest are legion.

The good news is that there is a lot we can do to reverse the symptoms of autism and ADHD. This will be discussed in the follow-up to this book, *Reversing Autism* (pending completion by author).

So, don't give up hope.

The truth will eventually "get its pants on," as Winston Churchill put it, and with the help of non-conflicted politicians and a committed electorate, allow it to overtake the Big Lies (*"There is no autism epidemic; we don't know what causes autism, but it isn't immunizations or mercury; the immunization program is perfectly safe,"* etc.).

> *"Our remedies oft in ourselves do lie…"*
>
> *— William Shakespeare,* All's Well that Ends Well

---

2   http://www.ageofautism.com/2015/01/dachel-media-update-vax-clemantis-in-deserto.html?utm_source=feedburner&utm_medium=e mail &utm_campaign=Feed percent3A+ ageofautism+ percent28AGE+OF+AUTISM percent29

Appendix to Autism Uncensored

Appendix I
References (From ARI)

Research Documenting Biomedical Problems in Autism - February 2009.

The following index links to citations describing emerging findings in autism research.

A. Autism and the Gastrointestinal System

1. Afzal, N. et al. "Constipation with acquired megarectum in children with autism." *Pediatrics*. 2003 Oct; 112(4):939-42.

2. Arvilommi, H., Isolauri, E., Kalliomäki, M., Poussa, T., Salminen, S. "Probiotics and prevention of atopic disease: 4-year follow-up of a randomised placebo-controlled trial." *Lancet*. 2003; 361(9372):1869-71.

3. Ashwood, P. et al. "Intestinal lymphocyte populations in children with regressive autism: evidence for extensive mucosal immunopathology." J Clin Immunol. 2003 Nov; 23(6):504-17.

4. Ashwood, P., Wakefield, A.J. "Immune activation of peripheral blood and mucosal CD3+ lymphocyte cytokine profiles in children with autism and gastrointestinal symptoms." *J Neuroimmunol*. 2006 Apr; 173(1-2):126-34.

5. Balzola, F., Barbon, V., Repici, A., Rizzetto, M. "Panenteric IBD-like disease in a patient with regressive autism shown for the first time by the wireless capsule enteroscopy: another piece in the jigsaw of this gut-brain syndrome?" *Am J Gastro*. 2005; 979-981.

6. Balzola, F. et al. "Autistic enterocolitis: confirmation of a new inflammatory bowel disease in an Italian cohort of patients." *Gastroenterology*. 2005; 128:Suppl.2; A-303.

7. Balzola, F. et al. "Autistic Enterocolitis in childhood: the early evidence of the later Crohn's disease in autistic adulthood?" *Gastroenterology*. April 2007; Vol 132, N. 4, suppl 2 W 1100 A 660.

8. Balzola, F. et al. "Beneficial behavioural effects of IBD therapy and gluten/casein-free diet in an Italian cohort of patients with autistic enterocolitis followed over one year." *Gastroenterology*. April 2006; Vol 130 Number 4 suppl. 2 S1364 A-21.

9. Biller, J.A., Katz, A.J., Flores, A.F., Buie, T.M., Gorbach, S.L. "Treatment of recurrent Clostridium difficile colitis with Lactobacillus GG." *J Pediatr Gastroenterol Nutr*. 1995 Aug; 21(2):224-6.

10. Billoo, A.G., Memon, M.A., Khaskheli, S.A. et al. "Role of probiotic Saccharomyces boulardii in management and prevention of diarrhea." *World J Gastroenterol.* 2006; 12:4557-4560.

11. Black, C. Kaye, J.A., Jick, H. "Relation of childhood gastrointestinal disorders to autism: nested case-control study using data from the UK General Practice Research Database." *BMJ.* 2002 Aug 24; 325(7361):419-21.

12. Binstock, T. "Intra-monocyte pathogens delineate autism subgroups." *Med Hypotheses.* 2001 Apr; 56(4):523-31.

13. Binstock, T. "Anterior insular cortex: linking intestinal pathology and brain function in autism-spectrum subgroups." *Med Hypotheses.* 2001; 57(6):714-7.

14. Borruel, N. et al. "Increased mucosal tumour necrosis factor alpha production in Crohn's disease can be down-regulated ex vivo by probiotic bacteria." *Gut.* 2002 Nov; 51(5):659-64.

15. Bousvaros, A. et al; and the Members of the Challenges in Pediatric IBD Study Groups. "Challenges in pediatric inflammatory bowel disease." *Inflamm Bowel Dis.* 2006 Sep; 12(9):885-913.

16. Buchman, A.L. et al. "Hyperbaric oxygen therapy for severe ulcerative colitis." *J Clin Gastroenterol.* 2001 Oct; 33(4):337-9.

17. Buts, J.P., De Keyser, N. "Effects of Saccharomyces boulardii on intestinal mucosa." *Dig Dis Sci.* 2006 Aug; 51(8):1485-92.

18. Cade, R. et al. "Autism and schizophrenia: intestinal disorders." *Nutritional Neuroscience.* 2000; 3:57-72.

19. Cade, J.R. et al. "Autism and schizophrenia linked to malfunctioning enzyme for milk protein digestion." *Autism.* Mar 1999.

20. Czerucka, D. et al. "Experimental effects of Saccharomyces boulardii on diarrheal pathogens." *Microbes Infect.* 2002; 4(7): p. 733-9.

21. DeFelice, M.L. et al. "Intestinal cytokines in children with pervasive developmental disorders." *Am J Gastroenterol.* 2003; 98(8):1777-82.

22. del Giudice, M.M., Brunese, F.P. "Probiotics, prebiotics, and allergy in children: what's new in the last year?" *J Clin Gastroenterol.* 2008 Sep; 42 Suppl 3 Pt 2:S205-8.

23. D'Eufemia, P. et al. "Abnormal intestinal permeability in children with autism." *Acta Paediatr.* 1996 Sep; 85(9):1076-9.

24. Fedorak, R.N., Madsen, K.L. "Probiotics and the management of inflammatory bowel disease." *Inflamm Bowel Dis.* 2004 May; 10(3):286.

25. Forsberg, G. et al. "Presence of bacteria and innate immunity of intestinal epithelium in childhood celiac disease." *Am J Gastroenterol.* 2004 May; 99(5):894-904.

26. Furlano, R.I. et al. "Colonic CD8 and gamma delta T-cell infiltration with epithelial damage in children with autism." *J Pediatr.* 2001 Mar; 138(3):366-72.

27. Ghosh, S. et al. "Probiotics in inflammatory bowel disease: is it all gut flora modulation?" *Gut.* 2004 May; 53(5):620-2.

28. Gonzalez, L., Lopez, K., Navarro, D., Negron, L., Flores, L., Rodriguez, R., Martinez, M., Sabra, A. "Endoscopic and Histological Characteristics of the digestive mucosa in autistic children with gastrointestinal symptoms." *Arch Venez Pueric Pediatr.* 69; 1:19-25.

29. Gottschall, Elaine G. *Breaking the Vicious Cycle: Intestinal Health Through Diet.* Ontario: Kirkton Press, 1994.

30. Hadjivassiliou, M. et al. "Does cryptic gluten sensitivity play a part in neurological illness?" *Lancet.* 1996 Feb 10; 347(8998):369-71.

31. Hart, A.L. et al. "Modulation of human dendritic cell phenotype and function by probiotic bacteria." *Gut.* 2004 Nov; 53(11):1602-9.

32. Haskey, N., Dahl, W.J. "Synbiotic therapy: a promising new adjunctive therapy for ulcerative colitis." *Nutr Rev.* 2006 Mar; 64(3):132-8.

33. Hassall, E. "Decisions in diagnosing and managing chronic gastroesophageal reflux disease in children." *J Pediatr.* 2005 Mar; 146(3 Suppl):S3-12.

34. Homan, M., Baldassano, R.N., Mamula, P. "Managing complicated Crohn's disease in children and adolescents." *Nat Clin Pract Gastroenterol Hepatol.* 2005 Dec; 2(12):572-9.

35. Horvath, K. et al. "Gastrointestinal abnormalities in children with autistic disorder." *J Pediatr.* 1999 Nov; 135(5):559-63.

36. Horvath, K., Perman, J.A. "Autism and gastrointestinal symptoms." *Curr Gastroenterol Rep.* 2002 Jun; 4(3):251-8.

37. Horvath, K., Perman, J.A. "Autistic disorder and gastrointestinal disease." *Curr Opin Pediatr.* 2002 Oct; 14(5):583-7.

38. Iacono, G. et al. "Intolerance of cow's milk and chronic constipation in children. *N Engl J Med.* 1998 Oct 15; 339(16):1100-4.

39. Işeri, S.O., Sener, G., Sağlam, B., Gedik, N., Ercan, F., Yeğen, B.C. "Oxytocin ameliorates oxidative colonic inflammation by a neutrophil-dependent mechanism." *Peptides.* 2005 Mar; 26(3):483-91.

40. Kawashima, H. et al. "Detection and sequencing of measles virus from peripheral mononuclear cells from patients with inflammatory bowel disease and autism." *Dig Dis Sci.* 2000 Apr; 45(4):723-9.

41. Koch, T.R. et al. "Induction of enlarged intestinal lymphoid aggregates during acute glutathione depletion in a murine model." *Dig Dis Sci.* 2000; 45(11): 2115-21.

42. Kruis, W. "Antibiotics and probiotics in inflammatory bowel disease." *Aliment Pharmacol Ther.* 2004 Oct; 20 Suppl 4:75-8.

43. Kuddo, T., Nelson, K.B. "How common are gastrointestinal disorders in children with autism." *Curr Opin Pediatr.* 2003; 15(3):339-343.

44. Kushak, R., Winter, H., Farber, N., Buie, T. "Gastrointestinal symptoms and intestinal disaccharidase activities in children with autism." Abstract of presentation to the North American Society of Pediatric Gastroenterology, Hepatology, and Nutrition, Annual Meeting, October 20-22, 2005; Salt Lake City, Utah.

45. Levy, S. et al. "Children with autistic spectrum disorders. I: Comparison of placebo and single dose of human synthetic secretin." *Arch. Dis. Child.* 2003; 88:731-736.

46. Lewis, J.D. et al. "An open-label trial of the PPAR-gamma ligand rosiglitazone for active ulcerative colitis." *Am J Gastroenterol.* 2001 Dec; 96(12):3323-8.

47. Liu, Z., Li, N., Neu, J. "Tight junctions, leaky intestines, and pediatric diseases." *Acta Paediatr.* 2005 Apr; 94(4):386-93.

48. Macdonald, A. "Omega-3 fatty acids as adjunctive therapy in Crohn's disease." *Gastroenterol Nurs.* 2006 Jul-Aug; 29(4):295-301.

49. Melmed, R.D., Schneider, C.K., Fabes, R.A. "Metabolic markers and gastrointestinal symptoms in children with autism and related disorders." *J Pediatr Gastroenterol Nutr* 2000; 31(suppl 2)S31-32.

50. Ménard, S., Candalh, C., Bambou, J.C., Terpend, K., Cerf-Bensussan, N., Heyman M. "Lactic acid bacteria secrete metabolites retaining anti-inflammatory properties after intestinal transport." *Gut.* 2004 Jun; 53(6):821-8.

51. Parracho, H.M., Bingham, M.O., Gibson, G.R., McCartney, A.L. "Differences between the gut microflora of children with autistic spectrum disorders and that of healthy children." *J Med Microbiol.* 2005 Oct; 54(Pt 10):987-91.

52. Qin, H.L., Shen, T.Y., Gao, Z.G., Fan, X.B., Hang, X.M., Jiang, Y.Q., Zhang, H.Z. "Effect of lactobacillus on the gut microflora and barrier function of rats with abdominal infection." *World J Gastroenterol.* 2005 May 7; 11(17):2591-6.

53. Quigley, E.M., Hurley, D. "Autism and the gastrointestinal tract." *Am J Gastroenterol.* 2000 Sep; 95(9):2154-6. Reichelt, K.L., Knivsberg, A.M. "Can the pathophysiology of autism be explained by the nature of the discovered urine peptides?" *Nutr Neurosci.* 2003 Feb; 6(1):19-28.

54. Reichelt, K.L. et al. "Probable Etiology and Possible Treatment of Childhood Autism." *Brain Dysfuntion.* 1991; 4:308-319.

55. Rimland, B. "Secretin treatment for autism." *N Engl J Med.* 2000; 342(16): 1216-7; author reply 1218.

57. Romano, C. et al. "Usefulness of omega-3 fatty acid supplementation in addition to mesalazine in maintaining remission in pediatric Crohn's disease: a double-blind, randomized, placebo-controlled study." *World J Gastroenterol.* 2005 Dec 7; 11(45):7118-21.

58. Salminen, S., Isolauri, E., Salminen, E. "Clinical uses of probiotics for stabilizing the gut mucosal barrier: successful strains and future challenges." *Antonie Van Leeuwenhoek.* 1996 Oct; 70(2-4):347-58.

59. Sandler, R.H. et al. "Short-term benefit from oral vancomycin treatment of regressive-onset autism." *J Child Neurol.* 2000 Jul; 15(7):429.

60. Schneider, C.K., Melmed, R.D., Barstow, L.E., Enriquez, F.J., Ranger-Moore, J., Ostrem, J.A. "Oral Human Immunoglobulin for Children with Autism and Gastrointestinal Dysfunction: A Prospective, Open-Label Study." *J Autism Dev Disord.* 2006 Jul 15.

61. Sido, B., Hack, V., Hochlehnert, A., Lipps, H., Herfarth, C., Droge, W. "Impairment of intestinal glutathione synthesis in patients with inflammatory bowel disease." *Gut.* 1998 Apr; 42(4):485-92.

62. Sienkiewicz-Szapka, E. et al. "Transport of bovine milk derived opioid peptides across a Caco-2 monolayer." *Int Dairy J.* 2008

63. Song, Y., Liu, C., Finegold, S.M. "Real-time PCR quantitation of clostridia in feces of autistic children." *Appl Environ Microbiol.* 2004 Nov; 70(11):6459-65.

64. Sougioultzis, S. et al. "Saccharomyces boulardii produces a soluble anti-inflammatory factor that inhibits NF-kappaB-mediated IL-8 gene expression." *Biochem Biophys Res Commun.* 2006 Apr 28; 343(1):69-76.

65. Sturniolo, G.C. et al. "Zinc supplementation tightens 'leaky gut' in Crohn's disease." *Inflamm Bowel Dis.* 2001. 7(2): p. 94-8.

66. Surawicz, C.M. "Probiotics, antibiotic-associated diarrhoea and Clostridium difficile diarrhoea in humans." *Best Pract Res Clin Gastroenterol.* 2003 Oct; 17(5):775-83.

67. Taylor, B., Miller, E., Lingam, R., Andrews, N., Simmons, A., Stowe, J. "Measles, mumps, and rubella vaccination and bowel problems or developmental regression in children with autism: population study." *BMJ.* 2002 Feb 16; 324(7334):393-6.

68. Torrente, F., Anthony, A. "Focal-enhanced gastritis in regressive autism with features distinct from Crohn's disease and helicobacter Pylori gastritis." *Am J Gastroenterol.* 2004 Apr; 99(4):598-605.

69. Torrente, F. et al. "Small intestinal enteropathy with epithelial IgG and complement deposition in children with regressive autism." *Mol Psychiatry.* 2002; 7(4):375-82, 334.

70. Uhlmann, V. et al. "Potential viral pathogenic mechanism for new variant inflammatory bowel disease." *Mol Pathol.* 2002 Apr; 55(2):84-90.

71. Valicenti-McDermott, M. et al. "Frequency of gastrointestinal symptoms in children with autistic spectrum disorders and association with family history of autoimmune disease." *J Dev Behav Pediatr.* 2006 Apr; 27(2 Suppl):S128-36.

72. Valicenti-McDermott, M.D., McVicar, K., Cohen, H.J., Wershil, B.K., Shinnar, S. "Gastrointestinal symptoms in children with an autism spectrum disorder and language regression." *Pediatr Neurol.* 2008 Dec; 39(6):392-8.

73. Wakefield, A.J., Ashwood, P., Limb, K., Anthony, A. "The significance of ileo-colonic lymphoid nodular hyperplasia in children with autistic spectrum disorder." *Eur J Gastroenterol Hepatol.* 2005 Aug; 17(8):827-36.

74. Wakefield, A.J. et al. "Ileal-lymphoid-nodular hyperplasia, non-specific colitis, and pervasive developmental disorder in children." *Lancet.* 1998;28 351(9103):637-41.

75. Wakefield, A.J. "Enterocolitis, autism and measles virus." *Mol Psychiatry.* 2002; 7 Suppl 2:S44-6.

76. Wakefield, A.J. "The gut-brain axis in childhood developmental disorders." *J Pediatr Gastroenterol Nutr.* 2002 May-Jun; 34 Suppl 1:S14-7.

77. Wakefield, A.J. et al. "Review article: the concept of entero-colonic encephalopathy, autism and opioid receptor ligands." *Aliment Pharmacol Ther.* 2002; 16(4):663-74.

78. Wakefield, A.J. et al. "Enterocolitis in children with developmental disorders." *Am J Gastroenterol.* 2000 Sep; 95(9):2285-95.

79. Wakefield, A.J. et al. "Autism, viral infection and measles-mumps-rubella vaccination." *Isr Med Assoc J.* 1999 Nov; 1(3):183-7.

80. Wakefield, A.J. "MMR vaccination and autism." *Lancet.* 1999 Sep 11; 354(9182):949-50.

81. Welch, M.G., Welch-Horan, T.B., Anwar, M., Anwar, N., Ludwig, R.J., Ruggiero, D.A. "Brain effects of chronic IBD in areas abnormal in autism and treatment by single neuropeptides secretin and oxytocin." *J Mol Neurosci* 2005; 25(3):259-74.

82. White, J.F. "Intestinal pathophysiology in autism." *Exp Biol Med (Maywood).* 2003 Jun; 228(6):639-49.

83. Whiteley, P., Shattock, P. "Biochemical aspects in autism spectrum disorders: updating the opioid-excess theory and presenting new opportunities for biomedical intervention." *Expert Opin Ther Targets.* 2002 Apr; 6(2):175-83.

B. Autism and Biomedical Treatment

1. Goin-Kochel, R.P., Mackintosh, V.H., Myers, B.J. "Parental reports on the efficacy of treatments and therapies of their children with autism spectrum disorders." *Res Autism Spectr Disord*. 2009, doi:10.1016/j.rasd.2008.11.001.

2. O'Hara, N.H., Szakacs, G.M. "The recovery of a child with autism spectrum disorder through biomedical interventions." *Altern Ther Health Med*. 2008 Nov-Dec; 14(6):42-4.

C. Nutritional Deficiencies, Supplements, & Diet

1. Adams, J.B., Holloway, C. "Pilot study of a moderate dose multivitamin/mineral supplement for children with autistic spectrum disorder." *J Altern Complement Med*. 2004 Dec; 10(6):1033-9.

2. Adams, J.B., George, F., Audhya, T. "Abnormally high plasma levels of vitamin B6 in children with autism not taking supplements compared to controls not taking supplements." *J Altern Complement Med*. 2006 Jan-Feb; 12(1):59-63.

3. Aldred, S. et al. "Plasma amino acid levels in children with autism and their families." *J Autism Dev Disord*. 2003 Feb; 33(1):93-7.

4. Amminger, G.P., Berger, G.E., Schafer, M.R., Klier, C., Friedrich, M.H., Feucht, M. "Omega-3 Fatty Acids Supplementation in Children with Autism: A Double-blind Randomized, Placebo-controlled Pilot Study." *Biol Psychiatry*. 2006 Aug 22.

5. Andersen, I.M. et al. "Melatonin for Insomnia in Children With Autism Spectrum Disorders." *J Child Neurol*. 2008 Jan 8. 65. Arnold, G.L. et al. "Plasma amino acids profiles in children with autism: potential risk of nutritional deficiencies." *J Autism Dev Disord*. 2003 33(4):449-54.

6. Ashkenazi, A., Levin, S., Krasilowsky, D. "Gluten and autism." *Lancet*. 1980 Jan 19; 1(8160):157.

7. Baker, S.B., Worthley, L.I. "The essentials of calcium, magnesium and phosphate metabolism: part I. Physiology." *Crit Care Resusc*. 2002 Dec; 4(4):301-6.

8. Barthelemy, C. et al. "Biological and clinical effects of oral magnesium and associated magnesium-vitamin B6 administration on certain disorders observed in infantile autism." *Therapie*. 1980 Sep-Oct; 35(5):627-32.

9. Bolman, W.M., Richmond, J.A. "A double-blind, placebo-controlled, crossover pilot trial of low dose dimethylglycine in patients with autistic disorder." *J Autism Dev Disord*. 1999 Jun; 29(3):191-4.

10. Bruni, O. et al. "L -5-Hydroxytryptophan treatment of sleep terrors in children." *Eur J Pediatr*. 2004 Jul; 163(7):402-7.

11. Bubenik, G.A. et al. "Prospects of the clinical utilization of melatonin." *Biological Signals and Receptors*. 1998; 7:195-219.

12. Bu, B., Ashwood, P., Harvey, D., King, I.B., Water, J.V., Jin, L.W. "Fatty acid compositions of red blood cell phospholipids in children with autism." *Prostaglandins Leukot Essent Fatty Acids*. 2006 Apr; 74(4):215-21.

13. Carlton, R et al. "Rational dosages of nutrients have a prolonged effect on learning disabilities." *Alternative Therapies*. 2000; 6:85-91.

14. Christison, G.W., Ivany, K. "Elimination diets in autism spectrum disorders: any wheat amidst the chaff?" *J Dev Behav Pediatr*. 2006 Apr; 27(2 Suppl):S162-71.

15. Connors, S.L., Crowell, D.E. "Secretin and autism: the role of cysteine." *J Am Acad Child Adolesc Psychiatry*. 1999 Jul; 38(7):795-6.

16. Curtis, L.T., Patel, K. "Nutritional and environmental approaches to preventing and treating autism and attention deficit hyperactivity disorder (ADHD): a review." *J Altern Complement Med.* 2008 Jan-Feb; 14(1):79-85.

17. Dolske, M.C., Spollen, J., McKay, S., Lancashire, E., Tolbert, L. "A preliminary trial of ascorbic acid as supplemental therapy for autism." *Prog Neuropsychopharmacol Biol Psychiatry.* 1993 Sep; 17(5):765-74.

18. Elder, J.H. "The gluten-free, casein-free diet in autism: an overview with clinical implications." *Nutr Clin Pract.* 2008 Dec-2009 Jan; 23(6):583-8.

19. El Idrissi, A. et al. "Prevention of epileptic seizures by taurine." *Adv Exp Med Biol.* 2003; 526:515-25.

20. Erdeve, O. et al. "The probiotic effect of Saccharomyces boulardii in a pediatric age group." *J Trop Pediatr.* 2004 Aug; 50(4):234-6.

21. Fernstrom, J.D. "Can nutrient supplements modify brain function?" *Am J Clin Nutr.* 2000 Jun; 71(6 Suppl):1669S-75S.

22. Finegold, S.M. et al. "Gastrointestinal microflora studies in late-onset autism." *Clin Infect Dis.* 2002; 35 (Suppl 1):S6-S16.

23. Giannotti, F., Cortesi, F., Cerquiglini, A., Bernabei, P. "An open-label study of controlled-release melatonin in treatment of sleep disorders in children with autism." *J Autism Dev Disord.* 2006 Aug; 36(6):741-52.

24. Gill, H.S., Rutherfurd, K.J., Prasad, J., Gopal, P.K. "Enhancement of natural and acquired immunity by Lactobacillus rhamnosus (HN001), Lactobacillus acidophilus (HN017) and Bifidobacterium lactis (HN019)." *Br J Nutr.* 2000 Feb; 83(2):167-76.

25. Grattan-Smith, P.J., Wilcken, B., Procopis, P.G., Wise, G.A. "The neurological syndrome of infantile cobalamin deficiency: developmental regression and involuntary movements." *Mov Disord.* 1997 Jan; 12(1):39-46.

26. Herbert, V. "Detection of malabsorption of vitamin B12 due to gastric or intestinal dysfunction." *Semin Nucl Med.* 1972 Jul; 2(3):220.

27. Ishizaki, A., Sugama, M., Takeuchi, N. "Usefulness of melatonin for developmental sleep and emotional/behavior disorders—studies of melatonin trial on 50 patients with developmental disorders." *No To Hattatsu.* 1999 Sep; 31(5):428-37.

28. Jonas, C., Etienne, T., Barthelemy, C., Jouve, J., Mariotte, N. "Clinical and biochemical value of Magnesium + vitamin B6 combination in the treatment of residual autism in adults." *Therapie.* 1984 Nov-Dec; 39(6):661-9.

29. Jory, J., McGinnis, W.R. "Red-Cell Trace Minerals in Children with Autism." *Am J Biochem Biotechnol.* 2008; 4(2): 101-104.

30. Kern, J.K., Miller, V.S., Cauller, P.L., Kendall, P.R., Mehta, P.J., Dodd, M. "Effectiveness of N,N-dimethylglycine in autism and pervasive developmental disorder." *J Child Neurol.* 2001 Mar; 16(3):169-73.

31. Kleijnen, J., Knipschild, P. "Niacin and vitamin B6 in mental functioning: a review of controlled trials in humans." *Biol Psychiatry.* 1991 May 1; 29(9):931-41.

32. Knivsberg, A.M. et al. "A randomised, controlled study of dietary intervention in autistic syndromes." *Nutr Neurosci.* 2002 Sep; 5(4): 251-61.

33. Knivsberg, A.M. et al. "Reports on dietary intervention in autistic disorders." *Nutr Neurosci.* 2001; 4(1):25-37.

34. Kozielec, T., Starobrat-Hermelin, B. "Assessment of magnesium levels in children with attention deficit hyperactivity disorder (ADHD)." *Magnes Res.* 1997 Jun; 10(2):143-8.

35. Lelord, G., Muh, J.P., Barthelemy, C., Martineau, J., Garreau, B., Callaway, E. "Effects of pyridoxine and magnesium on autistic symptoms—initial observations." *J Autism Dev Disord.* 1981 Jun; 11(2):219-30.

36. Lelord, G., Callaway, E., Muh, J.P. "Clinical and biological effects of high doses of vitamin B6 and magnesium on autistic children." *Acta Vitaminol Enzymol.* 1982; 4(1-2):27-44.

37. Liebscher, D.H., Liebscher, D.E. "About the misdiagnosis of magnesium deficiency." *J Am Coll Nutr.* 2004 Dec; 23(6):730S-1S.

38. Martineau, J., Barthelemy, C., Garreau, B., Lelord, G. "Vitamin B6, magnesium, and combined B6-Mg: therapeutic effects in childhood autism." *Biol Psychiatry.* 1985 May; 20(5):467-78.

39. Megson, M.N. "Is autism a G-alpha protein defect reversible with natural vitamin A?" *Med Hypotheses.* 2000 Jun; 54(6):979-83.

40. Moretti, R. et al. "Vitamin B12 and folate depletion in cognition: a review." *Neurol India.* 2004 Sep; 52(3):310-8.

41. Mousain-Bosc, M., Roche, M., Polge, A., Pradal-Prat, D., Rapin, J., Bali, J.P. "Improvement of neurobehavioral disorders in children supplemented with magnesium-vitamin B6. II. Pervasive developmental disorder-autism." *Magnes Res.* 2006 Mar; 19(1):53-62.

42. Mousain-Bosc, M., Roche, M., Rapin, J., Bali, J.P. "Magnesium VitB6 intake reduces central nervous system hyperexcitability in children." *J Am Coll Nutr.* 2004 Oct; 23(5):545S-548S.

43. Murch, S.H., Walker-Smith, J.A. "Nutrition in inflammatory bowel disease." *Baillieres Clin Gastroenterol.* 1998 Dec; 12(4):719-38.

44. Olmez, A. et al. "Serum selenium levels in acute gastroenteritis of possible viral origin." *J Trop Pediatr.* 2004 Apr; 50(2):78-81.

45. Pfeiffer, C.C., Braverman, E.R. "Zinc, the brain and behavior." *Biol Psychiatry.* 1982 Apr; 17(4):513-32.

46. Richardson, A.J. "Omega-3 fatty acids in ADHD and related neurodevelopmental disorders." *Int RevPsychiatry.* 2006 Apr; 18(2):155-2.

47. Rimland, B. "High dosage levels of certain vitamins in the treatment of children with severe mental disorders." In D. Hawkins & L. Pauling (Eds.) *Orthomolecular Psychiatry.* 1973 (pp. 513-538).

48. Rimland, B. "Vitamin B6 (and magnesium) in the treatment of autism." *Autism Research Review International.* 1987, Vol. 1, No. 4.

49. Rimland, B., Callaway, E., Dreyfus, P. "The effect of high doses of vitamin B6 on autistic children: a double-blind crossover study." *Am J Psychiatry.* 1978 Apr; 135(4):472-5.

50. Saavedra, J.M. "Use of probiotics in pediatrics: rationale, mechanisms of action, and practical aspects." *Nutr Clin Pract.* 2007 Jun; 22(3):351-65.

51. Salminen, S.J., Gueimonde, M., Isolauri, E. "Probiotics that modify disease risk." *J Nutr.* 2005 May; 135(5):1294-8.

52. Servin, A.L. "Antagonistic activities of lactobacilli and bifidobacteria against microbial pathogens." *FEMS Microbiol Rev.* 2004 Oct; 28(4):405-40.

53. Shoenthaler, S. et al. "The effect of vitamin-mineral supplementation on the intelligence of American schoolchildren: a randomized, double-blind, placebo-controlled trial." *J Altern Complement Med.* 2000; 6:19-29.

54. Starobrat-Hermelin, B., Kozielec, T. "The effects of magnesium physiological supplementation on hyperactivity in children with attention deficit hyperactivity disorder (ADHD). Positive response to magnesium oral loading test." *Magnes Res.* 1997 Jun; 10(2):149-56.

55. Stevens, L.J. et al. "Essential fatty acid metabolism in boys with attention-deficit hyperactivity disorder." *Am J Clin Nutr.* 1995; 62(4): 761-8.

56. Toskes, P.P. et al. "Vitamin B 12 malabsorption in chronic pancreatic insufficiency." *N Engl J Med.* 1971 Mar 25; 284(12):627-32.

57. Vancassel, S. et al. "Plasma fatty acid levels in autistic children." *Prostaglandins Leukot Essent Fatty Acids.* 2001 Jul; 65(1):1-7.

58. Van Gelder, N.M., Sherwin, A.L., Sacks, C., Anderman, F. "Biochemical observations following administration of taurine to patients with epilepsy." *Brain Res.* 1975 Aug 29; 94(2):297-306.

59. Walsh, W.J. et al. "Reduced violent behavior following biochemical therapy." *Physiol Behav.* 2004 Oct 15; 82(5):835-9.

60. Whiteley, P. et al. "Spot urinary creatinine excretion in pervasive developmental disorders." *Pediatr Int.* 2006 Jun; 48(3):292-7.

61. Wright, C.E. et al. "Taurine: biological update." *Annu Rev Biochem.* 1986; 55: 427-53.

62. Yorbik, O., Akay, C. et al. "Zinc status in autistic children." *J Trace Elem Exp Med.* 2004; 17(2):101-107.

63. Young, G., Conquer, J. "Omega-3 fatty acids and neuropsychiatric disorders." *Reprod Nutr Dev.* 2005 Jan-Feb; 45(1):1-28.

D. Autism and Detoxification

1. Adams, J.B., Romdalvik, J., Ramanujam, V.M.S., Legator, M.S. "Mercury, Lead, and Zinc in Baby Teeth of Children with Autism vs. Controls." *J Toxicol Environ Health.* 2007; 70(12):1046-51.

2. Adams, J.B., Romdalvik, J., Levine, K.E., Hu, L.W. "Mercury in first-cut baby hair of children with autism versus typically developing children." *Toxic Environ Chem.* 2008; 1-14, iFirst.

3. Alberti, A., Pirrone, P., Elia, M., Waring, R.H., Romano, C. "Sulphation deficit in 'low-functioning' autistic children: a pilot study. *Biol Psychiatry.* 1999 Aug 1; 46(3):420-4.

4. Aposhian, H.V., Maiorino, R.M., Dart, R.C., Perry, D.F. "Urinary excretion of meso-2,3-dimercaptosuccinic acid in human subjects." *Clin Pharmacol Ther.* 1989 May; 45(5):520-6.

5. Aremu, D.A., Madejczyk, M.S., Ballatori, N. "N-acetylcysteine as a potential antidote and biomonitoring agent of methylmercury exposure." *Environ Health Perspect.* 2008 Jan; 116(1):26-31.

6. Aschner, M., Syversen, T., Souza, D.O., Rocha. J.B. "Metallothioneins: mercury species-specific induction and their potential role in attenuating neurotoxicity." *Exp Biol Med (Maywood).* 2006 Oct; 231(9):1468-73.

7. Aw, T.Y., Wierzbicka, G., Jones, D.P. "Oral glutathione increases tissue glutathione in vivo." *Chem Biol Interact.* 1991; 80(1):89-97.

8. Aw, T.Y. "Intestinal glutathione: determinant of mucosal peroxide transport, metabolism, and oxidative susceptibility." *Toxicol Appl Pharmacol.* 2005 May 1; 204(3):320-8.

9. Bello, S.C. "Autism and environmental influences: review and commentary." *Rev Environ Health.* 2007; 22(2): 139-56.

10. Beversdorf, D.Q., Manning, S.E. et al. "Timing of prenatal stressors and autism." *J Autism Dev Disord.* 2005; 35(4): 471-8.

11. Blanusa, M. et al. "Chelators as antidotes of metal toxicity: therapeutic and experimental aspects." *Curr Med Chem.* 2005; 12(23):2771.

12. Burbacher, T.M., Shen, D.D., Liberato, N., Grant, K.S., Cernichiari, E., Clarkson, T. "Comparison of blood and brain mercury levels in infant monkeys exposed to methylmercury or vaccines containing thimerosal." *Environ Health Perspect.* 2005 Aug; 113(8):1015-21.

13. Desoto, M.C., Hitlan, R.T. "Blood Levels of Mercury Are Related to Diagnosis of Autism: A Reanalysis of an Important Data Set." *J Child Neurol.* 2007 Nov; 22(11):1308-1311.

14. Dringen, R., Hirrlinger, J. "Glutathione pathways in the brain." *Biol Chem.* 2003 384(4):505-16.

15. Edelson, S.B., Cantor, D.S. "Autism: xenobiotic influences. *Toxicol Ind Health.* 1998 Jul-Aug; 14(4):553-63.

16. Fonnum, F., Lock, E.A. "The contributions of excitotoxicity, glutathione depletion and DNA repair in chemically induced injury to neurones: exemplified with toxic effects on cerebellar granule cells." *J Neurochem.* 2004 Feb; 88(3):513-31.

17. Forman, J. et al. "A cluster of pediatric metallic mercury exposure cases treated with meso-2,3-dimercaptosuccinic acid (DMSA)." *Environ Health Perspect.* 2000 Jun; 108(6):575-7.

18. Golse, B., Debray-Ritzen, P., Durosay, P., Puget, K., Michelson, A.M. "Alterations in two enzymes: superoxide dismutase and glutathione peroxidase in developmental infantile psychosis (infantile autism)." *Rev Neurol* (Paris). 1978 Nov; 134(11):699-705.

19. Goth, S.R., Chu, R.A., Gregg, J.P., Cherednichenko, G., Pessah, I.N. "Uncoupling of ATP-mediated calcium signaling and dysregulated interleukin-6 secretion in dendritic cells by nanomolar thimerosal." *Environ Health Perspect.* 2006; 114(7):1083-91.

20. Goyer, R.A., Cherian, M.G., Jones, M.M., Reigart, J.R. "Role of chelating agents for prevention, intervention, and treatment of exposures to toxic metals." *Environ Health Perspect.* 1995 Nov; 103(11):1048-52. Grandjean, P., Landrigan, P.J. "Developmental neurotoxicity of industrial chemicals." *Lancet.* 2006 Dec 16; 368(9553):2167-78.

21. Graziano, J.H., Lolacono, N.J., Moulton, T., Mitchell, M.E., Slavkovich, V., Zarate, C. "Controlled study of meso-2,3-dimercaptosuccinic acid for the management of childhood lead intoxication." *J Pediatr.* 1992 Jan; 120(1):133-9.

22. Havarinasab, S., Hultman, P. "Organic mercury compounds and autoimmunity." *Autoimmunity Rev.* 2005; 4:270-275.

23. Havarinasab, S., Haggqvist, B., Bjorn, E., Pollard, K.M., Hultman, P. "Immunosuppressive and autoimmune effects of thimerosal in mice." *Toxicol Appl Pharmacol.* 2005 Apr 15; 204(2):109-21.

24. Hayes, J.D. et al. "Glutathione S-transferase polymorphisms and their biological consequences." *Pharmacology.* 2000 Sep; 61(3):154.

25. Holmes, A.S. et al. "Reduced levels of mercury in first baby haircuts of autistic children." *Int J Toxicol.* 2003 Jul-Aug; 22(4):277-85. Hornig, M. et al. "Neurotoxic effects of postnatal thimerosal are mouse-strain dependent." *Mol Psychiatry.* 2004 Sep; 9(9):833-45.

26. Hunjan, M.K., Evered, D.F. "Absorption of glutathione from the gastro-intestinal tract." *Biochim Biophys Acta.* 1985 May 14; 815(2):184.

27. Hurlbut, K.M. et al. "Determination and metabolism of dithiol chelating agents. XVI: Pharmacokinetics of 2,3-dimercapto-1-propanesulfonate after intravenous administration to human volunteers." *J Pharmacol Exp Ther.* 1994 Feb; 268(2):662-8.

28. Ip, P., Wong, V., Ho, M., Lee, J., Wong, W. "Mercury exposure in children with autistic spectrum disorder: case-control study." *J Child Neurol.* 2004 Jun; 19(6):431-4.

29. Kern, J.K., Jones, A.M. "Evidence of toxicity, oxidative stress, and neuronal insult in autism." J Toxicol Environ Health B Crit *Rev.* 2006 Nov-Dec; 9(6):485-99.

30. Kern, J.K. et al. "Sulfhydryl-reactive metals in autism." *J Toxicol Environ Health A.* 2007 Apr 15; 70(8):715-21. Kinney, D.K., Miller, A.M. et al. "Autism prevalence following prenatal exposure to hurricanes and tropical storms in Louisiana." *J Autism Dev Disord.* 2008; 38(3):481-8.

31. Lafleur, D.L. et al. "N-acetylcysteine augmentation in serotonin reuptake inhibitor refractory obsessive-compulsive disorder." *Psycho-pharmacology* (Berl). 2006 Jan; 184(2):254-6.

32. Lanphear, B.P. et al. "Low-level environmental lead exposure and children's intellectual function: an international pooled analysis." *Environ Health Perspect.* 2005 Jul; 113(7):894-9.

33. Lauterburg, B.H., Mitchell, J.R. "Therapeutic doses of acetaminophen stimulate the turnover of cysteine and glutathione in man." *J Hepatol.* 1987 Apr; 4(2):206-11.

34. Lonsdale, D., Shamberger, R.J., Audhya, T. "Treatment of autism spectrum children with thiamine tetrahydrofurfuryl disulfide: a pilot study." *Neuroendocrinol Lett.* 2002 Aug; 23(4):303-8.

35. Makani, S., Gollapudi, S., Yel, L., Chiplunkar, S., Gupta, S. "Biochemical and molecular basis of thimerosal-induced apoptosis in T cells: a major role of mitochondrial pathway." *Genes Immun.* 2002 Aug; 3(5):270-8.

36. Mayer, M., Noble, M. "N-acetyl-L-cysteine is a pluripotent protector against cell death and enhancer of trophic factor-mediated cell survival in vitro." *Proc Natl Acad Sci U S A.* 1994 Aug 2; 91(16):7496-500.

37. Miller, A.L. "Dimercaptosuccinic acid (DMSA), a non-toxic, water-soluble treatment for heavy metal toxicity." *Altern Med Rev.* 1998 Jun; 3(3):199-207.

38. Mutter, J., Naumann, J. et al. "Mercury and autism: accelerating evidence?" *Neuro Endocrinol Lett.* 2005; 26(5): 439-46.

39. "N-acetylcysteine." [No authors listed]. *Altern Med Rev.* 2000 Oct; 5(5):467-71.

40. Nataf, R., Skorupka, C., Amet, L., Lam, A., Springbett, A., Lathe, R. "Porphyrinuria in childhood autistic disorder: implications for environ-mental toxicity." *Toxicol Appl Pharmacol.* 2006 Jul 15; 214(2):99-108.

41. Oka, S., Kamata, H., Kamata, K., Yagisawa, H., Hirata, H. "N-acetylcysteine suppresses TNF-induced NF-kappaB activation through inhibition of IkappaB kinases." *FEBS Lett.* 2000 Apr 28; 472(2-3):196-202.

42. Palmer, R.F., Blanchard, S., Stein, Z., Mandell, D., Miller, C. "Environmental mercury release, special education rates, and autism disorder: an ecological study of Texas." *Health Place.* 2006 Jun; 12(2):203-9.

43. Palmer, R.F., Blanchard, S., Wood, R. "Proximity to point sources of environmental mercury release as a predictor of autism prevalence." *Health Place*. 2008 Feb 12.

44. Pasca, S.P., Nemes, B., Vlase, L., Gagyi, C.E., Dronca, E., Miu, A.C., Dronca, M. "High levels of homocysteine and low serum paraoxonase 1 arylesterase activity in children with autism." *Life Sci*. 2006 Apr 4; 78(19):2244-8. Pastore, A. et al. "Analysis of glutathione: implication in redox and detoxification." *Clin Chim Acta*. 2003 Jul 1; 333(1):19-39.

45. Planas-Bohne, F. "The effect of 2,3-dimercaptorpropane-1-sulfonate and dimercaptosuccinic acid on the distribution and excretion of mercuric chloride in rats." *Toxicology*. 1981; 19(3):275-8.

46. Rea, W.J., Didriksen, N., Simon, T.R., Pan, Y., Fenyves, E.J., Griffiths, B. "Effects of toxic exposure to molds and mycotoxins in building-related illnesses." *Arch Environ Health*. 2003 Jul; 58(7):399-405.

47. Rose, S., Melnyk, S. et al. "The frequency of polymorphisms affecting lead and mercury toxicity among children with autism." *Am J Biochem Biotechnol*. 2008; 4(2):85-94.

48. Shannon, M., Graef, J.W. "Lead intoxication in children with pervasive developmental disorders." *J Toxicol Clin Toxicol*. 1996; 34(2):177-81.

49. Sheehan, D. et al. "Structure, function and evolution of glutathione transferases: implications for classification of non-mammalian members of an ancient enzyme superfamily." *Biochem J*. 2001 Nov 15; 360(Pt 1):1-16.

50. Stangle, D.E. et al. "Succimer chelation improves learning, attention and arousal regulation in lead-exposed rats but produces lasting cognitive impairment in the absence of lead exposure." *Environ Health Perspect*. 30 October 2006.

51. Testa, B. et al. "Management of chronic otitis media with effusion: the role of glutathione." *Laryngoscope*. 2001 Aug; 111(8):1486-9.

52. Waly, M. et al. "Activation of methionine synthase by insulin-like growth factor-1 and dopamine: a target for neurodevelopmental toxins and thimerosal." *Mol Psychiatry*. 2004 Apr; 9(4):358-7.

53. Waring, R.H., Klovrza, L.V. "Sulphur metabolism in autism." *J Nutr Env Med*. 2000; 10:25-32.

54. Waring, R.H. et al. "Biochemical parameters in autistic children." *Dev Brain Dysfunction*. 1997; 10:40-43.

55. Westphal, G.A. et al. "Homozygous gene deletions of the glutathione S-transferases M1 and T1 are associated with thimerosal sensitization." *Int Arch Occup Environ Health*. 2000; 73(6):384-8.

56. Windham, G., Zhang, L., Gunier, R., Croen, L., Grether, J. "Autism Spectrum Disorders in Relation to Distribution of Hazardous Air Pollutants in the San Francisco Bay Area." *Environ Health Perspect*. 2006 Sep; 114(9):1438-44.

57. Woods, J.S. "Altered porphyrin metabolism as a biomarker of mercury exposure and toxicity." *Can J Physiol Pharmacol*. 1996; 74(2):210-5.

58. Woods, J.S. et al. "Studies on porphyrin metabolism in the kidney. Effects of trace metals and glutathione on renal uroporphyrinogen decarboxylase." *Mol Pharmacol*. 1984; 26(2):336-41.

59. Woods, J.S. et al. "Urinary porphyrin profiles as a biomarker of mercury exposure: studies on dentists with occupational exposure to mercury vapor." *J Toxicol Environ Health*. 1993; 40(2-3):235-46.

60. Woods, J.S. et al. "Quantitative measurement of porphyrins in biological tissues and evaluation of tissue porphyrins during toxicant exposures." *Fundam Appl Toxicol*. 1993. 21(3):291-7.

61. Zoroglu, S.S. et al. "Pathophysiological role of nitric oxide and adrenomedullin in autism." *Cell Biochem Funct.* 2003 Mar; 21(1):55-60.

E. Autism and the Brain

1. Ahlsen, G., Rosengren, L., Belfrage, M., Palm, A., Haglid, K., Hamberger, A., Gillberg, C. "Glial fibrillary acidic protein in the cerebrospinal fluid of children with autism and other neuropsychiatric disorders." *Biol Psychiatry.* 1993 May 15; 33(10):734-43.

2. Anderson, M.P., Hooker, B.S., Herbert, M.R. "Bridging from Cells to Cognition in Autism Pathophysiology: Biological Pathways to Defective Brain Function and Plasticity." *Am J Biochem Biotechnol.* 2008; 4(2): 167-176.

3. Bauman, M.L., Kemper, T.L. "Neuroanatomic observations of the brain in autism: a review and future directions." *Int J Dev Neurosci.* 2005; 23:183-7.

4. Connor, D.F., Fletcher, K.E., Swanson, J.M. "A meta-analysis of clonidine for symptoms of attention-deficit hyperactivity disorder." *J Am Acad Child Adolesc Psychiatry.* 1999 Dec; 38(12):1551-9.

5. Corbett, B.A., Mendoza, S. et al. "Cortisol circadian rhythms and response to stress in children with autism." *Psychoneuroendocrinology.* 2006; 31(1):59-68.

6. Dennog, C., Gedik, C., Wood, S., Speit, G. "Analysis of oxidative DNA damage and HPRT mutations in humans after hyperbaric oxygen treatment." *Mutat Res.* 1999 Dec 17; 431(2):351-9.

7. Dufour, F. et al. "Modulation of absence seizures by branched-chain amino acids: correlation with brain amino acid concentrations." *Neurosci Res.* 2001 Jul; 40(3):255-63.

8. Erickson, C.A., Posey, D.J., Stigler, K.A., Mullett, J., Katschke, A.R., McDougle, C.J. "A retrospective study of memantine in children and adolescents with pervasive developmental disorders." *Psychopharmacology* (Berl). 2006 Oct 3.

9. Filipek, P.A. et al. (2000). "Practice parameter: screening and diagnosis of autism: report of the Quality Standards Subcommittee of the American Academy of Neurology and the Child Neurology Society." *Neurology.* 55(4):468-79.

10. Friedman, S.D., Shaw, D.W., Artru, A.A., Richards, T.L., Gardner, J., Dawson, G., Posse, S., Dager, S.R. "Regional brain chemical alterations in young children with autism spectrum disorder." *Neurology.* 2003 Jan 14; 60(1):100-7.

11. Garbett, K., Ebert, P.J., Mitchell, A., Lintas, C., Manzi, B., Mirnics, K., Persico, A.M. "Immune transcriptome alterations in the temporal cortex of subjects with autism." *Neurobiol Dis.* 2008 Jun; 30(3):303-11.

12. Helms, A.K., Whelan, H.T., Torbey, M.T. "Hyperbaric oxygen therapy of cerebral ischemia." *Cerebrovasc Dis.* 2005; 20(6):417-26.

13. Helt, M. et al. "Can children with autism recover? If so, how?" *Neuropsychol Rev.* 2008 Dec; 18(4):339-66. Herbert, M. "Autism: A Brain disorder, or disorder that affects the brain?" *Clinical Neuropsychiatry.* 2006; 2:354-79.

14. Herbert, M.R. "Large brains in autism: the challenge of pervasive abnormality." *Neuroscientist.* 2005. 11(5): 417-40.

15. Hollander, E. et al. "Oxytocin Increases Retention of Social Cognition in Autism." *Biol Psychiatry.* 2006 Aug 10.

16. Hrdlicka, M. et al. "Not EEG abnormalities but epilepsy is associated with autistic regression and mental functioning in childhood autism." *Eur Child Adolesc Psychiatry.* 2004; 13(4):209-13.

17. Joiner, J.T. (Ed.). *The Proceedings of the 2nd International Symposium on Hyperbaric Oxygenation for Cerebral Palsy and the Brain-Injured Child*. Flagstaff, AZ: Best Publishing Company. (2002). King, B.H., Bostic, J.Q. "An update on pharmacologic treatments for autism spectrum disorders." *Child Adolesc Psychiatr Clin N Am*. 2006 Jan; 15(1):161-75.

18. López-Hurtado, E., Prieto, J.J. "A microscopic study of language-related cortex in autism. *Am J Biochem Biotechnol*. 2008; 4(2): 130. Lewine, J.D. et al. "Magnetoencephalographic patterns of epileptiform activity in children with regressive autism spectrum disorders." *Pediatrics*. 1999 Sep; 104(3 Pt 1):405-18.

19. MacFabe, D.F. et al. "Neurobiological effects of intraventricular propionic acid in rats: possible role of short chain fatty acids on the pathogenesis and characteristics of autism spectrum disorders." *Behav Brain Res*. 2007 Jan 10; 176(1):149-69.

20. McCracken, J.T. et al. "Risperidone in children with autism and serious behavioral problems." *N Engl J Med*. 2002; 347(5):314-21.

21. Mehler, M.F., Purpura, D.P. "Autism, fever, epigenetics and the locus coeruleus." *Brain Res Rev*. 2008 Nov 24. Ohnishi, T. et al. "Abnormal regional cerebral blood flow in childhood autism." *Brain*. 2000 Sep; 123 (Pt 9):1838-44.

22. Pardo, C.A., Eberhart, C.G. "The neurobiology of autism." *Brain Pathol*. 2007; 17(4):434-47.

23. Park, Y.D. "The effects of vagus nerve stimulation therapy on patients with intractable seizures and either Landau-Kleffner syndrome or autism." *Epilepsy Behav*. 2003 Jun; 4(3):286-90.

24. Plioplys, A.V., Greaves, A., Yoshida, W. "Anti-CNS antibodies in childhood neurologic diseases." *Neuropediatrics*. 1989; 20:93. Plioplys, A.V. "Autism: electroencephalogram abnormalities and clinical improvement with valproic acid." *Arch Pediatr Adolesc Med*. 1994 Feb; 148(2):220-2.

25. Posey, D.J., Puntney, J.I., Sasher, T.M., Kem, D.L., McDougle, C.J. "Guanfacine treatment of hyperactivity and inattention in pervasive developmental disorders: a retrospective analysis of 80 cases." *J Child Adolesc Psychopharmacol*. 2004 Summer; 14(2):233-41.

26. Ramaekers, V.T., Blau, N., Sequeira, J.M., Nassogne, M.C., Quadros, E.V. "Folate receptor autoimmunity and cerebral folate deficiency in low-functioning autism with neurological deficits." *Neuropediatrics*. 2007 Dec; 38(6):276-81.

27. Rockswold, G.L., Ford, S.E., Anderson, D.C., Bergman, T.A., Sherman, R.E. "Results of a prospective randomized trial for treatment of severely brain-injured patients with hyperbaric oxygen." *J Neurosurg*. 1992 Jun; 76(6):929-34.

28. Rossignol, D.A., Rossignol, L.W. "Hyperbaric oxygen therapy may improve symptoms in autistic children." *Med Hypotheses*. 2006; 67(2):216-28.

29. Ryu, Y.H. et al. "Perfusion impairments in infantile autism on technetium-99m ethyl cysteinate dimer brain single-photon emission tomography: comparison with findings on magnetic resonance imaging." *Eur J Nucl Med*. 1999 Mar; 26(3):253-9.

30. Sakoda, M., Ueno, S., Kihara, K., Arikawa, K., Dogomori, H., Nuruki, K., Takao, S., Aikou, T. "A potential role of hyperbaric oxygen exposure through intestinal nuclear factor-kappaB." *Crit Care Med*. 2004 Aug; 32(8):1722-9.

31. Shattock, P., Kennedy, A., Rowell, F., Berney, T. "Role of neuropeptides in autism and their relationship with classical neurotransmitters." *Brain Dysfunction*. 1990; 3:328-345.

32. Shultz, S.R., MacFabe, D.F. et al. "Intracerebroventricular injection of propionic acid, an enteric bacterial metabolic end-product, impairs social behavior in the rat: Implications for an animal model of autism." *Neuropharmacology.* 2008 May; 54(6):901-11.

33. Tharp, B.R. "Epileptic encephalopathies and their relationship to developmental disorders: Do spikes cause autism?" *Ment Retard Dev Disabil Res Rev.* 2004; 10(2):132-4.

34. Toda, Y., Mori, K., Hashimoto, T., Miyazaki, M., Nozaki, S., Watanabe, Y., Kuroda, Y., Kagami, S. "Administration of secretin for autism alters dopamine metabolism in the central nervous system." *Brain Dev.* 2006 Mar; 28(2):99-103.

35. Vargas, D.L., Nascimbene, C., Krishnan, C., Zimmerman, A.W., Pardo, C.A. "Neuroglial activation and neuroinflammation in the brain of patients with autism." *Ann Neurol.* 2005 Jan; 57(1)67-81.

36. Wang, X.F., Cynader, M.S. "Astrocytes provide cysteine to neurons by releasing glutathione." *J Neurochem.* 2000; 74(4):1434-42.

37. Welch, M.G., Ludwig, R.J., Opler, M., Ruggiero, D.A. "Secretin's role in the cerebellum: a larger biological context and implications for developmental disorders." *Cerebellum.* 2006; 5(1):2-6.

38. Yang, Z., Nandi, J., Wang, J., Bosco, G., Gregory, M., Chung, C., Xie, Y., Yang, X., Camporesi, E.M. "Hyperbaric oxygenation ameliorates indomethacin-induced enteropathy in rats by modulating TNF-alpha and IL-1beta production." *Dig Dis Sci.* 2006 Aug; 51(8):1426.

F. Viruses and Bacteria in Autism

1. Bradstreet, J.J., El Dahr, J.M., Anthony, A., Kartzinel, J.J., Wakefield, A.J. "Detection of measles virus genomic RNA in cerebrospinal fluid of children with regressive autism: a report of three cases." *J Am Phys Surg.* 2004; 9(2):38-45.

2. Caruso, J.M. et al. "Persistent preceding focal neurologic deficits in children with chronic Epstein-Barr virus encephalitis." *J Child Neurol.* 2000 Dec; 15(12):791-6.

3. Chess, S., Fernandez, P., Korn, S. "Behavioral consequences of congenital rubella." *J Pediatr.* 1978 Oct; 93(4):699-703.

4. DeLong, G.R. et al. "Acquired reversible autistic syndrome in acute encephalopathic illness in children." *Arch Neurol.* 1981 Mar; 38(3):191-4.

5. Dyken, P.R. "Neuroprogressive disease of post-infectious origin: a review of a resurging subacute sclerosing panencephalitis (SSPE)." *Ment Retard Dev Disabil Res Rev.* 2001; 7(3):217-25.

6. Ghaziuddin, M. et al. "Autistic symptoms following herpes encephalitis." *Eur Child Adolesc Psychiatry.* 2002 Jun; 11(3):142-6.

7. Gillberg, I.C. "Autistic syndrome with onset at age 31 years: herpes encephalitis as a possible model for childhood autism." *Dev Med Child Neurol.* 1991 Oct; 33(10):920-4.

8. Gillberg, C. "Onset at age 14 of a typical autistic syndrome. A case report of a girl with herpes simplex encephalitis." *J Autism Dev Disord.* 1986 Sep; 16(3):369-75.

9. Hornig, M., Weissenbock, H., Horscroft, N., Lipkin, W.I. "An infection-based model of neurodevelopmental damage." *Proc Natl Acad Sci USA.* 1999 Oct 12; 96(21):12102-7.

10. Hornig, M., Lipkin, W.I. "Infectious and immune factors in the pathogenesis of neurodevelopmental disorders: Epidemiology, hypotheses, and animal models." *Ment Retard Dev Disabil Res Rev.* 2001; 7(3):200-10.

11. Ivarsson, S.A. et al. "Autism as one of several disabilities in two children with congenital cytomegalovirus infection." *Neuropediatrics.* 1990 May; 21(2):102-3.

12. Libbey, J.E., Sweeten, T.L., McMahon, W.M., Fujinami, R.S. "Autistic disorder and viral infections." *J Neurovirol.* 2005 Feb; 11(1):1-10.

13. Nicolson, G.L., Gan, R., Nicolson, N.L., Haier, J. "Evidence for Mycoplasma ssp., Chlamydia pneunomiae, and human herpes virus-6 coinfections in the blood of patients with autistic spectrum disorders." *J Neurosci Res.* 2007 Apr; 85(5):1143-8.

14. O'Leary, J.J. et al. "Measles virus and autism." *Lancet.* 2000 Aug 26; 356(9231):772.

15. Pletnikov, M.V., Jones, M.L., Rubin, S.A., Moran, T.H., Carbone, K.M. "Rat model of autism spectrum disorders. Genetic background effects on Borna disease virus-induced developmental brain damage." *Ann N Y Acad Sci.* 2001 Jun; 939:318-9.

16. Singh, V.K., Jensen, R.L. "Elevated levels of measles antibodies in children with autism." *Pediatr Neurol.* 2003 Apr; 28(4):292-4.

17. Singh, V.K. et al. "Abnormal measles-mumps-rubella antibodies and CNS autoimmunity in children with autism." *J Biomed Sci.* 2002 Jul-Aug; 9(4):359-64.

18. Singh, V.K. et al. "Serological association of measles virus and human herpesvirus-6 with brain autoantibodies in autism." *Clin Immunol Immunopathol.* 1998; 89(1):105-8.

19. Stubbs, E.G., Budden, S.S., Burger, D.R., Vandenbark, A.A. "Transfer factor immunotherapy of an autistic child with congenital cytomega-lovirus." *J Autism Dev Disord.* 1980 Dec; 10(4):451-8.

20. Stubbs, E.G. et al. "Autism and congenital cytomegalovirus." *J Autism Dev Disord.* 1984 Jun; 14(2):183-9.

21. Sweeten, T.L., Posey, D.J., McDougle, C.J. "Brief report: autistic disorder in three children with cytomegalovirus infection." *J Autism Dev Disord.* 2004 Oct; 34(5):583-6.

22. Valsamakis, A. et al. "Altered virulence of vaccine strains of measles virus after prolonged replication in human tissue." *J Virol.* 1999; 73(10):8791-7.

G. Immune System Dysfunction and Treatment

1. Ashwood, P., Kwong, C., Hansen, R., Hertz-Picciotto, I., Croen, L., Krakowiak, P., Walker, W., Pessah, I.N., Van de Water, J. "Brief report: plasma leptin levels are elevated in autism: association with early onset phenotype?" *J Autism Dev Disord.* 2008 Jan; 38(1):169-75.

2. Ashwood, P. et al. "Spontaneous mucosal lymphocyte cytokine profiles in children with autism and gastrointestinal symptoms: mucosal immune activation and reduced counter regulatory interleukin-10." *J Clin Immunol.* 2004 Nov; 24(6):664-73.

3. Ashwood, P., Van de Water, J. "Is autism an autoimmune disease?" *Autoimmun Rev.* 2004 Nov; 3(7-8):557-62.

4. Ashwood, P. et al. "The immune response in autism: a new frontier for autism research." *J Leuk Biol.* 2006 Jul; 80:1-15.

5. Bayary, J. et al. "Intravenous immunoglobulin in autoimmune disorders: an insight into the immunoregulatory mechanisms." *Int Immunopharmacol.* 2006 Apr; 6(4):528-34.

6. Boris, M. et al. "Improvement in children treated with intravenous gamma globulin." *J Nutr Environmental Med.* Dec 2006; 15(4):1-8.

7. Boris, M. et al. "Effect of Pioglitazone treatment on behavioral symptoms in autistic children." *J Neuroinflammation.* 2007 Jan 5; 4:3.

8. Bradstreet, J.J., Smith, S., Granpeesheh, D., El-Dahr, J.M., Rossignol, D. "Spironolactone Might be a Desirable Immunologic and Hormonal Intervention in Autism Spectrum Disorders." *Med Hypotheses.* 2006 Dec 4.

9. Brandtzaeg, P. "Current Understanding of Gastrointestinal Immuno-regulation and Its Relation to Food Allergy." *Ann NY Acad Sci.* 2002; 964:14-45.

10. Braunschweig, D. et al. "Autism: Maternally derived antibodies specific for fetal brain proteins." *Neurotoxicology.* 2007 Nov 6.

11. Bray, T.M., Taylor, C.G. "Enhancement of tissue glutathione for antioxidant and immune functions in malnutrition." *Biochem Pharmacol.* 1994 Jun 15; 47(12):2113-23.

12. Cabanlit, M., Wills, S., Goines, P., Ashwood, P., Van de Water, J. "Brain-specific autoantibodies in the plasma of subjects with autistic spectrum disorder." *Ann N Y Acad Sci.* 2007 Jun; 1107:92-103.

13. Cave, S.F. "The history of vaccinations in the light of the autism epidemic." *Altern Ther Health Med.* 2008 Nov-Dec; 14(6):54-7.

14. Chinetti, G., Fruchart, J.C., Staels, B. "Peroxisome proliferators-activated receptors (PPAR): nuclear receptors at the crossroads between lipid metabolism and inflammation." *Inflamm Res.* 2000; 49:497-505.

15. Cohly, H.H., Panja, A. "Immunological findings in autism." *Int Rev Neurobiol.* 2005; 71:317-41.

16. Chmelik, E., Awadallah, N. et al. "Varied presentation of PANDAS: a case series." *Clin Pediatr (Phila).* 2004; 43(4): 379-82.

17. Connolly, A.M., Chez, M.G., Pestronk, A., Arnold, S.T., Mehta, S., Deuel, R.K. "Serum autoantibodies to brain in Landau-Kleffner variant, autism, and other neurologic disorders." *J Pediatr.* 1999 May; 134(5):607-13.

18. Croen, L.A., Grether, J.K., Yoshida, C.K., Odouli, R., Van de Water, J. "Maternal autoimmune diseases, asthma and allergies, and childhood autism spectrum disorders: a case-control study." *Arch Pediatr Adolesc Med.* 2005 Feb; 159(2):151-7.

19. Croonenberghs, J., Wauters, A., Devreese, K., Verkerk, R., Scharpe, S., Bosmans, E., Egyed, B., Deboutte, D., Maes, M. "Increased serum albumin, gamma globulin, immunoglobulin IgG, and IgG2 and IgG4 in autism." *Psychol Med.* 2002 Nov; 32(8):1457-63.

20. Croonenberghs, J. et al. "Activation of the inflammatory response system in autism." *Neuropsychobiology.* 2002; 45(1):1-6.

21. Cross, M.L. "Immune-signalling by orally-delivered probiotic bacteria: effects on common mucosal immuno-responses and protection at distal mucosal sites." *Int J Immunopathol Pharmacol.* 2004 May-Aug; 17(2):127-34.

22. Dalton, P. et al. "Maternal neuronal antibodies associated with autism and a language disorder." *Ann Neurol.* 2003 Apr; 53(4):533-7. DelGiudice-Asch, G., Simon, L., Schmeidler, J., Cunningham-Rundles, C., Hollander, E. "Brief report: A pilot open clinical trial of intravenous immunoglobulin in childhood autism." *J Autism Dev Disord.* 1999; 29(2):157-60.

23. Denney, D.R. et al. "Lymphocyte subsets and interleukin-2 receptors in autistic children." *J Autism Dev Disord.* 1996 Feb; 26(1):87-97.

24. Dietert, R.R., Dietert, J.M. "Potential for early-life immune insult including developmental immunotoxicity in autism and autism spectrum disorders: focus on critical windows of immune vulnerability." *J Toxicol Environ Health B Crit Rev.* 2008 Oct; 11(8):660-80.

25. Drakes, M., Blanchard, T., Czinn, S. "Bacterial probiotic modulation of dendritic cells." *Infect Immun.* 2004 Jun; 72(6):3299-309.

26. Droge, W., Breitkreutz, R. "Glutathione and immune function." *Proc Nutr Soc.* 2000 Nov; 59(4):595-600. El-chaar, G.M., Maisch, N.M., Augusto, L.M., Wehring, H.J. "Efficacy and safety of naltrexone use in pediatric patients with autistic disorder." *Ann Pharmacother.* 2006 Jun; 40(6):1086-95.

27. Engstrom, H.A., Ohlson, S., Stubbs, E.G., Maciulis, A., Caldwell, V., Odell, J.D., Torres, A.R. "Decreased Expression of CD95 (FAS/APO-1) on CD4+ T-lymphocytes from Participants with Autism." *J Dev Phys Disabil.* 2003 Jun 15; 2:155-163(9).

28. Ferrante, P., Saresella, M., Guerini, F.R., Marzorati, M., Musetti, M.C., Cazzullo, A.G. "Significant association of HLA A2-DR11 with CD4 naive decrease in autistic children." *Biomed Pharmacother.* 2003 Oct; 57(8):372-4.

29. Feinstein, D.L. "Therapeutic potential of peroxisome proliferator-activated receptor agonists for neurological disease." *Diabetes Technol Ther.* 2003; 5(1):67-73.

30. Fudenberg, H.H. "Dialysable lymphocyte extract (DLyE) in infantile onset autism: a pilot study." *Biotherapy.* 1996; 9(1-3):143-7.

31. Furlano, R.I. et al. "Autism and the immune system." *J Child Psychol Psychiatry.* 1997 Mar; 38(3):337-49. Griem, P. et al. "Allergic and autoimmune reactions to xenobiotics: how do they arise?" *Immunology Today.* 1998; 19:133-141.

32. Gao, H.M., Hong, J.S. "Why neurodegenerative diseases are progressive: uncontrolled inflammation drives disease progression." *Trends Immunol.* 2008 Aug; 29(8):357-65.

33. Geier, D.A., Geier, M.R. "A Clinical and Laboratory Evaluation of Methionine Cycle-Transsulfuration and Androgen Pathway Markers in Children with Autistic Disorders." *Horm Res.* 2006 Jul 5; 66(4):182-188.

34. Geier, D.A., Mumper, E., Gladfelter, B., Coleman, L., Geier, M.R. "Neurodevelopmental disorders, maternal Rh-negativity, and Rho(D) immune globulins: a multi-center assessment." *Neuro Endocrinol Lett.* 2008 Apr; 29(2):272-80.

35. Griem, P. et al. "Allergic and autoimmune reactions to xenobiotics: how do they arise?" *Immunology Today.* 1998; 19:133-141.

36. Gupta, S. "Immunological treatments for autism." *J Autism Dev Disord.* 2000 Oct; 30(5):475-9.

37. Gupta, S., Aggarwal, S., Heads, C. "Dysregulated immune system in children with autism: beneficial effects of intravenous immune globulin on autistic characteristics." *J Autism Dev Disord.* 1996 Aug; 26(4):439-52.

38. Gupta, S. et al. "Th1- and Th2-like cytokines in CD4+ and CD8+ T cells in autism." *J Neuroimmunol.* 1998 May 1; 85(1):106-9.

39. Hamilton, R.G. et al. "In vitro assays for the diagnosis of IgE-mediated disorders." *J Allergy Clin Immunol.* 114(2):213-25.

40. Hertz-Picciotto, I., Park, H.Y., Dostal, M., Kocan, A., Trnovec, T., Sram, R. "Prenatal exposures to persistent and non-persistent organic compounds and effects on immune system development." *Basic Clin Pharmacol Toxicol.* 2008 Feb; 102(2):146-54.

41. Jyonouchi, H. et al. "Evaluation of an association between gastrointestinal symptoms and cytokine production against common dietary proteins in children with autism spectrum disorders." *J Pediatr.* 2005 May; 146(5): 605-10.

42. Jyonouchi, H., Geng, L., Cushing-Ruby, A., Quraishi, H. "Impact of innate immunity in a subset of children with autism spectrum disorders: a case control study." *J Neuroinflammation.* 2008 Nov 21; 5(1):52.

43. Jyonouchi, H., Sun, S., Le, H. "Proinflammatory and regulatory cytokine production associated with innate and adaptive immune re-sponses in children with autism spectrum disorders and developmental regression." *J Neuro-immunol.* 2001 Nov 1; 120(1-2):170-9.

44. Jyonouchi, H., Sun, S., Itokazu, N. "Innate immunity associated with inflammatory responses and cytokine pro-duction against common dietary proteins in patients with autism spectrum disorder." *Neuropsychobiology.* 2002; 46(2):76-84.

45. Jyonouchi, H., Geng, L., Ruby, A., Zimmerman-Bier, B. "Dysregulated innate immune responses in young chil-dren with autism spectrum disorders: their relationship to gastrointestinal symptoms and dietary intervention." *Neuropsychobiology.* 2005; 51(2):77-85.

46. Kelly, G.S. "Bovine colostrums: a review of clinical uses." *Altern Med Rev.* 2003 Nov; 8(4):378-94.

47. Kidd, P.M. "Autism, an extreme challenge to integrative medicine. Part 2: medical management." *Altern Med Rev.* 2002 Dec; 7(6):472-99.

48. Kirjavainen, P.V. et al. "New aspects of probiotics--a novel approach in the management of food allergy." *Allergy.* 1999 Sep; 54(9):909.

49. Knickmeyer, R., Baron-Cohen, S., Raggatt, P., Taylor, K. "Foetal testosterone, social relationships, and restricted interests in children." *J Child Psychol Psychiatry.* 2005 Feb; 46(2):198-210.

50. Konstantareas, M.M., Homatidis, S. "Ear infections in autistic and normal children." *J Autism Dev Disord.* 1987 Dec; 17(4):585-94.

51. Koski, C.L., Patterson, J.V. "Intravenous immunoglobulin use for neurologic diseases." *J Infus Nurs.* 2006 May-Jun; 29(3 Suppl):S21-8.

52. Krause, I. et al. "Brief report: immune factors in autism: a critical review." *J Autism Dev Disord.* 2002 Aug; 32(4):337-45.

53. Li, X. et al. "Elevated immune response in the brain of autistic patients." *J Neuroimmunol.* 2009 Jan 19.

54. Lipkin, W.I., Hornig, M. "Microbiology and immunology of autism spectrum disorders." *Novartis Found Symp.* 2003; 251:129-43; discussion 144-8, 281-97.

55. Lucarelli, S. et al. "Food allergy and infantile autism." *Panminerva Med.* 1995 Sep; 37(3):137-41.

56. March, J.S. "Pediatric Autoimmune Neuropsychiatric Disorders Associated With Streptococcal Infection (PAN-DAS): implications for clinical practice." *Arch Pediatr Adolesc Med* 2004; 158(9):927-9.

57. Martin, L.A., Ashwood, P., Braunschweig, D., Cabanlit, M., Van de Water, J., Amaral, D.G. "Stereotypies and hyper-activity in rhesus monkeys exposed to IgG from mothers of children with autism." *Brain Behav Immun.* 2008 Feb 7.

58. Messahel, S. et al. "Urinary levels of neopterin and biopterin in autism." *Neurosci Lett*. 1998; 241(1):17-20.

59. McDonald, K.L., Huq, S.I., Lix, L.M., Becker, A.B., Kozyrskyj, A.L. "Delay in diphtheria, pertussis, tetanus vaccination is associated with a reduced risk of childhood asthma." *J Allergy Clin Immunol*. 2008.

60. Meffert, M., Baltimore, D. "Physiological Functions of brain NF-KB." *Trends in Neurosciences*. 2005; 28(1):37-43.

61. Meyer, U., Nyffeler, M., Engler, A., Urwyler, A., Schedlowski, M., Knuesel, I., Yee, B.K., Feldon, J. "The time of prenatal immune challenge determines the specificity of inflammation-mediated brain and behavioral pathology." *J Neurosci*. 2006 May 3; 26(18):4752-62.

62. Molloy, C. et al. "Elevated cytokine levels in children with autism spectrum disorder." *J Neuroimmunology*. 2006; 172:198-205.

63. Mouridsen, S.E., Rich, B., Isager, T., Nedergaard, N.J. "Autoimmune diseases in parents of children with infantile autism: a case-control study." *Dev Med Child Neurol*. 2008 Jun; 49(6):429-32.

64. Niehus, R., Lord, C. "Early medical history of children with autism spectrum disorders." *J Dev Behav Pediatr*. 2006 Apr; 27(2 Suppl):S120-7.

65. Okada, K. et al. "Decreased serum levels of transforming growth factor-beta1 in patients with autism." *Prog Neuropsychopharmacol Biol Psychiatry*. 2006 Oct 5.

66. Pardo, C.A. et al. "Immunity, neuroglia and neuroinflammation in autism." *Int Rev Psychiatry*. 2005 Dec; 17(6):485-95.

67. Patterson, P.H. "Immune involvement in schizophrenia and autism: Etiology, pathology and animal models." *Behav Brain Res*. 2008 Dec.

68. Pessah, I.N. et al. "Immunologic and neurodevelopmental susceptibilities of autism." *Neurotoxicology*. 2008.

69. Plioplys, A.V. "Intravenous immunoglobulin treatment of children with autism." *J Child Neurol*. 1998 Feb; 13(2):79-82.

70. Rampersad, G.C. et al. "Chemical compounds that target thiol-disulfide groups on mononuclear phagocytes inhibit immune mediated phagocytosis of red blood cells." *Transfusion*. 2005; 45(3):384-93.

71. Reichenberg, A. et al. "Cytokine-associated emotional and cognitive disturbances in humans." *Arch Gen Psychiatry*. 2001; 58(5):445.

72. Schneider, C.K., Melmed, R.D., Barstow, L.E., Enriquez, F.J., Ranger-Moore, J., Ostrem, J.A. "Oral Human Immunoglobulin for Children with Autism and Gastrointestinal Dysfunction: A Prospective, Open-Label Study." *J Autism Dev Disord*. 2006 Jul 15.

73. Scifo, R. et al. "Opioid-immune interactions in autism: behavioural and immunological assessment during a double-blind treatment with naltrexone." *Ann Ist Super Sanita*. 1996; 32(3):351-9.

74. Silva, S.C. et al. "Autoantibody repertoires to brain tissue in autism nuclear families." *J Neuroimmunol*. 2004 Jul; 152(1-2):176-82.

75. Singer, H.S. et al. "Antibrain antibodies in children with autism and their unaffected siblings." *J Neuroimmunol*. 2006 Sep; 178(1-2):149.

76. Singer, H.S. et al. "Antibodies against fetal brain in sera of mothers with autistic children." *J Neuroimmunol.* 2008 Feb; 194(1-2):165-72.

77. Singh, V.K. "Plasma increase of interleukin-12 and interferon-gamma. Pathological significance in autism." *J Neuroimmunol.* 1996 May; 66(1-2):143-5.

78. Singh, V.K. "Th1- and Th2-like cytokines in CD4+ and CD8+ T cells in autism." *J Neuroimmunol.* 1998 May 1; 85(1):106-9.

79. Singh, V.K. et al. "Circulating autoantibodies to neuronal and glial filament proteins in autism." *Pediatr Neurol.* 1997 Jul; 17(1):88-90.

80. Singh, V.K. et al. "Antibodies to myelin basic protein in children with autistic behavior." *Brain Behav Immun.* 1993 Mar; 7(1):97-103.

81. Singh, V.K., Singh, E.A., Warren, R.P. "Hyperserotoninemia and serotonin receptor antibodies in children with autism but not mental retardation." *Biol Psychiatry.* 1997 Mar 15; 41(6):753-5.

82. Singh, V.K., Rivas, W.H. "Prevalence of serum antibodies to caudate nucleus in autistic children." *Neurosci Lett.* 2004 Jan 23; 355(1-2):53-6.

83. Siragam, V., Crow, A.R., Brinc, D., Song, S., Freedman, J., Lazarus, A.H. "Intravenous immunoglobulin ameliorates ITP via activating Fc gamma receptors on dendritic cells." *Nat Med.* 2006 Jun; 12(6):688-92.

84. Stubbs, E.G. et al. "Depressed lymphocyte responsiveness in autistic children." *J Autism Child Schizophr.* 1977 Mar; 7(1):49-55.

85. Stubbs, E.G., Budden, S.S., Burger, D.R., Vandenbark, A.A. "Transfer factor immunotherapy of an autistic child with congenital cytomegalovirus." *J Autism Dev Disord.* 1980 Dec; 10(4):451-8.

86. Suh, J.H., Walsh, W.J., McGinnis, W.R., Lewis, A., Ames, B.N. "Altered Sulfur Amino Acid Metabolism In Immune Cells of Children Diagnosed With Autism." *Am J Biochem Biotechnol.* 2008; 4(2):105-113.

87. Swedo, S.E. et al. "Pediatric autoimmune neuropsychiatric disorders associated with streptococcal infections: clinical description of the first 50 cases." *Am J Psychiatry.* 1998 Feb; 155(2):264-71.

88. Swedo, S.E., Leonard, H.L., Rapoport, J.L. "The pediatric autoimmune neuropsychiatric disorders associated with streptococcal infection (PANDAS) subgroup: separating fact from fiction." *Pediatrics.* 2004 Apr; 113(4):907-11.

89. Swedo, S.E., Grant, P.J. "Annotation: PANDAS: a model for human autoimmune disease." *J Child Psychol Psychiatry.* 2005 Mar; 46(3):227-34.

90. Sweeten, T.L. et al. "Increased prevalence of familial autoimmunity in probands with pervasive developmental disorders." *Pediatrics.* 2003.

91. Sweeten, T.L., Posey, D.J., McDougle, C.J. "High blood monocyte counts and neopterin levels in children with autistic disorder." *Am J Psychiatry.* 2003 Sep; 160(9):1691-3.

92. Sweeten, T.L., Posey, D.J., Shankar, S., McDougle, C.J. "High nitric oxide production in autistic disorder: a possible role for interferon-gamma." *Bio Psychiatry.* 2004 Feb 15; 55(4):434-7.

93. Todd, R.D., Hickok, J.M., Anderson, G.M., Cohen, D.J. "Antibrain antibodies in infantile autism." *Biol Psychiatry.* 1988 Mar 15; 23(6):644-7.

94. Trajkovski, V., Ajdinski, L., Spiroski, M. "Plasma concentration of immunoglobulin classes and subclasses in children with autism in the Republic of Macedonia: retrospective study." *Croat Med J*. 2004 Dec; 45(6):746-9.

95. Vojdani, A. et al. "Low natural killer cell cytotoxic activity in autism: The role of glutathione, IL-2 and IL-15." *J Neuroimmunol*. 2008 Dec 15; 205(1-2):148-54.

96. Vojdani, A. et al. "Antibodies to neuron-specific antigens in children with autism: possible cross-reaction with encephalitogenic proteins from milk, Chlamydia pneumoniae and Streptococcus group A." *J Neuroimmunol*. 2002 Aug; 129(1-2):168-77.

97. Vojdani, A. et al. "Infections, toxic chemicals and dietary peptides binding to lymphocyte receptors and tissue enzymes are major instigators of autoimmunity in autism." *International J Immunopathol Pharmacology*. 2003; 16: 189-199.

98. Vojdani, A., O'Bryan, T., Green, J.A., Mccandless, J., Woeller, K.N., Vojdani, E., Nourian, A.A., Cooper, E.L. "Immune response to dietary proteins, gliadin and cerebellar peptides in children with autism." *Nutr Neurosci*. 2004 Jun; 7(3):151-61.

99. Todd, R.D., Hickok, J.M., Anderson, G.M., Cohen, D.J. "Antibrain antibodies in infantile autism." *Biol Psychiatry*. 1988 Mar 15; 23(6):644-7.

100. Trajkovski, V., Ajdinski, L., Spiroski, M. "Plasma concentration of immunoglobulin classes and subclasses in children with autism in the Republic of Macedonia: retrospective study." *Croat Med J*. 2004 Dec; 45(6):746-9.

101. Vojdani, A. et al. "Low natural killer cell cytotoxic activity in autism: The role of glutathione, IL-2 and IL-15." *J Neuroimmunol*. 2008 Dec 15; 205(1-2):148-54.

102. Vojdani, A. et al. "Antibodies to neuron-specific antigens in children with autism: possible cross-reaction with encephalitogenic proteins from milk, Chlamydia pneumoniae and Streptococcus group A." *J Neuroimmunol*. 2002 Aug; 129(1-2):168-77.

103. Vojdani, A. et al. "Infections, toxic chemicals and dietary peptides binding to lymphocyte receptors and tissue enzymes are major instigators of autoimmunity in autism." *International J Immunopathol Pharmacology*. 16:189-199, 2003.

104. Vojdani, A., O'Bryan, T., Green, J.A., Mccandless, J., Woeller, K.N., Vojdani, E., Nourian, A.A., Cooper, E.L. "Immune response to dietary proteins, gliadin and cerebellar peptides in children with autism." *Nutr Neurosci*. 2004 Jun; 7(3):151-61.

105. Vojdani, A. et al. "Heat shock protein and gliadin peptide promote development of peptidase antibodies in children with autism and patients with autoimmune disease." *Clin Diagn Lab Immunol*. 2004 May; 11(3):515-24.

106. Wakefield, A.J., Walker-Smith, J.A., Murch, S.H. "Colonic CD8 and gamma delta T-cell infiltration with epithelial damage in children with autism." *Pediatrics* 2001; 138:366-72.

107. Warren, R.P. et al. "Immune abnormalities in patients with autism." *J Autism Dev Disord*. 1986 Jun; 16(2):189.

108. Warren, R.P. et al. "Detection of maternal antibodies in infantile autism." *J Am Acad Child Adolesc Psychiatry*. 1990 Nov; 29(6):873-7.

109. Warren, R.P. et al. "Reduced natural killer cell activity in autism." *J Am Acad Child Adolesc Psychiatry*. 1987 May; 26(3):333-5.

110. Warren, R.P. et al. "Immunogenetic studies in autism and related disorders." *Mol Chem Neuropathol.* 1996 May-Aug; 28(1-3):77-81.

111. Wills, S. et al. "Autoantibodies in autism spectrum disorders (ASD)." *Ann N Y Acad Sci.* 2007 Jun; 1107:79-91.

112. Yonk, L.J. et al. "CD4+ helper T cell depression in autism." *Immunol Lett.* 1990 Sep; 25(4):341-5.

113. Youseff, S., Steinman, L. "At once harmful and beneficial: the dual properties of NFKB. *Nature Immunology.* 2006; 7(9):901-902.

114. Zimecki, M., Artym, J. "Therapeutic properties of proteins and peptides from colostrum and milk." *Postepy Hig Med Dosw.* 2005; 59:309-23.

115. Zimmerman, A.W. et al. "Maternal antibrain antibodies in autism." *Brain Behav Immun.* 2006 Oct 5.

116. Zimmerman, A.W. et al. "Cerebrospinal fluid and serum markers of inflammation in autism." *Pediatr Neurol.* 2005 Sep; 33(3):195.

H. Prevalence

1. Arvidsson, T., Danielsson, B., Forsberg, P. et al. "Autism in 3-6-year-old children in a suburb of Goteborg, Sweden." *Autism.* 1997; 1:163.

2. Baird, G. et al. "Prevalence of disorders of the autism spectrum in a population cohort of children in South Thames: the Special Needs and Autism Project (SNAP)." *Lancet.* 2006 Jul 15; 368(9531):210-5.

3. Barbaresi, W.J., Katusic, S.K., Colligan, R.C., Weaver, A.L., Jacobsen, S.J. "The incidence of autism in Olmsted County, Minnesota, 1976-1997: results from a population-based study." *Arch Pediatr Adolesc Med.* 2005 Jan; 159(1):37-44.

4. Bertrand, J. et al. "Prevalence of autism in a United States population: the Brick township, NJ, investigation." *Pediatrics.* 2001; 108:1155-61.

5. Blaxill, M.F. "What's going on? The question of time trends in autism." *Public Health Reports.* 2004 Nov; 119.6:536-551.

6. Blaxill, M.F. "Any changes in prevalence of autism must be determined." *BMJ.* 2002 Feb 2; 324(7332):296.

7. Blaxill, M.F., Baskin, D.S., Spitzer, W.O. "Blaxill, Baskin, and Spitzer on Croen et al. (2002), The changing prevalence of autism in California." *J Autism Dev Disord.* 2003 Apr; 33(2):223-6; discussion 227-9.

8. Bryson, S.E., Clark, B.S., Smith, I.M. "First report of a Canadian epidemiological study of autistic syndromes." *J Child Psychiatry.* 1988 Jul; 29(4)433-45.

9. Burd, L., Fisher, W., Kerbeshian, J. "A prevalence study of pervasive developmental disorders in North Dakota." *J Am Acad Child Adolesc Psychiatry.* 1987 Sep; 26(5):700-3.

10. Byrd, Robert. MIND Institute. "Report to the Legislature on the Principle Findings from The Epidemiology of Autism in California: A Comprehensive Pilot Study." UC Davis. 17 Oct 2002. www.dds.ca.gov/autism/pdf/study_final.pdf

11. California Department of Developmental Services. "Changes in the Population of Persons with Autism and Pervasive Developmental Disorders in California's Developmental Services System: 1987 through 1998." Report to the Legislature March 1, 1999:1-19.

12. Chakrabarti, S., Fombonne, E. "Pervasive developmental disorders in preschool children: confirmation of high prevalence." *Am J Psychiatry.* 2005 Jun; 162(6):1133-41.

13. Chang, H.L., Juang, Y.Y., Wang, W.T., Huang, C.I., Chen, C.Y., Hwang, Y.S. "Screening for autism spectrum disorder in adult psychiatric outpatients in a clinic in Taiwan." *Gen Hosp Psychiatry.* 2003 Jul-Aug; 25(4):284-8.

14. Charman, T. "The prevalence of autism spectrum disorders. Recent evidence and future challenges." *EurChild Adolesc Psychiatry.* 2002 Dec; 11(6):249-56.

15. Croen, L., Grether, J., Hoogstrate, J., Selvin, S. "The changing prevalence of autism in California." *J Autism Dev Disord.* 2002 Jun; 32(3):207-15.

16. Croen, L.A., Grether, J.K. "A Response to Blaxill, Baskin, and Spitzer on Croen et al. (2002), 'The Changing Prevalence of Autism in California.'" *J Autism Dev Disord.* 2003 Apr; 33:227-229(3).

17. Ganz, Michael. "The Costs of Autism." *Understanding Autism: From Basic Neuroscience to Treatment.* Eds. Steven O. Moldin, John L.R. Rubenstein. CRC Press, 2006

18. Gillberg, C., Wing, L. "Autism: not an extremely rare disorder." *Acta Psychiatr Scand.* 1999 Jun; 99(6):399-406.

19. Gillberg, C., Cederlund, M., Lamberg, K., Zeijlon, L. "Brief Report: 'The Autism Epidemic.' The registered prevalence of autism in a Swedish urban area." *J Autism Dev Disord.* 2006 Mar 28.

20. Hertz-Piccioto, I., Delwiche, L. "The rise in autism and the role of age at diagnosis." *Epidemiology.* 2009 Jan; 20(1):84-90.

21. Honda, H., Shimizu, Y., Imai, M., Nitto, Y. "Cumulative incidence of childhood autism: a total population study ofbetter accuracy and precision." *Dev Med Child Neurol.* 2005 Jan; 47(1):10-8.

22. Hoshino, Y. et al. "The epidemiological study of autism in Fukushima-ken." *Folia Psychiatr Neurol Jpn.* 1982; 36(2):115-24.

23. Icasiano, F., Hewson, P., Machet, P., Cooper, C., Marshall, A. "Childhood autism spectrum disorder in the Barwon region: a community based study." *J Pediatr Child Health.* 2004 Dec; 40(12):696-701.

24. Kielinen, M., Linna, S.L., Moilanen, I. "Autism in Northern Finland." *Eur Child Adolesc Psychiatry.* 2000 Sep; 9(3):162-7.

25. Kadesjo, B., Gillberg, C., Hagberg, B. "Brief report: autism and Asperger syndrome in seven-year-old children: a total population study." *J Autism Dev Disord.* 1999 Aug; 29(4):327-31.

26. Kirby, R.S., Brewster, M.A., Canino, C.U., Pavin, M. "Early childhood surveillance of developmental disorders by a birth defects surveillance system: methods, prevalence comparisons, and mortality patterns." *J Dev Behav Pediatr.* 1995 Oct; 16(5):318-26.

27. Lauritsen, M.B., Pedersen, C.B., Mortensen, P.B. "The incidence and prevalence of pervasive developmental disorders: a Danish population-based study." *Psychol Med.* 2004 Oct; 34(7):1339-46.

28. Lotter, V. "Epidemiology of autistic conditions in young children. I. Prevalence." *Soc. Psychiatry* 1966; 1:124-137.

29. Magnusson, P., Saemundsen, E. "Prevalence of autism in Iceland." *J Autism Dev Disord.* 2001 Apr; 31(2):153-63.

30. Nylander, L., Gillberg, C. "Screening for autism spectrum disorders in adult psychiatric outpatients: a preliminary report." *Acta Psychiatr Scand.* 2001 Jun; 103(6):428-34.

31. Powell, J.E. et al. "Changes in the incidence of childhood autism and other autistic spectrum disorders in preschool children from two areas of the West Midlands, UK." *Dev Med Child Neurol.* 2000 Sep; 42(9):624-8.

32. Ritvo, E.R., Freeman, B.J., Pingree, C., Mason-Brothers, A., Jorde, L., Jenson, W.R., McMahon, W.M., Petersen, P.B., Mo, A., Ritvo, A. "The UCLA-University of Utah epidemiologic survey of autism: prevalence." *Am J Psychiatry.* 1989 Feb; 146(2)194-9.

33. Scott, F.J., Baron-Cohen, S., Bolton, P., Brayne, C. "Brief report: prevalence of autism spectrum conditions in children aged 5-11 years in Cambridgeshire, UK." *Autism.* 2002 Sep; 6(3)231-7.

34. Smeeth, L., Cook, C., Fombonne, P.E., Heavey, L., Rodrigues, L.C., Smith, P.G., Hall, A.J. "Rate of first recorded diagnosis of autism and other pervasive developmental disorders in a United Kingdom general practice 1988 to 2001." *BMC Med.* 2004 Nov 9; 2:39.

35. Steffenberg, S., Gillberg, C. "Autism and autistic-like conditions in Swedish rural and urban areas: a population study." *Br J Psychiatry.* 1986 Jul; 149:81-7.

36. Szatmari, P. "Thinking about Autism, Asperger Syndrome and PDDNOS." *PRISME.* 2001. 34:24-34.

37. Wing, L., Potter, D. "The epidemiology of autistic spectrum disorders: Is the prevalence rising?" *Ment Retard Dev Disabil Res Rev.* 2002; 8(3):151-61.

38. Yazbak, F.E. "Autism in the United States: a perspective." *JPANDS.* 2003; 8:4:103-107.

39. Yeargin-Allsopp, M. et al. "Prevalence of autism in a US metropolitan area." *JAMA.* 2003 Jan 1; 289(1)49-55.

I. Genetics and Autism

1. Blasi, F., Bacchelli, E. et al. "SLC25A12 and CMYA3 gene variants are not associated with autism in the IMGSAC multiplex family sample." *Eur J Hum Genet.* 2006; 14(1):123-6.

2. Boris, M., Goldblatt, A., Galanko, J., James, J. "Association of MTHFR gene variants with autism." *J Am Phys Surg.* 2004; 9(4)106-8.

3. Brimacombe, M., Xue, M., Parikh, A. "Familial risk factors in autism." *J Child Neurol.* 2007 May; 22(5):593-7.

4. Campbell, D.B. et al. "A genetic variant that disrupts MET transcription is associated with autism." *Proc Natl Acad Sci U S A.* 2006 Oct 19.

5. Comi, A.M., Zimmerman, A.W., Frye, V.H., Law, P.A., Peeden, J.N. "Familial clustering of autoimmune disorders and evaluation of medical risk factors in autism." *J Child Neurol.* 1999 Jun; 14(6):388-94.

6. Folstein, S. and M. Rutter (1977). "Genetic influences and infantile autism." *Nature* 265(5596): 726-8.

7. Gregg, J.P. et al. "Gene expression changes in children with autism." *Genomics.* 2008 Jan; 91(1):22-29.

8. Herbert, M.R., Russo, J.P., Yang, S. et al. "Autism and environmental genomics." *Neurotoxicology.* 2006; 27(5):671-84.

9. Korvatska, E. et al. "Genetic and immunologic considerations in autism." *Neurobiol Dis.* 2002 Mar; 9(2):107-25.

10. Molloy, C.A. et al. "Familial autoimmune thyroid disease as a risk factor for regression in children with Autism Spectrum Disorder: a CPEA Study." *J Autism Dev Disord.* 2006 Apr; 36(3):317-24.

11. Pasca, S.P., Dronca, E., Kaucsar, T., et al. "One Carbon Metabolism Disturbances and the C667T MTHFR Gene Polymorphism in Children with Autism Spectrum Disorders." *J Cell Molec Med.* Aug 2008.

12. Persico, A.M. et al. "Adenosine deaminase alleles and autistic disorder: case-control and family-based association studies." *Am J Med Genet.* 2000 Dec 4; 96(6):784-90.

13. Szatmari, P. "Heterogeneity and the genetics of autism." *J Psychiatry Neurosci.* 1999 Mar; 24(2):159-65. Torres, A.R. et al. "The association and linkage of the HLA-A2 class I allele with autism." *Hum Immunol.* 2006 Apr-May; 67(4-5):346-1.

14. Ueland, P.M., Hustad, S., Schneede, J., Refsum, H., Vollset, S.E. "Biological and clinical implications of the MTH-FR C677T polymorphism." *Trends Pharmacol Sci.* 2001 Apr; 22(4):195-201.

15. Williams, T.A., Mars, A.E. et al. "Risk of autistic disorder in affected offspring of mothers with a glutathione S-transferase P1 haplotype." *Arch Pediatr Adolesc Med.* 2007; 161(4):356-61.

J. Autism and Mitochondria

1. Chugani, D.C., Sundram, B.S., Behen, M., Lee, M.L., Moore, G.J. "Evidence of altered energy metabolism in autistic children." *Prog Neuropsychopharmacol Biol Psychiatry.* 1999 May; 23(4):635-41.

2. Clark-Taylor, T., Clark-Taylor, B.E. "Is autism a disorder of fatty acid metabolism? Possible dysfunction of mitochondrial beta-oxidation by long chain acyl-CoA dehydrogenase." *Med Hypotheses.* 62(6):970-5.

18. Ehrhart, J., Zeevalk, G.D. "Cooperative interaction between ascorbate and glutathione during mitochondrial impairment in mesencephalic cultures." *J Neurochem.* 2003; 86(6):1487-97.

19. Fernandez-Checa, J.C. et al. "Oxidative stress: role of mitochondria and protection by glutathione." *Biofactors.* 1998; 8(1-2):7-11.

20. Filipek, P.A., Juranek, J. et al. "Relative carnitine deficiency in autism." *J Autism Dev Disord.* 2004; 34(6):615-23.

21. Filipek, P.A., Juranek, J. et al. "Mitochondrial dysfunction in autistic patients with 15q inverted duplication." *Ann Neurol.* 2003; 53(6):801-4.

22. Fillano, J.J., Goldenthal, M.J. et al. "Mitochondrial dysfunction in patients with hypotonia, epilepsy, autism, and developmental delay: HEADD syndrome." *J Child Neurol.* 2002; 17(6): 435-9.

23. Gargus, J.J., Imtiaz, F. "Mitochondrial energy-deficient endophenotype in autism." *Am J Biochem Biotechnol.* 2008; 4(2):198-207.

24. Graf, W.D., Marin-Garcia, J. et al. "Autism associated with the mitochondrial DNA G8363A transfer RNA(Lys) mutation." *J Child Neurol.* 2000; 15(6):357-61.

25. Holtzman, D. "Autistic spectrum disorders and mitochondrial encephalopathies." *Acta Paediatr.* 2008 Jul; 97(7):859-60.

26. Kidd, P.M. "Neurodegeneration from mitochondrial insufficiency: nutrients, stem cells, growth factors, and prospects for brain rebuilding using integrative management." *Altern Med Rev.* 2005 Dec; 10(4):268-93.

27. Lerman-Sagie, T. et al. "Should autistic children be evaluated for mitochondrial disorders." *J Child Neurol.* 2004; 19(5):379-81. Lombard, J. "Autism: a mitochondrial disorder?" *Med Hypotheses.* 1998; 50(6):497-500.

28. Oliveira, G., Ataide, A. et al. "Epidemiology of autism spectrum disorder in Portugal: prevalence, clinical characterization, and medical conditions." *Dev Med Child Neurol* 2007; 49(10): 726-33.

29. Oliveira, G., Diogo, L. et al. "Mitochondrial dysfunction in autism spectrum disorders: a population-based study." *Dev Med Child Neurol.* 2005; 47(3):185-9.

30. Poling, J.S. et al. "Developmental regression and mitochondrial dysfunction in a child with autism." *J Child Neurol.* 2006; 21(2):170-2.

31. Pons, R., Andreu, A.L. et al. "Mitochondrial DNA abnormalities and autistic spectrum disorders." *J Pediatr.* 2004; 144(1):81-5.

32. Ramoz, N., Reichert, J.G. et al. "Linkage and association of the mitochondrial aspartate/glutamate carrier SLC25A12 gene with autism." *Am J Psychiatry.* 2004; 161(4):662-9.

33. Rossignol, D.A., Bradstreet, J.J. "Evidence of mitochondrial dysfunction in autism and implications for treatment." *A J Biochem Biotechnol.* 2008; 4(2):208-217.

34. Segurado, R., Conroy, J. et al. "Confirmation of association between autism and the mitochondrial aspartate/glutamate carrier SLC25A12 gene on chromosome 2q31." *Am J Psychiatry.* 2005; 162(11):2182-4.

35. Silverman, J.M., Buxbaum, J.D. et al. "Autism-related routines and rituals associated with a mitochondrial aspartate/glutamate carrier SLC25A12 polymorphism." *Am J Med Genet B Neuropsychiatr Genet.* 2007.

36. Smith, M., Spence, M.A., Flodman, P. "Nuclear and mitochondrial genome defects in autisms." *Ann. N.Y. Acad. Sci.* 2009; 1151:102–132.

37. Trushina, E., McMurray, C.T. "Oxidative stress and mitochondrial dysfunction in neurodegenerative diseases." *Neuroscience.* 2007. 145(4):1233-48.

38. Tsao, C.Y., Mendell, J.R. "Autistic disorder in 2 children with mitochondrial disorders." *J Child Neurol.* 2007; 22(9):1121-3.

39. Weissman, J.R. et al. "Mitochondrial disease in autism spectrum disorder patients: a cohort analysis." *PLoS ONE.* 2008; 3(11):e3815.

K. Autism and Oxidative Stress

1. Abbott, L.C., Nahm, S.S. "Neuronal nitric oxide synthase expression in cerebellar mutant mice." *Cerebellum.* 2004; 3(3):141-51.

2. Anderson, M.P., Hooker, B.S. et al. "Bridging from cells to cognition in autism pathophysiology: biological pathways to defective brain function and plasticity." *A J Biochem Biotechnol.* 2008; 4(2):167-176.

3. Bell, J.G., MacKinlay, E.E. et al. "Essential fatty acids and phospholipase A2 in autistic spectrum disorders." *Prostaglandins Leukot Essent Fatty Acids.* 2004; 71(4):201-4.

4. Bell, J.G., Sargent, J.R. et al. "Red blood cell fatty acid compositions in a patient with autistic spectrum disorder: a characteristic abnormality in neurodevelopmental disorders?" *Prostaglandins Leukot Essent Fatty Acids.* 2000; 63(1-2):21-5.

5. Blaylock, R. "Interactions of cytokines, excitotoxins, and reactive nitrogen and oxygen species in autism spectrum disorders." *J Amer Nutr Assoc.* 2003; 6:21-35.

6. Boso, M., Emanuele, E. et al. "Alterations of circulating endogenous secretory RAGE and S100A9 levels indicating dysfunction of the AGE-RAGE axis in autism." *Neurosci Lett.* 2006; 410(3):169-73.

7. Chauhan, A., Chauhan, V. "Oxidative stress in autism." *Pathophysiology.* 2006; 13(3):171-81.

8. Chauhan, A., Chauhan, V. et al. "Oxidative stress in autism: increased lipid peroxidation and reduced serum levels of ceruloplasmin and transferrin—the antioxidant proteins." *Life Sci.* 2004; 75(21):2539-49.

9. Chauhan, A., Sheikh, A. et al. "Increased copper-mediated oxidation of membrane phosphatidylethanolamine in autism." *Am J Biochem Biotechnol.* 2008; 4(2):95-100.

10. Chauhan, V., Chauhan, A. et al. "Alteration in amino-glycerophospholipids levels in the plasma of children with autism: a potential biochemical diagnostic marker." *Life Sci.* 2004; 74(13):1635-43.

11. Chez, M.G., Buchanan, C.P. et al. "Double-blind, placebo-controlled study of L-carnosine supplementation in children with autistic spectrum disorders." *J Child Neurol.* 2002; 17(11):833-7.

12. Danfors, T., von Knorring, A.L. et al. "Tetrahydrobiopterin in the treatment of children with autistic disorder: a double-blind placebo-controlled crossover study." *J Clin Psychopharmacol.* 2005; 25(5):485-9.

13. Deth, R. et al. "How environmental and genetic factors combine to cause autism: A redox/methylation hypothesis." *Neurotoxicology.* 2008; 29(1):190-201.

14. Evans, T.A., Siedlak, S.L. et al. "The autistic phenotype exhibits a remarkably localized modification of brain protein by products of free radical-induced lipid oxidation." *Am J Biochem Biotechnol.* 2008; 4(2):61-72.

15. Flora, S.J., Pande, M., Kannan. G.M., Mehta. A. "Lead induced oxidative stress and its recovery following co-administration of melatonin or N-acetylcysteine during chelation with succimer in male rats." *Cell Mol Biol* (Noisy-le-grand). 2004; 50.

16. Jackson, M.J., Garrod, P.J. "Plasma zinc, copper, and amino acid levels in the blood of autistic children." *J 17. Autism Child Schizophr.* 1978; 8(2):203-8.

17. James, S.J., Cutler, P., Melnyk, S., Jernigan, S., Janak, L., Gaylor, D.W., Neubrander, J.A. "Metabolic biomarkers of increased oxidative stress and impaired methylation capacity in children with autism." *Am J Clin Nutr.* 2004 Dec; 80(6):1611-7.

18. James, S.J. et al. "Metabolic endophenotype and related genotypes are associated with oxidative stress in children with autism." *Am J Med Genet B Neuropsychiatr Genet.* 2006 Aug 17.

19. James, S.J., Slikker, W., Melnyk, S., New, E., Pogribna, M., Jernigan, S. "Thimerosal neurotoxicity is associated with glutathione depletion: protection with glutathione precursors." *Neurotoxicology.* 2005 Jan; 26(1):1-8.

20. James, S.J. et al. "Efficacy of methylcobalamin and folinic acid treatment on glutathione redox status in children with autism." *Am J Clin Nutr.* 2008 Dec 3.

21. Johannesson, T., Kristinsson, J. et al. "[Neurodegenerative diseases, antioxidative enzymes and copper. A review of experimental research.]" *Laeknabladid.* 2003; 89(9):659-671.

22. Johnson, S. "Micronutrient accumulation and depletion in schizophrenia, epilepsy, autism and Parkinson's disease?" *Med Hypotheses.* 2001; 56(5):641-5.

23. Jory, J., McGinnis, W.R. "Red-cell trace minerals in children with autism." *Am J Biochem Biotechnol.* 2008; 4(2):101-104.

24. Junaid, M.A., Kowal, D. et al. "Proteomic studies identified a single nucleotide polymorphism in glyoxalase I as autism susceptibility factor." *Am J Med Genet A.* 2004; 131(1):11-7.

25. Kazutoshi, N., Naoko, N., Emiko, T., Man, U., Miyuki, T., Kaori, S. "A Preliminary Study of Methylcobalamin Therapy in Autism." *J Tokyo Women's Medical University.* 2005; 75(3/4):64-69.

26. Keithahn, C., Lerchl, A. "5-hydroxytryptophan is a more potent in vitro hydroxyl radical scavenger than melatonin or vitamin C." *J Pineal Res.* 2005 Jan; 38(1):62-6.

27. MacFabe, D.F., Rodríguez-Capote, K. et al. "A novel rodent model of autism: intraventricular infusions of propionic acid increase locomotor activity and induce neuroinflammation and oxidative stress in discrete regions of adult rat brain." *Am J Biochem Biotechnol.* 2008; 4(2):146-166.

28. Mahadik, S.P., Scheffer, R.E. "Oxidative injury and potential use of antioxidants in schizophrenia." *Prostaglandins Leukot Essent Fatty Acids.* 1996 Aug; 55(1-2):45-54.

29. McGinnis, W.R. "Oxidative stress in autism." *Altern Ther Health Med.* 2004; 10(6):22-36; quiz 37, 92.

30. McGinnis, W.R. "Oxidative stress in autism." *Altern Ther Health Med.* 2005; 11(1):19.

31. McGinnis, W.R. "Could oxidative stress from psychosocial stress affect neurodevelopment in autism?" *J Autism Dev Disord.* 2007; 37(5):993-4.

32. Miller, D.M., Woods, J.S. "Urinary porphyrins as biological indicators of oxidative stress in the kidney. Interaction of mercury and cephaloridine." *Biochem Pharmacol.* 1993; 46(12):2235-41.

33. Ming, X., Stein, T.P., Brimacombe, M., Johnson, W.G., Lambert, G.H., Wagner, G.C. "Increased excretion of a lipid peroxidation biomarker in autism." *Prostaglandins Leukot Essent Fatty Acids.* 2005 Nov; 73(5):379-84.

34. Ming, X. et al. "Evidence of Oxidative Stress in Autism Derived from Animal Models." *Am J Biochem Biotechnol.* 2008; 4(2):218-225.

35. Ng, F., Berk, M. et al. "Oxidative stress in psychiatric disorders: evidence base and therapeutic implications." *Int J Neuropsychopharmacol.* 2008; 1-26.

36. Pasca, S.P., Nemes, B. et al. "High levels of homocysteine and low serum paraoxonase 1 arylesterase activity in children with autism." *Life Sci.* 2006; 78(19):2244-8.

37. Reiter, R.J., Tan, D.X., Burkhardt, S. "Reactive oxygen and nitrogen species and cellular and organismal decline: amelioration with melatonin." *Mech Ageing Dev.* 2002 Apr 30; 123(8):1007-19.

38. Ross, M.A. "Could oxidative stress be a factor in neurodevelopmental disorders?" *Prostaglandins Leukot Essent Fatty Acids.* 2000; 63(1-2):61-3.

39. Rossignol, D.A., Rossignol, L.W. "The effects of hyperbaric oxygen therapy on oxidative stress, inflammation, and symptoms in children with autism: an open-label pilot study." *BMC Pediatr.* 2007; 7(1):36.

40. Sajdel-Sulkowska, E.M., Lipinski, B. et al. "Oxidative stress in autism: elevated cerebellar 3-nitrotyrosine levels." *Am J Biochem Biotechnol.* 2008; 4(2):73-84.

41. Sierra, C., Vilaseca, M.A. et al. "Oxidative stress in Rett syndrome." *Brain Dev.* 2001; 23 Suppl 1:S236-9.

42. Sogut, S., Zoroglu, S.S. et al. "Changes in nitric oxide levels and antioxidant enzyme activities may have a role in the pathophysiological mechanisms involved in autism." *Clin Chim Acta.* 2003; 331(1-2):111-7.

43. Sokol, D.K., Chen, D. et al. "High levels of Alzheimer beta-amyloid precursor protein (APP) in children with severely autistic behavior and aggression." *J Child Neurol.* 2006; 21(6):444-9.

44. Suh, J.H., Walsh, W.J. et al. "Altered sulfur amino acid metabolism in immune cells of children diagnosed with autism." *Am J Biochem Biotechnol.* 2008; 4(2):105-113.

45. Tchantchou, F., Graves, M., Shea, T.B. "Expression and activity of methionine cycle genes are altered following folate and vitamin E deficiency under oxidative challenge: modulation by apolipoprotein E-deficiency." *Nutr Neurosci.* 2006 Feb-Apr; 9(1-2):17-24.

46. Torsdottir, G., Hreidarsson, S. et al. "Ceruloplasmin, superoxide dismutase and copper in autistic patients." *Basic Clin Pharmacol Toxicol.* 2005; 96(2):146-8.

47. Yao, Y., Walsh, W.J. et al. "Altered vascular phenotype in autism: correlation with oxidative stress." *Arch Neurol.* 2006; 63(8):1161-4.

48. Yorbik, O., Sayal, A., Akay, C., Akbiyik, D.I., Sohmen, T. "Investigation of antioxidant enzymes in children with autistic disorder." *Prostaglandins Leukot Essent Fatty Acids.* 2002 Nov; 67(5):341-3.

49. Zoroglu, S.S., Armutcu, F. et al. "Increased oxidative stress and altered activities of erythrocyte free radical scavenging enzymes in autism." *Eur Arch Psychiatry Clin Neurosci.* 2004: 254(3):143-7.

Appendix II
The Transmethylation Cycle

Transmethylation: The passing of the methyl group (CH3-) from one molecule to another.

Transsulfuration: The passing of a sulfur or sulfur hydrogen (SH-) group from one molecule to another.

Folate (folic acid-<u>inactive</u>) → dihydrofolate (DHF) → tetrahydrofolate (THF) ⮂ methylene-THF (5, 10-CH2-THF) →methyl-THF-<u>active</u> (5, CH3-THF).

Folic acid → DHF

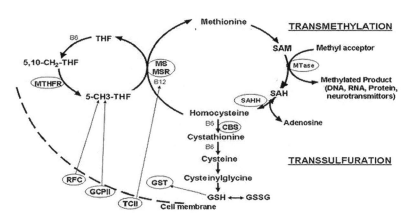

Figure A.1. An overview of the pathways involved in folate-dependent methionine transmethylation and transsulfuration.

Folic acid is first enzymatically converted to dihydrofolic acid (DHF) and then to tetra hydro folic acid (THF), which then is enzymatically converted with the help of vitamin B6 (as P5P) to methylenetetrahydrofolate (5,10-CH2-THF).

Methylene-tetrahydrofolate-reductase (MTHFR) catalyzes the synthesis of 5-methyltetrahydrofolate (5-CH3-THF), the active form of folic acid, from 5,10,methylenetetrahydrofolfate (5,10-CH-THF).

The methyl group from 5-CH3THF is transferred initially to cobalamin (vitamin B12), which then transfers it to homocysteine to regenerate methionine via the *folate/B12-dependent* methionine synthase (MS) reaction. Methionine synthase reductase (MSR) maintains the B12 cofactor in a reduced state for optimal MS activity.

Methionine is then activated to S-adenosylmethionine (SAM), the major methyl donor for multiple cellular methyltransferase (MTase) reactions. After methyl group transfer, SAM is converted to SAH (S-adenosyl homocysteine) which is further metabolized to homocysteine and adenosine by a reversible reaction catalyzed by SAH hydrolase (SAHH).

Homocysteine may be permanently removed from the methionine cycle by irreversible conversion to cystathionine by *B6-dependent (as P5P)* cystathionine beta synthase (CBS) which initiates the transsulfuration pathway.

Cystathionine is subsequently converted to cysteine, the rate limiting amino acid for the synthesis of the tripeptide, glutathione (Glutamine-Cysteine-Glycine). Reduced *active* glutathione (GSH) is in dynamic equilibrium with the oxidized (*inactive*) disulfide GSSG form of glutathione.

Reduced folates (the various forms of folic acid) are transported from the plasma into the cell by the reduced folate carrier (RFC). Transport of folate into the intestinal mucosa is mediated by glutamate carboxypepsidase II (GCPII). Vitamin B12 is transported into the cell bound to the B12 transport protein transcobalmin II (TCII). (GST) is the enzyme glutathione S-transferase. *Note that the vitamin B6 in these reactions is not pyridoxine (inactive) but the active form: pyridoxine 5-phosphate (P5P).*

Am J Med Genet B Neuropsychiatr Genet. Author manuscript; available in PMC 2008 December 27.

Published in final edited form as:

Am J Med Genet B Neuropsychiatr Genet. 2006 December 5; 141B(8): 947–956. doi: 10.1002/ajmg.b.30366.

Appendix III
The Criteria for Diagnosing Autism and Related Disorders

1. Diagnostic Criteria for 299.00 Autistic Disorder; DSM-IV

(I) A total of six (or more) items from (A), (B), and (C), with at least two from (A), and one each from (B) and (C)

(A) qualitative impairment in social interaction, as manifested by at least two of the following:

1. Marked impairments in the use of multiple nonverbal behaviors such as eye-to-eye gaze, facial expression, body posture, and gestures to regulate social interaction.

2. Failure to develop peer relationships appropriate to developmental level.

3. A lack of spontaneous seeking to share enjoyment, interests, or achievements with other people, (e.g., by a lack of showing, bringing, or pointing out objects of interest to other people).

4. A lack of social or emotional reciprocity (note: in the description, it gives the following as examples: not actively participating in simple social play or games, preferring solitary activities, or involving others in activities only as tools or "mechanical" aids).

(B) qualitative impairments in communication as manifested by at least one of the following:

1. A delay in, or total lack of, the development of spoken language (not accompanied by an attempt to compensate through alternative modes of communication such as gesture or mime)
2. In individuals with adequate speech, marked impairment in the ability to initiate or sustain a conversation with others
3. Stereotyped and repetitive use of language or idiosyncratic language
4. A lack of varied, spontaneous make-believe play or social imitative play appropriate to developmental level

(C) restricted repetitive and stereotyped patterns of behavior, interests, and activities, as manifested by at least two of the following:

1. An encompassing preoccupation with one or more stereotyped and restricted patterns of interest that is abnormal either in intensity or focus
2. An apparently inflexible adherence to specific, nonfunctional routines or rituals
3. A stereotyped and repetitive motor mannerisms (e.g. hand or finger flapping or twisting, or complex whole-body movements)
4. persistent preoccupation with parts of objects

(II) Delays or abnormal functioning in at least one of the following areas, with onset prior to age 3 years:

(A) social interaction
(B) language as used in social communication
(C) symbolic or imaginative play

(III) The disturbance is not better accounted for by Rett's Disorder or Childhood Disintegrative Disorder.

2. ICD-10 Criteria for "Childhood Autism"[1]

A. Abnormal or impaired development is evident before the age of 3 years in at least one of the following areas:

1. Receptive or expressive language as used in social communication;

2. The development of selective social attachments or of reciprocal social interaction;

3. Functional or symbolic play

B. A total of at least six symptoms from (1), (2), and (3) must be present, with at least two from (1) and at least one from each of (2) and (3)

1. Qualitative impairments in social interaction are manifest in at least two of the following areas:

a. Failure adequately to use eye-to-eye gaze, facial expression, body postures, and gestures to regulate social interaction;

b. Failure to develop (in a manner appropriate to mental age, and despite ample opportunities) peer relationships that involve a mutual sharing of interests, activities, and emotions;

c. A lack of socio-emotional reciprocity as shown by an impaired or deviant response to other people's emotions; or lack of modulation of behavior according to social context; or a weak integration of social, emotional, and communicative behaviors;

d. A lack of spontaneous seeking to share enjoyment, interests, or achievements with other people (e.g., a lack of showing, bringing, or pointing out to other people objects of interest to the individual).

2. Qualitative abnormalities in communication as manifest in at least one of the following areas:

a. A delay in or total lack of, development of spoken language that is not accompanied by an attempt to compensate through the use of gestures or mime as an alternative mode of communication (often preceded by a lack of communicative babbling);

b. A relative failure to initiate or sustain conversational interchange (at whatever level of language skill is present), in which there is reciprocal responsiveness to the communications of the other person;

c. Stereotyped and repetitive use of language or idiosyncratic use of words or phrases;

d. A lack of varied spontaneous make-believe play or (when young) social imitative play

3. Restricted, repetitive, and stereotyped patterns of behavior, interests, and activities are manifested in at least one of the following:

---

1   World Health Organization. (1992). *International classification of diseases: Diagnostic criteria for research* (10th edition). Geneva, Switzerland: Author.

a. An encompassing preoccupation with one or more stereotyped and restricted patterns of interest that are abnormal in content or focus; or one or more interests that are abnormal in their intensity and circumscribed nature though not in their content or focus;

b. Apparently compulsive adherence to specific, nonfunctional routines or rituals;

c. Stereotyped and repetitive motor mannerisms that involve either hand or finger flapping or twisting or complex whole body movements;

d. Preoccupations with part-objects of non-functional elements of play materials (such as their odor, the feel of their surface, or the noise or vibration they generate).

C. The clinical picture is not attributable to the other varieties of pervasive developmental disorders; specific development disorder of receptive language (F80.2) with secondary socio-emotional problems, reactive attachment disorder (F94.1) or disinhibited attachment disorder (F94.2); mental retardation (F70-F72) with some associated emotional or behavioral disorders; schizophrenia (F20.-) of unusually early onset; and Rett's Syndrome (F84.12)

3. ICD-10 Criteria for Asperger Syndrome

ICD-10 Diagnostic Criteria for Research: F84.5 - Asperger Syndrome[2]

Reference

Another list of diagnostic criteria was developed by Christopher Gillberg

Comparison of ICD-10 and Gillberg's Criteria for Asperger Syndrome

Leekam, Susan et al *Autism*, Vol. 4, No. 1, 11-28 (2000); DOI: 10.1177/1362361300004001002

4. ICD-10 Criteria for ADHD (Attention Deficit/Hyperactivity Disorder

F90 Hyperkinetic disorders

(1) often fails to give close attention to details, or makes careless errors in school work, work, or other activities;

(2) often fails to sustain attention in tasks or play activities;

(3) often appears not to listen to what is being said to him or her;

(4) often fails to follow through on instructions or to finish school work, chores, or duties in the workplace (not because of oppositional behavior or failure to understand instructions);

(5) is often impaired in organizing tasks and activities;

(6) often avoids or strongly dislikes tasks, such as homework, that require sustained mental effort;

(7) often loses things necessary for certain tasks and activities, such as school assignments, pencils, books, toys, or tools;

(8) is often easily distracted by external stimuli;

(9) is often forgetful in the course of daily activities.

---

2   World Health Organization. (1992). International classification of diseases: Diagnostic criteria for research (10th edition). Geneva, Switzerland: Author. (pg.186-187).

G2 Hyperactivity

At least three of the following symptoms of hyperactivity have persisted for at least six months, to a degree that is maladaptive and inconsistent with the developmental level of the child:

(1) often fidgets with hands or feet or squirms on seat;

(2) leaves seat in classroom or in other situations in which remaining seated is expected;

(3) often runs about or climbs excessively in situations in which it is inappropriate (in adolescents or adults, only feelings of restlessness may be present);

(4) is often unduly noisy in playing or has difficulty in engaging quietly in leisure activities;

(5) Exhibits a persistent pattern of excessive motor activity that is not substantially modified by social context or demands

G3 Impulsivity

At least one of the following symptoms of impulsivity has persisted for at least six months, to a degree that is maladaptive and inconsistent with the developmental level of the child:

(1) often blurts out answers before questions have been completed;

(2) often fails to wait in lines or await turns in games or group situations;

(3) Often interrupts or intrudes on others (eg butts into others' conversations or games);

(4) Often talks excessively without appropriate response to social constraints

G4

Onset of the disorder is no later than the age of seven years

G5 Pervasiveness

The criteria should be met for more than a single situation, e.g. the combination of inattention and hyperactivity should be present both at home and at school, or at both school and another setting where children are observed, such as a clinic. (Evidence for cross-situationality will ordinarily require information from more than one source; parental reports about classroom behavior, for instance, are unlikely to be sufficient.)

G6

The symptoms in G1 and G3 cause clinically significant distress or impairment in social, academic, or occupational functioning

G7

The disorder does not meet the criteria for pervasive developmental disorders (F84.-), manic episode (F30.-), depressive episode (F32.-), or anxiety disorders (F41.-)

Comment

Many authorities also recognize conditions that are sub-threshold for hyperkinetic disorder. Children who meet criteria in other ways but do not show abnormalities of hyperactivity/impulsiveness, may be recognized as showing attention deficit; conversely, children who fall short of criteria for attention problems but meet criteria in other respects may be recognized as showing activity disorder. In the same way, children who meet criteria for only one situation (e.g. only the home or only the classroom) may be regarded as showing a home-specific or classroom-specific disorder. These conditions are not yet included in the main classification because of insufficient empirical predictive validation, and because many children with sub-threshold disorders show other syndromes (such as Oppositional Defiant Disorder, F91.3) and should be classified in the appropriate category

F90.0 Disturbance of activity and attention

The general criteria for hyperkinetic disorder (F90) must be met, but not those for conduct disorders (F91.–)

F90.1 Hyperkinetic Conduct Disorder

The general criteria for both hyperkinetic disorder (F90) and conduct disorders (F91.–) must be met

F90.8 Other hyperkinetic disorder

F90.9 Hyperkinetic disorder, unspecified

This residual category is not recommended and should be used only when there is a lack of differentiation between F90.0 and F90.1 but the overall criteria for F90.– are fulfilled

From: International Statistical Classification of Diseases and Related Health Problems (ICD-10), 10th edition, (1992), The World Health Organization; Avenue Appia 20, 1211 Geneva 27, Switzerland.

Table A-3.1. The Abbreviated Connor's Scale for Diagnosing ADHD
http://www.neurotransmitter.net/adhdscales.html is a link for free rating scales.
Connor's Abbreviated Rating Scale is shown below, a total of more than 15 is suggestive of ADD/ADHD:

Name: Date:	Not at all (0)	Just a little (1)	Pretty much (2)	Very much (3)
Restless and overactive				
Excitable, impulsive				
Disturbs other children				
Fails to finish things. Short attention span				
Constantly fidgeting				
Inattentive, easily distracted				
Demands must be met immediately Easily frustrated				
Cries often and easily				
Mood changes quickly and drastically				
Temper outbursts, explosive and unpredictable behavior				

SNAP Checklist Better than ACTeRS: The Swanson, Nolan, and Pelham (SNAP) checklist from the Diagnostic and Statistical Manual of Mental Disorders, revised 3rd edition (DSM-III-R) has been shown to have a sensitivity and specificity in excess of 94% to distinguish hyperactive, inattentive, and impulsive children with ADHD from those without ADHD. This was based on criteria in the DSM-III-R. The DSM-IV SNAP checklist (available at www.adhd.net/snap-iv-form.pdf; scoring at www.adhd.net/snap-iv-instructions.pdf), based on the newer diagnostic criteria, has not been adequately evaluated

Adult ADHD Rating Scales Oversensitive: Adult ADHD is estimated between 0.3% and 5% of the population, a huge range. Researchers examined the diagnostic and screening utility of three ADHD scales (Adult Rating Scale [ARS],

Attention-Deficit Scales for Adults [ADSA], and Symptom Inventory for ADHD) in 82 adults presenting for ADHD evaluation. All three instruments were sensitive to the presence of symptoms in adults with ADHD (supposedly correctly identifying 78% to 92% of patients with ADHD), but a high proportion of individuals with non-ADHD diagnoses screened positive (incorrectly identifying between 36% and 67% of non-ADHD patients).[3]

3   Screening and diagnostic utility of self-report attention deficit hyperactivity disorder scales in adults. McCann, B.S., Roy-Byrne, P. *Compr Psychiatry.* 2004 May-Jun;45(3):175-83. Ed:

Appendix IV
Comparing Mercury Poisoning Symptoms with those of Autism

From Autism Research Institute Web Site Autism: A Unique Type of Mercury Poisoning. Sallie Bernard (sbernard@ nac.net); Albert Enayati, B.S., Ch.E., M.S.M.E. Teresa Binstock Heidi Roger; Lyn Redwood, R.N., M.S.N., C.R.N.P.; Woody McGinnis, M.D. Copyright 2000 by ARC Research; 14 Commerce Drive; Cranford, NJ 07016; April 3, 2000 Revision of April 21, 2000.

Table A-4.1. Summary Comparison of Characteristics of Autism & Mercury Poisoning

Mercury Poisoning	Autism
Psychiatric Disturbances	
Social deficits, shyness, social withdrawal	Social deficits, social withdrawal, shyness
Depression, mood swings; mask face	Depressive traits, mood swings; flat affect
Anxiety	Anxiety
Schizoid tendencies, OCD traits	Schizophrenic & OCD traits; repetitiveness
Lacks eye contact, hesitant to engage others	Lack of eye contact, avoids conversation
Irrational fears	Irrational fears
Irritability, aggression, temper tantrums	Irritability, aggression, temper tantrums
Impaired face recognition	Impaired face recognition
Speech, Language & Hearing Deficits	
Loss of speech, failure to develop speech	Delayed language, failure to develop speech
Dysarthria; articulation problems	Dysarthria; articulation problems
Speech comprehension deficits	Speech comprehension deficits
Verbalizing & word retrieval problems	Echolalia; word use & pragmatic errors
Sound sensitivity	Sound sensitivity
Hearing loss; deafness in very high doses	Absent to profound hearing loss
Poor performance on language IQ tests	Poor performance on verbal IQ tests
Sensory Abnormalities	
Abnormal sensation in mouth & extremities	Abnormal sensation in mouth & extremities
Sound sensitivity	Sound sensitivity

Mercury Poisoning	Autism
Abnormal touch sensations; touch aversion	Abnormal touch sensations; touch aversion
Vestibular abnormalities	Vestibular abnormalities
Motor Disorders	
Involuntary jerking movements - arm flapping, ankle jerks, myoclonal jerks, choreiform movements, circling, rocking	Stereotyped movements - arm flapping, jumping, circling, spinning, rocking; myoclonal jerks; choreiform movements
Deficits in eye-hand coordination; limb apraxia; intention tremors	Poor eye-hand coordination; limb apraxia; problems with intentional movements
Gait impairment; ataxia - from incoordination & clumsiness to inability to walk, stand, or sit; loss of motor control	Abnormal gait and posture, clumsiness and incoordination; difficulties sitting, lying, crawling, and walking
Difficulty chewing or swallowing	Difficulty chewing or swallowing
Unusual postures; toe walking	Unusual postures; toe walking
Cognitive Impairments	
Borderline intelligence, mental retardation - some cases reversible	Borderline intelligence, mental retardation - sometimes "recovered"
Poor concentration, attention, response inhibition	Poor concentration, attention, shifting attention
Uneven performance on IQ subtests	Uneven performance on IQ subtests
Verbal IQ higher than performance IQ	Verbal IQ higher than performance IQ
Poor short-term, verbal & auditory memory	Poor short-term, auditory & verbal memory
Poor visual and perceptual motor skills, impairment in simple reaction time	Poor visual and perceptual motor skills, lower performance on timed tests
Difficulty carrying out complex commands	Difficulty carrying out multiple commands
Word-comprehension difficulties	Word-comprehension difficulties
Deficits in understanding abstract ideas & symbolism; degeneration of higher mental powers	Deficits in abstract thinking & symbolism, understanding other mental states, sequencing, planning & organizing
Unusual Behaviors	
Stereotyped sniffing (rats)	Stereotyped, repetitive behaviors
ADHD traits	ADHD traits
Agitation, unprovoked crying, grimacing, staring spells	Agitation, unprovoked crying, grimacing, staring spells
Sleep difficulties	Sleep difficulties
Eating disorders, feeding problems	Eating disorders, feeding problems
Self injurious behavior, e.g. head banging	Self injurious behavior, e.g. head banging
Poor eye contact, impaired visual fixation	Poor eye contact, problems in joint attention
Visual impairments, blindness, near-sightedness, decreased visual acuity	Visual impairments, inaccurate/slow saccades; decreased rod functioning
Light sensitivity, photophobia	Over-sensitivity to light
Blurred or hazy vision	Blurred vision
Constricted visual fields	Not described

Mercury Poisoning	Autism
Physical Disturbances	
Increase in cerebral palsy; hyper- or hypotonia; abnormal reflexes; decreased muscle strength, especially upper body; incontinence; problems chewing, swallowing, salivating	Increase in cerebral palsy; hyper- or hypotonia; decreased muscle strength, especially upper body; incontinence; problems chewing and swallowing
Rashes, dermatitis/dry skin, itching, burning	Rashes, dermatitis, eczema, itching
Autonomic disturbance: excessive sweating, poor circulation, elevated heart rate	Autonomic disturbance: unusual sweating, poor circulation, elevated heart rate
Gastro-intestinal Disturbances	
Gastroenteritis, diarrhea; abdominal pain, constipation, colitis?	Diarrhea, constipation, gaseousness, abdominal discomfort, colitis
Anorexia, weight loss, nausea, poor appetite	Anorexia; feeding problems/vomiting
Lesions of ileum & colon; increased gut permeability	Leaky gut syndrome
Inhibits dipeptidyl peptidase IV, which cleaves casomorphin	Inadequate endopeptidase enzymes needed for breakdown of casein & gluten
Abnormal Biochemistry	
Binds -SH groups; blocks sulfate transporter in intestines, kidneys	Low sulfate levels
Has special affinity for purines & pyrimidines	Purine & pyrimidine metabolism errors lead to autistic features
Reduces availability of glutathione, needed in neurons, cells & liver to detoxify heavy metals	Low levels of glutathione; decreased ability of liver to detoxify heavy metals
Causes significant reduction in glutathione peroxidase and glutathione reductase	Abnormal glutathione peroxidase activities in erythrocytes
Disrupts mitochondrial activities, especially in brain	Mitochondrial dysfunction, especially in brain
Immune Dysfunction	
Sensitivity due to allergic or autoimmune reactions; sensitive individuals more likely to have allergies, asthma, autoimmune-like symptoms, especially rheumatoid-like ones	More likely to have allergies and asthma; familial presence of autoimmune diseases, especially rheumatoid arthritis; IgA deficiencies
Can produce an immune response in CNS	On-going immune response in CNS
Causes brain/MBP autoantibodies	Brain/MBP autoantibodies present
Causes overproduction of Th2 subset; kills/inhibits lymphocytes, T-cells, and monocytes; decreases NK T-cell activity; induces or suppresses IFNg & IL-2	Skewed immune-cell subset in the Th2 direction; decreased responses to T-cell mitogens; reduced NK T-cell function; increased IFNg & IL-12
CNS Structural Pathology	
Selectively targets brain areas unable to detoxify or reduce Hg-induced oxidative stress	Specific areas of brain pathology; many functions spared
Damage to Purkinje and granular cells	Damage to Purkinje and granular cells
Accumulates in amygdala and hippocampus	Pathology in amygdala and hippocampus
Causes abnormal neuronal cytoarchitecture; disrupts neuronal migration & cell division; reduces NCAMs	Neuronal disorganization; increased neuronal cell replication, increased glial cells; depressed expression of NCAMs
Progressive microcephaly	Progressive microcephaly and macrocephaly

Mercury Poisoning	Autism
Brain stem defects in some cases	Brain stem defects in some cases
Abnormalities in Neuro-chemistry	
Prevents presynaptic serotonin release & inhibits serotonin transport; causes calcium disruptions	Decreased serotonin synthesis in children; abnormal calcium metabolism
Alters dopamine systems; peroxidine deficiency in rats resembles mercurialism in humans	Possibly high or low dopamine levels; positive response to peroxidine (lowers dopamine levels)
Elevates epinephrine & norepinephrine levels by blocking enzyme that degrades epinephrine	Elevated norepinephrine and epinephrine
Elevates glutamate	Elevated glutamate and aspartate
Leads to cortical acetylcholine deficiency; increases muscarinic receptor density in hippocampus & cerebellum	Cortical acetylcholine deficiency; reduced muscarinic receptor binding in hippocampus
Causes demyelinating neuropathy	Demyelination in brain
EEG Abnormalities / Epilepsy	
Causes abnormal EEGs, epileptiform activity	Abnormal EEGs, epileptiform activity
Causes seizures, convulsions	Seizures; epilepsy
Causes subtle, low amplitude seizure activity	Subtle, low amplitude seizure activities
Population Characteristics	
Effects more males than females	Male:female ratio estimated at 4:1
At low doses, only affects those genetically susceptible	High heritability - concordance for MZ twins is 90%
First added to childhood vaccines in 1930s	First "discovered" among children born in 1930s
Exposure levels steadily increased since 1930s with rate of vaccination, number of vaccines	Prevalence of autism has steadily increased from 1 in 2000 (pre1970) to 1 in 500 (early 1990s), higher in 2000.
Exposure occurs at 0 - 15 months; clinical silent stage means symptom emergence delayed; symptoms emerge gradually, starting with movement & sensation	Symptoms emerge from 4 months to 2 years old; symptoms emerge gradually, starting with movement & sensation

Appendix V
ARI's Parent Ratings of Therapies for Autism and Asperger's Disease

ARI Publ. 34/ February 2008
Parent Ratings of Behavorial Effects of Biomedical Interventions
Autism Research Institute
4182 Adams Avenue
San Diego, CA 92116 USA

The parents of autistic children represent a vast and important reservoir of information on the benefits—and adverse effects—of the large variety of drugs and other interventions that have been tried with their children. Since 1967 the Autism Research Institute has been collecting parent ratings of the usefulness of the many interventions tried on their autistic children.

The following data have been collected from the more than 26,000 parents who have completed our questionnaires designed to collect such information. For the purposes of the present table, the parents' responses on a six-point scale have been combined into three categories: "made worse" (ratings 1 and 2), "no effect" (ratings 3 and 4), and "made better" (ratings 5 and 6). The "Better:Worse" column gives the number of children who "Got Better" for each one who "Got Worse."

There are three sections: Special Diets, Drugs, and Biomedical/Non-Drug/Supplements.[1]

Table A-5.1. Special Diets

	Got Worse [A]	No Effect	Got Better	Better: Worse	No. of Cases [B]
Candida Diet	3%	41%	56%	19:1	941
Feingold Diet	2%	42%	56%	25:1	899
Gluten- /Casein-Free Diet	3%	31%	66%	19:1	2561
Removed Chocolate	2%	47%	51%	28:1	2021
Removed Eggs	2%	56%	41%	17:1	1386
Removed Milk Products/Dairy	2%	46%	52%	32:1	6360
Removed Sugar	2%	48%	50%	25:1	4187
Removed Wheat	2%	47%	51%	28:1	3774
Rotation Diet	2%	46%	51%	21:1	938
Specific Carbohydrate Diet	7%	24%	69%	10:1	278

Table A-5.2. Biomedical/Non-Drug/Supplements

	Got Worse [A]	No Effect	Got Better	Better: Worse	No. of Cases [B]
Calcium[E]:	3%	62%	35%	14:1	2097
Cod Liver Oil	4%	45%	51%	13:1	1681
Cod Liver Oil with Bethanecol	10%	54%	37%	3.8:1	126
Colostrum	6%	56%	38%	6.1:1	597
Detox. (Chelation)[C]:	3%	23%	74%	24:1	803
Digestive Enzymes	3%	39%	58%	17:1	1502
DMG	8%	51%	42%	5.4:1	5807
Fatty Acids	2%	41%	56%	24:1	1169
5 HTP	13%	47%	40%	3.1:1	343
Folic Acid	4%	53%	43%	11:1	1955
Food Allergy Treatment	3%	33%	64%	24:1	952
Hyperbaric Oxygen Therapy	5%	34%	60%	12:1	134
Magnesium	6%	65%	29%	4.6:1	301
Melatonin	8%	27%	65%	7.8:1	1105
Methyl B12 (nasal)	15%	29%	56%	3.9:1	48
Methyl B12 (subcutaneous)	7%	26%	67%	9.5:1	170
MT Promoter	13%	49%	38%	2.9:1	61
P5P (Vit. B6)	12%	37%	51%	4.2:1	529
Pepcid	12%	59%	30%	2.6:1	164
SAMe	16%	63%	21%	1.3:1	142
St. Johns Wort	18%	66%	16%	0.9:1	150
TMG	15%	43%	42%	2.8:1	803
Transfer Factor	10%	48%	42%	4.3:1	174
Vitamin A	2%	57%	41%	18:1	1127
Vitamin B3	4%	52%	43%	10.1:1	927
Vitamin B6 with Magnesium	4%	48%	48%	11:1	6634
Vitamin B12 (oral)	7%	32%	61%	8.6:1	98
Vitamin C	2%	55%	43%	19:1	2397
Zinc	2%	47%	51%	22.1:1	1989

Table A-5.3. Possible Adverse Effects of Prescription Drugs

	Got Worse [A]	No Effect	Got Better	Better: Worse	No. of Cases [B]
Adderall	43%	25%	32%	0.8:1	775
Amphetamine	47%	28%	25%	0.5:1	1312
Anafranil	32%	38%	30%	0.9:1	422
Antibiotics	33%	53%	15%	0.5:1	2163
Antifungals[C]: Diflucan	5%	38%	57%	11:1	653
Antifungals[C]: Nystatin	5%	44%	50%	9.7:1	1388
Atarax	26%	53%	22%	0.9:1	517
Benadryl	24%	50%	26%	1.1:1	3032
Beta Blocker	17%	51%	31%	1.8:1	286
Buspar	27%	45%	28%	1.0:1	400
Chloral Hydrate	41%	39%	20%	0.5:1	459
Clonidine	22%	31%	47%	2.1:1	1525
Clozapine	37%	44%	19%	0.5:1	155
Cogentin	19%	54%	27%	1.4:1	186
Cylert	45%	36%	20%	0.4:1	623
Deanol	15%	57%	28%	1.9:1	210
DepakeneD: Behavior:	25%	43%	32%	1.3:1	1071
Depakene[D]: Seizures	11%	33%	56%	4.8:1	705
Desipramine	34%	35%	31%	0.9:1	86
DilantinD: Behavior	28%	49%	23%	0.8:1	1110
DilantinD: Seizures	15%	37%	48%	3.3:1	433
Felbatol	20%	55%	25%	1.3:1	56
Fenfluramine	21%	52%	27%	1.3:1	477
Haldol	38%	28%	34%	0.9:1	1199
IVIG	10%	44%	46%	4.5:1	79
Klonapin[D]: Behavior	28%	42%	30%	1.0:1	246
KlonapinD: Seizures	25%	60%	15%	0.6:1	67
Lithium	24	45%	31%	1.3:1	463
Luvox	30%	37%	34%	1.1:1	220
Mellaril	29%	38%	33%	1.2:1	2097
Mysoline[D]: Behavior	41%	46%	13%	0.3:1	149
Mysoline[D]: Seizures	19%	56%	25%	1.3:1	78
Naltrexone	20%	46%	34%	1.8:1	302
Paxil	33%	31%	36%	1.1:1	416
Phenergan	29%	46%	25%	0.9:1	301
Phenobarbital[D]: Behavior	47%	37%	16%	0.3:1	1109
Phenobarbital[D]: Seizures	18%	43%	39%	2.2:1	520

	Got Worse [A]	No Effect	Got Better	Better: Worse	No. of Cases [B]
Prolixin	30%	41%	29%	1.1:1	105
Prozac	32%	32%	36%	1.1:1	1312
Risperidal	20%	26%	54%	2.8:1	1038
Ritalin	45%	26%	29%	0.7:1	4127
Secretin: Intravenous	7%	49%	44%	6.3:1	468
Secretin: Transdermal	10%	53%	37%	3.6:1	196
Stelazine	28%	45%	26%	0.9:1	434
Steroids	35%	33%	32%	0.9:1	132
Tegretol[D]: Behavior	25%	45%	30%	1.2:1	1520
Tegretol[D]: Seizures	13%	33%	54%	4.0:1	842
Thorazine	36%	40%	24%	0.7:1	940
Tofranil	30%	38%	32%	1.1:1	776
Valium	35%	41%	24%	0.7:1	865
Valtrex	6%	42%	52%	8.5:1	65
Zarontin[D]: Behavior	35%	46%	19%	0.6:1	153
Zarontin[D]: Seizures	19%	55%	25%	1.3:1	110
Zoloft	35%	33%	32%	0.9:1	500

Note: For seizure drugs: The first line shows the drug's behavioral effects;
the second line shows the drug's effects on seizures.

Appendix VI
Excipients in Today's Immunizations[1]

Table A-6.1. This list of vaccine ingredients indicates the culture media used in the production of common vaccines and the excipients they contain:[1][2]

Vaccine	Culture media	Excipients
Anthrax vaccine (BioThrax)	Puziss-Wright medium 1095, synthetic or semisynthetic	Aluminum Hydroxide, Amino Acids, Benzethonium Chloride, Formaldehyde or Formalin, Inorganic Salts and Sugars, Vitamins
BCG (Bacillus Calmette-Guérin) (Tice)	Synthetic or semisynthetic	Asparagine, Citric Acid, Lactose, Glycerin, Iron Ammonium Citrate, Magnesium Sulfate, Potassium Phosphate
DTaP (Daptacel)	Cohen-Wheeler or Stainer-Scholte media, synthetic or semisynthetic	Aluminum Phosphate, Ammonium Sulfate, Casamino Acid, Dimethyl-betacyclodextrin, Formaldehyde or Formalin, Glutaraldehyde, 2-Phenoxyethanol
DTaP (Infanrix)	Cohen-Wheeler or Stainer-Scholte media, Lathan medium derived from bovine casein, Linggoud-Fenton medium derived from bovine extract, synthetic or semisynthetic	Aluminum Hydroxide, Bovine Extract, Formaldehyde or Formalin, Glutaraldhyde, 2-Phenoxyethanol, Polysorbate 80
DTaP (Tripedia)	Cohen-Wheeler or Stainer-Scholte media, synthetic or semisynthetic	Aluminum Potassium Sulfate, Ammonium Sulfate, Bovine Extract, Formaldehyde or Formalin, Gelatin, Polysorbate 80, Sodium Phosphate, Thimerosal[3]
DTaP/Hib (TriHIBit)	Synthetic or semisynthetic	ALUMINUM Potassium Sulfate, Ammonium Sulfate, Bovine Extract, Formaldehyde or Formalin, Gelatin, Polysorbate 80, Sucrose, THIMEROSAL[3]
DTaP-IPV (Kinrix)	Synthetic or semisynthetic	ALUMINUM Hydroxide, Bovine Extract, Formaldehyde, Lactalbumin Hydrolysate, Monkey Kidney Tissue, Neomycin Sulfate, Polymyxin B, Polysorbate 80

---

1   from Wikipedia

Vaccine	Culture media	Excipients
DTaP-HepB-IPV (Pediarix)	Bovine protein, Lathan medium derived from bovine casein, Linggoud-Fenton medium derived from bovine extract, Monkey kidney tissue culture (Vero), synthetic or semisynthetic	ALUMINUM Hydroxide, ALUMINUM Phosphate, Bovine Protein, Lactalbumin Hydrolysate, Formaldehyde or Formalin, Glutaraldhyde, MONKEY KIDNEY TISSUE, Neomycin, 2-Phenoxyethanol, Polymyxin B, Polysorbate 80, Yeast Protein
DTaP-IPV/Hib (Pentacel)	Synthetic or semisynthetic	ALUMINUM Phosphate, Bovine Serum Albumin, Formaldehyde, Glutaraldhyde, MRC-5 DNA and Cellular Protein, Neomycin, Polymyxin B Sulfate, Polysorbate 80, 2-Phenoxyethanol
DT (diphtheria vaccine plus tetanus vaccine) (Sanofi)	Synthetic or semisynthetic	ALUMINUM Potassium Sulfate, Bovine Extract, Formaldehyde or Formalin, THIMEROSAL (multi-dose) or Thimerosal[3] (single-dose)
Hib vaccine (ACTHib)	Synthetic or semisynthetic	Ammonium Sulfate, Formaldehyde or Formalin, Sucrose
DT (Massachusetts)	Synthetic or semisynthetic	ALUMINUM Hydroxide, Formaldehyde or Formalin
HIB (PedvaxHib)	Synthetic or semisynthetic	ALUMINUM Hydroxyphosphate Sulfate
HIB/Hep B (Comvax)	Synthetic or semisynthetic, yeast or yeast extract	Amino Acids, ALUMINUM Hydroxyphosphate Sulfate, Dextrose, Formaldehyde or Formalin, Mineral Salts, Sodium Borate, Soy Peptone, Yeast Protein
Hep A (Havrix), Hepatitis A vaccine	Human diploid tissue culture, MRC-5	ALUMINUM Hydroxide, Amino Acids, Formaldehyde or Formalin, MRC-5, Cellular Protein, Neomycin Sulfate, 2-Phenoxyethanol, Phosphate Buffers, Polysorbate
Hep A (Vaqta), Hepatitis A vaccine	Human diploid tissue culture, MRC-5	ALUMINUM Hydroxyphosphate Sulfate, Bovine Albumin or Serum, DNA, Formaldehyde or Formalin, MRC-5 Cellular Protein, Sodium Borate
Hep B (Engerix-B), Hepatitis B vaccine	Yeast or yeast extract	ALUMINUM Hydroxide, Phosphate Buffers, THIMEROSAL,[3] Yeast Protein
Hep B (Recombivax), Hepatitis B vaccine	Yeast or yeast extract	ALUMINUM Hydroxyphosphate Sulfate, Amino Acids, Dextrose, Formaldehyde or Formalin, Mineral Salts, Potassium ALUMINUM Sulfate, Soy Peptone, Yeast Protein
HepA/HepB vaccine (Twinrix)	Human diploid tissue culture (MRC-5), yeast or yeast extract	ALUMINUM Hydroxide, ALUMINUM Phosphate, Amino Acids, Dextrose, Formaldehyde or Formalin, Inorganic Salts, MRC-5 Cellular Protein, Neomycin Sulfate, 2-Phenoxyethanol, Phosphate Buffers, Polysorbate 20, THIMEROSAL,[3]
Human Papillomavirus (HPV) (Gardasil)	Yeast or yeast extract	Amino Acids, Amorphous ALUMINUM Hydroxyphosphate Sulfate, Carbohydrates, L-histidine, Mineral Salts, Polysorbate 80, Sodium Borate, Vitamins
Influenza vaccine (Afluria)	Chicken embryo	Beta-Propiolactone, Calcium Chloride, Neomycin, Ovalbumin, Polymyxin B, Potassium Chloride, Potassium Phosphate, Sodium Phosphate, Sodium Taurodeoxychoalate.

Vaccine	Culture media	Excipients
Influenza vaccine (Fluarix)	Chicken embryo	Egg Albumin (Ovalbumin), Egg Protein, Formaldehyde or Formalin, Gentamicin, Hydrocortisone, Octoxynol-10, á-Tocopheryl Hydrogen Succinate, Polysorbate 80, Sodium Deoxycholate, Sodium Phosphate, THIMEROSAL[3]
Influenza vaccine (Flulaval)	Chicken embryo	Egg Albumin (Ovalbumin), Egg Protein, Formaldehyde or Formalin, Sodium Deoxycholate, Phosphate Buffers, THIMEROSAL,
Influenza vaccine (Fluvirin)	Chicken embryo	Beta-Propiolactone, Egg Protein, Neomycin, Polymyxin B, Polyoxyethylene 9-10 Nonyl Phenol (Triton N-101, Octoxynol 9), THIMEROSAL (multidose containers), Thimerosal[3] (single-dose syringes)
Influenza vaccine (Fluzone)	Chicken embryo	Egg Protein, Formaldehyde or Formalin, Gelatin, Octoxinol-9 (Triton X-100), THIMEROSAL (multidose containers)
Influenza vaccine (FluMist)	Chicken kidney cells, chicken embryo	CHICK KIDNEY CELLS, Egg Protein, Gentamicin Sulfate, Monosodium Glutamate, Sucrose Phosphate Glutamate Buffer
IPV (Ipol), Polio vaccine	Monkey kidney tissue culture (Vero cell)	Calf Serum Protein, Formaldehyde or Formalin, MONKEY KIDNEY TISSUE, Neomycin, 2-Phenoxyethanol, Polymyxin B, Streptomycin
Japanese encephalitis vaccine (JE-Vax)	MOUSE BRAIN CULTURE	Formaldehyde or Formalin, Gelatin, Mouse Serum Protein, Polysorbate 80,Thimerosal
Japanese encephalitis vaccine (Ixiaro)		ALUMINUM Hydroxide, Bovine Serum Albumin, Formaldehyde, Protamine Sulfate, Sodium Metabisulphite
Meningococcal vaccine (Menactra)	Mueller-Miller medium, Mueller-Minton medium, Watson-Scherp medium	Formaldehyde or Formalin, Phosphate Buffers Meningococcal (Menomune) Lactose, Thimerosal (10-dose vials only)
MMR vaccine (MMR-II)	Human diploid tissue culture (WI-38), Medium 199	Amino Acid, Bovine Albumin or Serum, Chick Embryo Fibroblasts, Human Serum Albumin, Gelatin, Glutamate, Neomycin, Phosphate Buffers, Sorbitol, Sucrose, Vitamins
MMRV vaccine (ProQuad)	Human diploid tissue cultures (MRC-5, WI-38), Medium 199	Bovine Albumin or Serum, Gelatin, Human Serum Albumin, Monosodium L-glutamate, MRC-5 Cellular Protein, Neomycin, Sodium Phosphate Dibasic, Sodium Bicarbonate, Sorbitol, Sucrose, Potassium Phosphate Monobasic, Potassium Chloride, Potassium Phosphate Dibasic
Pneumococcal vaccine (Pneumovax)	Bovine protein	Bovine Protein, PHENOL

Vaccine	Culture media	Excipients
Pneumococcal vaccine (Prevnar)	Soy peptone broth	Aluminum Phosphate, Amino Acid, Soy Peptone, Yeast Extract
Poliovirus inactivated (Poliovax), Polio vaccine	Human diploid tissue culture, MRC-5	?
Rabies vaccine (Imovax)	Human diploid tissue culture, MRC-5	Human Serum Albumin, Beta-Propiolactone, MRC-5 Cellular Protein, Neomycin, Phenol Red (Phenolsulfonphthalein), Vitamins
Rabies vaccine (RabAvert)	Rhesus fetal lung tissue culture, Chicken embryo	Amphotericin B, Beta-Propiolactone, Bovine Albumin or Serum, Chicken Protein, Chlortetracycline, Egg Albumin (Ovalbumin), Ethylene-diamine- Tetra-acetic Acid Sodium (EDTA), Neomycin, Potassium Glutamate
Rotavirus vaccine (RotaTeq)	MONKEY KIDNEY TISSUE CULTURE (VERO)	Cell Culture Media, Fetal Bovine Serum, Sodium Citrate, Sodium Phosphate, Monobasic Monohydrate, Sodium Hydroxide Sucrose, Polysorbate 80
Rotavirus vaccine (Rotarix)		Amino Acids, Calcium Carbonate, Calcium Chloride, D-glucose, Dextran, Ferric (III) Nitrate, L-cystine, L-tyrosine, Magnesium Sulfate, Phenol Red, Potassium Chloride, Sodium Hydrogen carbonate, Sodium Phosphate, Sodium L-glutamine, Sodium Pyruvate, Sorbitol, Sucrose, Vitamins, Xanthan
Td vaccine (Decavac)	Synthetic or semisynthetic	ALUMINUM Potassium Sulfate, Bovine Extract, Formaldehyde or Formalin, 2-Phenoxyethanol, Peptone, THIMEROSAL[3]
Td vaccine (Massachusetts)	Synthetic or semisynthetic	ALUMINUM Hydroxide, Aluminum Phosphate, Formaldehyde or Formalin, THIMEROSAL (some multidose containers)
Tdap vaccine (Adacel)	Synthetic or semisynthetic	ALUMINUM Phosphate, Formaldehyde or Formalin, Glutaraldehyde, 2- Phenoxyethanol
Tdap vaccine (Boostrix)	Fenton media with bovine casein, Lathan medium derived from bovine casein, Linggoud-Fenton medium derived from bovine extract, synthetic or semisynthetic	ALUMINUM Hydroxide, Bovine Extract, Formaldehyde or Formalin, Glutaraldehyde, Polysorbate 80
Typhoid (inactivated –Typhim Vi), Typhus vaccine	Synthetic or semisynthetic	Disodium Phosphate, Monosodium Phosphate, Phenol, Polydimethylsilozone, Hexadecyl-trimethylammonium Bromide
Typhoid (oral – Ty21a), Typhus vaccine	Bovine protein	Amino Acids, Ascorbic Acid, Bovine Protein, Casein, Dextrose, Galactose, Gelatin, Lactose, Magnesium Stearate, Sucrose, Yeast Extract
Vaccinia (ACAM2000)	Calf skin, Monkey kidney cell culture (Vero cell)	Glycerin, Human Serum Albumin, Mannitol, Monkey Kidney Cells, Neomycin, Phenol, Polymyxin B

Vaccine	Culture media	Excipients
Varicella vaccine (Varivax)	Human diploid tissue cultures, MRC-5 and WI-38	Bovine Albumin or Serum, Ethylenediamine-Tetra-acetic Acid Sodium (EDTA), Gelatin, Monosodium L-Glutamate, MRC-5 DNA and Cellular Protein, Neomycin, Potassium Chloride, Potassium Phosphate Monobasic, Sodium Phosphate Monobasic, Sucrose
Yellow fever vaccine (YF-Vax)	Chicken embryo	Egg Protein, Gelatin, Sorbitol
Zoster vaccine (Zostavax)	Human diploid tissue cultures, MRC-5, and WI-38	Bovine Calf Serum, Hydrolyzed Porcine Gelatin, Monosodium L-glutamate, MRC-5 DNA and Cellular Protein, Neomycin, Potassium Phosphate Monobasic, Potassium Chloride, Sodium Phosphate Dibasic, Sucrose

References

The initial list is based on information from the Centers for Disease Control and Prevention (CDC) and thus limited to U.S.-approved vaccines.

1. Vaccine Excipient & Media Summary, Part 1, CDC, April 2009
2. Vaccine Excipient & Media Summary, Part 2, CDC, April 2009
3. Note: Thimerosal content less than 0.3 mcg.

About the Author

Dr. Alan Schwartz is a retired, happily-married, holistically-oriented family practitioner with extensive experience evaluating and successfully treating children with autism and autism spectrum disorders using the biomedical approach pioneered by the late Dr. Bernie Rimland. He is a graduate of Cornell University and the State University of N.Y. Downstate Medical Center, and a former Associate Clinical Professor at the University of Kansas Medical School in Wichita.

He has lectured on a variety of medical topics and has been a guest speaker at an autism conference. He was invited to present the highly successful alternative medicine approach to treating attention deficit/hyperactivity disorder (ADHD) at the fourth annual Safe Harbor Conference in Glendale, California in 2005.

Dr. Schwartz' concerns regarding the dramatic recent increase in autism led to his investigations into the etiology of autism and autism spectrum disorders, which in turn led to the creation of this book.

Made in the USA
San Bernardino, CA
23 June 2017